Medical Imaging Contrast Agents: A Clinical Manual

Sukru Mehmet Erturk • Pablo R. Ros
Tomoaki Ichikawa • Suzan Saylisoy
Editors

Medical Imaging Contrast Agents: A Clinical Manual

Springer

Editors
Sukru Mehmet Erturk
Department of Radiology
Istanbul University School of Medicine
Istanbul
Turkey

Tomoaki Ichikawa
Departments of Diagnostic Radiology and Nuclear Medicine
Gunma University, Graduate School of Medicine
Maebashi
Gunma
Japan

Pablo R. Ros
Departments of Radiology and Pathology
Stony Brook University
Stony Brook, NY
USA

Suzan Saylisoy
Department of Radiology
Eskişehir Osmangazi University
Eskisehir
Turkey

ISBN 978-3-030-79255-8 ISBN 978-3-030-79256-5 (eBook)
https://doi.org/10.1007/978-3-030-79256-5

This Springer imprint is published by the registered company Springer Nature Switzerland AG
The registered company address is: Gewerbestrasse 11, 6330 Cham, Switzerland

Preface

On behalf of the Co-Editors of **Medical Imaging Contrasts Agents: A Clinical Manual**, I am delighted to put in your hands this comprehensive work that fills a gap in the armamentarium available to all interested in the use of contrasts agents in Radiology and Medical Imaging. These include all of us using medical imaging contrasts, such as radiologists, cardiologists, vascular surgeons, obstetricians, urologists, gastroenterologists, and their trainees, licensed independent providers (LIPs) such as physician assistants and nurse practitioners, medical physicists, medical imaging nurses, and pharmacists, radiology technologists, sonographers, clinicians frequently ordering medical imaging studies and in general all interested in the broad spectrum of medical imaging contrast agents and drugs.

A key element of this Manual is its comprehensiveness discussing in 26 chapters the different kinds of medical imaging drugs used in all medical imaging modalities, from radiography, including angiography and fluoroscopy-guided GI and GU studies, to Computed Tomography (CT), Magnetic Resonance Imaging (MRI), and ultrasound.

Further, organ-specific applications are reviewed, discussing contrast-enhanced imaging examinations of the liver, pancreas, GI tract, brain, breast, heart, chest, musculoskeletal system, and vessels (angiography).

Besides, this Manual dedicates chapters to unique clinical situations such as the use of medical imaging contrasts in pregnancy, lactation, and pediatrics.

The three major medical imaging drug groups are reviewed: (1) iodinated contrasts for ionizing radiation techniques such as radiography, fluoroscopy, and CT; (2) gadolinium, manganese, and iron-based contrasts for MRI; and (3) ultrasound contrasts.

The Manual discusses the chemical and pharmacokinetic properties for each group, their potential toxicity, and allergic reactions, including their treatment.

The editors assembled a magnificent cadre of 32 authors, recognized global class experts worldwide, from the United States, Germany, Japan, Spain, Turkey, and Latvia, making this Manual a truly international effort.

The Manual is not only comprehensive, but all materials are up-to-date and to-the-point using a direct, practical approach with a peer-peer style we believe addresses the "what you need to know" principle so desired among practicing clinicians.

In short, on behalf of the editors of **Medical Imaging Contrasts Agents: A Clinical Manual,** we are delighted that you are reading this preface since it indicates you are interested in this topic; we invite you to read it, trusting its contents are of help in your daily medical imaging practice.

Enjoy!!

Stony Brook, NY, USA Pablo R. Ros

Contents

Contrast Agents in Radiology: An Overview

1

Pablo R. Ros, Ibrahim Inan, and Sukru Mehmet Erturk

Contrast agents are like dressing in a salad, literally enhancing the effectiveness of imaging studies and becoming essential in the characterization and eventual diagnosis of pathology. Contrast agents are to radiology like stains are to pathology.

Contrast agents are chemical compounds allowing the visualization of specific anatomical structures of the human body in medical imaging and integral part to many imaging methods.

Contrasts were initially utilized to better visualize vascular structures and the gastrointestinal tract. Over time, they became a key, perhaps essential, component of medical imaging with their use extended to the evaluation of vascularization and perfusion of the tissue in solid organs, specifically using cross-sectional imaging techniques and enhanced visualization and characterization of focal lesions within these organs.

Iodine- and barium-containing compounds are frequently used in X-ray-based imaging modalities (radiography, fluoroscopy, computed tomography (CT), angiography), and gadolinium-containing compounds are utilized in magnetic resonance imaging (MRI). Depending upon the anatomical structure to be visualized, contrast agents can be administered in different ways, including intravenous, intra-arterial, intrathecal, oral and rectal routes.

The initial use of contrast agents took place immediately after the discovery of X-rays by Wilhelm Roentgen in 1895. It was early and clearly understood that elements with a high atomic number could provide radiopacity. The first documented use of contrast agents in humans dates back to 1896, only 1 year after Roentgen's discovery, when Teichmann's solution (iodine solution), a mixture of chalk, cinnabar, and paraffin, was applied to perform an angiogram of an amputated hand in Vienna [1]. However, these toxic compounds could still not be used in humans. The first use of contrast material in a living human resulted from an incidental event. Osborn et al. discovered that the urine of patients undergoing syphilis treatments with iodized compounds was radiopaque, and subsequently they obtained the first pyelogram in 1923 [2]. In the same year, Berberich and Hirsch performed the first femoral angiogram using strontium bromide for this purpose [3]. Femoral angiography using iodinated contrast agents followed suite in 1924 [4]. In 1927, the first carotid angiogram was acquired using sodium iodide by Dr. Moniz in Portugal [5]. On a parallel fashion, there was interest in opacifying the gastrointestinal tract, and in the early 1920s, barium compounds were

P. R. Ros
Case Western Reserve University, Cleveland, OH, USA

I. Inan
Centermed Imaging Center, Istanbul, Turkey

S. M. Erturk (✉)
Department of Radiology, Istanbul University School of Medicine, Istanbul, Turkey

S. M. Erturk et al. (eds.), *Medical Imaging Contrast Agents: A Clinical Manual*,
https://doi.org/10.1007/978-3-030-79256-5_1

initially tested in animals and eventually in humans as oral contrast agents by Dt. Cannon in the United States [6].

Once the use of iodine-based contrast agents became widespread, the new frontier evolved into reducing their toxicity. Synthetic iodopyridine derivatives were clinically available as therapeutic drugs in the mid-1920s and therefore used as the first contrast agents and were rapidly and commonly adopted worldwide [7]. In his study investigating different compounds and heavy metals, Moniz suggested in 1927 that a high molecular weight reduced the toxicity of iodized compounds, which contributed to the development and marketing of iodine-based contrast agents widespread intra-arterial used including cerebral and cardiac angiography. After WWII and the development of the atomic bomb, there was availability of nuclear power by-products, one of them was thorium dioxide, which was used widely as a vascular contrast under the trademark name of Thorotrast. This contrast was well accepted since Thorotrast had a much higher attenuation than iodine-based contrasts and could be used successfully intravascularly producing excellent vascular delineation with only a few mLs injected. Thorotrast was the contrast of choice for cerebral angiograms for a decade from the mid-1940s to the mid-1950s [5]. However, Thorotrast had major drawback; it is an alpha ray emitter with a very prolonged half-life and was picked up by the rethiculoendothelial system of the liver and spleen and not biodegradable. Thorotrast had carcinogenic effects, developing primarily angiosarcoma in the liver and spleen and other visceral neoplasms in the kidney and lung, and it was discontinued in the 1950s [7].

In the following years, benzene derivatives with increased radiopacity using more than one iodine particle in the same molecule gained popularity. When researchers realized that free amine caused toxicity, these derivatives were modified as acetyl and converted to modern iodinated contrast agents, which are still widely used [8]. The development of low-osmolality and non-ionic iodinated compounds with even a lower side effect profile, and compounds with a lower viscosity for high-dose and high-rate applications occurred in the last few decades [7, 9–12].

After the introduction of MR imaging in the early 1980s, gadopentetate dimeglumine was developed in Germany as a first extracellular contrast agent based on gadolinium [11, 13, 14]. Gadopentetate dimeglumine or gadolinium DTPA was a huge success and has become the widespread choice throughout the world [11, 14]. Organ-specific contrast agents were later developed based on manganese chelates and iron oxide particles to enhance the liver. Manganese-based contrasts are excreted by the hepatocytes into the biliary tree and iron oxide particle are uptaken by the liver Kupffer cells. Neither of these two specific contrasts was used clinically currently.

In 2006, the first case of nephrogenic systemic fibrosis (NSF) associated with gadolinium administration in patients with renal insufficiency was reported [11]. The FDA (Federal Drug Administration), the ACR (American College of Radiology), the EMEA (European Medicines Agency), and ESUR (European Society of Urogenital Radiology) among other entities established guidelines with recommendations and warnings on the use of gadolinium-based contrast agents [15]. A significant decrease in NSF cases was observed after increasing awareness about this issue and avoiding the use of gadolinium in high-risk patients [11].

Gadolinium is a highly toxic rare-earth metal containing seven unpaired electrons, which makes it ideal for MR imaging once chelated to avoid toxicity. Gadolinium DTPA compounds are spread extracellularly through aromatic side chains, do not cross the blood-brain barrier, and are excreted by the kidneys. Gadolinium compounds with long fatty chains such as Gd-EOB-DTPA82 and to a lesser degree Gd-BOPTA83 are metabolized by the liver in certain proportions and excreted via the bile ducts. Therefore, these molecules are liver-specific agents and are preferred for contrast enhancement of the liver parenchyma and evaluation of the biliary tract.

Gadofosveset trisodium was another contrast agent bound to albumin resulting in a prolonged intravascular presence and a distribution limited to the vascular space. It was preferred for the visualization of the vascular system as a blood pool agent and discontinued by the manufacturer in 2017 due to low demand [11, 16].

Currently, numerous nanoparticles conjugated with paramagnetic ions such as iron, gadolinium, and manganese with different shapes, sizes, and compositions are being developed. The common goal is to produce molecules that are tissue or organ specific and thus provide high contrast resolution for particular indications and have fewer side effects [17].

Contrast media involving micro-bubbles may be used in ultrasound imaging as a ubiquitous, portable, affordable, safe, and easily accessible imaging technique. The use of contrast media in ultrasonography was first reported in 1968. Albumin-bound coating was developed in 1984 to stabilize the micro-bubbles [18, 19]. These air bubbles, which are smaller than 7 μm, reach the systemic circulation through the pulmonary capillaries and are used to evaluate epicardium, intracardiac thrombus detection, characterization of pancreatic lesions in endoscopic ultrasonography, inflammatory bowel diseases, and solid organ trauma [20].

Today, contrast agents have a wide range of application areas. About 30% of MRI scans are performed using contrast agents [11]. Contrast agents are utilized to characterize lesions in solid organs; visualize vascular structures; follow up tumor activity; evaluate infections, abscesses, and other inflammatory diseases; and detect tissue perfusion. In addition, with the use of an appropriate contrast agent, it is possible to visualize any tubular structure, such as the hollow viscera of the gastrointestinal system, cerebrospinal fluid, salivary glands, breast ducts, and lymphatic vessels.

Despite radiology and its astonishing and ongoing technological advances, the clinical use of contrast agents remains a necessity; today, there is no other workable alternative. However, although the available contrast agents are reliable, their potential to trigger side effects is still of concern. NSF cases associated with gadolinium intravenous administration have not been reported for a long time; but this issue remains relevant. In recent years, gadolinium accumulation in different tissues such as the basal ganglia of the brain has raised questions even though its clinical importance is yet to be known [21–23].

The widespread use of contrast media in medical imaging has led to significant growth in the contrast media market and the emergence of a large medical imaging drug sector. Contrast media are used in approximately half of all radiological examinations. Considering the 76 million CT scans and 34 million MRI scans performed yearly in a worldwide basis, one can easily notice the size of this market.

Medical imaging drugs or contrast media history parallel that of radiology and have evolved as the specialty developing agents to enhance all modalities. The sector is strong with an annual business size estimated in $ 4.96 billion in 2018 and a predicted increase by 6.3% in the 2017–2021 period [24]. The size of the business is such that brings a strict and healthy competition of pharmaceutical industry in this sector, resulting in the discovery of new drugs with a lower side effect profile as one positive outcome of the competitive forces.

In conclusion, the use of contrast agents is indispensable in radiology, and it will remain as such in the foreseeable future. Contrast agents providing high contrast resolution without adverse side effects are the ultimate goal of all clinicians and researchers involved in this area.

References

1. Barton M, Grüntzig J, Husmann M, Rösch J. Balloon angioplasty—the legacy of Andreas Grüntzig, M.D. (1939-1985). Front Cardiovasc Med. 2014;1:15.
2. Osborne ED, Sutherland CG, Scholl AJ, Rowntree LG. Roentgenography of urinary tract during excretion of sodium iodid. J Am Med Assoc. 1923;80(6):368–73.
3. Berberich J, Hirsch S. Die röntgenographische Darstellung der Arterien und Venen am lebenden Menschen. J Mol Med. 1923;2(49):2226–8.
4. Brooks B. Intra-arterial injection of sodium iodid: preliminary report. J Am Med Assoc. 1924;82(13):1016–9.
5. Moniz E. Die cerebrale Arteriographie und Phlebographie. Vol. 70. Springer; 2013.
6. Bradley WG. History of medical imaging. Proc Am Philos Soc. 2008;152(3):349–61.

7. Quader MA, Sawmiller CJ, Sumpio BE. Radio contrast agents: history and evolution. In: Textbook of angiology. Springer; 2000. p. 775–83.
8. Hoey GB, Wiegert PE, Rands R. Organic iodine compounds as X-ray contrast media, vol. 76. Oxford: Pergamon Press; 1971.
9. Sovak M, Ranganathan R, Lang J, Lasser E. Concepts in design of improved intravascular contrast agents. In: Annales de radiologie. 1978.
10. Sovak M, Terry RC, Douglass JG, Schweitzer L. Primary carboxamides: nonionic isotonic monomers. Investig Radiol. 1991;26:S159–61.
11. Frenzel T, Lawaczeck R, Taupitz M, et al. Contrast media for x-ray and magnetic resonance imaging: development, current status and future perspectives. Investig Radiol. 2015;50(9):671–8.
12. Jost G, Pietsch H, Lengsfeld P, Hütter J, Sieber MA. The impact of the viscosity and osmolality of iodine contrast agents on renal elimination. Investig Radiol. 2010;45(5):255–61.
13. Weinmann H-J, Brasch RC, Press W-R, Wesbey GE. Characteristics of gadolinium-DTPA complex: a potential NMR contrast agent. Am J Roentgenol. 1984;142(3):619–24.
14. Rohrer M, Bauer H, Mintorovitch J, Requardt M, Weinmann H-J. Comparison of magnetic properties of MRI contrast media solutions at different magnetic field strengths. Investig Radiol. 2005;40(11):715–24.
15. Thomsen HS, Morcos SK. Contrast media and the kidney: European Society of Urogenital Radiology (ESUR) guidelines. Br J Radiol. 2003;76(908):513–8.
16. Khairnar S, More N, Mounika C, Kapusetti G. Advances in contrast agents for contrast-enhanced magnetic resonance imaging. J Med Imaging Radiat Sci. 2019;50(4):575–89.
17. Pellico J, Ellis CM, Davis JJ. Nanoparticle-based paramagnetic contrast agents for magnetic resonance imaging. Contrast Media Mol Imaging. 2019;2019:1845637.
18. Stride E, Segers T, Lajoinie G, et al. Microbubble agents: new directions. Ultrasound Med Biol. 2020;46(6):1326–43.
19. Fu J-W, Lin Y-S, Gan S-L, et al. Multifunctionalized microscale ultrasound contrast agents for precise theranostics of malignant tumors. Contrast Media Mol Imaging. 2019;2019:3145647.
20. Caschera L, Lazzara A, Piergallini L, et al. Contrast agents in diagnostic imaging: present and future. Pharmacol Res. 2016;110:65–75.
21. Olchowy C, Cebulski K, Łasecki M, et al. The presence of the gadolinium-based contrast agent depositions in the brain and symptoms of gadolinium neurotoxicity—a systematic review. PLoS One. 2017;12(2):e0171704.
22. American College of Radiology. ACR manual on contrast media. American College of Radiology; 2015.
23. Beckett KR, Moriarity AK, Langer JM. Safe use of contrast media: what the radiologist needs to know. Radiographics. 2015;35(6):1738–50.
24. Contrast Media Market Research Report-Global forecast till 2025. 2019. https://www.marketresearchfuture.com/reports/contrast-media-market-1284.

2 Chemistry, Physicochemical Properties and Pharmacokinetics of Iodinated Contrast Agents

Kevser Erol and Semra Yigitaslan

2.1 Introduction

Contrast agents (CAs) are expected not to have any pharmacological activity in the organism. Their basic role is to absorb X-rays. Therefore, sodium iodide is thought to be ideal from an absorption perspective—85% of the molecule is iodine—but not from a toxicity perspective. Iodine which atomic number is 53 and atomic weight is 127 is 3× denser than bone and 5× denser than soft tissue. It is essential for nutrition, abundant in thyroid and also a principal ingredient in the surgical scrub, betadine. Non-metallic iodine is commonly found in salt water swamps or brackish waters; in greyish-black, lustrous plates or granules. A halogen (group VII elements including fluorine, bromine and chlorine) iodine readily binds to salt. Iodine is proved as a satisfactory element for general use as an intravascular CA for radiography. Original "ionic" iodine contrasts were bound to sodium, calcium, magnesium or meglumine salts. The concentration of ionic contrast refers to the amount of salt in solution.

The iodine may be bound to either an organic (non-ionic) compound or an ionic compound. So, iodine-based CAs are basically classified as ionic or non-ionic. Both types are most commonly used in radiology because of their relatively harmless interaction with the body. Ionic agents were developed first and are still in widespread use depending on the requirements but may result in additional complications. Organic agents which covalently bind the iodine have fewer side effects as they do not dissociate into component molecules. Many of the side effects are due to the hyperosmolar solution being injected, i.e. they deliver more iodine atoms per molecule. The more iodine content means the more "dense" the X-ray effect is.

Iodine-based CAs are water-soluble. The most used iodinated organic molecules used for contrast include iohexol, iodixanol and ioversol. These CAs are sold commercially available as clear, colourless water solutions with the iodine concentration usually expressed as mgI/mL.

2.2 Physicochemical Properties

Iodinated CAs used for radiographic procedures today are unique pharmaceuticals. They are highly concentrated solutions that can be administered in high doses, because CAs possess a high safety profile and have special physicochemical properties. They are very hydrophilic and inert substances, which is illustrated by their extremely low propensity to bind with proteins.

K. Erol (✉)
Bahcesehir University School of Medicine, Istanbul, Turkey

S. Yigitaslan
Eskisehir Osmangazi University, Eskisehir, Turkey

S. M. Erturk et al. (eds.), *Medical Imaging Contrast Agents: A Clinical Manual*,
https://doi.org/10.1007/978-3-030-79256-5_2

Five physicochemical parameters are important in the development of iodinated contrast molecules: stability, solubility, hydrophylicity, osmolality and viscosity. Viscosity is the basic criterion rather than the others. Because all the criteria which contribute to improve solubility, osmolality and hydrophilicity affect inversely viscosity [1]. Organically bound iodine which is stable is much better tolerated if particularly shielded by hydrophilic groups [2].

Modern iodinated CAs mostly used in clinical practice can be divided into two basic classes based on their chemical structures. Monomeric agents are composed of a single tri-iodinated benzene ring, whereas dimeric agents consist of two covalently bonded tri-iodinated benzene rings.

The osmolality of a CA solution is proportional to the number of independent particles in the solution. Both the concentration of the CA (or any other constituents) and the temperature of the solution influence strongly the osmolality. The osmotic pressure of a CA preparation is expressed in milliosmol kg^{-1} water (mosm kg^{-1}), in megapascal (MPa) or in atmospheres (atm). CAs can be classified into three different groups, high-osmolar compounds with osmolalities in the order of 1500 mosm kg^{-1}, low-osmolar agents with 600–700 mosm kg^{-1} and isotonic substances with osmolalities similar to that of blood (300 mosm kg^{-1}). High osmolality may cause certain types of side effects such as pain at the injection site, cardiovascular effects (heart rate, blood pressure) and diuresis. The closer the osmolality is to that of blood, the lower is the overall side effect ratio [2].

The osmolalities and viscosities of these two classes are different. In regard to iodine concentrations, non-ionic monomers (low-osmolar CAs) have higher osmolalities and lower viscosities than non-ionic dimeric CAs (iso-osmolar CAs) in vitro. Small changes in concentration can cause large changes in CA viscosity, because the viscosity of CA increases exponentially, as a function of iodine concentration [3]. Monomeric CAs are formulated as iso-osmolar relative to human plasma, whereas iodixanol is currently the only iso-osmolar and dimeric CA commercially available for intravascular use. The viscosity of iodixanol is considerably higher than that of most other CAs. Therefore very thin catheters should not be used for injection. Its high viscosity might counteract the beneficial effects of the low osmolality [4]. Nowadays high-osmolar monomeric CAs are replaced by non-ionic low-osmolar agents because of their impractical intravascular usage [5].

Most modern CAs are non-ionic; therefore they do not dissociate in solution, but vary with regard to iodine content and physicochemical properties. Ionic CAs generally, but not always, possess higher osmolality and more side effects [6]. After the injection of ionic CAs, the molecule begins to dissociate by releasing ionic particles (+ cation and − anion) at a concentration 4–8 times higher than the particle content of blood (osmolality). High osmolality (2–8×) of a CA can change electrolyte balance. The osmolality and also the viscosity of CAs have been considered as important properties for renal tolerance [7].

2.3 History

Osborne et al. obtained an X-ray image of a urinary tract by using intravenous sodium iodide as early as 1923 [8]. Iodine has remained the most widely used element for intravenous injection as a radio-opaque agent ever since. Inorganic sodium iodide was found too toxic for routine use; thereafter the development of organic compounds has extended the clinical use of iodinated compounds [7]. Each development stage of CAs represents a progressive evolution of the original agents [3]. The first CAs were ionic tri-iodinated derivatives of benzoic acid, and their osmolalities were also high.

The historic development of X-ray CAs followed a logical consequence by moving from lipophilic to hydrophilic agents, from ionic (diatrizoate) to non-ionic drugs (iopromide), from inorganic iodide to organic mono-iodine compounds (Uroselectan A), from bis-iodine (Uroselectan B) to tris-iodine substances (diatrizoate) and from monomers (iopromide) to dimers (iotrolan). Hydrophilicity, osmolality and viscosity are directly related to the chemical structure of the CAs [2]. The first tri-iodinated CA was developed in the 1950s [9]. The first synthesised nonspecific hydrophilic iodinated CA was diatrizoic acid in 1953 [2]. Its osmolality is 5–7 times higher than that of plasma. Thereafter iothalamate, metrizoate and ioxithalamate were synthesised and marketed. These are also high-osmolar CAs.

The reduction of osmolality leads to reduce pain and haemodynamic disturbances of the injected solution. Metrizamide, which is synthesised by condensation of metrizoic acid and glucosamine, was the first non-ionic CA. But it was not appropriate to autoclave sterilisation while it was possible to be lyophilised. Iopamidol and iohexol were developed in the mid-1970s and then iobitridol. These are stable non-ionic CAs. Ioxaglic acid, derived from the synthesis of mono-carboxylic acid dimers, leads to reduce osmolality. It was used for interventional procedures because of its beneficial properties on platelet function and thrombin. Non-ionic iodinated CAs are the most widely used drugs in the radiological field to enhance X-ray procedures.

Non-ionic CAs were synthesised by substituting non-iodine parts of the benzoic ring with a non-ionising side chain. They are highly concentrated solutions [10] and are classified as high osmolality and low osmolality; the latter can be further subdivided as ionic or non-ionic [11]. Non-ionic CAs with low osmolality became popular in the late 1980s. They have fewer particles, and these characteristics caused to lower osmolality than ionic agents. The osmolalities of these non-ionised agents are two times higher than that of blood plasma, and they do not disrupt electrolyte balance. Their cost is significantly higher; however contrast reactions were observed fewer than ionic ones. Iotrolan and iodixanol as non-ionic dimers were synthesised to provide iso-osmolality with plasma in the 1990s.

However viscosity of these compounds is high. A series of compact dimers were characterised by a three-dimensionally distributed hydrophylicity due to the perpendicular ring conformation by hydroxylated amino groups and stabilisation of hydrophylicity. Therefore their viscosities were low [2].

2.3.1 Physicochemistry

The pharmacological and toxicological behaviours of CAs are dependent on their physicochemical characteristics. Therefore these features can guide the search for improved substances [2].

CAs are usually injected in high concentrations for most radiographic examinations [9]. Therefore, the commonly used solutions have a concentration of 1.5 mol/L (1.5 mol of CA per litre of solution). The physical properties of some CAs are summarised in Table 2.1. The osmolality which represents the ratio of CA to water molecules in the solution determines the osmotic pressure [12]. High viscosity is a property of these concentrated solutions although the solutions with high molarity do not always have high viscosity [13].

2.4 Characteristics of Ionic CAs

Iodine concentration of an agent measured in weight/volume determines **the radiopacity**. The concentration usually changes in ranges from 10 to 82, independent on its use. The other elements in the CA do not have radiopacity, but act as carriers of iodine. They provide to increase solubility and reduce the toxicity of the CA. Many products including iodine salts are expressed in the brand name: Renografin-60, Hexabrix 76, Isovue-200 and their concentrations are 20%.

The electrical charge (acid group) and the oxygen and nitrogen atoms in the side chains reduce the lipophilicity of triiodobenzene derivatives, while methyl groups in the side chains increase it. Low lipophilicity is expected for urography, angiography, CT and myelography. A correlation between lipophilicity and certain types of side effects of ionic CAs was found. This correlation was even more obvious when the degree of binding of the CAs to plasma proteins was measured rather than lipophilicity [14]. Non-ionic CAs are generally very hydrophilic, and their binding to plasma proteins is minor.

Iodine preparations are expected to be water-soluble and stay stable in solution and mix with blood. Products that do not meet this requirement are packages of a solute and a solvent.

Table 2.1 Physicochemical properties of iodinated contrast agents. Data have been collected from [2]

Agent	Compound type	Molecular weight	Concentration (mgI mL^{-1})	Osmolality (mosm kg^{-1})	Viscosity (mPas)
Diatrizoate	Ionic	810	306	1502	9.3[a]
Sodium diatrizoate	Ionic	614	300	1500	2.5[b]
Ioxaglate	Ionic	1269	300	584	7.8[b]
Iotalamate	Ionic	643	300	1500	5.2[b]
Iopentol	Non-ionic	835	300	835	6.5[b]
Iopamidol	Non-ionic	777	300	640	4.8[b]
Iohexol	Non-ionic	821	300	690	4.5[b]
Iopromide	Non-ionic	791	300	607	4.6[b]
Ioversol	Non-ionic	807	300	807	6[b]
Iotrolan	Non-ionic	1626	300	320	9.1[b]
Ioxilan	Non-ionic	805	300	585	9.4[a]
Iodixanol	Non-ionic	1550	320	290	20.7[a]

[a]At a temperature of 20 °C
[b]At a temperature of 37 °C

2.5 Viscosity

The viscosity of a CA provides its ability to flow and is given in millipascal × second (mPa s). The concentration of the CA and the temperature of the solution strongly influence the viscosity. Viscosity is increased by increasing concentration and decreasing temperature. The viscosity of CA determines and limits the maximal rate of injection. High viscosity leads to side effects. Low viscosity is essential, because the thickness of an agent particularly affects the easiness of a bolus injected and the rate of drip infusion.

The viscosity of iodixanol is considerably higher than that of most other CAs. Therefore it is less suited for injection in very thin catheters [7, 15]. Iosimenol, a non-ionic and dimeric CA, is iso-osmolar but exhibits a lower viscosity than iodixanol at the same concentration [16]. Moreover it was under development for use in cardiac angiography [17].

2.6 Osmolality

In general the water can cross from the capillary bed to maintain the balance because of higher blood pressure in capillary arteriole than the osmotic pressure in the tissue. The osmolality increases as a CA is injected. Blood entering the capillary bed is hypertonic to the fluid in the surrounding tissues. Extravascular fluid crosses the semi-permeable membrane of the capillary to provide isotonicity, causing hypervolemia. Fluid drawn from RBCs causes sickling. Epithelial cells lining the intimal wall are similarly affected and can lead to inflammation and thrombophlebitis. Flexibility of vessel walls allows vasodilation to accommodate against hypervolemia.

The osmotic pressure of a solution can be expressed in two different ways, osmolarity and osmolality. Osmolarity means the concentration of osmotically active particles in relation to the volume of a solution. In the case of nonelectrolytes, it is identical to molarity. Osmolality describes the concentration of solute per kg of water. It is nearly proportional to the number of freely mobile particles (molecules, ions) per kg water. The osmolality of CAs is dependent dominantly on the concentration and only slightly on the temperature. The osmolalities of different CAs can be diverse, even if they have the same concentration of iodine [14]. Therefore the osmolality of a solution is related to the ratio of solute particles to water molecules. When the osmolality of the injected drug is higher than plasma osmolality (300 mOsm/L), vascular entrance of interstitial water produces adverse reactions such as increase in blood viscosity, endothelial damage, hypervolaemia, vasodilatation, oedema with neurotoxicity, depressed myocardial contractility and systemic toxicity [18]. The number of particles in solution is the basic factor of toxicity. **Low toxicity** is essentially expected. But any preparation not natural to the body can be toxic to the body more or less, unlike as natural substances can be given in excess. The goal of used CAs is to keep adverse reactions to a minimum. Non-ionic CAs have lower osmolality and tend to have fewer side effects.

2.7 Chemical Composition of Ionic CA

The most important step in the synthesis of iodinated CAs is to add iodine into the molecule. Iodine is introduced either through substitution or by addition reactions. The benzene ring can be iodinated by a number of methods via the intermediate I^+, which will react with positions of the benzene ring activated by enough electronegative of neighbour groups. Normally, amine groups are used for the activation. An aqueous solution is used for achieving the active iodine ion (I^+). The last tri-iodinated compounds are usually less water-soluble than their precursors. Purification of the intermediates is easily by performing precipitation. The synthesis of ionic CAs is complete by following acylation of the amino groups. As a typical reaction scheme for an ionic monomer, the synthesis pathway for diatrizoate is given in Fig. 2.1.

The synthesis of non-ionic CAs is much more complicated. Because of the higher aqueous solubility of the intermediates, the purification processes are harder than the ionic ones. Its necessarily more expensive and sophisticated procedures are recrystallisation, extraction and/or chromatography.

2.7.1 Ionic CAs

Ionic tri-iodinated CAs are synthesised by using bisamino nitrophthalic acid or amino isophthalic acid as precursor. The nitro group is reduced to the amino moiety by hydrogenation and iodinated by iodine monochloride in aqueous solution. Therefore solubility decreases, and triiodobenzene precipitates from the solution and can be recrystallised. Amino functions are then acylated. The solubility of triiodobenzoic acid analogues was increased by esterification with meglumine or by conversion to sodium salt. These ionic CAs form both anions (containing iodine atoms) and cations (sodium or meglumine or a mixture of both) in solution. Only the anion carrying iodine atoms is radio-opaque; the cation is instrumental in forming the solution. Ionic monomeric CAs are fully saturated tri-iodinated benzoic acid derivatives such as diatrizoate, acetrizoate, metrizoate, iothalamate, iodamide and ioxitalamate.

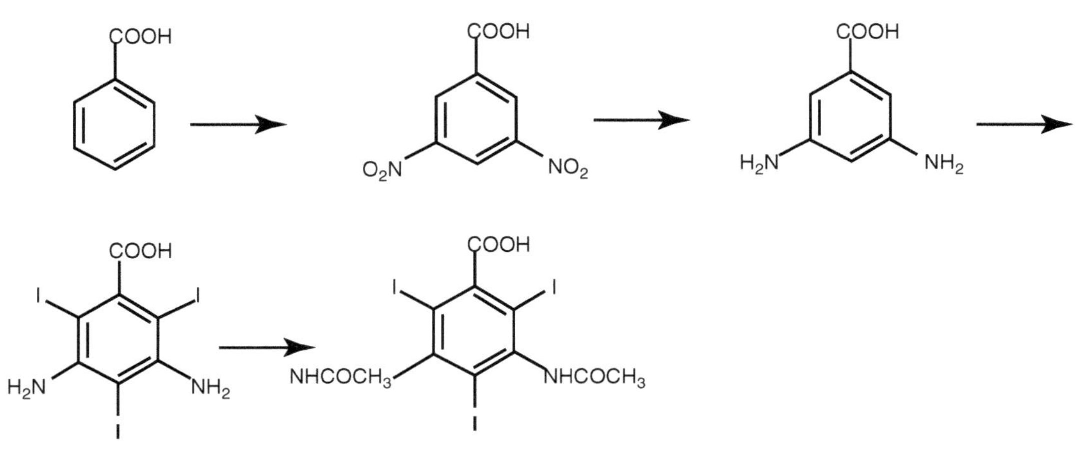

Fig. 2.1 Synthetic pathway to ionic contrast agents – reaction scheme for diatrizoate

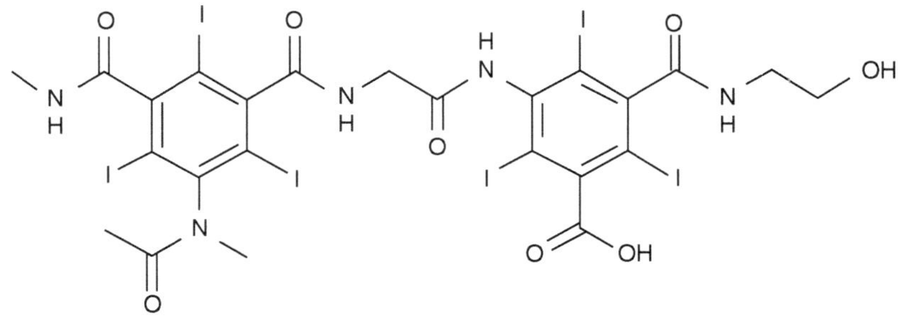

Fig. 2.2 The molecular structure of ioxaglate

The molecules completely dissociate in water into two parts (the anion containing iodine atoms and a cation). Their osmolalities are about five times that of blood. Therefore their adverse reactions and adverse effects are commonly expected occur [19, 20].

A new monoacidic dimer is ioxaglate and contains two tri-iodinated rings of benzoic acid. The dimer forms two particles containing three iodine molecules in solution after ionisation of its acid group. Therefore ioxaglate has an iodine-to-particle ratio of 6:2 or 3:1 (Fig. 2.2). Its configuration enables the CA to maintain low osmolality by requiring only one cation to balance the single anion and also providing an adequate iodine concentration [9]. It is the only compound in low-osmolar ionic CAs. Its osmolality is similar to that of the non-ionic monomers [5].

2.7.2 Non-ionic CAs

2.7.2.1 Low-Osmolar Non-ionic CAs

The first derivative of iothalamic acid dimers was iocarmate. It was found less neurotoxic than the other CAs. However the synthesis of metrizamide, water-soluble CA, provided improvement in imaging spinal lesions. There was a better patient tolerance of these non-ionic CAs with low osmolality. Their adverse effects and adverse reactions were significantly reduced [21]. However, myelography performed with metrizamide produced adverse effects. But the modification of the metrizamide side chains lessened these adverse effects. The second generation of non-ionic monomers are iohexol, iopamidol, iopromide, ioversol, ioxilan, iomeron, iobitridol, iopentol and iobitridol. These are much more stable, soluble and less toxic. None of them dissociate in solution and provide three iodine atoms to one osmotically active particle, producing an iodine-to-particle ratio of 3:1. Their osmolalities are less than half of the osmolalities of high-osmolar agents. The iodine concentrations of some radio-opaque CAs such as iopamidol, iohexol, ioxaglate, iotrol and iopromide are approximately 3 mol/L. Their physiological effects produced in conventional film-based angiography are significantly light. Certain techniques such as computed tomography and digital subtraction angiography can achieve good contrast with a substantially lower iodine concentration. They have low short-term intravenous toxicity [22–25] and fewer adverse effects [9]. Non-ionic CAs have usually solubility problem in water, while iopamidol and iohexol are more soluble. Such non-ionic CAs with lower osmolality are better tolerated, have fewer adverse effects and are less toxic [26, 27]. Studies of acute toxicity show low acute intravenous toxicity, e.g. 50% lethal dose (LD50) of iopamidol was 20 g/kg and that of iohexol was 25 g/kg [23, 24, 28]. Moreover, non-ionic CAs have a reduced potential for interactions because better masking of the hydrophobic core by hydrophilic side chains and their lack of charge provide them greater hydrophilicity and get them more inert and less toxic than low-osmolality ionic agents [9].

Non-ionic monomeric CAs such as iopamidol, iohexol, ioversol, iopromide and iopentol are synthesised by increasing the length of the substituted side groups. Therefore this kind of substitution increased their molecular weights and reduced osmolalities without changing the iodine concentration. Their osmolalities are about 600 mOsm/kg H_2O, at a concentration of 300 mgI/mL [5].

2.7.2.2 Iso-osmolar Non-ionic CAs

These agents are isotonic with blood (300 mOsm/kg H_2O) and do not dissociate in solution. Their examples are isomendol, iotrolan, iodixanol and GE-145. Therefore, an ionic CA, ioxaglate with a low osmolality, takes place an intermediate position between the conventional (ionic) and the more recent (non-ionic) compounds [9, 29]. It has six atoms of iodine per molecule, which dissociates into two ions, like the non-ionic preparations [30]. Metrizamide which is similar to ioxaglate needs to be lyophilised because of its instability in solution [31]. Thus it has not now been used anymore.

2.8 Atropisomerism

Atropisomerism has a different property of creating molecular chirality as a result of hindered rotation about a bond axis. Therefore, it is considered as a (noncovalent) molecular dissymmetry depending on temperature. Iomeprol, iopamidol and iopromide are non-ionic iodinated contrast agents (NICAs) characterised by an extensive atropisomer chirality [32]. They are commonly used for radiological analyses such as urography, angiography and myelography [2]. These CAs are purchased commercially as highly concentrated aqueous solutions but relatively low osmolality and viscosity. A high amount of iodine in a molecule can provide an efficient radiopacity, because the quality of image depends on the iodine concentration [33, 34]. Therefore iodine contents of these CAs are about 50% of the weight. Iodine covalently bound to organic molecules is also nontoxic. Atropisomer chirality may affect properties such as pharmacokinetics and toxicity. The generic molecular structure of NICAs consists of a fully substituted aromatic ring (Fig. 2.3) with three iodine atoms covalently linked in positions 2, 4 and 6. Positions 1, 3 and 5 are substituted with three hydrophilic side chains attached to the benzene ring by amidic bonds via the amino group (position 1) or the carbonyl group (positions 3 and 5). The main role of the side chains is to (1) increase the water solubility (relevant for image quality), 2.7 (2) increase their biocompatibility and (3) aid their clearance [35].

The rate of atropisomer interconversion is extremely slow (of the order of years), and the compounds obtained by this kind of atropisomer interconversion are called "formally chiral" compounds and can be regarded as thermodynamically distinct species that can be isolated as pure substances and stored as individual formulations. However NICAs are used only as diagnostic molecules without any biological or therapeutic activity. Thus, a mixture of atropisomer forms can also be used without danger at a concentration level above the solubility limit of each individual species. Consequently, the concentrated solution is not metastable because of being prevented interconversionally.

2.9 Pharmacokinetics

Many radio-opaque CAs may be administered either intravenously or intra-arterially and sometimes orally for diagnostic procedures. Modern iodinated CAs can be used almost anywhere in the body. They can also be used intrathecally (as in diskography of the spine) and intra-abdominally.

Iodine CAs are used for the following diagnostic procedures:

- Contrast CTs
- Angiography (*arterial investigations*)
- Venography (*venous investigations*)
- VCUG (*voiding cystourethrography*)
- HSG (*hysterosalpingogram*)
- IVU (*intravenous urography*)

The iodine molecule effectively absorbs X-rays and permits an excellent visualisation of the anatomical structure with no accompanying toxicity or an alteration in physiological functions. **Iodinated CAs** increase the visibility of vascular structures and organs such as the urinary tract, uterus and fallopian tubes during radiographic procedures. It also causes a metallic taste in the mouth of the patient.

After intravascular injection they diffuse across vessel walls into the interstitial compartment until equilibrium is reached with the vascular space because of high capillary

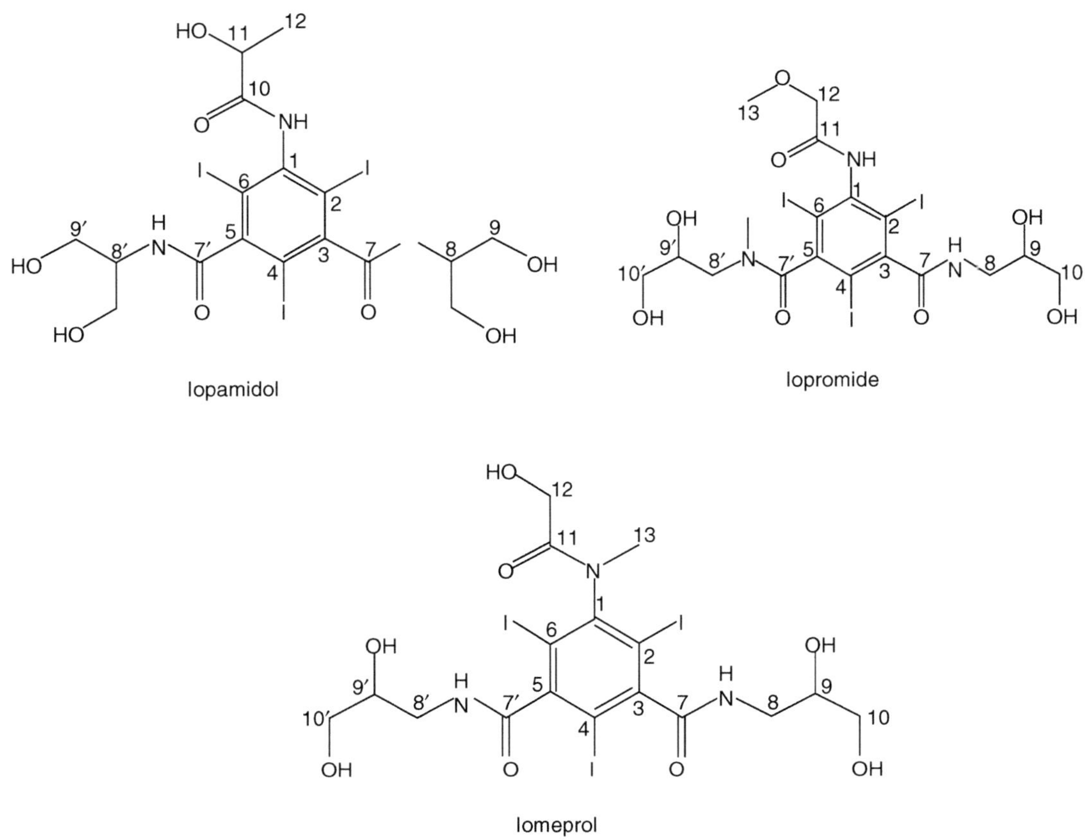

Fig. 2.3 Molecular structure of iopamidol, iopromide and iomeprol. The numbers refer to carbon atoms. The symmetrical side arms are important for atropisomerism of these molecules

permeability. But it is not possible to enter into an intact blood-brain barrier, the blood cells or tissues. They can minimally bind to plasma protein. Therefore the pharmacokinetics of iodinated CAs may be represented by a two-compartment model which consists of the central compartment, blood and the secondary compartment, extracellular space, in both of which the CA is distributed [9, 36]. Iodinated agents always reach rapidly to peak plasma concentrations, and there is a good agreement with contrast enhancement of the blood, liver, spleen and other organs [37]. Therefore the plasma iodine concentration profile is biphasic. The first phase is due to the rapid diffusion of the CA from the plasma compartment into the interstitial compartment and the second phase corresponds to slow urinary excretion [38].

Consequently most modern iodinated CAs are either mono- or dimeric (i.e. based on one or two benzene rings) and non-ionic (i.e. they do not dissociate in solution). They are all based on tri-iodinated benzene molecules. All of them vary with regard to iodine content and physicochemical properties. Their viscosities and, in particular, osmolalities have important roles on renal tolerance.

2.10 Absorption

Iodinated CAs are usually employed for intravenous, intra-arterial and intrathecal injections [30]. Calcium iopodate is highly lipophilic and can be administered orally. It is strongly bound to plasma albumin which limits the tissue transfer to its unbound form. Therefore the agent is almost totally retained in the compartment of the distribution of albumin [39]. After intestinal absorption, it is metabolised by glucuroconjugation and biliary concentration, well reabsorbed in the duodenum and eliminated. However, when iopamidol or meglumine iothalamate is used for endoscopic retrograde cholangiopancreatography, a significant systemic transfer is sometimes observed and anaphylactic reactions could also happen [40].

2.11 Distribution

The peak concentration of iodine occurs rapidly in the aorta after the bolus injection of CAs [37]. The agents with low osmolality create higher concentrations than the compounds with high osmolality. Therefore a better tissue contrast can be obtained by using them. The differences may be in the hepatic enhancement profiles of the iodinated agents. The histological structure (necrotic zones) and vascularisation differences usually delay the maximum contrast enhancement time in a pathological tissue.

The different CAs diffuse to extracellular fluid with an equivalent volume. The calculated parameters obtained from the studies on children and healthy volunteers are similar to those of other low-osmolar non-ionic CAs independent of the dose given. Lipid solubilities of CAs are low, except the biliary agents. This property can explain that the molecules distribute in body fluid to the same extent as inulin. Only small amounts of CAs can enter the cells [9]. They do not pass the intact blood-brain barrier, the interior of blood cells or tissues but enter the cerebrospinal fluid [30]. Non-ionic low-osmolar compounds cannot transfer across the placental barrier. It was reported that only 0.7% of administered dose for iobitridol and 1.6% for iohexol were excreted in milk [41]. Meglumine iotraxate and meglumine ioglycamate can pass into the bile at high concentrations. Distribution kinetics of all contrast molecules are similar. Diagnostic procedures are based on the distribution of the contrast molecules to normal and abnormal tissues of the organs [9]. The dose of a CA, distribution volume of the tissue, blood flow, capillary permeability and diffusivity can affect the diagnostic procedures.

2.11.1 Plasma Protein Binding

The biliary CAs can bind to plasma proteins. There is no substitution on their benzene rings. Meglumine iotraxate bounds to plasma proteins less than dipiodone and meglumine ioglycamate.

The only CAs which do bind to plasma proteins are biliary CAs. The reason of binding is the absence of substitution on the benzene ring of these agents. But acidosis increases and alkalosis decreases binding to plasma protein. On the other hand, protein binding of all CAs with substituted benzene ring is negligible, because of minor hydrophobic binding on albumin. After the rapid intravenous injection of non-protein bound CA, the osmotic effects can cause to the attraction of fluid into vascular space that can result in a transient drop in packed cell volume [9].

2.12 Metabolism

CAs are considered not to be metabolised and basically eliminated by kidneys in an unchanged form. Iopromide, ioxaglic acid, ioxitalamic acid and iohexol were shown to be eliminated as unchanged forms [9]. It was reported that biliary excretion and transmucosal excretion in the small bowel are the major extra-renal pathway for certain agents, especially in cases of renal failure. The amount of extra-renally excreted CA increases as renal function decreases. If there is combined renal and hepatic diseases, alternative routes such as saliva, sweat and tears can help in the elimination. The biliary excretion of all CAs was less than 5% but except for metrizoate and ioxaglate [9].

2.13 Elimination

Most of iodinated CAs are highly water-soluble and eliminated in an unmetabolised form by glomerular filtration without secretion into the renal tubules in patients with normal kidney function. They are eliminated like inulin or Cr-EDTA, which are markers used for the evaluation of glomerular filtration rate [9]. Therefore iothalamate and iohexol have also been used as markers of glomerular filtration because of their specific renal elimination [36]. It has been reported that tubular transport processes can have a role in kidney elimination, but less than 5% of the amount is eliminated by glomerular filtration. Active tubular excretion for ionic monomers and tubular reabsorption for non-ionic molecules or monoacid dimers was also demonstrated. They have minimal hepatic elimination, negligible excretion in saliva, tears or sweat and no transport into blood-brain barrier [9, 36]. Their elimination half-life varies from 45 min to 2 h, with near-complete excretion within 24 h in patients without renal failure [36]. It has been reported that hepatic elimination of this kind of iodinated CAs slowly increased and total elimination delayed in patients with significant renal failure. Therefore this prolonged half-life can be considered as a function of the degree of renal insufficiency.

Total excretion is similar for all CAs after intravenous injection, but the nature of the molecule can affect urinary concentration [21]. It was noted that there were smaller differences in urine concentration between meglumine and sodium salts. These substances can negatively influence the glomerular filtration rate. It was demonstrated that prolonged elimination of iso-osmolar iodinated radiocontrast agent in children <6 months of age is related to renal immaturity [42].

2.14 Conclusion

The blood concentrations of CAs vary according to their physicochemical properties. The more hydrophylicity of non-ionic agents leads to the higher blood concentrations due to the greater initial enhancements in the parenchymal organs, liver, kidney and pancreas as well as in the brain and heart, compared to the ionic ones. Monomers and dimers tend to give the same enhancement if they contain the same amount of iodine. The ideal CA is expected to give enhancement of the body region of interest without adverse reactions. The agents with low osmolality seem to improve the general tolerance such as flushing, pain and cardiovascular side effects.

References

1. Eloy R, Corot C, Belleville J. Contrast media for angiography: physicochemical properties, pharmacokinetics and biocompatibility. Clin Mater. 1991;7(2):89–197.
2. Krause W, Schneider PW. Chemistry of X-ray contrast agents. In: Krause W, editor. Contrast agents II: optical, ultrasound, X-ray and radiopharmaceutical imaging. Berlin, Heidelberg: Springer; 2002. p. 107–50.
3. Jost G, et al. The impact of the viscosity and osmolality of iodine contrast agents on renal elimination. Invest Radiol. 2010;45(5):255–61.
4. Jost G, et al. Changes of renal water diffusion coefficient after application of iodinated contrast agents: effect of viscosity. Invest Radiol. 2011;46(12):796–800.
5. Grainger RG. Intravascular contrast media—the past, the present and the future. Mackenzie Davidson Memorial Lecture, April 1981. Br J Radiol. 1982;55(649):1–18.
6. Zhai L, et al. Non-ionic iodinated contrast media related immediate reactions: a mechanism study of 27 patients. Leg Med (Tokyo). 2017;24:56–62.
7. Voeltz MD, et al. The important properties of contrast media: focus on viscosity. J Invasive Cardiol. 2007;19(3):1a–9a.
8. Osborne ED, et al. Roentgenography of urinary tract during excretion of sodium iodid. J Am Med Assoc. 1923;80(6):368–73.
9. Bourin M, Jolliet P, Ballereau F. An overview of the clinical pharmacokinetics of x-ray contrast media. Clin Pharmacokinet. 1997;32(3):180–93.
10. Idee JM, et al. Allergy-like reactions to iodinated contrast agents. A critical analysis. Fundam Clin Pharmacol. 2005;19(3):263–81.
11. Bumbacea RS, et al. Immediate and delayed hypersensitivity reactions to intravascular iodine based radiocontrast media—an update. Pneumologia. 2013;62(1):47–51.
12. Deutsch AL, et al. Effects of low osmolality contrast materials on coronary hemodynamics, myocardial function, and coronary sinus osmolality in normal and ischemic states. Invest Radiol. 1982;17(3):284–91.
13. Morris TW, Kern MA, Katzberg RW. The effects of media viscosity on hemodynamics in selective arteriography. Invest Radiol. 1982;17(1):70–6.
14. Speck U. Physicochemical properties of water-soluble contrast media. In: X-ray contrast media. Berlin, Heidelberg: Springer; 2018.

15. Seeliger E, et al. Contrast-induced kidney injury: mechanisms, risk factors, and prevention. Eur Heart J. 2012;33(16):2007–15.
16. Riefke B, et al. ICJ 3393: a new Iodinated nonionic low osmolal dimer with low viscosity as contrast agent for X-ray. Acad Radiol. 2002;9(Suppl 1):S178–81.
17. Meurer K, Kelsch B, Hogstrom B. The pharmacokinetic profile, tolerability and safety of the iodinated, non-ionic, dimeric contrast medium Iosimenol 340 injection in healthy human subjects. Acta Radiol. 2015;56(5):581–6.
18. Bettmann MA, Morris TW. Recent advances in contrast agents. Radiol Clin North Am. 1986;24(3):347–57.
19. Ansell G, et al. The current status of reactions to intravenous contrast media. Invest Radiol. 1980;15(6 Suppl):S32–9.
20. Shehadi WH, Toniolo G. Adverse reactions to contrast media: a report from the Committee on Safety of Contrast Media of the International Society of Radiology. Radiology. 1980;137(2):299–302.
21. Spataro RF. Newer contrast agents for urography. Radiol Clin North Am. 1984;22(2):365–80.
22. Salvesen S. Acute intravenous toxicity of iohexol in the mouse and in the rat. Acta Radiol Suppl. 1980;362:73–5.
23. Shaw DD, Potts DG. Toxicology of iohexol. Invest Radiol. 1985;20(1 Suppl):S10–3.
24. Sovak M, Siefert HM, Ranganathan R. Combined methods for assessment of neurotoxicity: testing of new nonionic radiographic media. Invest Radiol. 1980;15(6 Suppl):S248–53.
25. Mutzel W, Speck U. Tolerance and biochemical pharmacology of iopromide. Fortschr Geb Rontgenstr Nuklearmed. 1983;118:11–7.
26. Widrich WC, et al. Iopamidol: a non-ionic contrast agent for peripheral arteriography. Radiology. 1982;145(1):53–5.
27. Wolf GL, et al. New angiographic agents with less fibrillatory propensity. Invest Radiol. 1981;16(4):320–3.
28. Salvesen S. Acute toxicity tests of metrizamide. Acta Radiol Suppl. 1973;335:5–13.
29. McClennan BL. Low-osmolality contrast media: premises and promises. Radiology. 1987;162(1 Pt 1):1–8.
30. Sage MR. Kinetics of water-soluble contrast media in the central nervous system. AJR Am J Roentgenol. 1983;141(4):815–24.
31. Haavaldsen J. Iohexol. Acta Radiol Suppl. 1980;362:9–11.
32. Thomsen HS, Morcos SK. Radiographic contrast media. BJU Int. 2000;86(Suppl 1):1–10.
33. Krasuski RA, Sketch MH Jr, Harrison JK. Contrast agents for cardiac angiography: osmolality and contrast complications. Curr Interv Cardiol Rep. 2000;2(3):258–66.
34. Yamauchi T, Furui S, Harasawa A, Ishimura M, Imai T, Hayashi T. Optimum iodine concentration of contrast material through microcatheters: hydrodynamic analysis of experimental results. Phys Med Biol. 2002;47:2511–23.
35. Fontanive L, et al. Myelography iodinated contrast media. I. Unraveling the atropisomerism properties in solution. Mol Pharm. 2015;12(6):1939–50.
36. Weisbord SD, Palevsky PM. Iodinated contrast media and the role of renal replacement therapy. Adv Chronic Kidney Dis. 2011;18(3):199–206.
37. Kormano M, Spataro RF, Soimakallio S, Wiljasalo M. Comparison of contrast enhancement pharmacokinetics of contrast media in clinical patients. In: Amiel M, editor. Contrast media in radiology. Berlin, Heidelberg: Springer; 1982. p. 314–8.
38. Gardeur D, et al. Pharmacokinetics of contrast media: experimental results in dog and man with CT implications. J Comput Assist Tomogr. 1980;4(2):178–85.
39. Herve F, et al. Drug binding in plasma. A summary of recent trends in the study of drug and hormone binding. Clin Pharmacokinet. 1994;26(1):44–58.
40. Carstensen F, Wurbs D. [Contrast medium resorption in ERCP]. Z Gastroenterol. 1993;31(6):369–75.
41. Bourrinet P, et al. Transplacental passage and milk excretion of iobitridol. Invest Radiol. 1995;30(3):156–8.
42. Johnson WH Jr, et al. Iodixanol pharmacokinetics in children. Pediatr Cardiol. 2001;22(3):223–7.

Nephrotoxicity of Iodinated Contrast Agents

3

Suzan Saylisoy and Sukru Mehmet Erturk

3.1 Introduction

This chapter discusses terminology, incidence, diagnosis, pathogenesis, associated risk factors, and preventive measures and treatment of nephrotoxicity of iodinated contrast agents.

3.2 Terminology

Post-contrast acute kidney injury (PC-AKI) is often defined as acute renal impairment within 48 h following exposure to intravascular iodinated contrast agents (ICAs) [1]. It can occur regardless of whether ICAs are the cause of renal degeneration. Contrast-induced nephropathy (CIN) is defined as acute renal impairment caused by renal degeneration due to ICA exposure [2]. Therefore, the two terms are not synonymous, with CIN belonging to the subgroup of PC-AKI and being a causative diagnosis [3]. After exposure to intravascular ICAs, serum creatinine usually increases within the first 24–48 h, reaches its peak in 3–5 days, and returns to values similar to the baseline within 1–3 weeks. In most cases, it is asymptomatic and has no significant clinical manifestation [4]. However, in rare cases, oliguria or anuria and irreversible kidney damage occur [5]. Basic workup of such cases includes clinical evaluation, urine output, urine analysis, and kidney imaging [6].

3.3 Incidence

CIN accounts for about 11% of the total AKI cases [7]. Its incidence can be strongly influenced by imaging modality, risk factors, and the type and dose of the ICA used. CIN mainly occurs after exposure to an ICA during coronary or peripheral angiography, but recent data show that modern radiographic procedures do not result in a significant increase in CIN incidence [3]. ICA exposure following cardiac or peripheral angiography differs from that of diagnostic imaging in that in the former, the injection is intra-arterial and the dose of ICA is concentrated and abrupt. In the general population without risk factors, the incidence of CIN is very low, but the risk increases with increasing comorbidity. The most important risk factor is pre-existing severe renal insufficiency (SCr level $\geq$ 1.5 mg/dL), in which the CIN incidence reaches 12–27%. In the presence of diabetic nephropathy, CIN is reported to have an incidence of 50% [8].

S. Saylisoy (✉)
Department of Radiology, Eskişehir Osmangazi University, Eskisehir, Turkey

S. M. Erturk
Department of Radiology, Istanbul University School of Medicine, Istanbul, Turkey

S. M. Erturk et al. (eds.), *Medical Imaging Contrast Agents: A Clinical Manual*,
https://doi.org/10.1007/978-3-030-79256-5_3

3.4 Diagnosis and Biomarkers

There is no standard definition of CIN. In the past, CIN was defined as a relative change in the baseline serum creatinine (>25–50%) or absolute elevation compared to the baseline serum creatinine (>0.5–2 mg/dL) within 72 h after ICA administration [9]. Exclusion of other causes of AKI (prerenal/renal/postrenal) is crucial for the diagnosis of CIN [10]. In 2004, the Acute Dialysis Quality Initiative (ADQI) proposed a standardized definition system for CIN, namely, the RIFLE system (Risk, Injury, Failure, Loss, ESKD), which was modified in 2007 by the Acute Kidney Injury Network (AKIN) group and called the AKIN system (Table 3.1) [11, 12]. The American College of Radiology (ACR)'s Manual on Contrast Media (version 10.2) recommended using the AKIN [Acute Kidney Injury Network] criteria to define CIN. According to the AKNI criteria, a serum creatinine increase of >0.3 mg/dL or ≥50% (≥1.5 times) or a urine output of ≤0.5 mL/kg/h for at least 6 h that occurs within 48 h after exposure to an ICA indicates the presence of CIN [9, 13]. Recently, some providers have been searching for rapid strip test-based methods for the quick measurement of serum creatinine in patients that need to undergo contrast-enhanced radiological studies [14].

Although the serum creatinine concentration is commonly used as a measure of renal function, it has certain limitations. For example, there is often a delay between the time of kidney injury and the increase in serum creatinine, which delays the diagnosis [8]. Serum creatinine is also an unreliable biomarker of renal function changes since it can be influenced by several non-renal factors, such as age, gender, nutritional status, volume status, hyper-catabolism, muscle mass, and concomitant use of other drugs [3]. Changes in serum creatinine concentration are not parallel to those in the effective glomerular filtration rate (eGFR). Normal serum creatinine levels are maintained until GFR or creatinine clearance is reduced by almost 50%. Therefore, there is a need for new specific predictive biomarkers to facilitate the early diagnosis of CIN. This will allow not only early identification of patients at risk for CIN but also timely medical treatment. Biomarkers either reflect a change in renal function (e.g., cystatin C) or represent renal damage (e.g., neutrophil gelatinase-associated lipocalin). Most of these biomarkers are available for post-contrast exposure; however, prediction before contrast exposure is more valuable in clinical practice [15].

Serum cystatin C, a 13-kDa cysteine proteinase inhibitor, could be used as a reliable marker for the identification of CIN. This protein is normally filtered by the glomerulus, reabsorbed by the tubules where it is almost completely catabolized, but it is not excreted at the tubular level.

Table 3.1 RIFLE and AKIN criteria for AKI diagnosis

RIFLE; class AKIN; stage	GFR and creatinine criteria RIFLE	 AKIN	 Urine output criteria
RIFLE: Risk AKIN: Stage 1	Increase in creatinine ≥1.5 × baseline or decrease in GFR ≥ 25%	Increase in creatinine ≥0.3 mg/dL or ≥150–200% of baseline	UO < 0.5 mL/kg per h × 6 h
RIFLE: Injury AKIN: Stage 2	Increase in SCr ≥ 2.0 × baseline or decrease in GFR ≥ 50%	Increase in creatinine ≥200–300% of baseline	UO < 0.5 mL/kg per h × 12 h
RIFLE: Failure AKIN: Stage 3	Increase in creatinine ≥3.0 × baseline or creatinine ≥4.0 mg/dL or decrease in GFR ≥ 75%	Increase in creatinine ≥150–200% of baseline or increase in creatinine ≥4 mg/dL with an increase of ≥0.5 mg/dL	UO < 0.3 mL/kg per h × 24 h or anuria × 12 h
RIFLE: Loss	Complete loss of kidney function >4 weeks		
RIFLE: End-stage kidney disease	>3 months		

Cystatin C is not normally found in urine; therefore, its urinary presence indicates a tubular disease. Cystatin C levels are less influenced by non-renal variables than serum creatinine. Normal serum cystatin C levels are <1 mg/L (<75 nmol/L) and increase after ICA exposure. The combination of serum cystatin C and serum creatinine could be beneficial for risk stratification and prediction of prognosis in patients exposed to ICAs [16, 17].

Natriuretic peptides [NPs] are a family of vasoactive peptides released in response to hypervolemic and hypertensive states [18]. The NP family consists of three important structurally related but genetically distinct natriuretic peptides: atrial natriuretic peptide (ANP), B-type natriuretic peptide (BNP), and C-type natriuretic peptide (CNP). BNP and N-terminal pro-brain natriuretic peptide (NT-proBNP) have been established as reliable markers for diagnosis and risk stratification in heart failure patients. Recently, it has also been shown that these cardiac neurohormone levels are also associated with accelerated progression of chronic kidney disease. Therefore, high BNP or NT-proBNP levels can be considered as markers of cardiorenal syndromes [16, 18].

Serum neutrophil gelatinase-associated lipocalin (NGAL), a small circulating protein, covalently bound to gelatinase from human neutrophils, is released after tubular damage. Urinary NGAL levels are a good diagnostic marker for predicting CIN. In patients with CIN, NGAL levels rise within 2–4 h. For the diagnosis of CIN, a cut-off value of 150 ng/mL has been established [19].

Urinary kidney injury molecule-1 (Kim-1), a transmembrane protein, is not normally present in healthy kidneys, but is expressed in dedifferentiated proximal tubule cells after AKI; thus, it can be useful for early diagnosis [20]. **Procalcitonin**, a novel marker for systemic inflammatory conditions, has recently been shown to predict CIN in patients with acute coronary syndrome [21]. **The ratio of urinary albumin/creatinine** might be a predictor of CIN [22]. **Urinary cyclic guanosine monophosphate (cGMP)** concentrations are influenced by renal function, making such biomarkers promising [23]. However, there is no standardized cut-off value for the diagnosis of CIN due to the lack of data on clinical outcomes.

3.5 Risk Factors

Determination of risk factors related to CIN facilitates identification of patients at increased risk of this condition. Various risk factors have been described that increase the risk for the development of CIN following ICA administration. These can be classified as intrinsic [patient-related] and extrinsic (procedural/contrast-related).

3.5.1 Patient-Related Risk Factors

Pre-existing chronic kidney disease [CKD] and diabetes mellitus are two important patient-related risk factors. However, recent studies concluded that there was an increased incidence of CIN in diabetes only when renal function was impaired (GFR < 30 mL/min/1.73 m^2). The calculated eGFR is much better at assessing renal function than serum creatinine [24]. The European Renal Best Practice together with the Kidney Disease: Improving Global Outcomes (KDIGO) guidelines suggests that the threshold at which the actual risk of CIN increases could be lowered to 45 mL/min/1.73 m^2 [13, 25]. Other established patient-related risk factors include advanced age (≥70 years), dehydration, anemia, vascular disease, hypertension, coronary heart disease, congestive heart failure, smoking, and concomitant use of other drugs, such as metformin, non-steroidal anti-inflammatory drugs (NSAIDs), diuretics, and calcium channel blockers [26]. CIN is rarely seen in children, and advanced age is associated with a higher risk of CIN. Elderly people usually present with impaired kidney function and other comorbidities [27]. Patients with ST-elevation myocardial infarction can develop CIN even in the absence of a pre-existing CKD [28]. Anemia has also been identified as a factor independently associated with CIN. Patients with multiple myeloma are considered to have an increased risk of CIN due to myeloma proteins in the kidney tubules. However, recent research suggests that contrast studies can be safely performed in myeloma patients with normal renal function if there is no dehydration [29].

According to guidelines of the ACR, risk factors that may require a renal function assessment prior to intravascular ICA administration include (1) age $\geq$ 60 years, (2) history of renal disease (dialysis, kidney transplant, single kidney, renal cancer, renal surgery), (3) history of hypertension requiring medical treatment, (4) history of diabetes mellitus, and (5) using metformin or metformin-containing drug combinations. For patients who do not have any of these factors, it is not necessary to determine the baseline serum creatinine level prior to ICA administration for routine intravascular studies [9].

3.5.2 Procedure-Related Risk Factors

Extrinsic factors include type and the amount of ICM, route of administration, and the number of ICA exposures.

Type of ICM The type of ICM has also been reported to affect the incidence of CIN. The renal toxicity of ICA is mainly related to its osmolality, ionicity, viscosity, and iodine content. Non-ionic contrast media are less nephrotoxic than ionic contrast media [30]. Frequently available ICM are benzoic acid derivatives with three iodine atoms. High-osmolality contrast media (HOCM) with up to eight times osmolality of plasma, frequently used in the past, is now only used for non-vascular radiology studies since they cause serious adverse effects related to the high osmolality. Today, low-osmolality contrast media (LOCM) and iso-osmolar contrast media (IOCM) are widely used, and they are also less nephrotoxic than HOCM [31].

Viscosity is responsible for vascular resistance. Viscosity increases from high to low levels of IOCMs. Therefore, a lower osmolality of ICA means higher viscosity. High viscosity results in increased viscosity of the renal ultrafiltrate and thus is parallel to increased resistance to the renal tubular flow, eventually leading to tubular damage [32].

The KDIGO guidelines suggest the use of LOCM or IOCM instead of HOCM; however, there is no recommendation on the preference of IOCM over LOCM due to the lack of data [13]. However, the CIN Consensus Working Panel stated that non-ionic IOCM should be used for coronary angiography studies in high-risk patient population, especially in the presence of severe renal impairment with an eGFR of <30 mL/min, while IOCM or LOCM can be used for ICA administration [33].

Dose of ICM A number of studies have shown that the nephrotoxic effect is proportional to the volume of the ICM in intra-arterial administration. Previous studies reported that the administered volume is directly related to risk, which is increased by 12% per 100 mL of ICM. Brown et al. proposed formula of "maximal allowable contrast (MAC) dose" (contrast volume limit [mL = 5 × bodyweight {kg}]/[88.4 × SCr {μmol/L}]), which correlated with the development of CIN. However, CIN can also occur with small (30 mL) volumes of ICA, which excludes a threshold effect [34].

Route of Administration The route of ICM administration has been reported as a risk factor. The incidence of CIN following intra-arterial administration in coronary angiographic procedures is compared to intravenous administration. The suggested mechanism behind an increased risk after intra-arterial administration is that when the contrast is administered into the abdominal aortorenal arteries, higher amount of arterial contrast directly enters the kidneys. The risk of CIN is lower if the contrast is administered below the origin of renal arteries; thus, the lowest risk is seen after intravenous administration [35]. The reported incidence of CIN following contrast-enhanced computed tomography (CT) ranges from 2 to 12% [36]. However, recent studies questioned the direct relationship between intravenous CM administration and CIN. In the majority of studies, there was a similar incidence of CIN between the contrast-enhanced and non-enhanced CT groups [2].

Number of ICA Exposures Administration of multiple doses of intravascular ICA within a short period of time is a well-documented risk factor for CIN. The dosing intervals should not be shorter than 24 h except in emergencies since the elimination of ICA from the body takes approximately 20 h, provided that the patient has normal renal function [3]. Repeated exposure in patients with CKD should be delayed to allow time for renal recovery.

3.5.3 Risk Scoring Systems

Several researchers have been working on the use of risk scores to guide preventive strategies, of which the most comprehensive is the Mehran risk score (Table 3.2). The analysis of 8357 patients receiving an ICM during percutaneous coronary interventions was undertaken, and patient-related and procedure-related variables were used to quantify the risk of CIN. The incidence of CIN was reported as 7.5% in patients with a Mehran score of ≤5 and 57.3% in those with a score of ≥16 [37].

3.6 Pathogenesis

The pathogenesis of CIN is multi-factorial and is not fully understood. Several distinct but interacting mechanisms including medullary ischemia, formation of reactive oxygen species, and direct tubular cell toxicity are implicated [38].

Medullary Ischemia ICM induces renal vasoconstriction through endothelin, changes in the intracellular calcium concentration of smooth muscle cells, and adenosine [in contrast to its effects on the heart, adenosine causes vasoconstriction in the kidneys]. Inhibition of vasodilatation due to a reduction in the intrarenal production of vasodilators nitric oxide and prostacyclin may also contribute to the pathogenesis of CIN. As a result, the renal blood flow to the medulla and GFR is reduced, followed by renal medullary ischemia [1, 39].

Table 3.2 Mehran contrast nephropathy risk score

Risk factor	Score
Hypotension	5
Congestive cardiac failure	5
Intra-aortic balloon pump	5
Age > 75 years	4
Serum creatinine	4
Diabetes mellitus	3
Anemia	4
eGFR < 60 mL/min/1.74 cm^2	2
Contrast media volume	1 per 100 cc

Formation of Reactive Oxygen Species Reactive oxygen species (ROS), such as superoxide (O_2 −), hydrogen peroxide (H_2O_2), and hydroxyl radical (OH−), are actively involved in inflammatory reactions. ROS are released during renal parenchymal hypoxia induced by ICAs. ROS constrict renal microcirculation and indirectly affect renal vascular tone by mediating the effects of other vasoconstrictors, stimulating the production of vasoconstrictors, and modulating the actions of vasodilators, such as nitric oxide. ROS are harmful to glomerular cells by increasing the membrane permeability, and they lead to the development of apoptosis [1, 38, 40].

Direct Tubular Cell Toxicity All types of ICA exhibit in vitro cytotoxic effects, and renal tubular epithelial cells present signs of severe cell damage or apoptosis when exposed to ICM. The cytotoxic effect of iodine to bacteria is well known, and iodine has been used as an antiseptic agent for medical procedures for decades. Loss of cell membrane integrity caused by the interaction of iodine with amino acids found in cell membrane proteins is responsible for the direct toxic effect on renal tubular cells. ICAs can also increase renal tubular viscosity in vitro, resulting in tubular obstruction and elevated interstitial pressure [40].

3.7 Prevention

Identification of patients at risk is an important step in the prevention of CIN. Current guidelines recommend that high-risk patients should be identified to plan appropriate preventive strategies. General recommendations are explained below.

3.7.1 Avoiding the Use of ICM or Limiting the ICM Volume

Although there is controversial data concerning the relationship between ICM dose and nephrotoxicity, there does seem to be a directly proportional dose-toxicity correlation. Using the lowest possible dose of the contrast agent to obtain the necessary diagnostic information may be the easiest way of reducing the risk of CIN. In addition, recent studies showed that the combined use of low-voltage, high-pitch acquisition and iterative reconstruction algorithms could provide diagnostic image quality at a very low ICM volume, such as 20–30 mL [41].

3.7.2 Choosing Alternative Imaging Modalities

In patients at high risk of CIN, alternative imaging modalities, e.g., ultrasonography, noncontrast CT, carbon dioxide angiography, and magnetic resonance imaging, should be considered prior to ICM administration. Gadolinium-based contrast agents can be used in patients at risk of CIN but should be avoided in those that are on dialysis or have severe renal impairment, especially stage 4 or 5 chronic kidney disease due to the concerns of nephrogenic systemic fibrosis [3].

3.7.3 Stopping Nephrotoxic Drugs

It is recommended to stop the use of nephrotoxic drugs, such as NSAIDs and cyclosporine A, 48 h before ICM exposure [42].

3.7.4 Hydration

Preprocedural hydration has been proven to be one of the easiest and most cost-effective measures to prevent CIN. Hydration reduces the toxic effects of ICM by reducing the concentration of the agent in the renal medulla, activity of the renin-angiotensin system, release of vasoconstrictors, and production of ROS. Hydration also leads to vasodilation in the renal medulla, probably mediated by an increase in the production of prostacyclin. Hydration with isotonic electrolyte solutions decreases the time of interaction between ICM and renal tubular cells due to the increased tubular flow by inhibiting the absorption of water and salt [43].

Oral hydration can be considered as a simple and harmless way to perform preventive hydration prior to ICM administration. However, the effects of oral hydration for CIN prevention are still unclear. A small recent meta-analysis of six randomized controlled trials showed that oral hydration with prespecified volume expansion is as effective as intravenous hydration for CIN prevention [44]. On the contrary, some studies reported that oral hydration was less effective [9]. The ideal volume and infusion rate are not well known. The fluid volume should be determined after a careful evaluation of the body fluid volume, since an excessive increase in the body fluid volume after the development of CIN is itself considered a risk factor for the progression of kidney dysfunction. The total hydration volume can be doubled by utilizing a left ventricular end-diastolic pressure-guided hydration scheme, without compromising patient safety [45].

For intravenous hydration, isotonic fluids are preferred (Lactated Ringer's solution or 0.9% NaCl). ACR recommends the use of 0.9% saline at 100 mL/h, beginning 6–12 h before ICA administration and continuing 4–12 h after the procedure, but this can only be performed in an inpatient setting [9, 46]. The guidelines of the European Society of Urogenital Radiology (ESUR) suggest that the prophylactic hydration regimen should comprise intravenous administration of 1.0–1.5 mL/kg/h fluid for at least 6 h before and after ICA administration [47]. According to the guidelines of the European Society of Cardiology/European Association for Cardio-Thoracic Surgery, the patients with chronic kidney disease undergoing diagnostic catheterization should receive preventive hydration with isotonic saline, starting 12 h prior to angiography and continuing for at least 24 h afterward [48].

The data from meta-analyses comparing hydration with sodium bicarbonate and sodium chloride provided contradictory results [49]. One meta-analysis showed that sodium bicarbonate hydration was not inferior to periprocedural saline hydration in terms of renal safety and might be more cost-effective. However, administration of bicarbonate may pose a risk to certain individuals, such as those with electrolyte imbalance. The most widely used sodium bicarbonate administration protocol is 3 mL/kg/h for 1 h before ICM administration, followed by 1 mL/kg/h for 6 h after this procedure [50].

Intravenous hydration beginning 6–12 h before and continuing 4–12 h after the procedure is better than bolus administration at the time of injection; however, it may not be feasible in urgent contrast-enhanced studies [3]. In an emergent setting, intravenous volume expansion should be initiated as early as possible prior to ICA administration.

Diuretics [mannitol or furosemide] are sometimes combined with hydration. If furosemide is used in addition to intravenous saline solution, an exacerbation of renal dysfunction is seen [51]. Neither mannitol nor furosemide is recommended to reduce the CIN risk [9]. However, according to the guidelines of the European Society of Cardiology/European Association for Cardio-Thoracic Surgery, furosemide combined with hydration can be preferred over standard hydration in patients at very high risk for CIN or in those where prophylactic hydration cannot be accomplished before the procedure. The proposed protocol is initially a 250 mL intravenous bolus of normal saline over 30 min (reduced to 150 mL in case of left ventricle dysfunction), followed by an intravenous bolus (0.25–0.5 mg/kg) of furosemide [48].

The ESUR guidelines also recommend adopting an appropriate CIN prevention strategy for contrast-enhanced CT based on patients' eGFR. According to this, if eGFR is ≥45 mL/min/1.73 m^2, no precaution is required; however, in the eGFR range of 30–45 mL/min/1.73 m^2, intravenous hydration should be arranged for inpatients, and oral hydration for outpatients in cases where intravenous hydration cannot be appropriately performed. Intravenous saline is also recommended for patients on metformin with an eGFR <45 mL/min/1.73 m^2; if eGFR is <30 mL/min/1.73 m^2, a consultant radiologist should determine whether an effective clinical evaluation can be performed without ICM administration. If ICM administration is considered necessary, then intravenous hydration should be initiated [47].

3.7.5 Pharmacological Premedication

In order to reduce the risk of CIN, several other strategies have been investigated. The current evidence is limited and conflicting for most drugs, including *N*-acetylcysteine (NAC), furosemide, mannitol, ascorbic acid, theophylline, dopamine, calcium channel blockers, atrial natriuretic peptide, L-arginine, prostaglandin E1, and endothelin receptor antagonists [52]. ICM administration can cause an increase in ROS production. Therefore, the antioxidant properties of several pharmacological agents, including NAC, ascorbic acid, statins, and recently phosphodiesterase type 5 inhibitors, have been investigated to decrease the incidence of CIN [53].

Sodium bicarbonate has been proposed as an effective method of hydration due to its alkalinizing properties. Urine alkalinization can also reduce the pH-dependent formation of methemoglobin (Fe^{3+}) in tubular casts, with the production of free radicals being catalyzed by ferrous ion. The main nephroprotective effect of sodium bicarbonate is a reduction in oxidative stress by urine alkalinization. Bicarbonate can also directly scavenge peroxynitrite generated from nitric oxide [52, 53]. The PRESERVE study is currently conducted with the aim to definitively answer these questions on the prevention of CIN in high-risk patients undergoing coronary or noncoronary angiography [54]. Some meta-analyses showed that intravenous volume expansion with sodium bicarbonate was superior compared to normal saline, while other meta-analyses questioned the efficacy of the ESUR guidelines' recommendation to perform hydration with isotonic saline or sodium bicarbonate (3 mL/kg/h for 1 h before contrast medium followed by 1 mL/kg/h for 6 h after) in order to reduce the incidence of CIN. However, according to the guidelines of the European Society of Cardiology/European Association for Cardio-Thoracic Surgery, infusion of 0.84% sodium bicarbonate instead of standard hydration is not indicated for patients with moderate-to-severe chronic kidney disease undergoing coronary angiography or multidetector computed tomography [48].

***N*-Acetyl cysteine (NAC)**, an acetylated derivative of the amino acid cysteine, is a cheap, easily available, and safe supplement, not associated with any serious adverse effects (except the risk of anaphylactic reaction at a high intravenous dose) [52, 53]. The use of NAC is generally not contraindicated because it rarely induces drug interactions. Its nephroprotective effects can be attributed to its antioxidant properties by restoring the reduced intracellular pool of the natural antioxidant glutathione, direct free radical scavenging, and/or interaction with ROS, as well as prevention of contrast-induced renal cell apoptosis. In addition to its antioxidant properties, NAC can also exhibit vasodilatory effects by stabilizing nitric oxide or even by increasing nitric oxide production. Moreover, the sulfhydryl group of NAC can decrease angiotensin-converting enzyme, leading to a reduction in angiotensin II production.

NAC is available in both oral and intravenous formulations. Some centers have used a NAC scheme for prophylaxis. A trial concluded that NAC (at 600 mg orally twice daily, prior to and after contrast administration) combined with hydration (0.45% saline intravenously), prevents renal function. Subsequently, NAC was studied at higher doses orally (1200 mg twice daily for 48 h) and intravenously (the total dose ranging from 2400 mg to 150 mg/kg) [55]. However, widely conflicting results were obtained concerning whether NAC reduced the risk of CIN. ESUR concluded that there is not sufficient evidence regarding the efficacy of NAC to recommend its routine clinical use. Therefore, NAC is no longer recommended by guidelines for CIN prevention [47].

Ascorbic acid is a safe, well-tolerated, and readily available antioxidant agent that has been extensively investigated in the prevention of oxidative stress-related diseases due to its antioxidant function. It has been recommended that oral ascorbic acid administration (3 g orally given 2 h before the procedure and 2 g on the night and in the morning after the procedure) against the development of CIN. However, conflicting results have been reported in terms of the ability of ascorbic acid to reduce the incidence of CIN [52].

Statins are readily available and relatively inexpensive. The efficacy of statins for CIN prevention seems to be related to their non-lipid lowering (pleiotropic) effects on factors contributing to CIN progression, such as improving endothelial function, maintaining nitric oxide production, reducing inflammatory and immuno-modulatory processes, and oxidative stress and platelet adhesion, which may contribute to beneficial effects on nephroprotection even in the short term. However, some of the statins, such as rosuvastatin and atorvastatin, may not have the same effect [52, 53].

There are controversial data regarding the preventive effects of statins in CIN prophylaxis. The ESC guidelines recommend the short-term use of high-dose therapy, such as rosuvastatin 40/20 mg or atorvastatin 80 mg or simvastatin 80 mg for CKD cases prior to cardiac catheterization or CECT [48].

Phosphodiesterase 5 inhibitors (sildenafil, tadalafil, vardenafil, and avanafil) are often used to treat erectile dysfunction in humans by inducing the vasodilatory effect of the released nitric oxide; thus, they can provide protection against CIN. These drugs selectively inhibit cGMP-specific phosphodiesterase type 5 which metabolizes cGMP, the main mediator of nitric oxide inducing smooth muscle relaxation and vasodilatation. However, the endogenous vasodilator nitric oxide is crucial for medullary oxygenation and improving regional blood flow. A decrease in nitric oxide availability can increase the hypoxic insult and contribute to the development of CIN [56]. Prophylactic administration of a phosphodiesterase 5 inhibitor before and after

ICM administration provides a simple and rational approach to reduce the risk of CIN [52, 53]. The protective effect of such drugs [mainly sildenafil and recently tadalafil] on renal ischemia-reperfusion injury has been investigated in animal models. Sildenafil showed anti-apoptotic effects in experimental ischemia-reperfusion renal injury. The drug was administered before ICM infusion and repeatedly thereafter. Treatment with sildenafil was associated with a lower degree of histological injury and attenuation in the markers of CIN. These data suggest that sildenafil has a promising effect on the prevention of CIN [56].

3.8 Treatment

3.8.1 Medical Treatment

Some studies showed that early renal replacement therapy might reduce mortality and complication rates in patients with CIN. According to the current ESUR guidelines, there is no evidence that hemodialysis protects patients with impaired renal function from CIN [47].

Many clinical studies reported the effects of drugs used to treat CIN. Medications, such as loop diuretics, low-dose dopamine, or human ANP, have not yet been proven to facilitate recovery from CIN or prevent the progression of kidney dysfunction [53].

B-type natriuretic peptide released by myocardium under increased wall stress causes vasodilation, reduction in cardiac preload and afterload, and inhibition of cardiac remodeling, the renin-angiotensin-aldosterone system, sympathetic nervous system, and release of adenosine and endothelin. BNP also directly affects renal function by increasing GFR and decreasing sodium reabsorption in the proximal tubule and collecting duct. It has been shown that the infusion of lyophilized recombinant human BNP with isotonic saline reduces the incidence of CIN [57].

Theophylline or fenoldopam for prophylaxis should not be the standard of care based on the current published evidence [45, 53, 54].

3.8.2 Intrarenal Drug Infusion

The effects of intrarenal infusion of various agents have been investigated to increase the potential efficacy of pharmacological agents. A bifurcated catheter (Benephit catheter, AngioDynamics, Latham, NY, USA) was used for the dual direct renal infusion of fenoldopam. It was shown that this drug improves the renal blood flow but not the CIN rate when used intravenously. It was concluded that dual intrarenal infusion was associated with a lower CIN incidence [58]. The practicality and efficacy of this approach should be supported by further studies.

3.8.3 Remote Ischemic Conditioning

This is a therapeutic strategy in which a vascular bed in the same or a different organ by creating brief episodes of non-lethal ischemia and reperfusion which leads to production of endogenous autacoids, such as adenosine, opioids, and bradykinin, that activate protein kinases to inhibit the opening of the mitochondrial permeability transition pore which plays a critical role in tissue necrosis reduces the generation of harmful ROS and attenuates inflammation [59]. Some studies showed that RIC [four cycles of 5 min inflation and 5 min deflation using a standard pressure cuff to induce transient repetitive arm ischemia/reperfusion], immediately before coronary angiography, markedly decreased the incidence of CIN in patients with CKD [60].

3.8.4 Forced Diuresis

The combined use of diuretics and hydration to reduce CIN has been generally associated with worse clinical outcomes, probably due to the difficulty in adjusting hydration, intravascular volume, and urine volume [61]. In this context, the RenalGuard™ system (PLC Medical Systems, Milford, MA) was developed to manage a real-time automated fluid balance by continuously measuring furosemide-induced diuresis and replacing it with matched isotonic intravenous hydration. The underlying mechanism is that limiting the contrast-nephron exposure time while maintaining the renal blood flow could prevent the occurrence of CIN [62].

3.8.5 Automated Contrast Injection Systems

Mechanical strategies to prevent CIN have also been attempted. The use of an automated ICM injection system has been proposed as a means of limiting the volume of the administered contrast and thus reducing the incidence of CIN. However, although a large-scale study demonstrated that automated injection systems reduced the contrast volume by less than 3%, observational studies did not report any reduction in the incidence of CIN [63].

3.8.6 Device-Based Approach

Elimination of contrast before kidney exposure can be targeted. For this purpose, two methods have been used in coronary imaging, involving the removal of ICM either from the coronary sinus before exiting the heart and penetrating into the general circulation or from the general circulation by hemodialysis (HD) or hemofiltration [64]. The use of prophylactic continuous venovenous hemofiltration in patients with CKD undergoing complex PCI [from 4–8 h before to 18–24 h after the procedure] has been demonstrated to decrease the incidence of CIN. On the other hand, despite the well-established efficacy of HD in eliminating the contrast agent from the blood, hemodialysis has not been found associated with a decrease in the risk of CIN [65].

A device developed to attenuate the loss of contrast caused by reflux by changing the contrast injection pressure profile (AVERT, Osprey Medical, Minneapolis, MN) was shown to decrease contrast volumes by approximately 40%. The CINCORTM system (Osprey Medical, St. Paul, MN), innovated to prevent CIN, removes contrast-laden blood during and shortly after intracoronary ICM injection by means of balloon occlusion and aspiration of the coronary sinus [66].

3.8.7 Renal Cooling

Due to the potential protective effects of cooling on oxidative tissue injury, whether systemic hypothermia is effective in preventing CIN in patients with CKD has been investigated in the COOL RCN trial. The study showed that therapy could be used safely in patients undergoing angiography; however, there was no clear beneficial effect on the rates of CIN [67].

3.9 Metformin

Patients using metformin are at risk for lactic acidosis when receiving an ICA. If renal dysfunction occurs due to the ICA, metformin accumulation may occur and cause lactic acidosis. According to the ACR guidelines, metformin should be stopped at the time of an examination or procedure involving the use of an intravascular ICA, withheld for 48 h after the procedure, and reinstated only after renal function has been reevaluated and found to be normal [9]. However, there is no indication to postpone the examination if the patient takes a dose of metformin in the morning of the procedure [1–3].

References

1. van der Molen AJ, Reimer P, Dekkers IA, Bongartz G, Bellin MF, Bertolotto M, et al. Post-contrast acute kidney injury—part 1: definition, clinical features, incidence, role of contrast medium and risk factors: recommendations for updated ESUR Contrast Medium Safety Committee guidelines. Eur Radiol. 2018;28:2845–55.
2. Meinel FG, De Cecco CN, Schoepf UJ, Katzberg R. Contrast-induced acute kidney injury: definition, epidemiology, and outcome. Biomed Res Int. 2014;2014:859328.
3. Modi K, Gupta M. Contrast-induced nephropathy. Treasure Island: StatPearls Publishing; 2019.
4. Goldfarb S, McCullough PA, McDermott J, Gay SB. Contrast-induced acute kidney injury:

specialty-specific protocols for interventional radiology, diagnostic computed tomography radiology, and interventional cardiology. Mayo Clin Proc. 2009;84:170–9.
5. Makris K, Spanou L. Acute kidney injury: definition, pathophysiology and clinical phenotypes. Clin Biochem Rev. 2016;37:85–98.
6. Ostermann M, Joannidis M. Acute kidney injury 2016: diagnosis and diagnostic workup. Crit Care. 2016;20:299.
7. Mitchell AM, Jones AE, Tumlin JA, Kline JA. Incidence of contrast-induced nephropathy after contrast-enhanced computed tomography in the outpatient setting. Clin J Am Soc Nephrol. 2010;5:4–9.
8. Mohammed NM, Mahfouz A, Achkar K, Rafie IM, Hajar R. Contrast-induced nephropathy. Heart Views. 2013;14:106–16.
9. American College of Radiology. ACR manual on contrast media v10.2. Reston: American College of Radiology; 2016.
10. Hertzberg D, Rydén L, Pickering JW, Sartipy U, Holzmann MJ. Acute kidney injury-an overview of diagnostic methods and clinical management. Clin Kidney J. 2017;10:323–31.
11. Chawla LS, Bellomo R, Bihorac A, Goldstein SL, Siew ED, Bagshaw SM, et al. Acute Disease Quality Initiative Workgroup 16. Acute kidney disease and renal recovery: consensus report of the Acute Disease Quality Initiative (ADQI) 16 Workgroup. Nat Rev Nephrol. 2017;13:241–57.
12. Mehta RL, Kellum JA, Shah SV, Molitoris BA, Ronco C, Warnock DG, et al. Acute Kidney Injury Network. Acute Kidney Injury Network: report of an initiative to improve outcomes in acute kidney injury. Crit Care. 2007;11:R31.
13. KDIGO clinical practice guideline for acute kidney injury Kidney Int Suppl. 2012;2:S1–138.
14. Namasivayam S, Kalra MK, Torres WE, Small WC. Adverse reactions to intravenous iodinated contrast media: a primer for radiologists. Emerg Radiol. 2006;12:210–5.
15. Owen RJ, Hiremath S, Myers A, Fraser-Hill M, Barrett BJ. Canadian Association of Radiologists consensus guidelines for the prevention of contrast-induced nephropathy: update 2012. Can Assoc Radiol J. 2014;65:96–105.
16. Andreucci M, Faga T, Riccio E, Sabbatini M, Pisani A, Michael A. The potential use of biomarkers in predicting contrast-induced acute kidney injury. Int J Nephrol Renovasc Dis. 2016;9:205–21.
17. Zaffanello M, Franchini M, Fanos V. Is serum Cystatin-C a suitable marker of renal function in children? Ann Clin Lab Sci. 2007;37:233–40.
18. Kurtul A, Duran M, Yarlioglues M, Murat SN, Demircelik MB, Ergun G, et al. Association between N-terminal pro-brain natriuretic peptide levels and contrast-induced nephropathy in patients undergoing percutaneous coronary intervention for acute coronary syndrome. Clin Cardiol. 2014;37:485–92.
19. Albeladi FI, Algethamy HM. Urinary neutrophil gelatinase-associated lipocalin as a predictor of acute kidney injury, severe kidney injury, and the need for renal replacement therapy in the intensive care unit. Nephron Extra. 2017;7:62–77.
20. Yin C, Wang N. Kidney injury molecule-1 in kidney disease. Ren Fail. 2016;38:1567–73.
21. Kurtul A, Murat SN, Yarlioglues M, Duran M, Ocek AH, Celik IE, et al. Procalcitonin as an early predictor of contrast-induced acute kidney injury in patients with acute coronary syndromes who underwent percutaneous coronary intervention. Angiology. 2015;66:957–63.
22. Wang C, Ma S, Deng B, Lu J, Shen W, Jin B, et al. The predictive value of the product of contrast medium volume and urinary albumin/creatinine ratio in contrast-induced acute kidney injury. Ren Fail. 2017;39:555–60.
23. Chaykovska L, Heunisch F, von Einem G, Hocher CF, Tsuprykov O, Pavkovic M, et al. Urinary cGMP predicts major adverse renal events in patients with mild renal impairment and/or diabetes mellitus before exposure to contrast medium. PLoS One. 2018;13:e0195828.
24. Nyman U, Almén T, Aspelin P, Hellström M, Kristiansson M, Sterner G. Contrast-medium-induced nephropathy correlated to the ratio between dose in gram iodine and estimated GFR in ml/min. Acta Radiol. 2005;46:830–42.
25. Ad-Hoc Working Group of ERBP, Fliser D, Laville M, Covic A, Fouque D, Vanholder R, Juillard L, Van Biesen W. A European Renal Best Practice (ERBP) position statement on the Kidney Disease Improving Global Outcomes (KDIGO) clinical practice guidelines on acute kidney injury: part 1: definitions, conservative management and contrast-induced nephropathy. Nephrol Dial Transplant. 2012;27:4263–72.
26. Evola S, Lunetta M, Macaione F, Fonte G, Milana G, Corrado E, et al. Risk factors for contrast induced nephropathy: a study among Italian patients. Indian Heart J. 2012;64:484–91.
27. Abdel-Kader K, Palevsky P. Acute kidney injury in the elderly. Clin Geriatr Med. 2009;5:331–58.
28. Jain T, Shah S, Shah J, Jacobsen G, Khandelwal A. Contrast-induced nephropathy in STEMI patients with and without chronic kidney disease. Crit Pathw Cardiol. 2018;17:25–31.
29. Stacul F, Bertolotto M, Thomsen HS, Pozzato G, Ugolini D, Bellin MF, Bongartz G, Clement O, Heinz-Peer G, van der Molen A, Reimer P, Webb JAW, ESUR Contrast Media Safety Committee. Iodine-based contrast media, multiple myeloma and monoclonal gammopathies: literature review and ESUR Contrast Media Safety Committee guidelines. Eur Radiol. 2018;28:683–91.
30. Seeliger E, Sendeski M, Rihal CS, Persson PB. Contrast-induced kidney injury: mechanisms, risk factors, and prevention. Eur Heart J. 2012;33:2007–15.

31. Bottinor W, Polkampally P, Jovin I. Adverse reactions to iodinated contrast media. Int J Angiol. 2013;22:149–54.
32. Fähling M, Seeliger E, Patzak A, Persson PB. Understanding and preventing contrast-induced acute kidney injury. Nat Rev Nephrol. 2017;13:169–80.
33. McCullough PA, Stacul F, Becker CR, Adam A, Lameire N, Tumlin JA, Davidson CJ, CIN Consensus Working Panel. Contrast-Induced Nephropathy (CIN) Consensus Working Panel: executive summary. Rev Cardiovasc Med. 2006;7:177–97.
34. Brown JR, Robb JF, Block CA, Schoolwerth AC, Kaplan AV, O'Connor GT, Solomon RJ, Malenka DJ. Does safe dosing of iodinated contrast prevent contrast-induced acute kidney injury? Circ Cardiovasc Interv. 2010;3:346–50.
35. Karlsberg RP, Dohad SY, Sheng R, Iodixanol Peripheral CTA Study Investigator Panel. Contrast-induced acute kidney injury (CI-AKI) following intra-arterial administration of iodinated contrast media. J Nephrol. 2010;23:658–66.
36. Tao SM, Wichmann JL, Schoepf UJ, Fuller SR, Lu GM, Zhang LJ. Contrast-induced nephropathy in CT: incidence, risk factors and strategies for prevention. Eur Radiol. 2016;26:3310–8.
37. Mehran R, Aymong ED, Nikolsky E, Lasic Z, Iakovou I, Fahy M, et al. A simple risk score for prediction of contrast-induced nephropathy after percutaneous coronary intervention: development and initial validation. J Am Coll Cardiol. 2004;44:1393–9.
38. Cronin RE. Contrast-induced nephropathy: pathogenesis and prevention. Pediatr Nephrol. 2010;25:191–204.
39. Ultramari FT, Bueno Rda R, da Cunha CL, de Andrade PM, Nercolini DC, Tarastchuk JC, et al. Contrast media-induced nephropathy following diagnostic and therapeutic cardiac catheterization. Arq Bras Cardiol. 2006;87:378–90.
40. Hossain MA, Costanzo E, Cosentino J, Patel C, Qaisar H, Singh V, Khan T, et al. Contrast-induced nephropathy: pathophysiology, risk factors, and prevention. Saudi J Kidney Dis Transpl. 2018;29:1–9.
41. Hu X, Ma L, Zhang J, Li Z, Shen Y, Hu D. Use of pulmonary CT angiography with low tube voltage and low-iodine-concentration contrast agent to diagnose pulmonary embolism. Sci Rep. 2017;7:12741.
42. Andreucci M, Faga T, Pisani A, Sabbatini M, Russo D, Michael A. Prevention of contrast-induced nephropathy through a knowledge of its pathogenesis and risk factors. Sci World J. 2014;2014:823169.
43. Geenen RW, Kingma HJ, van der Molen AJ. Contrast-induced nephropathy: pharmacology, pathophysiology and prevention. Insights Imaging. 2013;4:811–20.
44. Agarwal SK, Mohareb S, Patel A, Yacoub R, DiNicolantonio JJ, Konstantinidis I, et al. Systematic oral hydration with water is similar to parenteral hydration for prevention of contrast-induced nephropathy: an updated meta-analysis of randomised clinical data. Open Heart. 2015;2:e000317.
45. Faggioni M, Mehran R. Preventing contrast-induced renal failure: a guide. Interv Cardiol. 2016;11:98–104.
46. Weisbord SD, Palevsky PM. Prevention of contrast-induced nephropathy with volume expansion. Clin J Am Soc Nephrol. 2008;3:273–80.
47. Kolh P, Windecker S. ESC/EACTS myocardial revascularization guidelines 2014. Eur Heart J. 2014;35:3235–6.
48. Brown JR, Pearlman DM, Marshall EJ, Alam SS, MacKenzie TA, Recio-Mayoral A, et al. Meta-analysis of individual patient data of sodium bicarbonate and sodium chloride for all-cause mortality after coronary angiography. Am J Cardiol. 2016;118:1473–9.
49. Zoungas S, Ninomiya T, Huxley R, Cass A, Jardine M, Gallagher M, et al. Systematic review: sodium bicarbonate treatment regimens for the prevention of contrast-induced nephropathy. Ann Intern Med. 2009;151:631–8.
50. Gleeson TG, Bulugahapitiya S. Contrast-induced nephropathy. AJR Am J Roentgenol. 2004;183:1673–89.
51. Briguori C, Marenzi G. Contrast-induced nephropathy: pharmacological prophylaxis. Kidney Int Suppl. 2006;100:S30–8.
52. Pattharanitima P, Tasanarong A. Pharmacological strategies to prevent contrast-induced acute kidney injury. Biomed Res Int. 2014;2014:236930.
53. Weisbord SD, Gallagher M, Kaufman J, Cass A, Parikh CR, Chertow GM, et al. Prevention of contrast-induced AKI: a review of published trials and the design of the prevention of serious adverse events following angiography (PRESERVE) trial. Clin J Am Soc Nephrol. 2013;8:1618–31.
54. Dósa E, Heltai K, Radovits T, Molnár G, Kapocsi J, Merkely B, et al. Dose escalation study of intravenous and intra-arterial N-acetylcysteine for the prevention of oto- and nephrotoxicity of cisplatin with a contrast-induced nephropathy model in patients with renal insufficiency. Fluids Barriers CNS. 2017;14:26.
55. Windecker S, Kolh P, Alfonso F, et al. Authors/Task Force members. 2014 ESC/EACTS guidelines on myocardial revascularization: the task force on myocardial revascularization of the European Society of Cardiology (ESC) and the European Association for Cardio-Thoracic Surgery (EACTS) developed with the special contribution of the European Association of Percutaneous Cardiovascular Interventions (EAPCI). Eur Heart J. 2014;35:2541–619.
56. Lauver DA, Carey EG, Bergin IL, Lucchesi BR, Gurm HS. Sildenafil citrate for prophylaxis of nephropathy in an animal model of contrast-induced acute kidney injury. PLoS One. 2014;9:e113598.
57. Liu JM, Xie YN, Gao ZH, Zu XG, Li YJ, Hao YM, Chang L. Brain natriuretic peptide for prevention of contrast-induced nephropathy after percutaneous coronary intervention or coronary angiography. Can J Cardiol. 2014;30:1607–12.
58. Talati S, Kirtane AJ, Hassanin A, Mehran R, Leon MB, Moses JW, et al. Direct infusion of fenoldopam into the renal arteries to protect against contrast-

induced nephropathy in patients at increased risk. Clin Exp Pharmacol Physiol. 2012;39:506–9.
59. Zhou F, Song W, Wang Z, Yin L, Yang S, Yang F, et al. Effects of remote ischemic preconditioning on contrast induced nephropathy after percutaneous coronary intervention in patients with acute coronary syndrome. Medicine (Baltimore). 2018;97:e9579.
60. Heusch G, Bøtker HE, Przyklenk K, Redington A, Yellon D. Remote ischemic conditioning. J Am Coll Cardiol. 2015;65:177–95.
61. Majumdar SR, Kjellstrand CM, Tymchak WJ, Hervas-Malo M, Taylor DA, Teo KK. Forced euvolemic diuresis with mannitol and furosemide for prevention of contrast-induced nephropathy in patients with CKD undergoing coronary angiography: a randomized controlled trial. Am J Kidney Dis. 2009;54:602–9.
62. Katoh H, Nozue T, Horie K, Sozu T, Inoue N, Michishita I. Renal Guard system to prevent contrast-induced acute kidney injury in Japanese patients with renal dysfunction; RESPECT KIDNEY study. Cardiovasc Interv Ther. 2019;34:105–12.
63. Call J, Sacrinty M, Applegate R, Little W, Santos R, Baki T, et al. Automated contrast injection in contemporary practice during cardiac catheterization and PCI: effects on contrast-induced nephropathy. J Invasive Cardiol. 2006;18:469–74.
64. Stub D, Duffy SJ, Kaye DM. Device-based therapy in the prevention of contrast-induced nephropathy. Interv Cardiol Clin. 2014;3:421–8.
65. Guastoni C, Bellotti N, Poletti F, Covella P, Gidaro B, Stasi A, et al. Continuous venovenous hemofiltration after coronary procedures for the prevention of contrast-induced acute kidney injury in patients with severe chronic renal failure. Am J Cardiol. 2014;113:588–92.
66. Susantitaphong P, Eiam-Ong S. Nonpharmacological strategies to prevent contrast-induced acute kidney injury. Biomed Res Int. 2014;2014:463608.
67. Stone GW, Vora K, Schindler J, Diaz C, Mann T, Dangas G, Best P, Cutlip DE, COOL-RCN Investigators. Systemic hypothermia to prevent radiocontrast nephropathy [from the COOL-RCN Randomized Trial]. Am J Cardiol. 2011;108:741–6.

Adverse Reactions to Iodinated Contrast Agents

4

Suzan Saylisoy and Sukru Mehmet Erturk

4.1 Introduction

Iodinated contrast agents (ICAs) are the most widely used drugs in diagnostic radiology. In the United States, more than 50 million computed tomography (CT) studies are performed every year with approximately half of these studies involving the use of intravenous (IV) ICAs [1]. There has also been an increase in the utilization of intra-arterial ICAs in cardiac catheterization and percutaneous coronary interventions. However, these agents are not completely safe and may present with adverse reactions (ARs) to ICAs that are divided into general and organ-specific, such as contrast-induced nephropathy and encephalopathy [2]. General ARs are further classified as acute (occurring within 1 h of administration) and late (occurring from 1 h to 1 week after administration) [3–5].

It is important for radiologists, interventional cardiologists, and referring physicians to be aware of possible ARs to ICAs and their management. The decision to use ICAs should be made after obtaining an appropriate history for each patient, considering the clinical benefits of contrast-enhanced imaging, and risks of using or avoiding ICAs. The general policy of ICA use to obtain the required diagnostic clinical data from radiological studies should be the lowest dose, concentration, and number of injections [5].

The purpose of this chapter is to increase readers' familiarity in recognizing and managing ARs and review the classification, incidence, pathogenesis, risk factors, clinical features, treatment, and prevention of ARs to ICAs.

4.2 General Adverse Reactions

General ARs are classified as acute (occurring within 1 h of administration) and late (occurring from 1 h to 1 week after administration) [3–5]. ARs are also further divided into three categories according to their severity (mild, moderate, or severe). **Mild reactions** have a short duration and are self-limiting, and they generally do not require specific treatment. **Moderate and severe reactions** manifest serious degrees of reactions requiring immediate management. Almost all life-threatening ICA reactions occur within the first 20 min after an ICA injection [6].

4.2.1 Acute Adverse Reactions

Acute ARs (AARs) are classified as either allergy-like or chemotoxic (physiologic). This classification is important for the proper

S. Saylisoy (✉)
Department of Radiology, Eskişehir Osmangazi University, Eskisehir, Turkey

S. M. Erturk
Department of Radiology, Istanbul University School of Medicine, Istanbul, Turkey

S. M. Erturk et al. (eds.), *Medical Imaging Contrast Agents: A Clinical Manual*,
https://doi.org/10.1007/978-3-030-79256-5_4

management of patients experiencing different types of reactions (e.g., those who experience allergy-like reactions may require premedication before contrast-enhanced studies, but those who experience physiologic reactions do not) [3–5].

The incidence of AARs (allergy-like and chemotoxic) associated with intravascular administration of ICAs is low and significantly reduced by changes in the use of ionic high-osmolality contrast media (HOCM) to nonionic low-/iso-osmolality ICAs [7]. The use of HOCM for intravascular purposes is now very rare or even none due to its greater AR profile compared to low-/iso-osmolality ICAs. Low-/iso-osmolality ICAs are associated with a very low AAR rate, and most are not life-threatening. The incidence of AARs ranges from 0.2 to 0.7% [8].

4.2.1.1 Allergy-Like Reactions

Allergy-like reactions present with symptoms ranging from urticaria to an anaphylactoid process that resemble allergic reactions, but they are not actually allergies. The etiology of these reactions is not completely understood. Allergy-like ARs are likely to be independent of dose and concentration above a certain unknown threshold [9, 10].

Pathophysiologic explanations for allergy-like reactions include activation of mast cells and basophils releasing histamine and other mediators, activation of contact and complement systems, conversion of L-arginine into nitric oxide, activation of the XII coagulation and system leading to the production of bradykinin, and development of "pseudoantigens" [4]. The increase in the size and complexity of the contrast molecule may induce the histamine release from basophils. It is generally accepted that most allergy-like ARs are not associated with an increased IgE [10]. This probably explains why patients who have not previously been exposed to ICAs can still have similar reactions to those with a history of such exposure. However, skin and intradermal tests are positive in the minority of individuals, suggesting an IgE-mediated etiology [11]. Although allergy-like ARs after an ICA injection do not necessarily mean that the patient will experience a recurrent reaction next time an ICA is injected, a previous AR remains to be the best predictor of a future AR, with a probability of a recurrent reaction ranging from 8 to 25% [12]. Additives or contaminants, such as calcium-chelating substances and substances separated from rubber stoppers in bottles or syringes, are believed to contribute to certain allergy-like reactions. The treatment of an allergy-like ICA reaction is the same as that of an equivalent allergic reaction [4].

4.2.1.2 Chemotoxic Reactions

Chemotoxic (physiologic) reactions are related to specific molecular properties that directly lead to chemotoxicity, osmotoxicity (ARs due to hyperosmolality), or molecular binding to certain activators. These reactions frequently depend on the dose and concentration and include reactions, such as contrast-induced encephalopathy (CIE), cardiac arrhythmias, and cardiogenic pulmonary edema. Most of those reactions are mild, and severe chemotoxic ARs are rare with a rate of approximately one to four reactions per 10,000 patients [13].

Vasovagal reactions are relatively common and characterized by bradycardia and hypotension [3, 9]. Although their pathogenesis is not completely known, increased vagal tone caused by the central nervous system is thought to be the reason. Vasovagal reactions may also be anxiety-related and may occur while obtaining informed consent during the insertion of a needle or catheter for contrast medium injection or during intravascular ICA administration. Although most vagal reactions are mild and self-limited, a close patient observation is recommended until symptoms are completely resolved [3].

Risk Factors

The risk of ARs to ICAs increases due to several predisposing factors. It is important to identify all predisposing factors in a patient before ICA administration to reduce the risk of ARs.

Allergies

A previous allergy-like reaction to ICAs is the most important risk factor for recurrent allergy-like ARs. Patients with a history of ARs to ICAs have five times greater risk of an allergy-like AR when exposed to the same class of ICAs again. However, there is no cross-reactivity between different classes of contrast agents. A previous reaction to a gadolinium-based contrast medium does not necessarily mean that there will be a future reaction to ICAs [4, 13]. Atopic individuals (especially those with multiple severe allergies) and asthmatics also have an increased risk for allergy-like ARs. Unrelated allergy history increases the risk of an allergy-like AR two to three times [13, 14]. In the use of ICAs, shellfish or povidone-iodine allergies are not considered to constitute a greater risk than other allergies. However due to the modest level of increased risk, ICA restriction or premedication is not recommended in the presence of other indications, such as allergic reactions to other substances (including shellfish or ICAs from another class e.g., gadolinium-based iodinated), asthma, seasonal allergies, or multiple drug and food allergies [4].

Beta-Blockers

The effect of beta-blockers on ARs to ICAs is controversial. According to Lang et al., the incidence of an allergy-like reaction to ICAs is increased in patients taking beta-blockers [15]. Conversely, in another study, Greenberger et al. reported that beta-blockers did not increase the risk of allergy-like reactions to ICAs [16]. However, the use of beta-blockers reduces the patient's responsiveness to epinephrine treatment.

Age and Gender

Newborns, infants, children, and the elderly have lower reaction rates than middle-aged patients [4]. ARs are more common in people aged between 20 and 50 years and are less frequent above 50 years; however, these reactions tend to be more severe in the elderly. Male patients have lower reaction rates than female patients [2].

Sickle Cell Trait/Disease

Increased sickling of erythrocytes in patients with sickle cell anemia may occur following an IV administration of ICAs. However, there is no evidence to support this finding in the use of modern ICAs [17].

Pheochromocytoma

There is no evidence that an IV administration of modern ICAs increases the risk of a hypertensive crisis in patients with pheochromocytoma [4].

Myasthenia Gravis

The relationship between IV administration of ICA and myasthenic exacerbation in patients with myasthenia gravis is not clear [4].

Hyperthyroidism

Thyrotoxicosis may develop following ICA administration in patients with a history of hyperthyroidism, but this complication is rare. Therefore, ICA restriction or premedication based on a history of hyperthyroidism is not recommended. However, there are two exceptions to this. First, in patients with acute thyroid storm, ICA should not be used since it can potentiate thyrotoxicosis. Second, in patients considering radioactive iodine therapy or those undergoing radioactive iodine imaging of the thyroid gland, the use of ICA may prevent uptake of treatment and diagnostic dose [18, 19]. If ICA is to be given, a washout period is recommended to minimize this interaction. The ideal washout period is 3–4 weeks for patients with hyperthyroidism and 6 weeks for those with hypothyroidism [4].

Premedication

The radiologist should weigh the benefits of contrast-enhanced imaging against the risk of ARs before ICA administration. If the urgency of a contrast-enhanced examination outweighs the benefits of prophylaxis, regardless of duration, ICA is required to be administered to a high-risk patient without premedication.

The history of a previous severe AR is considered a relative contraindication to the future use of the same class of ICAs. In such circumstances, switching ICAs within the same class (e.g., one iodinated medium for another) may help reduce the likelihood of future ARs [20]. The effect of switching ICAs may be actually greater than that of premedication alone, but combining premedication with altered ICAs seems to have the greatest impact [4].

Corticosteroids can be given to reduce the risk of an allergy-like reaction or decrease the severity of ARs. However, premedication does not prevent all ARs [3]. Oral premedication is preferred for IV premedication in most settings due to its lower cost, greater convenience, and presence of more supportive evidence in the literature [4, 19]. Addition of a non-selective antihistamine (e.g., diphenhydramine) orally or intravenously 1 h prior to the administration of ICA may reduce the frequency of urticaria, angioedema, and respiratory symptoms. However, the use of selective antihistamines has not been well studied [4].

The minimum premedication time required for efficacy is not known [3]. Lasser et al. showed that in average-risk patients, one dose of 32 mg oral methylprednisolone 2 h before intravascular HOCM administration was not effective, while two doses administered at 2 and 12 h before ICA administration were effective [20]. There is no evidence to support the premedication duration of 2 h or less (oral or intravascular, corticosteroid- or antihistamine-based). An intravascular corticosteroid procedure lasting at least 4–5 h may be effective [4].

Elective premedication (12- or 13-h oral premedication) may be considered in outpatients with previous allergy-like ARs or ARs of unknown type to the same class of ICAs (e.g., iodinated-iodinated), emergency cases, or inpatients with previous allergy-like ARs or unknown-type ARs to the same class of ICAs (e.g., iodinated-iodinated), in whom the use of premedication is not anticipated to delay care or treatment. There are two types of elective premedication regimens recommended by the American College of Radiology (ACR) Manual on Contrast Media (version 10.3):

1. Prednisone-based (orally 50 mg prednisone at 13 h, 7 h, and 1 h before ICA administration)
2. Methylprednisolone-based (orally 32 mg methylprednisolone at 12 h and 2 h before ICA administration)

In option 1, 50 mg intravenous, intramuscular, or oral diphenhydramine can be added to these regimens 1 h before ICA administration. If a patient cannot take oral medication, option 1 can be modified by substituting each dose of oral prednisone by 200 mg IV hydrocortisone [4].

Accelerated IV premedication may be considered in outpatients with a previous allergy-like or unknown-type contrast reaction to the same class of contrast medium (e.g., iodinated-iodinated) who has arrived for a contrast-enhanced examination but has not been premedicated and whose examination cannot be easily postponed, emergency patients or inpatients with a previous allergy-like or unknown-type contrast reaction to the same class of contrast medium (e.g., iodinated-iodinated), in whom the use of 12- or 13-h premedication is anticipated to adversely delay care or treatment. There are three types of elective premedication regimens recommended by the American College of Radiology (ACR) Manual on Contrast Media (version 10.3):

1. Methylprednisolone sodium succinate (e.g., Solu-Medrol®) 40 mg IV or hydrocortisone sodium succinate (e.g., Solu-Cortef®) 200 mg IV immediately and then every 4 h until ICA administration, plus diphenhydramine 50 mg IV 1 h prior to ICA. This regimen usually takes 4–5 h.
2. Dexamethasone sodium sulfate (e.g., Decadron®) 7.5 mg IV immediately and then every 4 h until ICA administration, plus diphenhydramine 50 mg IV 1 h before contrast medium administration. This regimen may be useful in patients with an allergy to methylprednisolone and is usually 4–5 h in duration [4].
3. Methylprednisolone sodium succinate (e.g., Solu-Medrol®) 40 mg IV or hydrocortisone sodium succinate (e.g., Solu-Cortef®) 200 mg IV, plus diphenhydramine 50 mg IV, each 1 h before ICA administration.

   These regimens with a duration less than 4–5 have no evidence of efficacy. It may be considered in emergent situations when there are no alternatives.

Premedication in Patients Undergoing Chronic Corticosteroid Therapy

The premedication dose may be modified in patients who are receiving chronic corticosteroid therapy. If corticosteroid premedication is being used, a guiding principle is to reduce the dose of the chosen premedication dose regimen in an amount equivalent to the chronic therapeutic corticosteroid dose of the patient. If the patient is on simple replacement corticosteroid therapy, the premedication dosing regimen may not need to be adjusted [4].

Benefits of Premedication

It has been shown that premedication of patients with average risk prior to HOCM administration reduces the likelihood of AARs of all severity levels. However, HOCM is no longer used for IV purposes. Another randomized study showed that premedication prior to low-/iso-osmolality ICA administration reduced the likelihood of mild ARs, but there was no sufficient evidence suggesting its efficacy in preventing moderate or severe reactions or reaction-related deaths. However, many experts believe that premedication reduces the likelihood of ARs in high-risk patients receiving low-/iso-osmolality ICAs [4].

Risks of Premedication

The direct risks of premedication are small and include transient leukocytosis, transient (24–48 h) and generally asymptomatic hyperglycemia (non-diabetics, +20–80 mg/dL; diabetics, +100–150 mg/dL), and a questionable infection risk. Diphenhydramine may cause drowsiness and should not be taken shortly before using a tool. Some patients experience allergies to the drugs used in premedication. The greatest risk of premedication is indirect and is related to the delay in radiological diagnosis due to the multi-hour duration of premedication [4].

Breakthrough Contrast Reactions

All ARs cannot be prevented by premedication. Allergy-like ARs that occur despite premedication are called "breakthrough reactions." In patients premedicated due to the history of an AR, the breakthrough reaction rate is 2.1%, which is three to four times the usual reaction rate in the general population [21]. A prior breakthrough reaction does not mean a repeat breakthrough reaction. Chemotoxic reactions are not reduced by premedication and are not considered as breakthrough reactions, even if they occur after premedication [4].

Treatment

An emergency cart with facilities for airway management, oxygen and masks, intravenous fluids, and appropriate drugs should always be available immediately and must be regularly checked. The optimal treatment of ICA reactions begins with a well-designed action plan and well-trained staff who are competent in both rapid recognition and treatment strategies [3, 4, 9].

Basic emergency equipment and medications required to treat ARs should be easily accessible. These should include equipment necessary to evaluate a patient, such as a stethoscope, blood pressure/pulse meter, and pulse oximeter, as well as medications necessary to treat a patient, such as sterile saline for intravenous injection, diphenhydramine, beta-agonist inhaler (e.g., albuterol), epinephrine, atropine, oxygen, intubation equipment, and a cardiac defibrillator. When evaluating a patient for possible ARs, an immediate evaluation should be undertaken concerning the patient's appearance, voice, breathing, pulse strength and rate, and blood pressure [3–6, 9].

Mild reactions (both allergy-like and non-allergy-like) usually do not require medical treatment. Observation for 20–30 min or as long as needed to ensure clinical stability or recovery is generally sufficient for any patient with a mild allergy-like reaction. Sometimes, treatment with an antihistamine may be initiated for mild symptomatic allergy-like cutaneous contrast reactions, but this is often not necessary. Many mild reactions resolve during an observation period without treatment [12]. Most moderate and all severe reactions require prompt and aggressive treatment (Table 4.1) [3–6, 9, 19].

4.2.2 Late Adverse Reactions

A late AR (LAR) is defined as a reaction occurring 1 h to 1 week after ICA administration, and it generally develops between 3 h and 2 days [2–4]. Although the reactions actually are related to the

Table 4.1 Treatment of general acute adverse reactions to ICA

Symptom	Management
Hives (urticaria)	• **Mild**; no treatment often needed, consider diphenhydramine(Benadryl®, 1 mg/kg PO/IM/IV, max 50 mg) • **Moderate**; monitor vitals, consider diphenhydramine(Benadryl®, 1 mg/kg PO/IM/IV, max 50 mg) • **Severe**; monitor vitals, consider diphenhydramine(Benadryl®, 1 mg/kg PO/IM/IV, max 50 mg)
Diffuse erythema	• **Normotensive**; no treatment often needed • **Hypotensive**; IV 0.1 mL/kg (a dilution of 1 ampoule (1 mL) of epinephrine 1:1000 with 9 mL water)
Laryngeal edema	– Epinephrine SC or IM 0.1–0.3 mL (= 0.1–0.3 mg) (1:1000), if hypotensive, IV 1 mL (=0.1 mg) (1:10,000) epinephrine; can repeat as needed up to 1 mg – 6–10 L/min O_2 by mask
Bronchospasm	– Monitor vitals – O_2 by mask 6–10 L/min – Beta-agonist inhalers, 2–3 puffs; repeat up to three times – Beta-agonist nebulization (5 mg in 2 mL of saline) – If the bronchospasm is progressive, epinephrine SC or IM 0.1–0.3 mL (=0.1–0.3 mg) (1:1000); can repeat as needed up to 1 mg – Call for emergency response team for severe bronchospasm or if O_2 saturation <88% persists
Hypotension with tachycardia	– Elevate legs >60° or Trendelenburg position – Monitor vitals – O_2 by mask 6–10 L/min – Rapid large volumes of IV isotonic Ringer's lactate or normal saline – If unresponsive, epinephrine SC or IM 0.1–0.3 mL (=0.1–0.3 mg) (1:1000) can repeat as needed up to 1 mg – Call for emergency response team if still poorly responsive
Hypotension with bradycardia (vagal reaction)	– Elevate legs 60° or more (preferred) or Trendelenburg position – Monitor vitals – O_2 by mask 6–10 L/min – Rapid large volumes of IV isotonic Ringer's lactate or normal saline – If unresponsive, atropine 0.6–1 mg IV slowly—repeat up to 2–3 mg in adult
Severe hypertension	– Monitor vitals – O_2 by mask 6–10 L/min – Labetalol 20 mg, IV, slow infusion – Nitroglycerine 0.4-mg tablet, sublingual (may repeat × 3) – Diuretics—furosemide (Lasix®) 20–40 mg IV, slow push – Call for emergency response team if still poorly responsive – For pheochromocytoma—phentolamine 5 mg IV
Seizures or convulsions	– Lateral decubitus position to avoid aspiation – Monitor vitals – O_2 by mask 6–10 L/min – Consider diazepam (Valium®) 5 mg or more or midazolam (Versed®) 0.5–1 mg IV
Pulmonary edema	– Elevate torso; rotating tourniquets (venous compression) – Monitor vitals – 6–10 L/min O_2 by mask – Diuretics—furosemide (Lasix®) 20–40 mg IV, slow push – Call for emergency response team
Anaphylactoid generalized reaction	– Call for emergency response team – Ensure patients airvays – Elevate legs – O_2 by mask 6–10 L/min – IV fluid replasman (normal saline or ringer lactate) – Hydrocortisone 500 mg IV – Epinephrine (1:1000), 0.5 mL IV

ICA, reactions can be attributed to the underlying disease process. The recognition of LARs can be difficult due to the longer time interval between ICA administration and occurrence of symptoms. Although the pathogenesis of LARs is not completely understood, it appears that many are T-cell-mediated reactions. These are generally self-limiting skin reactions that resolve within 3–7 days [4, 10]. The majority of these skin reactions are T-cell-mediated allergic reactions. Various late non-cutaneous symptoms and signs have also been reported, including headache, nausea, dizziness, fever, arm pain, and gastrointestinal disorders. Examples of mild LARs are pruritus, urticaria, exanthema, nausea and vomiting, and headache. Moderate reactions, e.g., urticaria, facial edema, and bronchospasm, are more pronounced and commonly require medical management. Severe reactions, such as diffuse erythema with hypotension and cardiopulmonary arrest, are generally life-threatening [3, 9].

The types of late cutaneous reactions and their frequencies are similar to those associated with many other drugs. Cutaneous reactions usually show typical features of late hypersensitivity reactions, including exanthematous rashes, positive skin tests, and dermal perivascular lymphocyte infiltration together with eosinophils on skin biopsy [13]. Other cutaneous symptoms are urticaria, erythema, purpuric lesions, blisters, vesicles, angioedema, facial edema, and Stevens-Johnson syndrome. Systemic symptoms, e.g., fever and leukocytosis, may also accompany the disease. In most cases, cutaneous reactions are mild or moderate. Severe late reactions that require hospital treatment and/or lead to persistent disability or death have been reported, but they are very rare. A severe form of LARs is acute generalized exanthematous pustulosis (AGEP), characterized by the sudden appearance of dozens to hundreds of sterile, punctate pustules arising on a bed of erythema and edema. This rash is more prominent in skin folds [3, 4, 22].

4.2.2.1 Risk Factors

It has been reported that the incidence of LARs is between 0.5 and 14% [4]. There are many factors that predispose individuals to the development of LARs. A previous reaction to ICAs is an important predisposing factor that increases the risk by 1.7–3.3 times [3]. However, there is no apparent relationship between the occurrence of AARs and LARs. An allergy history is another risk factor that increases the risk by approximately two times [3, 4, 23, 24]. LARs are more common in young adults and women. Coexisting diseases, especially renal disease, but also including cardiac and liver disease and diabetes mellitus seem to be other predisposing factors for LARs. The increased incidence of LARs in patients receiving interleukin-2 (IL-2) immunotherapy is well documented. Cutaneous reactions may be more severe in individuals with systemic lupus erythematosus [13]. Cutaneous ARs may also occur at an increased frequency in certain seasons (April to June). The dimeric group may have a higher rate of LARs than the monomeric group [9]. In addition, there is a higher incidence of LARs in the iso-osmolar group (12.3%) than in the low osmolar group (8.4%).

Prophylaxis and Treatment

Patients with a history of a hypersensitivity reaction to ICAs are at increased risk for another reaction after re-exposure to ICAs. Compared to the response that occurs within 2–10 days at first exposure, re-exposure to ICAs generally results in a faster and more severe response that occurs within 1–2 days, which is consistent with an allergic drug reaction with a sensitization phase [24]. There is no clear consensus about the effect of corticosteroids and/or antihistamines on LARs, but some researchers have recommended using these agents. ACR, in the ACR Manual on ICA, Version 10.3, states that the efficacy of corticosteroids and antihistamines in preventing a contrast reaction is unknown [4]. The Safety Committee of the European Society of Urogenital Radiology (ESUR) recommends that patients with a history of a late cutaneous reaction after receiving ICAs, those with a major drug or contact allergy, and those who have received interleukin-2 are to be warned about the possibility of LARs and instructed to contact a doctor. An alternative contrast medium should be chosen along with steroid prophylaxis in cases with a history of moderate to severe LARs. However, given the similarity in molecular structures of all currently used contrast agents, these patients will still be at an increased risk of LARs [3].

ACR, in the ACR Manual on ICA, Version 10.3, states that most cases require no or minimal therapy due to the self-limited nature of LARs. Although mild general reactions are self-limiting, when they occur, the intravenous access must be retained, and the patient should be observed until complete recovery. With the exception of severe reactions, such as AGEP, Stevens-Johnson syndrome, and toxic epidermal necrolysis, the treatment of LARs is generally supported with antihistamines (chlorpheniramine maleate 4–8 mg orally or 10–20 mg IV slowly administered over 2 min) and corticosteroids or both for skin conditions, antipyretics for fever, antiemetics for nausea, oxygen and salbutamol for wheezing, and fluid resuscitation for hypotension. If manifestations are progressive or widespread, consultation with an allergist and/or dermatologist may be useful [4, 25].

4.3 Organ-Specific Adverse Effects

4.3.1 Salivary Gland Adverse Effects

Iodine mumps (iodine-related sialoadenopathy or salivary gland swelling) are characterized by the acute or delayed painless enlargement of salivary glands induced by ICAs. This disorder presents predominantly in parotid and submandibular glands [26]. Occasionally, the thyroid lacrimal or other glands are also involved. It may be seen as bilateral or unilateral. The pathogenesis of iodide mumps is not yet clear, but it is presumably secondary to toxic accumulation of iodide in salivary glands with a high iodide concentration. The course of iodide mumps is self-limiting, and treatment is not necessary [26, 27].

4.3.2 Central Nervous System Adverse Effects

Contrast-induced encephalopathy (CIE) is an acute and transient neurological disturbance occurring within minutes to hours after an IV, intra-arterial, or intrathecal ICA exposure. It may present with headache, vomiting, seizure, encephalopathy, aphasia motor and sensory disturbances, and vision disturbances, including cortical blindness and ophthalmoplegia [28]. Possible risk factors for CIE include hypertension with impaired cerebral autoregulation, direct injection into the cerebral circulation, intracranial pathology, diabetes mellitus, renal impairment, administration of a large volume of ICA, percutaneous coronary interventions, and history of ARs [29]. Disruption of the brain-blood barrier and direct neurotoxic effect caused by ICAs is believed to be potential mechanisms. Some authors hypothesize that osmolarity causes meningeal irritation. However, the role of immune-mediated factors has not been excluded.

After intrathecal administration, ICAs diffuse from the cisterna into the parenchyma, reaching the maximum effect within 5–24 h after injection. The most common minor ARs after myelography with ICAs are headache, nausea, vomiting, and dizziness. Aseptic meningitis and meningoencephalitis are also considered as complications associated with myelography with nonionic ICAs [30].

CIE is a diagnosis of exclusion and should be considered in the differential diagnosis of acute neurologic deficit that occurs after radiological procedures involving ICAs. Radiological signs, such as cerebral edema and cortical enhancement, are of great importance in the diagnostic process. These signs may be seen as unilateral. Symptoms resolve completely within 24–48 h. Prognosis is excellent even in comatose patients, and supportive management is sufficient.

4.3.3 Gastrointestinal Tract Adverse Effects

Bowel angioedema due to the IV administration of ICAs can be easily diagnosed based on its characteristic CT findings and clinical symptoms. The predilection location of ICA-associated bowel angioedema is the small bowel, particularly the proximal segment. The pathogenesis of this condition is not clear but is thought to be similar to that of other ICA-associated immediate hypersensitivity reactions. ICA-associated bowel angioedema can manifest with mild symptoms, such as abdominal discomfort, abdominal pain, and vomiting. While the bowel wall is normal in non-enhanced images, segmental circumferential wall thickening of the proximal small bowel is detected after contrast administration compared with precontrast images. The differential diagnosis includes inflammatory and ischemic bowel diseases, as well as neoplasia [31].

4.3.4 Hepatic Adverse Effects

The elevation of the liver enzymes subsequent into biliary administration has been reported [32].

4.3.5 Pancreatic Adverse Effects

Contrast-enhanced CT is widely used to confirm the diagnosis and establish the severity of acute pancreatitis. Intravenous ICA administration lengthens the duration of pancreatitis and increases the incidence of local or systemic complications, particularly in those with a body mass index of 25 or greater. The harmful effects of ICAs in experimental models have been attributed to the pancreatic blood reduction induced by these agents [33].

4.3.6 Musculoskeletal Adverse Effects

Acute polyarthropathy is a late contrast reaction rarely reported after ICA administration. This reaction may be more frequent in patients with renal dysfunction [34].

ICAs are also used for various intradiscal injections, such as discography and endoscopic spinal surgery. ICAs are cytotoxic to human disc cells in a dose- and time-dependent manner [35].

Malignant hyperthermia occurs when certain physiologically active compounds act on defective skeletal and cardiac muscle cells. Malignant hyperthermia has characteristically complicated the administrations of anesthetics but is being triggered by drugs used in other diagnostic activities [36].

4.3.7 Pulmonary Adverse Effects

The lung is an important target organ of the effects of ICAs. Pulmonary circulation is the first important vascular bed to receive ICAs following an intravenous injection and during the venous return after an arteriographic exam. The pulmonary ARs to the IV use of ICAs include bronchospasm, pulmonary edema, and increased pulmonary arterial blood pressure [37].

The pathogenesis of non-cardiogenic pulmonary edema is not clear, and it is not known whether this represents a physiologic or allergy-like reaction. Such pulmonary edemas can be caused by mediator release and complement activation, resulting in endothelial damage or by a direct irritant effect of the drug on the lungs. The primary emergency treatment is oxygen with continuous positive airway pressure or invasive ventilation with positive and expiratory pressure [38].

4.3.8 Cardiovascular Adverse Effects

Cardiac ARs are more common in angiocardiography than IV administration of ICAs. In patients with an underlying cardiac disease, cardiovascular effects are more frequent and significant. Cardiac arrhythmias, depressed myocardial contractility, and cardiogenic pulmonary edema are very rare. These reactions are probably related to either ICA-related hyperosmolality or calcium binding leading to functional hypocalcemia [39]. Kounis syndrome (also called allergic angina) is a cardiac complaint after ICA administration. All classes of ICAs are vasoactive and can induce both vasodilatation and vasoconstriction. Osmolality and the chemical structure of ICAs appear to determine their vasoactive effects [40].

4.4 Adverse Reactions After ICA Administration by Other Routes

Oral and rectal ICAs are used for the imaging of the gastrointestinal system. Oral agents are also occasionally used for the opacification of the biliary tree. Two commercial water-soluble HOCMs specifically designed for gastrointestinal tract opacification are widely used [Gastrografin® (Bracco Diagnostics, Inc.; Princeton, NJ) and Gastroview (Covidien; Hazelwood, MO)]. These HOCMs are hypertonic and draw fluid into the lumen of the bowel, leading to further hypovolemia and hypotension. In some children and older adults, the loss of plasma fluid may be sufficient to cause a shock-like condition. In this case, ICAs can be diluted with water. Low-osmolality contrast media (LOCM) draw less fluid into the bowel lumen [41].

HOCM can cause life-threatening pulmonary complications if aspirated. Low-/iso-osmolality ICAs can reduce the possibility of contrast-related pneumonitis in patients at risk of aspiration [42].

Allergy-like reactions can occur even due to small amounts of ICA absorbed from the gastrointestinal tract after oral or rectal administration. A small volume of ICA (approximately 1–2%) is absorbed and then excreted into the urinary tract. If mucosal inflammation, mucosal infection, or intestinal obstruction is present, the absorbed amount of ICA may increase [13].

ICAs are directly administered into the biliary and pancreatic ductal systems during endoscopic retrograde cholangiopancreatography (ERCP) studies of the biliary tree. Small amounts of these agents may be absorbed, resulting in a systemic exposure. Allergy-like reactions can be seen after ERCP [43].

4.5 Adverse Reactions After ICA Administration in Pregnant or Potentially Pregnant Women

When ICAs are administered at usual clinical doses, they cross the human placenta and enter the fetus in measurable quantities. After entering the fetal blood flow, these agents are excreted into amniotic fluid by urine and swallowed by the fetus. Then, a small amount is absorbed by the gut of the fetus [44]. The fetal thyroid plays a crucial role in the development of the central nervous system. There are a few reports of hypothyroidism in newborns after the administration of an ICA during pregnancy; however, these only developed following amniofetography with a fat-soluble ICA, which was used in the past to detect congenital malformations. Intravascular administration of ICAs does not affect the short-term neonatal thyroid-stimulating hormone, possibly because the amount of excess iodide in fetal circulation is small and temporary. Given all available data and routine assessment of all newborns for congenital hypothyroidism by the measurement of TSH levels at birth, no additional examination is needed [45].

Most ICAs are classified as category B (animal reproductive studies have failed to demonstrate a risk to the fetus, and there are not sufficient well-controlled studies in pregnant cases) by the FDA. It is not recommended to withhold the use of ICAs in pregnant or potentially pregnant patients when ICAs are needed for diagnostic purposes.

Although it is not possible to suggest that ICAs present a definite risk to the fetus, there is no sufficient evidence to conclude that they do not pose such risk. ACR, in the ACR Manual on ICA, Version 10.3, recommends that an ICA be given to pregnant patients only when (1) the requested diagnostic information cannot be obtained via alternative modalities, such as ultrasound, (2) it is necessary for the health of the patient and the fetus to obtain information through such procedures, and (3) it is not advisable to wait to obtain this information until the patient is no longer pregnant [4].

Before ICA administration, both referring physicians and pregnant patients with prior allergy-like reactions to ICAs should be informed about the possible risks and benefits of premedications being used, as well as alternative diagnostic options. Preventive strategies and treatment of ARs in pregnant patients are generally similar to those of ARs employed for non-pregnant adults. Antihistamines (diphenhydramine) and corticosteroids (most commonly prednisone and methylprednisolone) are mostly used as premedication in patients at risk of allergy-like ARs. Diphenhydramine is classified as category B by the FDA. Prednisone and dexamethasone are classified as category C by the FDA (animal reproduction studies have shown an adverse effect on the fetus, and there are no sufficient and well-controlled studies in pregnant cases, but potential benefits may justify the use of the drug in pregnant women despite possible risks). These agents cross the placenta. However, most of these agents are metabolized within the placenta before reaching the fetus, and therefore they are not associated with teratogenicity in humans. Nevertheless, sporadic cases of fetal adrenal suppression have been reported. Methylprednisolone constitute a small risk for the fetus in terms of the development of a cleft lip if used prior to 10 weeks of gestation [3, 4].

4.6 Adverse Reactions After ICA Administration in Breastfeeding Women

Less than 1% of ICAs is excreted into breast milk, of which only 1% is absorbed by the infant's intestine. Therefore, the expected systemic dose absorbed by the infant from the breast milk is less than 0.01% of the intravascular dose administered to the mother. This is less than 1% of the recommended dose for an infant. The risk of either direct toxic or allergy-like manifestations caused by swallowed ICAs in the infant is extremely low [46]. According to ACR Manual on ICA, Version 10.3 recommendations, it is safe for the mother and infant to continue breastfeeding after ICA administration. If the mother is concerned about any possible adverse effects on the infant, she can avoid breastfeeding for 24 h. The plasma half-life of IV-administered ICA is approximately 2 h, with nearly 100% being removed from the blood stream in patients with normal renal functions within 24 h. However, the taste of milk may be altered if it contains ICAs [4].

4.7 Adverse Reactions After ICA Administration in Oncologic Patients

The effect of cytotoxic agents on the risk of ARs to IV injections of ICAs is not well known. Among cancer patients, concomitant treatment with taxanes appears to be a risk factor for ICA-related ARs [47]. Methotrexate (MTX), a widely used anticancer agent, and IV ICAs used for radiographic studies can both cause acute renal failure. Their combined exposure may place patients at higher risk for renal failure. IVICAs should be avoided in patients receiving high-dose MTX [48].

4.8 Safe Injection of ICAs

Due to the risk of clot formation, it is important to avoid admixture of blood and ICAs in syringes and catheters for a long time. In general, the admixture of ICAs and any medication should be avoided unless it is known to be safe. However, heparin can be combined with ICAs [4].

4.8.1 Warming ICAs

There is controversial data concerning whether warmed ICAs reduce the AR rates. However, many institutions warm ICAs to human body temperature (37 °C) before routine clinical intravascular using an external incubator in which bottles of ICA are placed [49]. As the temperature of an injected ICA increases, there is a decrease in its dynamic viscosity. Therefore, a warmed ICA is less viscous than an ICA at room temperature. When a warmed ICA is manually injected or power-injected into a catheter, there will be less resistance compared to an unwarmed ICA. Extrinsic warming of ICAs can be useful to minimize complications and improve vascular opacification in the following circumstances: (1) high-rate (>5 mL/s) IV low-osmolality ICM power injections, (2) injections of viscous iodinated contrast (e.g., iopamidol 370 and presumably other ICAs with a similar or higher viscosity), (3) direct arterial injections through small-caliber catheters (5 French or smaller), and (4) intravenously injected agents for arterial studies in which timing and peak enhancement are critical [4].

4.8.2 Fasting Before Examination

Fasting has an impact on vomiting or nausea after ICA exposure. Most diagnostic imaging centers ask patients to fast for 4–6 h before contrast-enhanced imaging. Previous studies have shown that prolonged fasting can be harmful. In addition, manufacturer of ICAs claims that there is no special preparation needed before examination [50].

4.9 Extravasation of ICAs

Extravasation may occur during both hand and power injections. Risk factors for extravasation include infants, elderly, and chronically ill and debilitated patients; venous thrombosis, multiple venous puncture attempts, tourniquets, prior radiation therapy, or extensive surgery (e.g., axillary lymph node dissection); and injections on the dorsum of hands, feet, or ankles. Clinical presentation includes burning pain, tenderness, edema, and erythema. Majority of patients that develop extravasation recover without significant sequelae. Severe injury can cause blistering, sloughing off of the skin, and compartment syndrome. The last is the result of mechanical compression due to the extravasation of larger volumes of ICAs; however, it has also been observed after the extravasation of relatively small volumes, especially in less capacitive areas, such as over the ventral or dorsal surfaces of the wrists. On physical examination, the extravasation site may be edematous, erythematous, and tender. To prevent potential complications of ICA extravasation, the patient should be instructed to notify the technologist in case of any change in sensation, including increasing pain or swelling at the injection site. In such cases, injection should be discontinued [4, 13, 51].

If the patient is asymptomatic or if there are only mild symptoms, an appropriate evaluation and clinical follow-up are usually sufficient. Extremity should be initially elevated to reduce capillary hydrostatic pressure. Cold application may be helpful for relieving pain or the size of any subsequent ulceration at the injection site. Heat has been found to improve absorption of extravasation, as well as blood flow, particularly distal to the injection site. Outpatients suffering from ICA extravasation should be released from the radiology department only after an initial period of close observation for 2–4 h. The patient should be given clear instructions for further medical care and report any pain, swelling, paresthesia, decreased finger movements (active or passive), skin ulceration, and other neurological features or circulatory symptoms. An immediate surgical consultation is indicated if one or more of the following signs or symptoms develop in patients: progressive swelling or pain; altered tissue perfusion as evidenced by reduced capillary filling change in sensation in the affected limb; worsening of active or passive range of motion of the elbows, wrists, or fingers; skin ulceration or blistering; and an extravasated ICA volume of more than 30 mL for ionic ICAs or 100 mL for nonionic ICAs [52].

4.10 Conclusion

In conclusion, prior to ICA administration, an adequate evaluation should be performed to identify predisposing risk factors. Prompt recognition and treatment of acute ARs are crucial. Due to their pivotal roles in this process, radiologists should be aware of all predisposing factors, clinical presentation, and management of ARs to ICAs.

References

1. Chand RB, Maharjan S, Pant DK, Paudel S. The incidence of adverse reaction to contrast media in computed tomography scan. J Inst Med. 2013;35:33–6.

2. Namasivayam S, Kalra MK, Torres WE, Small WC. Adverse reactions to intravenous iodinated contrast media: a primer for radiologists. Emerg Radiol. 2006;12:210–5.
3. European Society of Urogenital Radiology. Contrast media guidelines version 9.0.
4. ACR, American College of Radiology. ACR manual on contrast media version 10.3. 2018.
5. Mruk B. Renal safety of iodinated contrast media depending on their osmolarity-current outlooks. Pol J Radiol. 2016;81:157–65.
6. Iyer RS, Schopp JG, Swanson JO, Thapa MM, Phillips GS. Safety essentials: acute reactions to iodinated contrast media. Can Assoc Radiol J. 2013;64:193–9.
7. Roh S, Laroia A. Practicing safe use of nonionic, low-osmolarity iodinated contrast. Appl Radiol. 2015;44:16–9.
8. Seong JM, Choi NK, Lee J, Chang Y, Kim YJ, Yang BR, Jin XM, Kim JY, Park BJ. Comparison of the safety of seven iodinated contrast media. J Korean Med Sci. 2013;28:1703–10.
9. Bottinor W, Polkampally P, Jovin I. Adverse reactions to iodinated contrast media. Int J Angiol. 2013;22:149–54.
10. Morzycki A, Bhatia A, Murphy KJ. Adverse reactions to contrast material: a Canadian update. Can Assoc Radiol J. 2017;68:187–93.
11. Brockow K, Romano A, Aberer W, Bircher AJ, Barbaud A, Bonadonna P, et al. European Network of Drug Allergy and the EAACI interest group on drug hypersensitivity. Skin testing in patients with hypersensitivity reactions to iodinated contrast media—a European multicenter study. Allergy. 2009;64:234–41.
12. Bettmann MA. Frequently asked questions: iodinated contrast agents. Radiographics. 2004;24(Suppl 1):S3–10.
13. Beckett KR, Moriarity AK, Langer JM. Safe use of contrast media: what the radiologist needs to know. Radiographics. 2015;35:1738–50.
14. Kobayashi D, Takahashi O, Ueda T, Deshpande GA, Arioka H, Fukui T. Risk factors for adverse reactions from contrast agents for computed tomography. BMC Med Inform Decis Mak. 2013;13:18.
15. Lang DM, Alpern MB, Visintainer PF, Smith ST. Increased risk for anaphylactoid reaction from contrast media in patients on beta-adrenergic blockers or with asthma. Ann Intern Med. 1991;115:270–6.
16. Greenberger PA, Patterson R, Tapio CM. Prophylaxis against repeated radiocontrast media reactions in 857 cases. Adverse experience with cimetidine and safety of beta-adrenergic antagonists. Arch Intern Med. 1985;145:2197–200.
17. Campbell KL, Hud LM, Adams S, Andrel J, Ballas SK, Feldman AM, Axelrod D. Safety of iodinated intravenous contrast medium administration in sickle cell disease. Am J Med. 2012;125:e11–6.
18. Lee SY, Rhee CM, Leung AM, Braverman LE, Brent GA, Pearce EN. A review: radiographic iodinated contrast media-induced thyroid dysfunction. J Clin Endocrinol Metab. 2015;100:376–83.
19. Han S, Yoon SH, Lee W, Choi YH, Kang DY, Kang HR. Management of adverse reactions to iodinated contrast media for computed tomography in Korean referral hospitals: a survey investigation. Korean J Radiol. 2019;20:148–57.
20. Lasser EC, Berry CC, Mishkin MM, Williamson B, Zheutlin N, Silverman JM. Pretreatment with corticosteroids to prevent adverse reactions to nonionic contrast media. AJR Am J Roentgenol. 1994;162:523–6.
21. Amrol DJ. Pretreatment to prevent radiocontrast reactions during CT procedures. AJR Am J Roentgenol. 2015;205:77.
22. Egbert RE, De Cecco CN, Schoepf UJ, McQuiston AD, Meinel FG, Katzberg RW. Delayed adverse reactions to the parenteral administration of iodinated contrast media. AJR Am J Roentgenol. 2014;203:1163–70.
23. Hosoya T, Yamaguchi K, Akutsu T, Mitsuhashi Y, Kondo S, Sugai Y, Adachi M. Delayed adverse reactions to iodinated contrast media and their risk factors. Radiat Med. 2000;18:39–45.
24. Mavromatis K, Rab ST. Radiographic contrast media. Interventional cardiology. 2nd ed. McGraw-Hill Education. 2018.
25. Macy EM. Current epidemiology and management of radiocontrast-associated acute- and delayed-onset hypersensitivity: a review of the literature. Perm J. 2018;22:17–072.
26. Lucarelli A, Perandini S, Borsato A, Strazimiri E, Montemezzi S. Iodinated contrast-induced sialadenitis: a review of the literature and sonographic findings in a clinical case. J Ultrason. 2018;18:359–64.
27. Federici M, Guarna T, Manzi M, Della Longa G, Di Renzi P, Bellelli A. Swelling of the submandibular glands after administration of low-osmolarity contrast agent: ultrasound findings. J Ultrasound. 2008;11:85–8.
28. Spina R, Simon N, Markus R, Muller DW, Kathir K. Contrast-induced encephalopathy following cardiac catheterization. Catheter Cardiovasc Interv. 2017;1:257–68.
29. Kahyaoğlu M, Ağca M, Çakmak EÖ, Geçmen Ç, İzgi İA. Contrast-induced encephalopathy after percutaneous peripheral intervention. Turk Kardiyol Dern Ars. 2018;46:140–2.
30. Kelley BC, Roh S, Johnson PL, Arnold PM. Malignant cerebral edema following CT myelogram using Isovue-M 300 intrathecal nonionic water-soluble contrast: a case report. Radiol Res Pract. 2011;2011:212516.
31. Seo N, Chung YE, Lim JS, Song MK, Kim MJ, Kim KW. Bowel angioedema associated with iodinated contrast media: incidence and predisposing factors. Invest Radiol. 2017;52:514–21.
32. Meyer-Burg J, Kater F. [Significance of serum transaminase changes following application of tri-iodinated, biliary contrast media]. Dtsch Med Wochenschr. 1970;95:1444–6.

33. Carmona-Sánchez R, Uscanga L, Bezaury-Rivas P, Robles-Díaz G, Suazo-Barahona J, Vargas-Vorácková F. Potential harmful effect of iodinated intravenous contrast medium on the clinical course of mild acute pancreatitis. Arch Surg. 2000;135:1280–4.
34. Donnelly PK, Williams B, Watkin EM. Polyarthropathy—a delayed reaction to low osmolality angiographic contrast medium in patients with end stage renal disease. Eur J Radiol. 1993;17:130–2.
35. Kim KH, Park JY, Park HS, Kuh SU, Chin DK, Kim KS, Cho YE. Which iodinated contrast media is the least cytotoxic to human disc cells? Spine J. 2015;15:1021–7.
36. Mozley PD. Malignant hyperthermia following intravenous iodinated contrast media. Report of a fatal case. Diagn Gynecol Obstet. 1981;3:81–6.
37. Morcos SK. Review article: effects of radiographic contrast media on the lung. Br J Radiol. 2003;76:290–5.
38. Pincet L, Lecca G. Acute pulmonary edema induced by non-ionic low-osmolar radiographic contrast media. Open Access Emerg Med. 2018;10:75–9.
39. Hayakawa K, Okuno Y, Fujiwara K, Shimizu Y. Effect of iodinated contrast media on ionic calcium. Acta Radiol. 1994;35:83–7.
40. Böhm I. Kounis syndrome in a patient with allergy to iodinated contrast media. Int J Cardiol. 2011;151:102–3.
41. Ott DJ, Gelfand DW. Gastrointestinal contrast agents. Indications, uses, and risks. JAMA. 1983; 249:2380–4.
42. Torigian DA, Ramchandani P. Radiology secrets plus E-Book Yazar. 4th ed. Elsevier; 2016.
43. Pan JJ, Draganov PV. Adverse reactions to iodinated contrast media administered at the time of endoscopic retrograde cholangiopancreatography (ERCP). Inflamm Allergy Drug Targets. 2009;8:17–20.
44. Niemann T, Nicolas G, Roser HW, Müller-Brand J, Bongartz G. Imaging for suspected pulmonary embolism in pregnancy-what about the fetal dose? A comprehensive review of the literature. Insights Imaging. 2010;1:361–72.
45. Bourjeily G, Chalhoub M, Phornphutkul C, Alleyne TC, Woodfield CA, Chen KK. Neonatal thyroid function: effect of a single exposure to iodinated contrast medium in utero. Radiology. 2010;256:744–50.
46. Singh N, McLean K. Five things to know about intravascular contrast media for imaging in breastfeeding women. CMAJ. 2012;184:E775.
47. Farolfi A, Della Luna C, Ragazzini A, Carretta E, Gentili N, Casadei C, Aquilina M, Barone D, Minguzzi M, Amadori D, Nanni O, Gavelli G. Taxanes as a risk factor for acute adverse reactions to iodinated contrast media in cancer patients. Oncologist. 2014;19:823–8.
48. Harned TM, Mascarenhas L. Severe methotrexate toxicity precipitated by intravenous radiographic contrast. J Pediatr Hematol Oncol. 2007;29:496–9.
49. Zhang B, Liu J, Dong Y, Guo B, Lian Z, Yu H, Luo X, Mo X, Zhang L, Huang W, Ouyang F, Li X, Liang C, Zhang S. Extrinsic warming of low-osmolality iodinated contrast media to 37°C reduced the rate of allergic-like reaction. Allergy Asthma Proc. 2018;39:e55–63.
50. Barbosa PNVP, Bitencourt AGV, Tyng CJ, Cunha R, Travesso DJ, Almeida MFA, Chojniak R. Preparative fasting for contrast-enhanced CT in a cancer center: a new approach. AJR Am J Roentgenol. 2018;210:941–7.
51. Chew FS. Extravasation of iodinated contrast medium during CT: self-assessment module. AJR Am J Roentgenol. 2010;195(6 Suppl):S80–5.
52. Lewis PJ, McNulty NJ. Oxford American Handboolk Of Radiology. 1st ed. Oxford University Press. 2013.

5 Dose Reduction Strategies for Iodinated Contrast Agents: Low-Tube Voltage and Iterative Reconstruction

Hiroyuki Morisaka

5.1 Introduction

Although the risk of acute kidney injury after intravenous injection of an iodinated contrast agent during computed tomography (CT) has remained controversial [1], administration of the lowest possible contrast agent dose is recommended for maintenance of diagnostic results [2]. Furthermore, the possible risk of amplifying double-stranded DNA damage and radiation absorption by the tissues due to the presence of an iodinated contrast agent has been proposed [3, 4]; the possibility that the level of risk depends on the administered dose has been reported as well [5].

One of the effective ways of reducing the amount of an iodinated contrast agent used in clinical CT imaging is through the use of a lower-tube voltage peak (kVp), such as 80–100 kVp (relative to a standard 120 kVp). This is because a lower-tube voltage peak positions the peak energy spectra of CT close to the iodine k-edge, which causes greater X-ray attenuation by iodine and results in improvement of contrast enhancement. However, a drawback of this method is an increase in image noise and image degradation because conventional filtered back projection (FBP) reconstruction is based on some mathematic assumptions of the CT system that differ from the actual CT acquisition situations, which leads to higher image noise and artifacts at reduced radiation dose of the low-tube-voltage CT acquisition. To overcome this limitation of FBP, iterative reconstruction (IR) techniques, which repeat the image reconstruction several times to estimate these mathematic assumptions better and generate images with lower noise, were developed and introduced for use in clinical CT imaging in combination with low-tube-voltage CT (Fig. 5.1) [6, 7].

This chapter will describe (a) how dose reduction of contrast agents can be achieved with low-tube-voltage CT scanning while maintaining image quality and diagnostic performance, (b) drawbacks to be considered when reducing the amount of contrast agent in low-tube-voltage CT, and (c) available options for image noise reduction in low-tube-voltage CT.

5.2 Dose Reduction of Contrast Agents in Low-Tube-Voltage CT

A tube voltage of approximately 63 kVp is the voltage at which the fraction of photons in the energy around the k-edge of iodine at 33.2 keV is highest [8], which means the effective energy spectra of 63 kVp is close to the k-edge of iodine. Although simple use of a low-tube volt-

H. Morisaka (✉)
Saitama Medical University, International Medical Center, Hidaka, Saitama, Japan

S. M. Erturk et al. (eds.), *Medical Imaging Contrast Agents: A Clinical Manual*,
https://doi.org/10.1007/978-3-030-79256-5_5

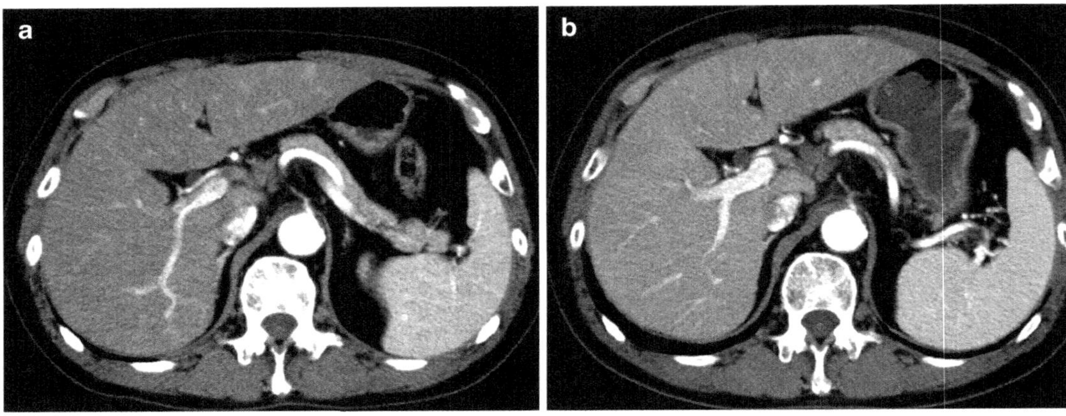

Fig. 5.1 (**a**) An upper abdominal 80-kilo-volt-peak (kVp) CT image generated with a 50% reduction of the contrast agent dose and (**b**) a 120-kVp CT image generated with a standard 600 mgI/kg contrast agent during the hepatic arterial phase, showing comparable contrast enhancement in the aorta, portal vein, inferior vena cava, and liver parenchyma. By using hybrid IR in the 80-kVp CT image, image quality is also comparable with that of the 120-kVp CT image

age close to 63 kVp, e.g., 70 or 80 kVp, is actually effective for increasing iodine contrast enhancement, there is an inherent limitation with this technique, particularly when attempting to apply it in patients with a higher body mass [8]. Another way to improve iodine contrast enhancement is to use a low-tube voltage monochromatic spectral image, which is "virtually" created from the data acquired by dual-energy CT scanning [9]. Varying monochromatic energy levels, from 40 to 100 keV, can be created by processing the data acquired at two different tube voltages, e.g., 80 and 140 kVp. Monochromatic spectral imaging at 40–50 keV, close to the k-edge of iodine at 33.2 keV, is effective for iodine contrast enhancement, in which inherently higher image noise of low-tube voltage image is offset by blending low image noise of high-tube voltage image data.

This does not necessarily suggest that you can reduce the amount of contrast agent uniformly for all patients or all organs in low-voltage CT. The dose reduction of a contrast agent is dependent on the target organ and target lesion that is to be detected. Dose reduction of contrast agents has been attempted in various body parts including coronary, pulmonary, cerebral, and other vascular structures and in solid organs such as the liver.

5.2.1 Coronary CT Angiography

An 80-kVp prospective electrocardiography-gated cardiac CT angiography performed with a 60% reduction of the contrast agent dose (data was reconstructed by hybrid IR or knowledge-based IR) demonstrated higher contrast-to-noise ratio and an image quality comparable to a standard 120 kVp CT [10]. In an animal experiment using minipigs, a 50% reduction of the contrast agent dose in an 80-kVp CT and a 38% reduction in a 100-kVp CT achieved by using hybrid IR showed a contrast-to-noise ratio and subjective image quality comparable to those of a standard 120 kVp CT [11].

5.2.2 Pulmonary CT Angiography

In a prospective randomized trial, an 80-kVp pulmonary CT angiography done with a 25% reduction of the contrast agent dose generated a subjective image quality and diagnostic confidence comparable to those of a standard iodine dose protocol in patients with pulmonary embolism [12]. Further reduction of the contrast agent dose, from 50% up to 85%, can be achieved by using virtual monochromatic or monoenergetic spectral imaging at 40–50 keV [13, 14].

5.2.3 Other Vascular Structures

In cerebral CT angiography, 80- and 100-kVp CT performed with a 43% reduction of the contrast agent dose showed a diagnostic accuracy in the detection of cerebral aneurysms comparable to that of a standard 120-kVp CT [15]. In renal CT angiography, an 80-kVp CT done with a 33% reduction of the contrast agent dose demonstrated a quantitative and qualitative image quality comparable to that of a standard 120-kVp CT angiography. Furthermore, by combining a bolus tracking technique and a saline chaser, a 52% reduction of the contrast agent dose could be accomplished, and a satisfactory image quality can be generated [16].

5.2.4 Hepatic Dynamic CT

In hepatocellular carcinoma (HCC), for which the early enhancement of the arterial phase image and subsequent wash-out during the delayed phase is diagnostic, more than 600 mgI/kg of iodine has been recommended for a standard 120-kVp CT because sufficient tumor-to-liver contrast (more than 40 Hounsfield units (HU)) or hepatic parenchymal enhancement (more than 50 HU) could be accomplished by using more than 600 mgI/kg of contrast agent [17]. In the 80-kVp CT with hybrid IR, a 50% reduction of the contrast agent dose provided a quantitative and qualitative image quality comparable to those of a standard dose protocol in patients with HCC [18, 19] (Fig. 5.2).

Based on the reports of previous studies, in practice, contrast agent dose can easily be reduced further in vascular structure assessment than in the assessment of solid organs given the same tube voltage because a strongly contrast-enhanced vascular structure is less affected by image noise than solid organs. In low-voltage CT, the contrast agent dose can be reduced by 30–50% in the assessment of vascular structures and in hypervascular HCC by using the IR technique. The percentage of dose reduction required for a contrast agent is usually predefined in low-tube-voltage CT as in previous studies, and results showed comparable or higher qualitative and quantitative image quality to those of the standard CT. However, it is difficult to determine the minimum quantity of contrast agent required in low-tube-voltage CT that provides an equivalent or non-inferior diagnostic performance compared to that of the standard CT.

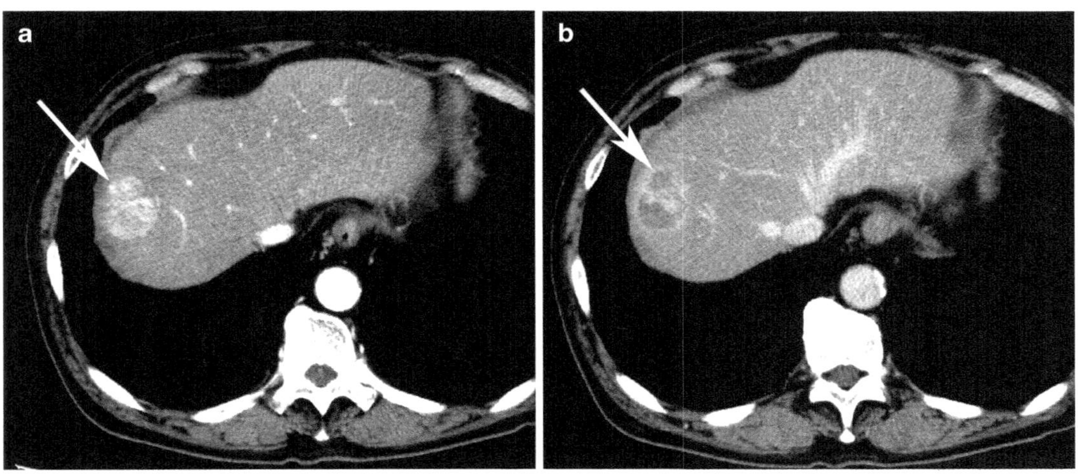

Fig. 5.2 An upper abdominal 80-kVp CT image generated with 50% reduction of the contrast agent dose in a patient with hepatocellular carcinoma during the (**a**) hepatic arterial phase and (**b**) delayed phase showing a heterogeneous early enhancement of the liver tumor (arrow) on the arterial phase image and subsequent washout during the delayed phase, which is diagnostic for hepatocellular carcinoma

5.3 Effect of Decreased Flow Rate on Contrast Enhancement

5.3.1 Basics of Contrast Agent Injection Protocol

Firstly, the effect of injection rate, duration, and total amount of contrast agent on the contrast enhancement of the aorta, which is assessed as the aortic peak enhancement on the time density curve, actively investigated both in vitro and in vivo, will be summarized.

In general, the time between the arrival of the contrast agent at the aorta and the trigger threshold (threshold value in bolus tracking technique, 100–150 HU) is 6–8 s when the contrast agent is administered within 25–35 s. The scan delay from the trigger is usually set at 10 s, and the scan duration is 10–15 s; the peak of aortic enhancement can be caught during scanning (Fig. 5.3). As the total amount of contrast agent is increased, aortic peak enhancement proportionally increases when the injection duration is fixed at 25–35 s (usually 30 s) [20]. Injection rate has a greater positive effect on aortic peak enhancement than the total amount of contrast agent. When the contrast dose is fixed, a higher injection rate with decreased injection duration (less than 30 s) can provide a higher aortic peak enhancement along with a narrow time window for the aortic peak [20] (Fig. 5.4). A narrow time window for the aortic peak makes is easier to overshoot the optimal scan timing for aortic peak enhancement. Therefore, fixed injection duration from 25 to 35 s is more important for keeping up the optimal time window for aortic peak enhancement than increasing injection rate. Optimal injection duration provides a "right shoulder" on the time density curve, while an insufficient injection duration leads to a "sloping shoulder" (Fig. 5.4).

5.3.2 Effect of Decreased Flow Rate on Contrast Enhancement

In the era of low-voltage CT, the amount of contrast agent used can be effectively reduced, thereby leading to a lower injection rate or injection duration. In terms of aortic peak enhancement, contrast dose can be reduced by about 20% in 100-kVp acquisition and 40–50% in 80-kVp acquisition compared with a standard 120-kVp CT. Here, let us consider the situation of liver dynamic CT for a patient weighing 60 kg: an optimal body-tailored contrast dose is 600 mgI/kg for a standard 120-kVp CT, and the required total amount of contrast agent is 120 mL of a contrast agent with a 300 mgI/mL concentration and 97 mL for a 370 mgI/mL concentration. Injection duration is set at 30 s, and

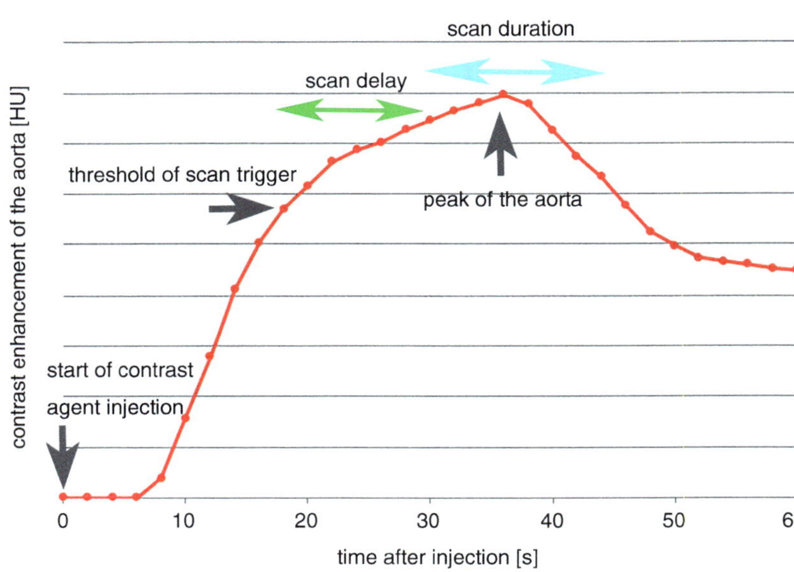

Fig. 5.3 Time density curve of the abdominal aorta: in general, the contrast agent arrives at the aorta 6–8 s after the start of injection if the contrast agent is administered within 25–35 s. The scan delay from the trigger (threshold value in bolus tracking technique, 100–150 HU) is usually set at 10 s (green double arrow bar), and the scan duration is 10–15 s (blue double arrow bar); the peak of aortic enhancement can be caught during scanning

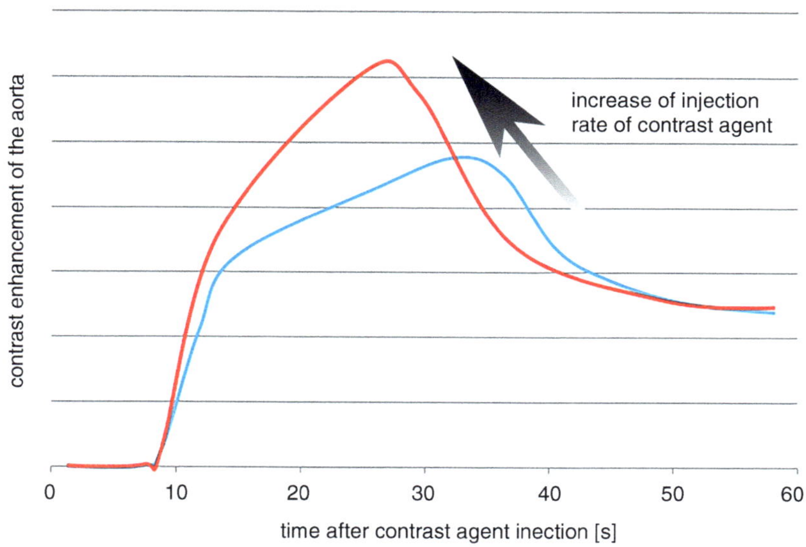

Fig. 5.4 Effect of injection rate given the same contrast agent dose: increased injection rate leads to an increased aortic peak enhancement along with decreased injection duration (less than 30 s), which provides a narrow time window for the aortic peak

injection rate will be 4 mL/s for 300 mgI/mL and 3.2 mL/s for 370 mgI/mL. These conditions can be efficient for an optimal time density curve of the aorta and the liver and will facilitate proper diagnosis. When a low-voltage CT, e.g., 80 kVp, is applied to this patient, the contrast agent dose can be reduced by 40%, that is, 72 mL for 300 mgI/mL and 58 mL for 370 mgI/mL, and the injection rate will be 2.4 mL/s and 1.9 mL/s. Such a low injection rate, especially less than 2.0 mL/s, is an "uncharted territory" for a standard 120-kVp dynamic liver CT. Although fixed injection duration is more important for aortic peak enhancement than injection rate as discussed previously, the effect of the lower injection rate on aortic peak enhancement should be considered. In the experiment of dynamic flow phantom, a flow rate lower than 2.0 mL/s decreased the aortic peak enhancement compared to a standard 3.0 mL/s, given the same total iodine dose (Fig. 5.5).

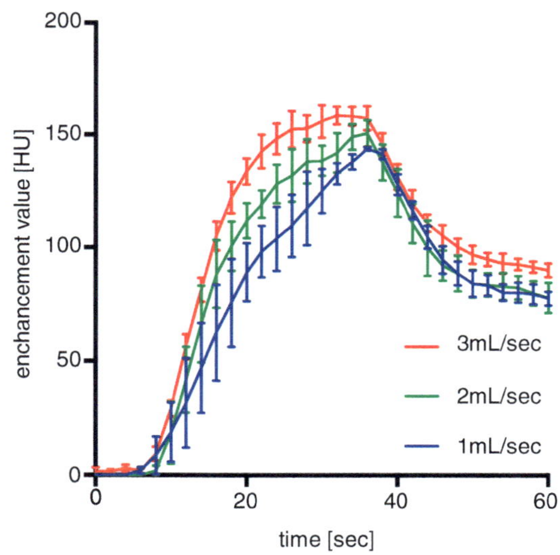

Fig. 5.5 Effect of injection rate given the same contrast agent dose and fixed injection duration: Flow rate less than 2.0 mL/s decreases aortic peak enhancement compared to a standard 3.0 mL/s given with the same total iodine dose and fixed injection duration. Furthermore, the slope before aortic peak enhancement becomes steeper as the injection rates decrease and the time window for the aortic peak becomes narrower

5.3.3 Other Techniques for Improving Contrast Enhancement in Low-Voltage CT

The fixed injection duration method has been widely accepted because it is simple and easy to use. Aside from a fixed injection method, another approach for more effective contrast enhancement, the multi-bolus injection technique, has been investigated. The goal of using the multi-bolus injection technique is to prolong the optimal scan duration for aortic enhancement. Various multi-bolus injection protocols in which small intermittent boli of contrast agent and saline are combined have been investigated. In low-voltage CT angiography, optimized multi-bolus injection protocol provides a significantly longer time window for diagnostic aortic enhancement (more than 200 HU) compared with that of a single bolus injection [21]. Despite the benefit of the multi-bolus injection technique, it has not been widely used because of the complexity of injection protocol.

Another optional technique for an efficient contrast enhancement is the use of a saline chaser. The aim of the saline chaser is to avoid accumulation of the contrast material in the injecting tube and in the venous system between the injection site and the right atrium; in other words, move the remaining contrast agent in the "dead space" to the right atrium. Adding the saline chaser has been shown to reduce the contrast agent dose by about 20%. Increased saline chaser injection rate provides significantly higher peak aortic enhancement values and longer time window for aortic peak enhancement compared with no saline chaser protocol [22].

5.4 Iterative Reconstruction in Low-Tube-Voltage CT

5.4.1 From Filtered Back Projection to Deep Learning Reconstruction

From its introduction in 1972, CT images were reconstructed by simple analytic methods such as FBP, in which images were reconstructed from projection data (sinograms) by applying a high-pass filter followed by a backward projection step with a limited model and some simple assumptions. FBP has been accepted due to its short reconstruction time and high image quality; however, because there is a direct relationship between image noise and radiation exposure, deteriorated image quality could be the outcome in patients with larger body size or in the low radiation dose acquisition, in which less photons reach the CT detector (Fig. 5.6a).

In the early 2000s, advanced iterative reconstruction (IR) algorithm was developed along with a computational advancement, in which a sinogram-based or image domain-based approach was applied. Raw data or image data are iteratively filtered to reduce artifact or image noise, following a backward projection applied for reconstruction. This hybrid IR provides image noise reduction with a clinically acceptable reconstruction time (Fig. 5.6b).

A full-type or model- or knowledge-based IR (MBIR) algorithm in which raw data are projected backward into the image space followed by image data projected forward to compute artificial raw data has been developed as well. The forward projection of MBIR algorithms can produce a physically precise data acquisition process including system geometry and noise models, and the process of backward and forward projection is repeated until the difference between true and artificial raw data is minimized. MBIR can reduce image noise extensively (Fig. 5.6c); however, computational heavy load and longer reconstruction time are drawbacks of iteration of MBIR.

Deep learning-based reconstruction (DLR) was released by Canon Medical Systems in 2018. It incorporates deep convolutional neural network processes into the reconstruction flow with hybrid IR images and high-dose MBIR images acting as training pairs by which statistical features that differentiate signal from noise and artifacts could be learned in the training process and then be updated in the deep convolutional neural network kernel [23]. DRL provides an image quality comparable to that produced with the MBIR algorithm but with a shorter reconstruction time and is robust over the radiation exposure shortage than MBIR algorithm (Fig. 5.6d).

5.4.2 Index for Image Quality Assessment in Low-Tube-Voltage CT

Image noise in CT is a random variation of CT attenuation values of reconstructed images and is produced by the CT detector and electronic circuit. The standard deviation of noise is simple to measure; it is widely used as a convenient index

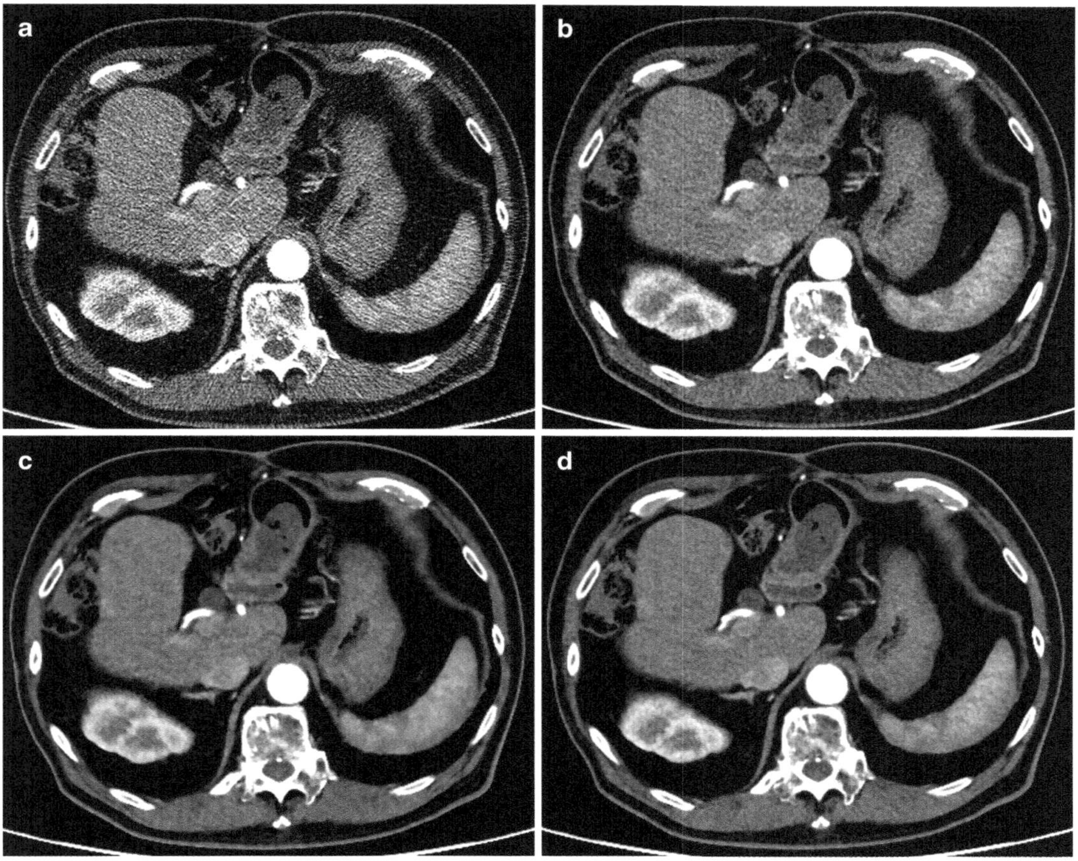

Fig. 5.6 An upper abdominal CT image with reduced radiation exposure (6 mGy) reconstructed with (**a**) filtered back projection (FBP), (**b**) hybrid iterative reconstruction (IR), (**c**) model-based IR (MBIR), and (**d**) deep learning-based reconstruction (DLR). Image noise in the FBP image is prominent but is suppressed in other reconstructions. MBIR leads to a relative increase of the low-spatial frequency component of noise and results in a more mottled texture or a "cartoon-like" appearance of the reconstructed image, whereas DRL can decrease more of the low-spatial frequency component of noise compared to MBIR, so the sharpness of the image is balanced in the DRL image

of image quality, and it provides a gross predictive value for object detectability. In low-voltage CT, the number of photons captured by the CT detector is inherently smaller than that captured in a standard dose CT at a given tube current; therefore, reconstructed images of low-voltage CT have a relatively high image noise. Contrast-to-noise ratio (CNR) is a simple measure used to assess image quality just like a signal-to-noise ratio, but CNR subtracts off a term before taking the ratio and can be an objective metric essentially matched to the observer's visual detectability. However, images reconstructed by a soft tissue kernel tend to have lower image noise and a high CNR, whereas images reconstructed by a sharp contrast kernel tend to have a higher image noise and low CNR, even in a same visual detectability. It should be noted that CNR is not completely matched to subjective visual detectability; therefore, radiation dose reduction based on image noise or CNR alone is debatable and has room for discussion; a task-based image quality assessment especially for low contrast detectability should be considered instead [24].

The standard deviation of noise, though simple to use, provides no information about the spatial characteristics of image noise. The noise power spectrum (NPS) characterizes both the

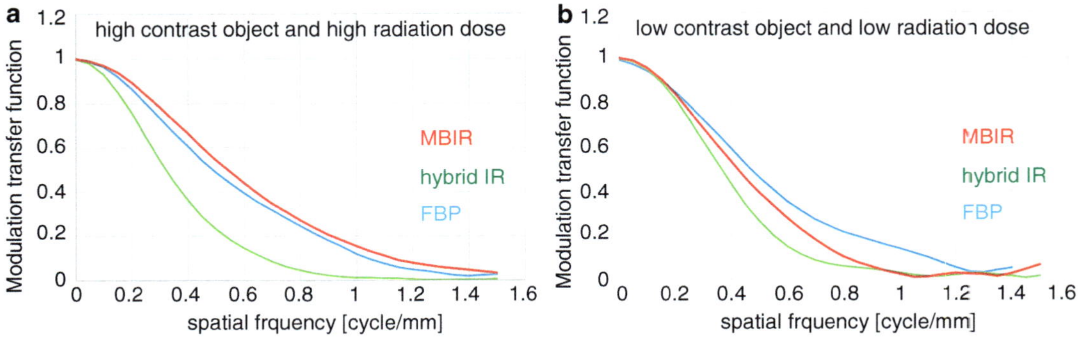

Fig. 5.7 Modulation transfer function (MTF) analysis of FBP, hybrid IR, and MBIR: (**a**) MTF of MBIR is superior to that of FBP for a high contrast structure (500 HU) and at high radiation exposure, whereas (**b**) MTF of MBIR is inferior to that of FBP for a low contrast structure (50 HU) and at low radiation exposure. Note that both MTF curves of FBP and hybrid IR are unchanged between the two conditions, whereas the MTF curves of MBIR are improved for a high contrast structure and at high radiation exposure. Dose and contrast dependence are unique characteristics of MBIR

magnitude and spatial frequency distribution of image noise, in which the Fourier transform is utilized on image noise to yield the variance of the noise power present at each spatial frequency. Value of integral of NPS over the full range of spatial frequency is equal to the standard deviation of image noise. The magnitude of the NPS reflects the degree of randomness at each spatial frequency, and the shape of the NPS curve reveals where the noise power is concentrated in frequency space. Low-frequency noise power produces an image with a mottled texture, whereas high-frequency noise power leads to a finely textured image. Image texture varies depending on the shape of the NPS curve even at the same standard deviation of image noise. Hybrid IR and MBIR reduce image noise by reducing the magnitude of the high-spatial frequency component of noise, which leads a relative increase of the low-spatial frequency component of noise and results in a more mottled texture or a "cartoon-like" appearance of the reconstructed image (Fig. 5.6c). Such image texture alteration provided by hybrid IR and MBIR may have an effect on visual detectability.

The modulation transfer function (MTF) is a Fourier metric of spatial resolution properties, in which the percentage of frequency domain (cycles/pixel) at a given frequency relative to that of the lowest frequency is plotted against the spatial frequency. A 50% MTF is a good indicator of image sharpness when comparing different reconstruction algorithms and scanners. Human visual detectability is insensitive to details of spatial frequency when MTF is less than 10%. In hybrid IR and MBIR reconstruction, MTF depends on contrast and noise due to non-linear image processing; therefore, an edge method is suitable for measuring MTF. MBIR has both contrast and radiation dose dependence on MTF, whereas FBP and hybrid IR have no such dependence on MTF. MBIR provides a higher spatial resolution compared to FBP and hybrid IR at a sufficient radiation dose and with high contrast structures (Fig. 5.7a), whereas the spatial resolution of MBIR is inferior to those of FBP and hybrid IR at an insufficient radiation dose and with low contrast structures (Fig. 5.7b). From the standpoint of MTF, the use of MBIR in low-voltage CT is discouraged because of its radiation dose dependency; hybrid IR or DLR is more suitable for low-voltage CT.

References

1. McDonald JS, McDonald RJ, Carter RE, Katzberg RW, Kallmes DF, Williamson EE. Risk of intravenous contrast material-mediated acute kidney injury: a propensity score-matched study stratified by baseline-estimated glomerular filtration rate. Radiology.

2014;271(1):65–73. https://doi.org/10.1148/radiol.13130775. Epub 2014/01/31. Cited in: Pubmed; PMID 24475854.
2. Nyman U, Ahlkvist J, Aspelin P, Brismar T, Frid A, Hellstrom M, Liss P, Sterner G, Leander P, Contrast Media Committee of the Swedish Society of Uroradiology and in collaboration with the Swedish Society of Nephrology (GS) and the Swedish Society of Diabetology (AF). Preventing contrast medium-induced acute kidney injury: side-by-side comparison of Swedish-ESUR guidelines. Eur Radiol. 2018;28(12):5384–95. https://doi.org/10.1007/s00330-018-5678-6. Epub 2018/08/23. Cited in: Pubmed; PMID 30132106.
3. Harbron R, Ainsbury EA, Bouffler SD, Tanner RJ, Eakins JS, Pearce MS. Enhanced radiation dose and DNA damage associated with iodinated contrast media in diagnostic X-ray imaging. Br J Radiol. 2017;90(1079):20170028. https://doi.org/10.1259/bjr.20170028. Epub 2017/08/24. Cited in: Pubmed; PMID 28830201.
4. Pathe C, Eble K, Schmitz-Beuting D, Keil B, Kaestner B, Voelker M, Kleb B, Klose KJ, Heverhagen JT. The presence of iodinated contrast agents amplifies DNA radiation damage in computed tomography. Contrast Media Mol Imaging. 2011;6(6):507–13. https://doi.org/10.1002/cmmi.453. Epub 2011/12/07. Cited in: Pubmed; PMID 22144029.
5. Deinzer CK, Danova D, Kleb B, Klose KJ, Heverhagen JT. Influence of different iodinated contrast media on the induction of DNA double-strand breaks after in vitro X-ray irradiation. Contrast Media Mol Imaging. 2014;9(4):259–67. https://doi.org/10.1002/cmmi.1567. Epub 2014/04/08. Cited in: Pubmed; PMID 24706609.
6. Padole A, Ali Khawaja RD, Kalra MK, Singh S. CT radiation dose and iterative reconstruction techniques. AJR Am J Roentgenol. 2015;204(4):W384–92. https://doi.org/10.2214/AJR.14.13241. Epub 2015/03/21. Cited in: Pubmed; PMID 25794087.
7. Willemink MJ, Noel PB. The evolution of image reconstruction for CT-from filtered back projection to artificial intelligence. Eur Radiol. 2019;29(5):2185–95. https://doi.org/10.1007/s00330-018-5810-7. Epub 2018/11/01. Cited in: Pubmed; PMID 30377791.
8. Huda W, Lieberman KA, Chang J, Roskopf ML. Patient size and x-ray technique factors in head computed tomography examinations. II. Image quality. Med Phys. 2004;31(3):595–601. https://doi.org/10.1118/1.1646233. Epub 2004/04/09. Cited in: Pubmed; PMID 15070259.
9. Grant KL, Flohr TG, Krauss B, Sedlmair M, Thomas C, Schmidt B. Assessment of an advanced image-based technique to calculate virtual monoenergetic computed tomographic images from a dual-energy examination to improve contrast-to-noise ratio in examinations using iodinated contrast media. Invest Radiol. 2014;49(9):586–92. https://doi.org/10.1097/RLI.0000000000000060. Epub 2014/04/09. Cited in: Pubmed; PMID 24710203.
10. Iyama Y, Nakaura T, Yokoyama K, Kidoh M, Harada K, Oda S, Tokuyasu S, Yamashita Y. Low-contrast and low-radiation dose protocol in cardiac computed tomography: usefulness of low tube voltage and knowledge-based iterative model reconstruction algorithm. J Comput Assist Tomogr. 2016;40(6):941–7. https://doi.org/10.1097/RCT.0000000000000440. Epub 2016/05/26. Cited in: Pubmed; PMID 27224224.
11. Van Cauteren T, Van Gompel G, Tanaka K, Verdries DE, Belsack D, Nieboer KH, Willekens I, Evans P, Macholl S, Verfaillie G, Droogmans S, de Mey J, Buls N. The impact of combining a low-tube voltage acquisition with iterative reconstruction on total iodine dose in coronary CT angiography. Biomed Res Int. 2017;2017:2476171. https://doi.org/10.1155/2017/2476171. Epub 2017/06/18. Cited in: Pubmed; PMID 28620616.
12. Szucs-Farkas Z, Megyeri B, Christe A, Vock P, Heverhagen JT, Schindera ST. Prospective randomised comparison of diagnostic confidence and image quality with normal-dose and low-dose CT pulmonary angiography at various body weights. Eur Radiol. 2014;24(8):1868–77. https://doi.org/10.1007/s00330-014-3208-8. Epub 2014/05/29. Cited in: Pubmed; PMID 24865694.
13. Meyer M, Haubenreisser H, Schabel C, Leidecker C, Schmidt B, Schoenberg SO, Henzler T. CT pulmonary angiography in patients with acute or chronic renal insufficiency: evaluation of a low dose contrast material protocol. Sci Rep. 2018;8(1):1995. https://doi.org/10.1038/s41598-018-20254-y. Epub 2018/02/02. Cited in: Pubmed; PMID 29386532.
14. Yuan R, Shuman WP, Earls JP, Hague CJ, Mumtaz HA, Scott-Moncrieff A, Ellis JD, Mayo JR, Leipsic JA. Reduced iodine load at CT pulmonary angiography with dual-energy monochromatic imaging: comparison with standard CT pulmonary angiography—a prospective randomized trial. Radiology. 2012;262(1):290–7. https://doi.org/10.1148/radiol.11110648. Epub 2011/11/16. Cited in: Pubmed; PMID 22084206.
15. Luo S, Zhang LJ, Meinel FG, Zhou CS, Qi L, McQuiston AD, Schoepf UJ, Lu GM. Low tube voltage and low contrast material volume cerebral CT angiography. Eur Radiol. 2014;24(7):1677–85. https://doi.org/10.1007/s00330-014-3184-z. Epub 2014/05/06. Cited in: Pubmed; PMID 24792591.
16. Kanematsu M, Goshima S, Kawai N, Kondo H, Miyoshi T, Watanabe H, Noda Y, Tanahashi Y, Bae KT. Low-iodine-load and low-tube-voltage CT angiographic imaging of the kidney by using bolus tracking with saline flushing. Radiology. 2015;275(3):832–40. https://doi.org/10.1148/radiol.14141457. Epub 2014/12/11. Cited in: Pubmed; PMID 25494297.
17. Ichikawa T, Okada M, Kondo H, Sou H, Murakami T, Kanematsu M, Yoshikawa S, Shiosakai K, Hayakawa A, Awai K, Yoshimitsu K, Yamashita Y. Recommended iodine dose for multiphasic contrast-enhanced mutidetector-row computed tomography imaging of liver for assessing hypervascular hepatocellular car-

cinoma: multicenter prospective study in 77 general hospitals in Japan. Acad Radiol. 2013;20(9):1130–6. https://doi.org/10.1016/j.acra.2013.05.003. Epub 2013/08/13. Cited in: Pubmed; PMID 23931427.
18. Noda Y, Kanematsu M, Goshima S, Kondo H, Watanabe H, Kawada H, Kawai N, Tanahashi Y, Miyoshi TRT, Bae KT. Reducing iodine load in hepatic CT for patients with chronic liver disease with a combination of low-tube-voltage and adaptive statistical iterative reconstruction. Eur J Radiol. 2015;84(1):11–8. https://doi.org/10.1016/j.ejrad.2014.10.008. Epub 2014/12/03. Cited in: Pubmed; PMID 25455414.
19. Goshima S, Kanematsu M, Noda Y, Kawai N, Kawada H, Ono H, Bae KT. Minimally required iodine dose for the detection of hypervascular hepatocellular carcinoma on 80-kVp CT. AJR Am J Roentgenol. 2016;206(3):518–25. https://doi.org/10.2214/AJR.15.15138. Epub 2016/02/24. Cited in: Pubmed; PMID 26901007.
20. Awai K, Nakayama Y, Nakaura T, Yanaga Y, Tamura Y, Hatemura M, Funama Y, Yamashita Y. Prediction of aortic peak enhancement in monophasic contrast injection protocols at multidetector CT: phantom and patient studies. Radiat Med. 2007;25(1):14–21. https://doi.org/10.1007/s11604-006-0095-1. Epub 2007/01/17. Cited in: Pubmed; PMID 17225048.
21. Benz MR, Szucs-Farkas Z, Froehlich JM, Stadelmann G, Bongartz G, Bouwman L, Schindera ST. Scan time adapted contrast agent injection protocols with low volume for low-tube voltage CT angiography: an in vitro study. Eur J Radiol. 2017;93:65–9. https://doi.org/10.1016/j.ejrad.2017.05.017. Epub 2017/07/03. Cited in: Pubmed; PMID 28668433.
22. Schindera ST, Nelson RC, Howle L, Nichols E, DeLong DM, Merkle EM. Effect of varying injection rates of a saline chaser on aortic enhancement in CT angiography: phantom study. Eur Radiol. 2008;18(8):1683–9. https://doi.org/10.1007/s00330-008-0911-3. Epub 2008/03/21. Cited in: Pubmed; PMID 18351346.
23. Akagi M, Nakamura Y, Higaki T, Narita K, Honda Y, Zhou J, Yu Z, Akino N, Awai K. Deep learning reconstruction improves image quality of abdominal ultra-high-resolution CT. Eur Radiol. 2019;29(11):6163–71. https://doi.org/10.1007/s00330-019-06170-3. Epub 2019/04/13. Cited in: Pubmed; PMID 30976831.
24. Solomon J, Marin D, Roy Choudhury K, Patel B, Samei E. Effect of radiation dose reduction and reconstruction algorithm on image noise, contrast, resolution, and detectability of subtle hypoattenuating liver lesions at multidetector CT: filtered back projection versus a commercial model-based iterative reconstruction algorithm. Radiology. 2017;284(3):777–87. https://doi.org/10.1148/radiol.2017161736. Epub 2017/02/09. Cited in: Pubmed; PMID 28170300.

Gastrointestinal Iodinated Contrast Agents

6

Suzan Saylisoy and Sukru Mehmet Erturk

6.1 Introduction

Oral contrast agents are classified as positive or neutral oral contrast agents. Positive oral contrast agents are used to opacify the bowel lumen and are divided into two categories: barium sulfate suspensions and water-soluble iodinated contrast media. Enterography using CT and MRI combines intravenous contrast and neutral or low-attenuation oral contrast agents to assess the small bowel in patients with known or suspected Crohn's disease and extraenteric structures. Suspected small-bowel polyps or cancer, vascular lesions of the small-bowel wall, and gastrointestinal bleeding are all common reasons for enterography. This chapter discusses physical properties, clinical uses, and adverse effects of oral contrast agents.

S. Saylisoy (✉)
Department of Radiology, Eskişehir Osmangazi University, Eskisehir, Turkey

S. M. Erturk
Department of Radiology, Istanbul University School of Medicine, Istanbul, Turkey

6.2 Positive Oral Contrast Agents

Positive oral contrast agents are administered to opacify the bowel lumen and thus to improve the differentiation of bowel from non-bowel structures [1]. The two main classes of positive oral contrast material are barium sulfate suspensions and water-soluble iodinated contrast media [2, 3].

Plain radiography is the first-line evaluation of various important diagnoses, such as bowel perforation, obstruction, volvulus, and colitis. When a detailed luminal evaluation is required, fluoroscopic barium or water-soluble single- or double-contrast studies are performed to investigate early mucosal changes and bowel transit time, discriminate between functional ileus and obstruction, and determine the cause of obstruction. However, recent rapid advances in both computed tomography (CT) and magnetic resonance imaging (MRI) are replacing fluoroscopic imaging for certain clinical indications. For example, CT colonography (CTC) allows visualizing the entire lumen and extra-colonic organs and providing higher sensitivity data in a dataset for cancer detection and higher patient acceptance compared to barium enema [4].

One of the major difficulties for radiologists who interpret gastrointestinal tract (GIT) studies is a gradual decrease in the number of commercially available sources of barium and iodinated contrast media specially developed for such purposes, as leading companies have started

S. M. Erturk et al. (eds.), *Medical Imaging Contrast Agents: A Clinical Manual*,
https://doi.org/10.1007/978-3-030-79256-5_6

consolidating their contrast agent portfolios due to reduction in use. Therefore, it is necessary to propose alternative contrast agents and imaging modalities, such as CT, MRI, and endoscopy, and radiologists may also need to substitute the contrast agent with a different formulation that is not specifically formulated, designed, or marketed for a gastrointestinal evaluation, for example, intravascular use [3].

6.2.1 Barium Sulfate

Barium sulfate is a white crystal solid structure with a chemical formula $BaSO_4$. It is insoluble in water. The forms used for imaging purposes are administered through various routes including oral, rectal, and direct injection into GIT (i.e., gastrostomy, enterostomy, and colostomy) and direct injection via catheters [3]. Barium compounds are primarily preferred because of their white appearance and high density. Commercial forms are mixed with sweeteners, as well as other substances, such as pectin, sorbitol, and agar-agar, all of which are discarded from GIT. Barium sulfate is not absorbed by the intact mucosa.

There are many brands of barium sulfate available for clinical use. The major US manufacturers are E-Z-Em (Lake Success, NY; http://www.ezem.com/) and Tyco Healthcare (Mansfield, MA; Mallinckrodt subsidiary and Lafayette products, Hazelwood, MO; http://imaging.mallinckrodt.com/). Oral barium sulfate contrast agents are available in powder or liquid forms; powders must be reconstituted with water, and liquids must be diluted [5].

6.2.1.1 Physical Properties of Barium Sulfate

Many studies have investigated the relationship between the physical characteristics of oral barium sulfate preparations, such as plasticity, viscosity, density, and thixotropy, and its ability to coat the colonic wall [5]. Some barium sulfate preparations are plastic, which means that a certain amount of shear stress is required to induce the flow, beyond which stress and shear are proportional [6]. The relationship between viscosity and shear rate varies greatly among barium sulfate formulations [7]. It has been found that plastic substances are more useful for double-contrast studies than their pseudoplastic counterparts [6]. Radiologists frequently describe barium sulfate suspensions as "thick" and "thin," but these terms should not be confused with two distinctly different properties: viscosity and density. Although the thickness may be due to increased viscosity, these suspensions may not be very radiodense, while thin preparations may have low viscosity but have a large percentage of barium. Therefore, when characterizing suspensions, it is better to describe both viscosity and density Double-contrast examinations use formulations with either high viscosity and medium density or low viscosity and high density to leave a layer of contrast with high radiographic density on the mucosa. High-viscosity preparations produce an opaque coating, but this may be non-uniform and obscure fine detail. In addition, if the viscosity is too high, the patient may not be able to swallow the contrast agent, and it may not spread across the mucosa [5]. Increasing the concentration of barium sulfate or combining it with various compounds can increase the viscosity of oral contrast agents. Magnesium has been found to improve mucosal coating, which is not related to the increase in viscosity [8]. There is a good correlation between viscosity and thixotropy, which is the tendency of a compound to harden if undisturbed. Thixotropy occurs due to the structural breakdown and subsequent accumulation of particles in barium sulfate suspensions. Residual magnesium in the bowel lumen may increase the thixotropy of barium sulfate contrast agents, which can contribute to mucosal coating seen in double-contrast barium enemas after the administration of magnesium-containing purgatives [5, 8].

6.2.1.2 Additives

Without additives, barium sulfate is unable to coat the mucosa, which results in flocculation.

Inert salts, including salts of alkali metals; ammonium salts of poly-acid monomers; citric and tartaric salts of sodium, potassium, and ammonium; and EDTA salt of sodium, can be added as deflocculants to prevent flocculation, which interacts inversely with mucosal coating and alters the effective size of barium particles.

To keep the barium in solution through weak bonds formed and to extend the shelf-life of liquid preparations, stabilizer (suspending) agents, such as sodium carboxymethyl cellulose, pectin, magnesium aluminum silicate, naturally and artificially occurring gums (hydrophilic colloids), long-chain organic molecules, acacia, tragacanth, and gelatin starch, are added. Removal of gums allows sedimentation of large particles into mucosal folds. Some suspending agents may increase viscosity and improve adhesion.

Dispersants, including surface-active agents and strongly ionic substances, such acid rate or polyphosphate ions, are largely responsible for the ability of barium sulfate preparations to mix with other fluids, to opacify fluid in GIT, and to coat the mucosa.

Wetting ability refers to the tendency of a liquid to form a thin, uniform film on a surface instead of pulling away from large areas. Natural and artificial gums added as suspension agents may act as wetting agents. Drying is prevented by adding humectants, such as sorbitol and mannitol, at isotonic concentrations with the colon.

Antifoaming agents, such as simethicone and siloxane, are usually added to the barium sulfate suspensions to prevent bubbling. To improve the taste and acceptability for the patient, sugar, saccharin, and other flavoring agents can also be utilized [5].

Magnesium is poorly absorbed by the bowel; therefore, the use of magnesium-containing purgatives before barium enema leaves many of these ions in the lumen of the colon. Magnesium increases the viscosity of barium suspensions and results in an improved mucosal coating [5, 8].

6.2.1.3 Advantages of Barium over Iodinated Contrast Agents

Barium sulfate is the preferred agent for opacification of GIT for fluoroscopic studies due to its mucosal coating properties and high contrast effects. Barium agents offer a better coating of the bowel wall by providing superior delineation of mucosal detail than iodinated agents [3]. The higher attenuation of barium agents is also potentially useful for detection of small leaks that are not visible with iodinated contrast agents. In addition, barium agents are more resistant to dilution than iodinated agents, which allows delayed imaging in the setting of slow transit time; however, due to the risk of development of barium concretions, caution should be taken in the case of prolonged transit time [3, 9].

6.2.1.4 Imaging of GIT Using Barium Enema

The ratio of weight/volume (w/v) varies according to the GIT passage speed, anatomical conditions, and the procedure. In general, 40% w/v is sufficient for small intestinal examinations, and 85% w/v barium for colon examinations. Instead of defined formulas, optimal image quality is obtained by adjusting the concentration and quantity [10].

Barium swallow studies continue to be the main examination method of dysphagia, allowing direct evaluation and inspection of the esophageal mucosa and gastroesophageal junction: an objective assessment of esophageal contractility, reflux, and presence of strictures, pouches, and hiatal hernias. In upper GIT examinations, the patient's morning fasting is adequate. During this examination, the patient ingests barium and carbex (effervescent granules) to provide a double-contrast (gas and barium) view of the stomach [4].

Small bowel follow-through barium studies are undertaken for the evaluation of abdominal pain, diarrhea, and diseases manifesting with mucosal abnormalities, such as celiac disease and Crohn's disease. The patient is asked to drink approximately 500 mL of barium diluted with water and liquid metoclopramide. These studies have been progressively replaced with CT and MR enterography, as well as enteroscopy and capsule endoscopy [4, 10].

Double-contrast enema studies are used to investigate the symptoms of the lower GIT malignancies, such as a change in bowel habits, anemia, and unexplained weight loss. In these cases, medical colon cleansing should be performed. The patient is asked to follow a low-residue diet for 48 h prior to the examination with a cathartic bowel preparation. Barium is instilled through a rectal tube to coat the colonic mucosa, followed by application of gas to distend the colon. One thousand to two thousand milliliters (85–100%) of barium w/v suspension is recommended for double-contrast examinations of the colon [3, 4, 10].

Barium sulfate can also stop bleeding in colon diverticular disease, but should not be used after surgery or in cases with suspected perforation [11].

6.2.1.5 Side Effects

Most side effects are not allergic reactions. The frequently encountered symptoms are nausea, vomiting, and abdominal discomfort [12]. Unabsorbed barium does not cause severe allergic reactions, but a small amount of barium is known to pass into intestinal mucosal cells during GIT examinations. Allergy-like (anaphylactoid) reactions to enteric barium are rarely seen either caused by the barium itself or various additives and medical devices used to deliver the barium [3]. Allergic reactions can develop in a wide spectrum from urticaria to severe anaphylactic reactions. There are very rare cases of barium encephalopathy. Vasovagal reflex development is also infrequently reported in double-contrast colon radiography. In cases of prolonged transit time, barium sulfate may remain in the intestines for a long time and can cause the development of a barolith, which may need to be removed by surgery. In such cases, a water-soluble contrast agent is recommended [13]. Barium may trigger toxic dilatation of the colon [14]. The leakage of sterile barium into the peritoneal cavity leads to peritoneal irritation [9].

The effect of barium on the mediastinum is less known. The leakage of barium from the esophagus into the mediastinum can trigger an inflammatory reaction with subsequent granuloma and fibrosis development, but there is little to no evidence that barium in the mediastinum causes clinically significant mediastinitis [3].

Aspirated low-volume barium is typically removed from the airways by the ciliary action of normal bronchial epithelium, while the epithelium being damaged due to a bronchial disorder can delay this process. Aspiration of barium during upper GIT examinations can cause serious pneumonia and death, especially in patients with a significant underlying lung disease [12].

Bacteremia may occur during and after contrast media enemas. Barium enema has been reported to be associated with transient bacteremia [15].

Following bile surgery or sphincteroplasty, orally ingested barium commonly refluxes into the biliary tree. Normally, gravity and the physiologic bile flow lead to emptying of the refluxed barium into the bowel. However, if the barium is not drained out of the biliary tree immediately, over distention of the bile ducts can occur, with the potential to develop suppurative cholangitis, choledocholiths, or disseminated intravascular coagulation [16].

Intravasation of barium is a serious condition with 55% mortality. Pulmonary embolism, disseminated intravascular coagulation, sepsis, and severe hypotension can also be observed [17].

6.2.2 Water-Soluble Iodinated Contrast Agents

Water-soluble contrast agents are available in different formulations, including HOCM and LOCM at different concentrations and volumes, and in different packaging. Gastrografin (diatrizoate meglumine and diatrizoate sodium; Bracco Diagnostics Inc., Monroe Township, NJ) and Gastroview (diatrizoate meglumine and diatrizoate sodium; Mallinckrodt, Raleigh, NC) are FDA-approved water-soluble HOCM specifically designed for enteric opacification in the small bowel and colon. These agents include 660 mg/mL diatrizoate meglumine and 100 mg/mL diatrizoate sodium. The resulting solution contains 367 mg of iodine per milliliter. Cystografin "Dilute" and Cysto-Conray II containing approximately 85 mgI/mL are marketed for cystourethrography and can also be used for rectal administration without mixing or dilution [3].

HOCM and LOCM supplied for intravenous use can also be administered safely orally, rectally, or through the enteric tube at full strength or diluted. This use is usually "off label," except for Omnipaque (iohexol; GE Healthcare, Princeton, NJ), which has an FDA-approved indication for oral use in select concentrations. When administered rectally, the concentration of iodinated contrast agents depends on a variety of factors, including whether the study is performed for diagnostic or therapeutic purposes. When used as an enema, the recommended dilution for adults is 240 mL (88 g iodine) in 1000 mL of tap water, thus providing 88 mg iodine per milliliter (mgI/mL) of solution. Water-soluble HOCM have also been successfully used for the treatment of postoperative paralytic ileus and adhesive small bowel obstruction [3].

6.2.2.1 Computed Tomographic Colonography

CTC, also known as virtual colonoscopy, involves complete bowel preparation (similar to the double-contrast barium studies), followed by rectal gas insufflation and helical CT examination of the distended colon with an intravenous contrast in supine and prone positions. The resulting image dataset is then displayed at a workstation with complex image analysis software, which provides images obtained by conventional colonoscopy [4]. Oral contrast agents used during CTC can reduce false-positive and false-negative detections due to stool and iso-attenuating residual fluid. These agents can also eliminate the requirement for a clean colon, as opacified stool and residual fluid can be distinguished either electronically or visually from polyps and normal colonic mucosa. Clinical results show that the sensitivity of CTC for the detection of colorectal polyps and cancer exceeds that of a barium enema examination. Recent studies have shown that oral contrast agents often coat polyps with a preference for those at risk for villous histology, a characteristic of advanced polyps. This finding encourages the development of contrast agents that can predict polyps constituting at greater risk of progression to malignancy [4, 18].

6.2.2.2 Side Effects

The greatest safety problem with water-soluble iodinated contrast agents is the potential for aspiration into the lungs; if aspirated into the lungs, HOCM, such as Gastrografin or Gastroview, can lead to chemical pneumonia, respiratory failure, and life-threatening pulmonary edema [3, 9]. Therefore, HOCM solutions are contraindicated for oral administration in patients at risk for aspiration. If water-soluble contrast media are to be used in this patient group, LOCM should be preferred due to their lower risk of morbidity and mortality [3].

Hypertonic HOCM should also be avoided in patients with fluid and/or electrolyte imbalances, especially in very young or elderly patients with hypovolemia or dehydration. HOCM solutions lead to hypovolemia and hypotension in susceptible patients, due to fluid loss by drawing water into the lumen. Iso-low-osmolar iodinated contrast agents can be used to prevent fluid displacement in children who are thought to have perforation of GIT. In high-risk patients, the contrast agent can be diluted with water (1:4 ratio) [19].

Allergy-like reactions can occur even due to small amounts of iodinated contrast agents absorbed from GIT after oral or rectal administration. During this process, a small volume of ICA (approximately 1–2%) is absorbed and excreted into the urinary tract. If mucosal inflammation, mucosal infection, or intestinal obstruction is present, the absorbed amount of ICA can increase. The ACR Manual on Contrast Media does not provide any specific guidelines concerning premedication for nonvascular administration of iodinated contrast agents to individuals who have had a previous reaction to vascular administration of these agents [20]. However, the guidelines of the European Society of Urogenital Radiology 2014 suggest that physicians "take the same precautions as for intravascular administration." Therefore, some centers recommend premedication of sensitive patients. However, other centers consider that such reactions are too rare to justify premedication and thus do not use premedication as the standard of care [21].

6.2.2.3 Advantages of ICAs over Barium

Water-soluble HOCM studies are usually performed in the early postoperative period to assess anastomotic integrity. The preference over barium is a consequence of the potential of free intraabdominal barium to induce peritonitis [3].

Water-soluble HOCM can be safely and effectively used for therapeutic cleansing enemas in patients with fecal impaction or cystic fibrosis. The recommended dilution of Gastrografin or Gastroview (240 mL in 1000 mL of water) may be advantageous since this hypertonic solution is more likely to induce a fluid shift into the colon, facilitating fecal evacuation [22].

6.2.2.4 Advantages of LOCM over HOCM

LOCM reduce the risk of contrast-related pneumonitis in patients prone to aspiration. The taste of LOCM may be more acceptable, although this is more important when administered at full strength compared to when these agents are diluted for CT scanning. In addition, non-ionic LOCM (e.g., Omnipaque) cause less fluid shift into the bowel and less stimulation of peristalsis and have been reported to result in lower iodine absorption from the intact bowel [9].

An isotonic solution of a contrast medium can be prepared by substituting LOCM, such as Isovue (iopamidol; Bracco Diagnostics Inc., Monroe Township, NJ) or Optiray (ioversol; Mallinckrodt, Raleigh, NC) for Gastrografin. Isovue 300 and Optiray 300 contain 300 mgI/mL; therefore, adding a 400-mL bottle of Isovue 300 or Optiray 300 to a 1000-mL bag of saline or water results in a 1400-mL solution containing 120,000 mg of organically bound iodine or 85 mgI/mL (almost identical to the 88 mgI/mL of the proposed dilution of HOCM for enema administration) [3].

6.2.3 Suspicion of Perforation

Water-soluble contrast media are widely used to evaluate for anastomotic leaks in the postoperative GIT. These agents are preferred to barium for patients with suspected leaks because they are quickly absorbed from interstitial spaces and the peritoneal cavity, whereas barium will remain in these spaces indefinitely [9]. However, water-soluble contrast agents are less radiopaque than barium and less adherent to sites of leakage, limiting their ability to detect perforations, particularly small or subtle perforations. Therefore, water-soluble oral contrast media is recommended for initial use in any study in which a perforation is known or suspected. If no perforation is detected with water-soluble contrast agents, high-density barium should be applied to improve detection of esophageal leaks. When a leak is detected only with barium, the disadvantage of retained barium in the mediastinum is more than balanced by early diagnosis and treatment of an esophageal perforation [23].

6.3 Neutral Contrast Agents

Enterography with CT and MRI combines neutral or low-attenuation oral contrast agents with intravenous contrast in order to evaluate the small bowel in patients with known or suspected Crohn's disease and extraenteric structures. Other common indications for enterography include suspected small bowel polyps or malignancy, vascular lesions of the small bowel wall, and gastrointestinal bleeding [24–29]. For the assessment of small bowel disorders, sufficient luminal distension by luminal contrast agents is important [30]. For small bowel imaging, positive contrast agents are generally not preferred because they mask the enhancement of the mucosa and lesions such as neuroendocrine tumors. Neutral oral contrast agents, which are isodense to water on CT and are biphasic on MRI (i.e., hypointense on T1-weighted images and hyperintense on T2-weighted images) are preferred because these agents improve the visualization of abnormal mural enhancement, mural thickening and stratification, and penetrating complications. Neutral oral contrast offers additional benefits, including the absence of streak artefacts that often occur at CT from high-attenuation positive oral contrast [24–29].

Several different neutral oral contrast agents such as water, milk, sugar alcohols like mannitol or sorbitol, dilute barium solutions, locust bean gum/mannitol (LBM), psyllium, and polyethylene glycol have been studied for use in enterography [29–31].

There are several factors that influence bowel distension and wall imaging. A larger volume of oral contrast, if tolerated by the patient, would undoubtedly provide better bowel distension. The time to optimal distension of the terminal ileum is 51–72 min. Therefore, it is recommended that the oral contrast agent be ingested about 60 min before CT imaging [26]. Bowel distension is also affected by the fat content of the oral contrast agent ingested. An oral contrast agent with a high fat content would decrease bowel peristalsis and delay gastrointestinal emptying, resulting in better bowel distension. Osmolarity of the oral contrast agent is another parameter, as higher osmolarity can result in better degree of bowel distension [27].

Water is a feasible oral contrast agent, as it is safe, cheap, and well-tolerated. However, water is rapidly absorbed across the stomach and proximal small bowel, which results in inadequate luminal distention of the distal small bowel, which is the area most affected in Crohn's disease [31].

Milk is an effective, cheap agent and preferred by patients with fewer abdominal adverse effects. 3.8% milk contains fat that effectively reduces peristalsis and slows passage through the GIT, resulting in better bowel distension. In addition, 3.8% milk does not require the administration of a smooth muscle relaxant such as glucagon to achieve sufficient small bowel distension and therefore eliminates potentially undesirable side effects and additional costs [25].

Sugar alcohols such as sorbitol or mannitol provide distention of the small bowel because they effectively trap the fluid in the lumen and prevent reabsorption. Mannitol is an effective agent to produce distension of the bowel wall. Locust bean gum is used as thickener [30, 31].

Two neutral barium sulfate suspensions containing sorbitol and a thickening agent are commercially available: VoLumen and Breeza. **VoLumen** (a berry-flavored barium sulfate suspension, 0.1% w/v, 0.1% w/w; E-Z-EM, Inc., a Bracco-owned company, Lake Success, N.Y) that contains sorbitol and a gum provides excellent distention and excellent visualization of the bowel wall. Most enterography protocols require ingestion of 900–1350 mL (two to three bottles) of this low-Hounsfield-value barium suspension followed by variable amounts of water. However, the currently available barium- and sorbitol-based substances are poorly tolerated by patients. Complaints about taste and texture as well as about the large amount that is required are frequent. Products containing sugar alcohol have an osmotic laxative effect that can cause cramping or diarrhea. Some patients may experience subsequent constipation. These symptoms may be particularly poorly tolerated by patients with inflammatory bowel disease who often have abdominal pain or experience complications of the disease including strictures that may cause partial obstruction [20, 32]. **Breeza** (Beekley Medical, Bristol, Conn) is a lemon-lime-flavored beverage for neutral abdominal/pelvic imaging. These two contrast agents provide similar small bowel distention. Significantly higher taste and texture scores for Breeza may reflect better patient acceptance and tolerability [32].

Psyllium fiber is cheap and commercially available and has a favorable taste. It may be used for small bowel distension [33].

Polyethylene glycol has the same density as water. Its main characteristics are an agreeable flavor and lack of toxicity [34].

References

1. Winklhofer S, Lin WC, Wang ZJ, Behr SC, Westphalen AC, Yeh BM. Comparison of positive oral contrast agents for abdominopelvic CT. AJR Am J Roentgenol. 2019;212:1037–43.
2. Kielar AZ, Patlas MN, Katz DS. Oral contrast for CT in patients with acute non-traumatic abdominal and pelvic pain: what should be its current role? Emerg Radiol. 2016;23:477–81.
3. Federle MP, Jaffe TA, Davis PL, Al-Hawary MM, Levine MS. Contrast media for fluoroscopic examinations of the GI and GU tracts: current challenges and recommendations. Abdom Radiol. 2017;42:90–100.
4. Robinson C, Punwani S, Taylor S. Imaging the gastrointestinal tract in 2008. Clin Med. 2009;9:609–12.

5. O'Connor SD, Summers RM. Revisiting oral barium sulfate contrast agents. Acad Radiol. 2007;14:72–80.
6. Anderson W, Harthill JE, James WB, Montgomery D. Barium sulphate preparations for use in double contrast examination of the upper gastrointestinal tract. Br J Radiol. 1980;53:1150–9.
7. Cumberland DC. Optimum viscosity of barium suspension for use in the double contrast barium meal. Gastrointest Radiol. 1977;2:169–74.
8. Conry BG, Jones S, Bartram CI. The effect of oral magnesium-containing bowel preparation agents on mucosal coating by barium sulphate suspensions. Br J Radiol. 1987;60:1215–9.
9. Ott DJ, Gelfand DW. Gastrointestinal contrast agents. Indications, uses, and risks. JAMA. 1983;249:2380–4.
10. Laufer I, Levine MS. Double contrast gastrointestinal radiology. 2nd ed. Philadelphia: WB Saunders; 1992.
11. Matsuhashi N, Akahane M, Nakajima A. Barium impaction therapy for refractory colonic diverticular bleeding. AJR Am J Roentgenol. 2003;180:490–2.
12. Gelfand DW, Ott DJ, Hunt TH. Gastrointestinal complications of radiologic procedures. In: Meyers MA, Ghahremani GG, editors. Iatrogenic gastrointestinal complications. New York: Springer. p. 91–122.
13. Wylie R, Hyams JS, Kay M, editors. Pediatric gastrointestinal and liver disease. 5th ed. Philadelphia: Elsevier.
14. Goldberg HI. Letter: the barium enema and toxic megacolon: cause-effect relationship? Gastroenterology. 1975;68:617–8.
15. Butt J, Hentges D, Pelican G, Henstorf H, Haag T, Rolfe R, Hutcheson D. Bacteremia during barium enema study. AJR Am J Roentgenol. 1978;130:715–8.
16. Walsham A, Larsen J. Adverse effects of barium sulfate in the biliary tract. Diagn Interv Radiol. 2008;14:94–6.
17. O'Hara DE, Krakovitz EK, Wolferth CC. Barium intravasation during an upper gastrointestinal examination: a case report and literature review. Am Surg. 1995;61:330–3.
18. Levine MS, Yee J. History, evolution, and current status of radiologic imaging tests for colorectal cancer screening. Radiology. 2014;273:S160–80.
19. Eisenberg RL, Hedgcock MW, Shanser JD, Brenner RJ, Gedgaudas RK, Marks WM. Iodine absorption from the gastrointestinal tract during hypaque-enema examination. Radiology. 1979;133:597–9.
20. ACR, American College of Radiology. ACR manual on contrast media version 10.3. 2018.
21. ESUR. ESUR guidelines on contrast media 9.0. 2014.
22. Culp WC. Relief of severe fecal impactions with water-soluble contrast enemas. Radiology. 1975;115:9–12.
23. Rubesin SE, Levine MS. Radiologic diagnosis of gastrointestinal perforation. Radiol Clin North Am. 2003;41:1095–115.
24. Paulsen SR, Huprich JE, Fletcher JG, Booya F, Young BM, Fidler JL, et al. CT enterography as a diagnostic tool in evaluating small bowel disorders: review of clinical experience with over 700 cases. Radiographics. 2006;26:641–57.
25. Ilangovan R, Burling D, George A, Gupta A, Marshall M, Taylor SA. CT enterography: review of technique and practical tips. Br J Radiol. 2012;85:876–86.
26. Lim BK, Bux SI, Rahmat K, Lam SY, Liew YW. Evaluation of bowel distension and mural visualisation using neutral oral contrast agents for multidetector-row computed tomography. Singap Med J. 2012;53:732–6.
27. Griffin N, Grant LA, Anderson S, Irving F, Sanderson J. Small bowel MR enterography: problem solving in Crohn's disease. Insights Imaging. 2012;3:251–63.
28. Naeger DM, Chang SD, Kolli P, Shah V, Huang W, Thoeni RF. Neutral vs positive oral contrast in diagnosing acute appendicitis with contrast-enhanced CT: sensitivity, specificity, reader confidence and interpretation time. Br J Radiol. 2011;84:418–26.
29. Ajaj W, Goehde SC, Schneemann H, Ruehm SG, Debatin JF, Lauenstein TC. Oral contrast agents for small bowel MRI: comparison of different additives to optimize bowel distension. Eur Radiol. 2004;14:458–64.
30. Hashemi J, Davoudi Y, Taghavi M, Pezeshki Rad M, Moghadam AM. Improvement of distension and mural visualization of bowel loops using neutral oral contrasts in abdominal computed tomography. World J Radiol. 2014;6:907–12.
31. Wang YR, Yu XL, Peng ZY. Evaluation of different small bowel contrast agents by multi-detector row CT. Int J Clin Exp Med. 2018;8(9):16175–82.
32. Gottumukkala RV, LaPointe A, Sargent D, Gee MS. Comparison of three oral contrast preparations for magnetic resonance enterography in pediatric patients with known or suspected Crohn disease: a prospective randomized trial. Pediatr Radiol. 2019;49(7):889–96. https://doi.org/10.1007/s00247-019-04378-5.
33. Saini S, Colak E, Anthwal S, Vlachou PA, Raikhlin A, Kirpalani A. Comparison of 3% sorbitol vs psyllium fibre as oral contrast agents in MR enterography. Br J Radiol. 2014;87:20140100.
34. Minordi LM, Vecchioli A, Mirk P, Bonomo L. CT enterography with polyethylene glycol solution vs CT enteroclysis in small bowel disease. Br J Radiol. 2011;84:112–9.

Chemistry, Physicochemical Properties and Pharmacokinetics of Gadolinium-Based Contrast Agents

7

Semra Yigitaslan and Kevser Erol

Gadolinium (Gd^{3+}) is a rare-earth metal from the lanthanide (Ln) family of elements and has seven unpaired electrons. Gadolinium (atomic number $Z = 64$) has a standard atomic weight of 157.25. In addition to its medical uses, it is also used in compact discs, televisions, etc.).

Today, it is the major contrast agent used in MRI because of having a high magnetic moment and an unusually long electronic spin relaxation time [1, 2]. Unfortunately, free gadolinium is highly toxic. Because ionic radius of Gd^{3+} is close to that of Ca^{2+} (107.8 pm and 114 pm, respectively), it can block many voltage-gated calcium channels even at nano- or micromolar concentrations. This blockage results in the inhibition of several physiologic processes such as muscle contraction, transmission of neuronal signals and coagulation [3]. It can also result in several other adverse effects including splenic degeneration, central lobular necrosis of the liver and haematological abnormalities [4]. Therefore, it is mandatory to attach the Gd^{3+} with a suitable chelating agent to avoid its toxic effects to humans.

The 50% lethal dose (LD50, i.e. the dose required to kill 50% of the population) of the chelated Gd was found to be 50–100 times higher than that of free Gd^{3+} ions [5, 6]. Chelation improves the solubility in water and protects the tissues from the deleterious effects of Gd^{3+} ions; it also reduces the biotransformation and/or accumulation of the Gd^{3+} ions in the body by increasing the renal excretion rate [5, 7].

The Gd^{3+} has nine coordination sites which are the number of atoms or ligands directly bonding to the metal centre. Eight of these sites represent the bonds between Gd^{3+} and the chelating agent with the ninth is being coordinated with the oxygen atom of a water molecule. This ninth coordination site is necessary in enhancing the signal by the contrast agent in *T*1-weighed images [4, 8].

Chemical structure of the chelating agent determines the biochemical differences between the Gd-based contrast agents (GBCAs). The chelating agent is either linear or macrocyclic and electrically neutral (non-ionic) or charged (ionic). Generally, macrocyclic chelating agents are more stable than the linear and ionic linear chelates more than non-ionic linear chelates [3, 9]. To be used as a contrast agent safely, the chelating agent must be thermodynamically and, more importantly, kinetically stable [1].

Today, there are nine GBCAs approved by the EMEA (European Medicines Agency) and the FDA (US Food and Drug Administration) for use in humans [9]. Physiochemical and pharmacokinetic properties of some GBCAs are summarized in Table 7.1.

S. Yigitaslan (✉)
Eskisehir Osmangazi University School of Medicine, Eskisehir, Turkey

K. Erol
Bahcesehir University School of Medicine, Istanbul, Turkey

S. M. Erturk et al. (eds.), *Medical Imaging Contrast Agents: A Clinical Manual*, https://doi.org/10.1007/978-3-030-79256-5_7

Table 7.1 Physicochemical and pharmacokinetic properties of gadolinium-based contrast agents

Contrast agent, trade name	Molecular structure/charge	Conditional thermodynamic stability (pH 7.4; log K_{cond}) [31]	Kinetic stability (pH 7.4) [31, 32]	Relaxivity ($r1/r2$; 1.5 T) [37 °C; L/(mmol s)] [20]	Relaxivity ($r1/r2$; 3 T) [37 °C; L/(mmol s)] [20]	Osmolality (37 °C; mOsm/kg H_2O) [9, 33]	Viscosity (37 °C; cP) [9, 24]	Dissociation half-life (pH 1.0 and 25 °C) [34]	Elimination pathway [9, 23]	Recommended dose (mmol/kg of body weight) [23, 26]
Gd-DTPA, Gadopentetate dimeglumine, **Magnevist®**	Linear/ionic	18.4	5–7 days	3.9–4.3/3.8–5.4	3.5–3.9/4.3–6.1	1960	2.9	<5 s	Renal	0.1
Gd-BOPTA, Gadobenate dimeglumine, **MultiHance®**	Linear/ionic	18.4	N/A	6.0–6.6/7.8–9.6	5.2–5.8/10.0–12.0	1970	5.3	<5 s	Renal 96–98%; hepatic 2–4%	0.05–0.1
Gd-EOB-DTPA, Gadoxetic acid disodium, **Primovist®**	Linear/ionic	18.7	N/A	6.5–7.3/7.8–9.6	5.9–6.5/10.0–12.0	688	1.2	<5 s	Renal 50%; hepatic 50%	0.025
MS325, Gadofosveset, **Vasovist®**	Linear/ionic	18.9	N/A	18.0–20.0/32.0–36.0	9.4–10.4/56.0–64.0	825	2.1	<5 s	Renal 91%; hepatic 9%	0.03
Gd-DTPA-BMA, Gadodiamide, **Omniscan®**	Linear/non-ionic	14.9	5–7 days	4.0–4.6/4.2–6.2	3.8–4.2/4.7–6.5	789	1.4	<5 s	Renal	0.1
Gd-DTPA-BMEA, Gadoversetamide, **OptiMARK®**	Linear/non-ionic	15.0	N/A	4.4–5.0/4.3–6.1	4.2–4.8/5.0–6.8	1110	2.0	<5 s	Renal	0.1
Gd-DOTA, Gadoterate meglumine, **Dotarem®**	Macrocyclic/ionic	19.3	>1000 years	3.4–3.8/3.4–5.2	3.3–3.7/4.0–5.8	1350	2.0	338 h	Renal	0.1
Gd-HP-DO3A, Gadoteridol, ProHance®	Macrocyclic/non-ionic	17.2	>1000 years	3.9–4.3/4.2–5.8	3.5–3.9/4.8–6.6	630	1.3	3.9 h	Renal	0.1
Gd-BT-DO3A, Gadobutrol, **Gadovist®**	Macrocyclic/non-ionic	15.5	>1000 years	4.9–5.5/5.2–7.0	4.7–5.3/6.2–8.0	1603	5.0	43 h	Renal	0.1

All the macrocyclic agents in clinical use whether ionic or non-ionic are derived from a 12-member macrocyclic polyamino ring [9]. The ionic macrocyclic GBCA, gadoterate meglumine (Gd-DOTA), has four carboxylate side groups. However, in the non-ionic macrocyclic GBCA, gadoteridol (Gd-HP-DO3A), one carboxylate group is replaced with a hydroxypropyl group, resulting in a decrease in stability and binding constant [9, 10]. The replacement of hydroxypropyl group of gadoteridol with the 2,3-dihydroxy-(1-hydroxymethyl)-propyl group forms the gadobutrol (Gd-BT-DO3A) and results in further destabilization [11] (Fig. 7.1).

All ionic linear GBCAs including gadopentetate dimeglumine (Gd-DTPA), gadobenate dimeglumine (Gd-BOPTA), gadoxetic acid (Gd-EOB-DTPA) and gadofosveset (MS-325) have five carboxyl groups and three amino nitrogen atoms. The three negatively charged carboxyl groups are neutralized by Gd^{3+} ion. On the other hand, the remaining two negative charges of gadopentetate dimeglumine and gadobenate dimeglumine are neutralized by two meglumine (a sugar amine with 1+ charge from a quaternary amine) cations, while that of gadoxetic acid and gadofosveset are neutralized with Na^{+} ions [4, 9] (Fig. 7.1).

In the non-ionic linear GBCAs, consisting of gadoversetamide and gadodiamide, in addition to three amino nitrogen atoms, there are three instead of five carboxyl atoms and two non-ionic methyl amides. The binding of the two non-ionic methyl amides to Gd^{3+} is weaker compared to the carboxyl oxygen atoms, resulting in decreased stability in comparison to the ionic linear GBCAs [4, 9] (Fig. 7.1).

7.1 Physiochemical Properties

7.1.1 Stability

The stability of the chelating agents is described by thermodynamic stability reflecting the energy required to break the bonds between Gd^{3+} and chelating agent and kinetic stability reflecting the rate of this dissociation.

Thermodynamic stability can be quantitatively estimated by the thermodynamic stability constant (K_{therm}, measured at pH ~11, at which there are no ions competing with the chelating agent) and the conditional thermodynamic stability constant (K_{cond}, measured at pH 7.4) [3]. Because K_{cond} is measured at the physiological pH, K_{cond} is more useful to estimate the thermodynamic stability compared to the K_{therm}. The higher values of all these parameters reflect the higher stability of the GBCAs [3, 4, 8, 12].

Chemical structure has a significant correlation with the thermodynamic and kinetic stability. Ionic macrocyclic chelate (gadoterate meglumine) is the most stable GBCA and exhibits the highest dissociation rate. Besides, macrocyclic GBCAs do not require excess chelating agent in the preparation [12, 13]. On the other hand, non-ionic linear GBCAs (gadodiamide and gadoversetamide) are the least stable with the shortest dissociation half-life. Also, they require excess chelating agent in the preparation [14].

7.1.2 Transmetallation

The body fluids contain a variety of metal ions which can be exchanged with Gd^{3+} in the GBCAs. The endogenous ions important for transmetallation include zinc, iron, copper and calcium. However, because free iron and copper are found in very small amounts in the blood and calcium ions have a low affinity for organic ligands, probably it is mainly zinc that can be exchanged with a significant amount of Gd^{3+} [15, 16].

Transmetallation of Gd^{3+} with zinc forms a zinc chelate that will be excreted in urine. On the other hand, free Gd^{3+} attaches to endogenous anions and accumulates in tissues in an insoluble form [17]. Among those in clinical use, non-ionic linear GBCAs have been shown to induce an increase in urinary zinc excretion which was thought to be secondary to transmetallation [16, 18, 19].

7.1.3 Relaxivity

The efficacy of GBCAs is determined by their *T*1 and *T*2 relaxivities. GBCAs mainly shorten *T*1 relaxation time. There are several other factors

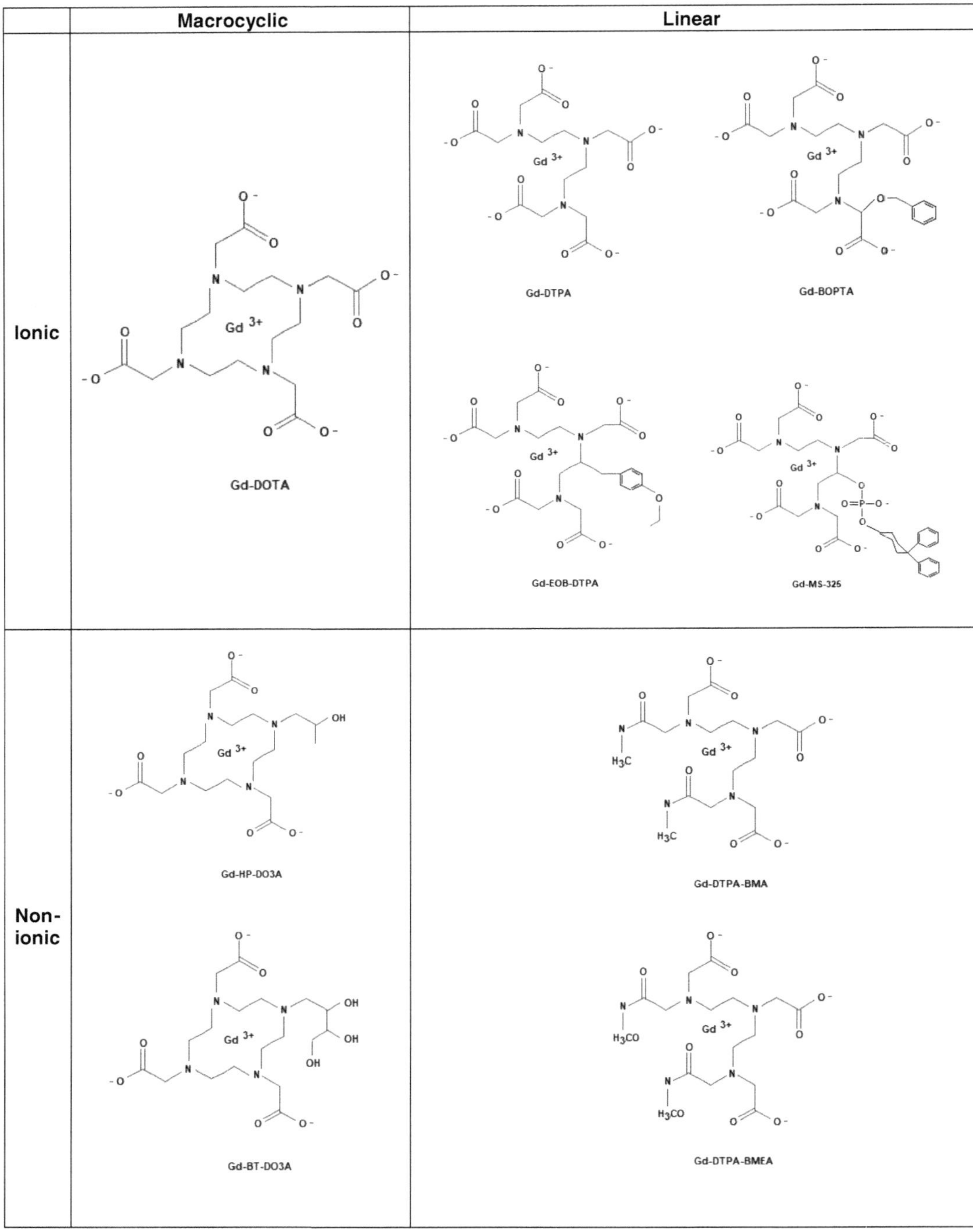

Fig. 7.1 Physicochemical and pharmacokinetic properties of gadolinium-based contrast agents

influencing relaxivity, including protein-binding affinity of the contrast agent, magnetic field strength and temperature [9, 20].

Relaxivity is quantitatively described by the equation of Solomon-Bloembergen-Morgan equations [21], where *T*1 refers to the longitudinal relaxation time, k is the constant for Gd^{3+}, r is the distance between Gd^{3+} and water proton and τc is the effective correlation time:

$$\frac{1}{T1} = k.\frac{1}{r6}.f(\mathrm{T}C)$$

In general, relativity has been suggested to decrease with increasing magnetic field strength and increasing temperature. On the other hand, relaxivity is more dependent on the magnetic field in the case of strongly binding of GBCAs to the macromolecules in the plasma, mainly to the albumin. However, it should be also noted that plasma proteins have a limited capacity to bind GBCAs which determine the concentration dependence of the relaxivity [9].

Of the GBCAs in clinical use, gadobutrol was found to provide the highest $T1$ shortening per volume of the contrast agent. Gadobutrol is also the only GBCA formulated with twofold concentration of Gd^{3+} compared to the others. The higher concentration and higher relaxivity of gadobutrol provide improved image enhancement [22].

7.1.4 Osmolality

Osmolality is defined as the concentration of dissolved particles present in the formulation of a contrast agent and expressed as osm/kg water. The osmolality is closely related to the ionicity of the contrast agent; the ionic GBCAs have a higher osmolality compared to the non-ionic ones. Because of low injection doses used for MRI, high osmolality of the ionic GBCAs results in only a slight increase in plasma osmolality. However, in cases where higher doses are required, non-ionic GBCAs with low osmolality should be preferred [23].

7.1.5 Viscosity

Viscosity is defined as the internal resistance within a fluid. Higher viscosity leads to increased resistance to flow. The viscosity is expressed as centipoise (cP), with the viscosities of plasma, and whole blood are 1.5 and 3 cP at 37 °C. On the other hand, viscosity of earlier GBCAs ranges from 1.3 to 2.9 cP at 37 °C. However, the so-called next-generation GBCA, gadobenate dimeglumine, has the highest viscosity of 5.3 cP at body temperature [24].

In fact, viscosity is generally not a significant concern when GBCAs are used in standard doses and injection rates. However, in the case of rapid injections and small catheters, viscosity should be taken into account [23].

7.2 Pharmacokinetics

The pharmacokinetic properties of most GBCAs are similar to that of iodine-based contrast agents. Most GBCAs except for three (gadoxetic acid, gadofosveset and gadobenate dimeglumine) are water-soluble, low molecular weight complexes rapidly diffusing into the extravascular space after intravenous injection (distribution half-life is about 5 min), do not go biotransformation and are eliminated mainly by the kidneys. In patients with normal renal function, more than 95% of these agents are excreted in urine within 24 h of the injection with a half-life of approximately 1.5 h [25, 26]. In patients with impaired renal functions, it can take several days or weeks for these agents to be cleared from the body. GBCAs can be removed from the body by haemodialysis or continuous ambulatory peritoneal dialysis with the latter is being less effective [27].

Gadobenate dimeglumine, gadoxetic acid and gadofosveset are eliminated from both kidneys and hepatobiliary system [28–30]. Of their injected doses, 2–4% of the gadobenate dimeglumine, 50% of the gadoxetic acid and 9% of the gadofosveset are eliminated from hepatobilier pathway [23].

GBCAs do not generally cross the blood-brain barrier nor bind to the proteins or receptors. These agents tend to accumulate in malign and inflammatory regions with abnormal vascularity and in the injured brain regions when blood-brain barrier is disrupted [26].

In clinical practice, the recommended dose for most GBCAs is 0.1 mmol/kg of body weight with a recommended injection rate of 0.5 mmol/

mL. Particularly when used in MR angiography and CNS imaging, up to 0.3 mmol/kg body weight may be used. Because of the protein binding, gadoxetic acid, gadofosveset and gadobenate dimeglumine are used in lower doses (0.025 mmol/kg, 0.03 mmol/kg and 0.05–0.1 mmol/kg, respectively) [23, 26].

References

1. De León-Rodríguez LM, Martins AF, Pinho MC, Rofsky NM, Sherry AD. Basic MR relaxation mechanisms & contrast agent design. J Magn Reson Imaging. 2015;42(3):545–65.
2. Caravan P, Ellison JJ, McMurry TJ, Lauffer RB. Gadolinium(III) chelates as MRI contrast agents: structure, dynamics, and applications. Chem Rev. 1999;99(9):2293–352.
3. Idée JM, Port M, Robic C, Medina C, Sabatou M, Corot C. Role of thermodynamic and kinetic parameters in gadolinium chelate stability. J Magn Reson Imaging. 2009;30:1249–58.
4. Dawson P. Gadolinium chelates: chemistry. In: Dawson P, Cosgrove DO, Grainger RG, editors. Textbook of contrast media. Oxford: Isis Medical Media; 1999. p. 291–6.
5. Cacheris WP, Quay SC, Rocklage SM. The relationship between thermodynamics and the toxicity of gadolinium complexes. Magn Reson Imaging. 1990;8(4):467–81.
6. Bousquet JC, Saini S, Stark DD, Hahn PF, Nigam M, Wittenberg J, Ferrucci JT Jr. Gd-DOTA: characterization of a new paramagnetic complex. Radiology. 1988;166(3):693–8.
7. Chang CA. Magnetic resonance imaging contrast agents. Design and physicochemical properties of gadodiamide. Invest Radiol. 1993;28(Suppl 1):S21–7.
8. Desreux JF, Gilsoul D. Chemical synthesis of paramagnetic complexes. In: Thomsen HS, Muller RN, Mattrey RF, editors. Trends in contrast media. Heidelberg: Springer; 1999. p. 161–9.
9. Hao D, Ai T, Goerner F, Hu X, Runge VM, Tweedle M. MRI contrast agents: basic chemistry and safety. J Magn Reson Imaging. 2012;36(5):1060–71.
10. Tweedle MF. Physicochemical properties of gadoteridol and other magnetic resonance contrast agents. Invest Radiol. 1992;27:S2–6.
11. Kumar K. Macrocyclic polyamino carboxylate complexes of Gd (III) as magnetic resonance imaging contrast agents. J Alloys Compd. 1997;249:163–72.
12. Morcos SK. Extracellular gadolinium contrast agents: differences in stability. Eur J Radiol. 2008;66(2):175–9.
13. Morcos SK. Nephrogenic systemic fibrosis following the administration of extracellular gadolinium based contrast agents: is the stability of the contrast agent molecule an important factor in the pathogenesis of this condition? Br J Radiol. 2007;80(950):73–6.
14. Kanda T, Oba H, Toyoda K, Kitajima K, Furui S. Brain gadolinium deposition after administration of gadolinium-based contrast agents. Jpn J Radiol. 2016;34(1):3–9.
15. Tweedle MF, Hagan JJ, Kumar K, Mantha S, Chang CA. Reaction of gadolinium chelates with endogenously available ions. Magn Reson Imaging. 1991;9(3):409–15.
16. Corot C, Idee JM, Hentsch AM, Santus R, Mallet C, Goulas V, Bonnemain B, Meyer D. Structure-activity relationship of macrocyclic and linear gadolinium chelates: investigation of transmetallation effect on the zinc-dependent metallopeptidase angiotensin-converting enzyme. J Magn Reson Imaging. 1998;8(3):695–702.
17. Gibby WA, Gibby KA, Gibby WA. Comparison of Gd DTPA-BMA (Omniscan) versus Gd HP-DO3A (ProHance) retention in human bone tissue by inductively coupled plasma atomic emission spectroscopy. Invest Radiol. 2004;39(3):138–42.
18. Laurent S, Elst LV, Muller RN. Comparative study of the physicochemical properties of six clinical low molecular weight gadolinium contrast agents. Contrast Media Mol Imaging. 2006;1(3):128–37.
19. Kimura J, Ishiguchi T, Matsuda J, Ohno R, Nakamura A, Kamei S, Ohno K, Kawamura T, Murata K. Human comparative study of zinc and copper excretion via urine after administration of magnetic resonance imaging contrast agents. Radiat Med. 2005;23(5):322–6.
20. Rohrer M, Bauer H, Mintorovitch J, Requardt M, Weinmann HJ. Comparison of magnetic properties of MRI contrast media solutions at different magnetic field strengths. Invest Radiol. 2005;40(11):715–24.
21. Bloembergen N, Morgan LO. Protein relaxation times in paramagnetic solutions, effects of electron spin relaxation. J Chem Phys. 1961;34:843–50.
22. Scott LJ. Gadobutrol: a review of its use for contrast-enhanced magnetic resonance imaging in adults and children. Clin Drug Investig. 2013;33(4):303–14.
23. Bellin MF, van der Molen AJ. Extracellular gadolinium-based contrast media: an overview. Eur J Radiol. 2008;66:160–7.
24. Lin SP, Brown JJ. MR contrast agents: physical and pharmacologic basics. J Magn Reson Imaging. 2007;25(5):884–99.
25. Oksendal AN, Hals PA. Biodistribution and toxicity of MR imaging contrast media. J Magn Reson Imaging. 1993;3(1):157–65.
26. Thomsen HS, Reimer P. Intravascular contrast media for radiography, CT, MRI and ultrasound. In: Adam A, Dixon AK, Gillard JH, Schaefer-Prokop CM, editors. Grainger & Allison's diagnostic radiology. Philadelphia: Elsevier; Churchill Livingstone; 2015. p. 31.
27. Joffe P, Thomsen HS, Meusel M. Pharmacokinetics of gadodiamide injection in patients with severe renal insufficiency and patients undergoing hemodialysis

or continuous ambulatory peritoneal dialysis. Acad Radiol. 1998;5(7):491–502.
28. Kirchin MA, Pirovano GP, Spinazzi A. Gadobenate dimeglumine (Gd-BOPTA). An overview. Invest Radiol. 1998;33(11):798–809.
29. Hamm B, Staks T, Mühler A, Bollow M, Taupitz M, Frenzel T, Wolf KJ, Weinmann HJ, Lange L. Phase I clinical evaluation of Gd-EOB-DTPA as a hepatobiliary MR contrast agent: safety, pharmacokinetics, and MR imaging. Radiology. 1995;195(3):785–92.
30. Rapp JH, Wolff SD, Quinn SF, Soto JA, Meranze SG, Muluk S, Blebea J, Johnson SP, Rofsky NM, Duerinckx A, Foster GS, Kent KC, Moneta G, Middlebrook MR, Narra VR, Toombs BD, Pollak J, Yucel EK, Shamsi K, Weisskoff RM. Aortoiliac occlusive disease in patients with known or suspected peripheral vascular disease: safety and efficacy of gadofosveset-enhanced MR angiography—multicenter comparative phase III study. Radiology. 2005;236(1):71–8.
31. Frenzel T, Lengsfeld P, Schirmer H, Hütter J, Weinmann HJ. Stability of gadolinium-based magnetic resonance imaging contrast agents in human serum at 37 degrees C. Invest Radiol. 2008;43(12):817–28.
32. Schmitt-Willich H. Stability of linear and macrocyclic gadolinium based contrast agents. Br J Radiol. 2007;80(955):581–2.
33. Kirchin MA, Runge VM. Contrast agents for magnetic resonance imaging: safety update. Top Magn Reson Imaging. 2003;14(5):426–35.
34. Port M, Idée JM, Medina C, Robic C, Sabatou M, Corot C. Efficiency, thermodynamic and kinetic stability of marketed gadolinium chelates and their possible clinical consequences: a critical review. Biometals. 2008;21(4):469–90.

Magnetic Resonance Imaging (MRI) and Contrast-Enhancing Agents

8

Ebru Erdal and Murat Demirbilek

8.1 Magnetic Resonance Imaging (MRI)

MRI is a technique that enables highly detailed images of the organs and tissues to be obtained by using a very powerful magnet and radio waves. MRI is a cross-sectional radiological examination method that doesn't use x-rays and doesn't involve ionizing radiation. The device scans hydrogen atoms to obtain images of the soft tissues in the body. When the patient is placed in a constant magnetic field, the protons in the body make a turn by showing parallel and antiparallel alignment in the direction of the magnet's vector. The radio waves created by magnetic fields cause distortions in the hydrogen atoms in the tissues. When the radio waves are cut off, the protons begin to release the energy they receive while returning to their previous position in the direction of the magnet, and this energy is converted into a signal by means of a receiver. The deviation that occurs for each tissue and in relation to the time to return to its former position is also different. The images are created with these signal differences [1, 2].

The hydrogen atom is excessive in tissues containing water and oil. Therefore, the use of MRI is more effective in the evaluation of solid organs such as the brain, musculoskeletal system and internal organs. Basically, two main sequences, T1-weighted and T2-weighted, are used in MRI. T1-weighted sequences allow for anatomic evaluation by providing excellent soft tissue contrast and resolution. In T2-weighted sequences, pathological signal intensity changes are distinguished [3, 4].

MRI should be able to distinguish abnormal lesions and their prolongation to the surrounding tissues as well as normal tissues. Therefore, contrast-enhancing agents have started to be used in MRI. In the early years when MRI was being used, it was thought that no contrast-enhancing agents were needed for MRI. However, studies have shown that the use of contrast-enhancing agents in MRI does not only provide dynamic physiological information between tissues, but also high anatomic detail can be obtained [5]. The purpose of using contrast-enhancing agents is to make the tissues more visible by making clear the density difference between tissues. In MRI, the contrast-enhancing agents used are not seen. Contrast-enhancing agents act by changing the proton behaviour or magnetic sensitivity of the tissue under the magnetic field. In other words, contrast-enhancing agents act by reducing

E. Erdal (✉)
Advanced Technologies Application and Research Center, Ankara Yıldırım Beyazıt University, Ankara, Turkey

M. Demirbilek
Department of Biology, Ankara Hacı Bayram Veli University, Ankara, Turkey
e-mail: mrt@hacettepe.edu.tr

S. M. Erturk et al. (eds.), *Medical Imaging Contrast Agents: A Clinical Manual*,
https://doi.org/10.1007/978-3-030-79256-5_8

T1 and T2 relaxation times [6]. Contrast-enhancing agents to be used in MRI should have certain properties. The contrast agents should be low cost and biocompatible, should not accumulate in the body and interact with different drugs or proteins when transported in the body and require no energy to excrete [7].

T1 Agents Gadolinium and manganese salts shorten T1 relaxation times in MRI. Thus, contrast-enhancing agents enable signal enhancement (hyperintensities) on T1-weighted images and consequently brighter (white) appearance of the tissues. The shortening in T1 is explained by "dipole-dipole interaction". Currently, there are seven approved gadolinium-based MR contrast agents used in the clinic [8].

T2 Agents T2 agents are contrast-enhancing agents containing iron oxide. These agents shorten the T2 or T2* relaxation time in MRI, resulting in loss of signal (hypointensity) on T2-weighted images and consequently a more black appearance of the tissues. T2 contrasting materials create a negative contrast in the tissues by impairing the magnetic homogeneity of the tissue. The shortening in T2 and T2* can be explained by the increase of inhomogeneity in the microscopic magnetic environment [9].

In recent years, new sequencing has been developed on T1- and T2-weighted images in MRI. However, the necessity of using contrast-enhancing agents has not lost its importance. Especially, contrasting images are preferred to non-contrasting images in the detection and characterization of liver lesions [10].

8.1.1 Gadolinium

Gadolinium is an important lanthanide with magnetic properties. A significant proportion of the substances used to enhance contrast in MRI are gadolinium-containing agents. Gadolinium-based drugs used in MRI applications allow to get contrast-enhanced and better quality imaging. The chemical symbol of gadolinium is "Gd". It is in the lanthanide series (rare-earth elements) in the 3B group of the periodic table. The atomic number is 64, the atomic weight is 157.25 and the density is 7.9 g/cm^3. Its melting point is 1313 °C and boiling point is 3273 °C. Gadolinium is superconducting and electropositive at temperatures below 810 °C.

Many of the paramagnetic materials used as contrast agents in MRI contain toxic metal ions. Therefore, in order to reduce toxicity, gadolinium is not applied in its natural form but is applied in a chelate form by attaching with a ligand. Gadolinium metal exhibits affinity to the ligands such as DTPA, DOTA, DTPA-BMA, HP-DO3A and BOPTA, and these bindings result in different formulations with different ligands. Gadolinium has strong neutron absorption ability [11, 12].

Gadolinium is a powerful magnet that shows ferromagnetic, paramagnetic and magnetocaloric properties at room temperature. The relative magnetic permeability of gadolinium is too much than 1 at temperatures below 17 °C and exhibits ferromagnetic properties. Relative magnetic permeability above room temperatures is greater than 1 and shows paramagnetic properties. That is, they can only protect magnetizations under magnetic field effect.

Relaxation determines the relaxation activity of a contrast agent. In this case, factors such as structure of the contrast material, heat and Larmor frequency are effective. The value of gadolinium is +3 and it has seven unpaired electrons. In this way, it is the most powerful paramagnetic element [13]. As the relativity increases, the interaction between the contrast agent and the adjacent water protons increases. This allows rapid relaxation of the protons and consequently the increase in signal intensity [14].

The resonance frequency of the paramagnetic gadolinium is very close to the hydrogen resonance frequency in MR devices. Thereby, it provides quality images as MR for the imaging applications of the internal structures of the body. Gadolinium can be given to the body by oral or injectable route. Gadolinium, rapidly absorbed by soft tissues, enables good imaging especially for tumour cells in MR applications. Gadolinium is a very ideal contrast material because it is not stored in the body and is ejected after a while.

Although gadolinium chelates are used as a contrast agent to reduce the toxic effect of gadolinium, side effects such as vomiting, hypotension, hives, allergic reactions, groin pain, laryngeal oedema, asthma, kidney damage and skin and connective tissue fibrosis (nephrogenic systemic fibrosis) may occur. The incidence of allergic side effects of contrast agents containing gadolinium is very low, such as 1 in 10,000 patients. The most important side effect is nephrogenic systemic fibrosis (NFS) disease [15].

8.1.2 Iron Oxide Nanoparticles

Magnetic iron oxide nanoparticle-based contrast agents are widely used as MRI contrast agents to reduce T2* relaxation times in imaging of the liver, spleen and bone marrow [16]. These agents include superparamagnetic iron oxides (SPIOs) with an average particle diameter greater than 50 nm and ultra-small superparamagnetic iron oxides (USPIOs) with an average particle diameter of less than 50 nm. SPIO structures have the general formula $Fe_2^{3+}O_3M^{2+}O$. M^{2+} is a divalent metal ion such as iron, manganese, nickel, cobalt or magnesium. SPIO is magnetite when the metal ion (M^{2+}) is iron (Fe^{2+}) [17]. There are different methods in the literature to prepare the iron oxide nanoparticles. In the last 10 years, it is possible to synthesize iron oxide nanoparticles of varying sizes ranging from a few nanometres to 10 nm. The iron oxide particle size of the contrast agents and therefore their physicochemical and pharmacokinetic properties vary depending on the method used. This affects the clinical application of the particles. Superparamagnetic agents act by increasing the relaxation times of both T1 and T2/T2* in MRI, and these particles can be detected at micromolar iron concentrations [18].

Some atoms have unpaired electrons due to the fact that the outer electron layers are not fully filled, and as a natural consequence, they have a net moment different from zero. When such materials are brought into a magnetic field, a strength is exerted on the atoms of matter to force the magnetic moments to take the magnetic field direction. According to their magnetizing behaviour, the materials are divided into diamagnetic, paramagnetic, ferromagnetic, ferrimagnetic and superparamagnetic. In ferromagnetic and ferrimagnetic materials, the saturation magnetization value is high, and when the external magnetic field applied to the structure is removed, the structure still shows a magnetization. Paramagnetic and superparamagnetic structures respond rapidly to an external magnetic field and exhibit high saturation magnetization, such as ferromagnetic and ferrimagnetic materials. However, no magnetization or magnetic moment is observed in the structure when the applied external magnetic field is removed [19].

After intravenous administration, the clinically approved SPIO particles are cleared from the blood by phagocytosis provided by the reticuloendothelial system (RES), so that the uptake of the particles in the liver, spleen, bone marrow and lymph nodes is observed. Magnetic nanoparticles show greater sensitivity in micromolar or nanomolar levels in MR applications compared to gadolinium complexes; therefore, they can be used as T2 MRI contrast agents. In particular, they are actively used in the imaging of the organs in the RES system.

Unlike gadolinium, iron is one of the most abundant metallic elements in living organisms and is required for various biological processes, including oxygen transport by haemoglobin and cellular respiration by redox enzymes. Following intracellular involvement, SPIOs are eluted in lysosomes. Degraded iron ions are used in biological functions by being metabolized to a soluble and non-magnetic iron form which becomes part of the normal iron pool (e.g. ferritin, haemoglobin) [20].

The toxicity, metabolism and pharmacokinetics of intravenously injected iron oxide nanoparticles have been well studied. Accordingly, many iron oxide nanoparticles have been approved for clinical use. For example, Feridex has been approved by the Food and Drug Administration (FDA) to detect liver lesions, and Combidex has been introduced in phase III clinical trials for imaging lymph node metastases (designed synthesis of uniformly sized iron oxide nanoparticles for efficient magnetic resonance imaging contrast agents).

8.1.3 Manganese Chelates

Manganese chelates also act by shortening the T1 relaxation time in MRI, such as gadolinium-based contrast-enhancing agents. Manganese chelates have clinical use for hepatocytes. In 1997, the name of Teslascan (Opacim), manganese dipyridoxyl diphosphate (MnDPDP) was started to be used in the clinic. In liver imaging, manganese chelates increase the signalling of hepatocytes in T1-weighted series. Tumour-containing tissues do not hold manganese chelates due to not containing hepatocyte and cause the contrast to be apparent between lesion and liver tissue [21].

8.1.4 CEST and PARACEST

In recent years, chemical shift-based agents are being developed to shorten the T1 relaxation time. Although there have been clinical applications and patented commercial products, they can be an alternative to overcome the disadvantages of Gd-based contrast agents. This new class of MR contrast agents is called chemical exchange saturation transfer (CEST or PARACEST) agents. CEST agents cause reduction in magnetization of the water signal by exchanging –NH, –OH or bound water protons of various biomolecules during MRI. These agents provide new opportunities and improve diagnosis by MRI, but they need further research and development [22, 23].

References

1. Herek D, Karabulut N. Manyetik rezonans görüntüleme. TTD Toraks Cerrahisi Bülteni. 2010;1:214–22.
2. Ananta JS, Godin B, Sethi R, Moriggi L, Liu X, Serda RE, Krishnamurthy R, Muthupillai R, Bolskar RD, Helm L. Geometrical confinement of gadolinium-based contrast agents in nanoporous particles enhances T 1 contrast. Nat Nanotechnol. 2010;5:815.
3. Bittner RC, Felix R. Magnetic resonance (MR) imaging of the chest: state-of-the-art. Eur Respir J. 1998;11:1392–404.
4. Müller NL. Computed tomography and magnetic resonance imaging: past, present and future. Eur Respir J. 2002;19:3s–12s.
5. Li J, You J, Wu C, Dai Y, Shi M, Dong L, Xu K. T1–T2 molecular magnetic resonance imaging of renal carcinoma cells based on nano-contrast agents. Int J Nanomed. 2018;13:4607.
6. Shellock FG, Kanal E. Safety of magnetic resonance imaging contrast agents. J Magn Reson Imaging. 1999;10:477–84.
7. Kirchin MA, Runge VM. Contrast agents for magnetic resonance imaging: safety update. Top Magn Reson Imaging. 2003;14:426–35.
8. Adam G, Dammer M, Bohndorf K, Christoph R, Fenke F, Günther RW. Rheumatoid arthritis of the knee: value of gadopentetate dimeglumine-enhanced MR imaging. AJR Am J Roentgenol. 1991;156:125–9.
9. Shokrollahi H. Contrast agents for MRI. Mater Sci Eng C. 2013;33:4485–97.
10. Lu J, Ma S, Sun J, Xia C, Liu C, Wang Z, Zhao X, Gao F, Gong Q, Song B. Manganese ferrite nanoparticle micellar nanocomposites as MRI contrast agent for liver imaging. Biomaterials. 2009;30:2919–28.
11. Weishaupt D, Köchli VD, Marincek B. How does MRI work?: an introduction to the physics and function of magnetic resonance imaging. Berlin Heidelberg: Springer Science & Business Media; 2008.
12. Greenberg SA. Zinc transmetallation and gadolinium retention after MR imaging: case report. Radiology. 2010;257:670–3.
13. Bellin M-F. MR contrast agents, the old and the new. Eur J Radiol. 2006;60:314–23.
14. Zhou Z, Lu Z. Gadolinium-based contrast agents for magnetic resonance cancer imaging. Wiley Interdiscip Rev Nanomed Nanobiotechnol. 2013;5:1–18.
15. Schieda N, Blaichman JI, Costa AF, Glikstein R, Hurrell C, James M, Jabehdar Maralani P, Shabana W, Tang A, Tsampalieros A. Gadolinium-based contrast agents in kidney disease: a comprehensive review and clinical practice guideline issued by the Canadian Association of Radiologists. Can J Kidney Heal Dis. 2018;5:2054358118778573.
16. Na HB, Song IC, Hyeon T. Inorganic nanoparticles for MRI contrast agents. Adv Mater. 2009;21:2133–48.
17. Wang Y-XJ, Hussain SM, Krestin GP. Superparamagnetic iron oxide contrast agents: physicochemical characteristics and applications in MR imaging. Eur Radiol. 2001;11:2319–31.
18. Pouliquen D, Le Jeune JJ, Perdrisot R, Ermias A, Jallet P. Iron oxide nanoparticles for use as an MRI contrast agent: pharmacokinetics and metabolism. Magn Reson Imaging. 1991;9:275–83.
19. Alwi R, Telenkov S, Mandelis A, Leshuk T, Gu F, Oladepo S, Michaelian K. Silica-coated super paramagnetic iron oxide nanoparticles (SPION) as

biocompatible contrast agent in biomedical photoacoustics. Biomed Opt Express. 2012;3:2500–9.
20. Wang Y-XJ. Superparamagnetic iron oxide based MRI contrast agents: current status of clinical application. Quant Imaging Med Surg. 2011;1:35.
21. Earls JP, Bluemke DA. New MR imaging contrast agents. Magn Reson Imaging Clin N Am. 1999;7:255–73.
22. Sherry AD, Woods M. Chemical exchange saturation transfer contrast agents for magnetic resonance imaging. Annu Rev Biomed Eng. 2008;10:391–411.
23. Hancu I, Dixon WT, Woods M, Vinogradov E, Sherry AD, Lenkinski RE. CEST and PARACEST MR contrast agents. Acta Radiol. 2010;51:910–23.

9 Gadolinium-Based Contrast Agent Toxicity and Accumulation

Shintaro Ichikawa

9.1 Introduction

Until recent times, gadolinium-based contrast agents (GBCAs) have been widely used in daily practice since the first GBCA became available for clinical use in 1988. Due to their great utility as contrast agents, contrast-enhanced magnetic resonance imaging (MRI) has become an essential diagnostic tool in many areas and in the detection of many diseases. Gadolinium is a heavy metal that is toxic to humans; therefore, it is administered in a chelated form when it is used as a contrast agent. The chelation protects the human body from the toxicity of gadolinium and allows its rapid excretion. Thus, GBCAs are safe for the majority of patients except in very rare cases in which adverse reactions or nephrogenic systemic fibrosis (NSF) might occur. In 2014, Kanda et al. reported on the gadolinium accumulation in the brain [1], and many researchers conducted follow-up or further studies on this issue [2–6]. The results of these studies led to the reconsideration of the safety associated with GBCA administration. Recently, the knowledge on the safety of administering GBCAs has changed greatly. GBCAs are drugs used for diagnostic purposes; thus, extraordinary consideration is required in terms of their safety, and new information on this subject should constantly be updated. This chapter focuses on the features of different GBCAs, their levels of toxicity, and their abilities to accumulate in the human body based on the European Society of Urogenital Radiology (ESUR) Guidelines on Contrast Agents v10.0 [7].

S. Ichikawa (✉)
Department of Radiology, Hamamatsu University School of Medicine, Hamamatsu, Japan
e-mail: shintaro@hama-med.ac.jp

9.2 Features of GBCAs

Commercially available GBCAs are divided into two types depending on the structure of their chelation complex: linear and macrocyclic GBCAs. Moreover, there are two types of chelates based on their electrical properties: electrically neutral (nonionic) and charged (ionic). Thus, GBCAs can be classified into four types: ionic linear, nonionic linear, ionic macrocyclic, and nonionic macrocyclic GBCAs [8]. Further, GBCAs are also classified as extracellular or hepatocyte-specific GBCAs based on their hemodynamic interactions (Table 9.1). Macrocyclic GBCAs have macrocyclic polyamino rings that cage the gadolinium ion (Gd^{3+}) in a chemically stable structure. Linear GBCAs consist of a polyamino carboxylic acid molecule wrapped partially around the Gd^{3+} ion but not fully enclosing it. According to an in vitro study, the kinetic stability of GBCAs is as follows: nonionic linear GBCAs have low kinetic stability; ionic linear GBCAs, intermediate stability; and macrocyclic GBCAs, high stability,

S. M. Erturk et al. (eds.), *Medical Imaging Contrast Agents: A Clinical Manual*,
https://doi.org/10.1007/978-3-030-79256-5_9

Table 9.1 Commercially available GBCAs

Generic name	Brand name	Acronym	Charge	Structure	Approved dose (mmol/kg)
Extracellular GBCAs					
Gadopentetate dimeglumine	Magnevist®	Gd-DTPA	Ionic	Linear	0.1[a]
Gadodiamide	Omniscan®	Gd-DTPA-BMA	Nonionic	Linear	0.1[a]
Gadoteridol	ProHance®	Gd-HP-DO3A	Nonionic	Macrocyclic	0.1[a]
Gadoterate meglumine	Dotarem® Magnescope®	Gd-DOTA	Ionic	Macrocyclic	0.1[a]
Gadobutrol	Gadovist® Gadavist®	Gd-BT-DO3A	Nonionic	Macrocyclic	0.1[a]
Hepatocyte-specific GBCAs					
Gadobenate dimeglumine	MultiHance®	Gd-BOPTA	Ionic	Linear	0.05[b]
Gadoxetate disodium	Primovist® Eovist®	Gd-EOB-DTPA	Ionic	Linear	0.025[a]

[a]Data in Japan
[b]Data in other countries (not approved in Japan)

regardless of their charges [9]. On the other hand, a recently conducted in vivo study revealed that GBCAs demonstrated a lower kinetic stability than what was previously postulated [10]. This result may support the notion that Gd^{3+} ions get dechelated in the human body and that there is a possibility that this may be involved in gadolinium accumulation, which is described later in this chapter.

9.3 Adverse Reactions to GBCAs

The adverse reactions to GBCAs are classified into three types: acute adverse reactions, which occur within 1 h of GBCA administration; late adverse reactions, which occur between 1 h and 1 week after GBCA administration; and very late adverse reactions (such as NSF), which occur a few days to months (sometimes few years) after GBCA administration [11].

9.3.1 Acute Adverse Reactions

The symptoms of acute adverse reactions to GBCAs are quite varied and are summarized in Table 9.2 [7]. Acute reactions are classified into allergy-like, hypersensitivity reactions or chemotoxic responses. The incidence of acute adverse reactions to GBCAs is very low compared to those that occur in response to the iodine-based contrast media. For example, severe reactions have been reported, in the frequency of 0.02–0.1%, corresponding to iodinated contrast agents [12, 13], while a much lower frequency of around 0.00002–0.03% has been reported in relation to GBCAs [14–16]. Most of the acute allergic reactions that we may occasionally encounter in daily clinical practice are mild and self-limited. The risk factors for acute adverse reactions are as follows: a previous history of moderate or severe acute reactions to GBCAs or asthma or atopy requiring medical treatment. When administering GBCAs to patients who have experienced a previous acute reaction, a different type of GBCA from the one that they were administered before should be used. Premedication is not recommended while administering these agents because there is no good evidence of its effectiveness in preventing such reactions [7].

9.3.2 Late Adverse Reactions

Similar to other drug-induced eruptions, skin reactions can mainly occur as a late adverse reaction to iodine-based contrast media. Although it is said that late skin reactions have not been described after GBCA use in the ESUR guidelines [7]; the first case of a late adverse reaction to gadobutrol was reported recently [17].

Table 9.2 Acute adverse reactions to GBCAs

Severity	Hypersensitivity/allergy-like	Chemotoxic
Mild	Mild urticaria	Nausea/mild vomiting
	Mild itching	Warmth/chills
	Erythema	Anxiety
		Vasovagal reaction which resolves spontaneously
Moderate	Marked urticaria	Vasovagal reaction
	Mild bronchospasm	
	Facial/laryngeal edema	
Severe	Hypotensive shock	Arrhythmia
	Respiratory arrest	Convulsion
	Cardiac arrest	

9.3.3 Very Late Adverse Reactions

A very late adverse reaction in response to GBCA administration is NSF. The association between NSF and GBCAs was recognized in 2006 [18]. Up to 2–3 months after exposure to GBCAs, skin symptoms, such as pain, pruritus, swelling, and erythema, may develop, mainly affecting the lower limbs. Rarely, this can occur years after exposure. Further, the changes that occur at a later stage following these symptoms include fibrotic thickening of the skin and subcutaneous tissues; following this, in the most severe cases, the fibrosis gradually leads to joint contractures and, possibly, to immobility. The head and neck areas are usually spared. Rarely, NSF can progress to multi-organ fibrosis and death [19]. There is no curative treatment for this condition; thus, it is crucial to prevent the development of NSF. The exact pathogenesis of NSF is still unknown, but one of the main hypotheses put forward to account for this is the dechelation of Gd^{3+} ions due to renal dysfunction, which may cause the delayed excretion of GBCAs. All reports of NSF occur in patients with renal dysfunction; therefore, patients with renal dysfunction, particularly those who have an estimated glomerular filtration rate (eGFR) of <15 mL/min/1.73 m^2 or who are on dialysis, which are both risk factors for NSF, are at a high risk of developing this condition [7]. It is also important to note that the risk of developing NSF is significantly different depending on the specific GBCAs administered (Table 9.3) [7]. The estimated incidence of NSF in patients with severe renal failure are as follows: 3–18% in response to gadodiamide (Omniscan®) and 0.1–1%, to gadopentetate dimeglumine (Magnevist®). The European Medicines Agency (EMA) has suspended the intravenous use of these high risk GBCAs. The risk for developing NSF also increases with increasing doses of GBCAs; thus, the smallest dose of GBCAs that is necessary for a diagnostic result should be used for all patients.

Table 9.3 Risk classification of GBCAs for NSF

Risk	Contrast agents
Highest risk	Gadodiamide (Omniscan®)
	Gadopentetate dimeglumine (Magnevist®)
	Gadoversetamide (OptiMARK®)[a]
Intermediate risk	Gadobenate dimeglumine (MultiHance®)
	Gadoxetate disodium (Primovist®, Eovist®)
Lowest risk	Gadobutrol (Gadovist®, Gadavist®)
	Gadoterate meglumine (Dotarem®, Magnescope®)
	Gadoteridol (ProHance®)

[a]OptiMARK® has already been withdrawn from the European market

9.4 Gadolinium Accumulation in the Human Body

9.4.1 Gadolinium Accumulation in the Brain

In 2014, Kanda et al. demonstrated the presence of high signal intensity on T1-weighted images (T1WI) corresponding to the dentate nucleus and globus pallidus and its correlation with the number of previous administrations of linear GBCAs [1] (Fig. 9.1). With a history of more than five linear GBCA administrations, high signal intensity was observed in T1WIs of the dentate nucleus and globus pallidus. Gadolinium accumulation was confirmed in these structures in autopsy specimens [4, 20]. Many researchers have conducted follow-up or further studies to investigate this issue, and per their observations, high signal intensity has been reported after the use of linear GBCAs but not after using macrocyclic GBCAs due to the difference in their stability [21–24]. There is a report that a mild signal increase can be observed in the T1WIs even after very high cumulative doses of macrocyclic GBCAs [25]; however, it is a general perception that macrocyclic GBCAs, even at high doses, are unlikely to result in a high signal intensity in the T1WIs of the dentate nucleus and globus pallidus. In addition, different linear GBCAs also demonstrate differences in their stability. According to previ-

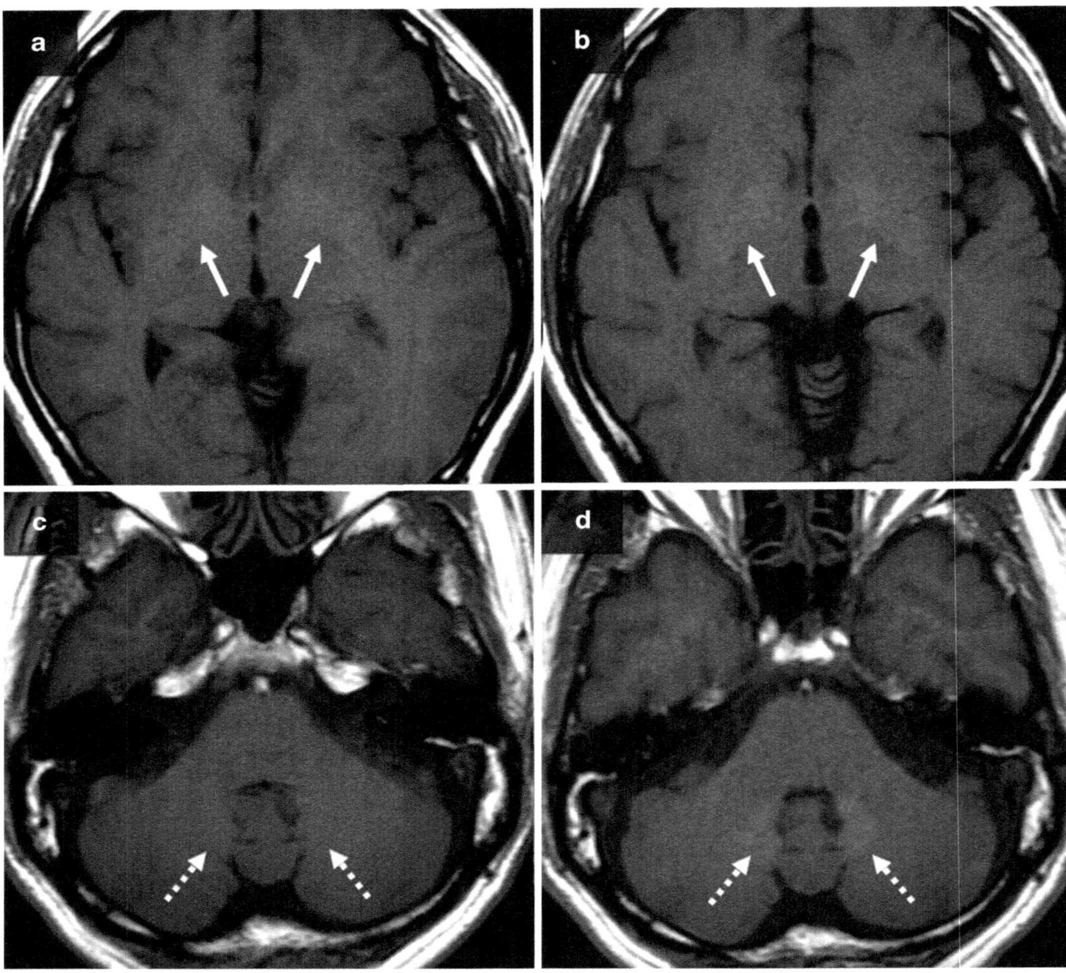

Fig. 9.1 T1-weighted images (T1WI) of a 59-year-old man who received administrations of gadodiamide (Omniscan®) nine times. (**a**, **c**) T1WI from his initial MRI (without the history of GBCA administration). (**b**, **d**) T1WI from his current MRI (with the history of gadodiamide administered nine times). The globus pallidus (arrows) and dentate nucleus (dashed arrows) regions show a higher intensity in the images (**b**) and (**d**) than in (**a**) and (**c**). The increase in the signal intensity corresponding to the dentate nucleus is more obvious than that of the globus pallidus

ous reports, the administration of gadobenate dimeglumine (Magnevist®) causes a high signal intensity in the dentate nucleus region on the T1WIs; but the intensity is of a smaller magnitude than that which is associated with other linear GBCAs [5, 6]. The high signal intensity observed in T1WIs is not limited to the dentate nucleus and globus pallidus but may also occur in other parts of the brain, such as the cerebral cortex, substantia nigra, red nucleus, thalamus, pulvinar, colliculi, superior cerebellar peduncle, caudate nucleus, putamen, etc. [26, 27].

Gadoxetate disodium (Primovist®, Eovist®) is a widely used hepatocyte-specific contrast agent. Gadoxetate disodium is also a linear GBCA; however, it contains half the concentration of gadolinium (0.25 mmol/mL) than that of extracellular GBCAs (0.50 mmol/mL), and its dosage of administration (0.1 mL/kg) is half of that of other GBCAs (0.2 mL/kg). Thus, investigations that are conducted using gadoxetate disodium involve only a quarter of the amount of gadolinium than those that are conducted using other types of GBCAs (extracellular GBCAs, 0.1 mmol/kg, vs. gadoxetate disodium, 0.025 mmol/kg). Moreover, gadoxetate disodium exhibits greater thermodynamic stability than some of the other linear GBCAs [28, 29]. Therefore, gadolinium accumulation in the brain after repeated gadoxetate disodium administrations may be expected to be significantly lower when compared to the levels of accumulation observed after other linear GBCAs are administered. According to previous reports, high signal intensity in T1WIs corresponding to the dentate nucleus was not observed with up to 15 previous administrations of gadoxetate disodium [30] (Fig. 9.2), and only a mild signal increase was observed in patients who were administered more than 15 doses of gadoxetate disodium [31].

9.4.2 Gadolinium Washout from the Brain

There are reports that patients whose T1WIs showed high signal intensity in the dentate nucleus region following multiple linear GBCAs administrations demonstrated a decreasing signal intensity on their T1WIs after they were switched to macrocyclic GBCAs for further follow-up MR examinations [32, 33]. These results suggest that the level of the gadolinium washout from the brain following the administration of macrocyclic GBCAs is greater than the level of gadolinium accumulation due to the administration of linear GBCAs. This hypothesis pertaining to the washout is consistent with a previous study on

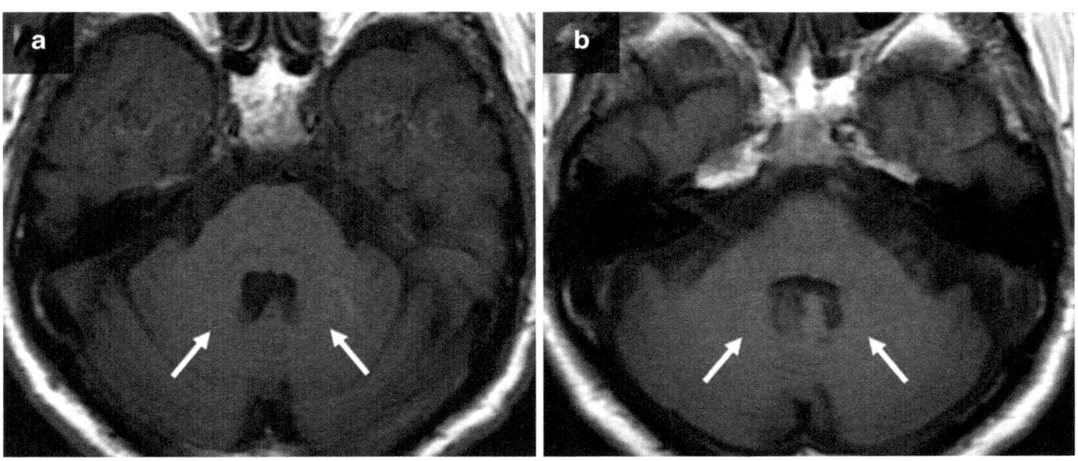

Fig. 9.2 T1-weighted images (T1WI) of a 75-year-old man who received administrations of gadoxetate disodium (Primovist®) nine times. (**a**) T1WI from his initial MRI (without the history of GBCA administration). (**b**) T1WI from his current MRI (with the history of nine gadoxetate disodium administrations). The dentate nucleus does not exhibit hyperintensity as seen in the T1WIs acquired before and after nine gadoxetate disodium administrations

animals that used inductively coupled plasma mass spectroscopy to measure the actual amount of gadolinium present in the brain. The gadolinium concentration in the rat brain at a 20-week timepoint after the GBCA administration was 50% less than that at the 1-week timepoint [34].

9.4.3 Mechanism of Gadolinium Accumulation in the Brain: The Glymphatic System

In this section we aim to answer the question on how GBCAs can enter the brain. The blood-brain barrier (BBB) is formed by the brain capillary endothelium and excludes almost 100% of drugs from the brain [35]. Several hypotheses regarding gadolinium accumulation in the brain have been published, such as the "metal transporter" [36] or "glymphatic system" [37] hypotheses; however, the theoretical basis for gadolinium accumulation and the mechanism behind it have not been fully elucidated. The "glymphatic system" is a coined phrase that combines "gl" from glia cells and "lymphatic" from the lymphatic system. According to this hypothesis, the perivascular spaces function as conduits via which the cerebrospinal fluid (CSF) flows into the brain parenchyma. The perivascular spaces around the arteries allow the CSF to enter the interstitial space of the brain tissue through water channels controlled by aquaporin 4. The CSF entering the interstitial space clears waste proteins from the tissue. It then flows into the perivascular spaces around the veins and is discharged outside the brain [37]. Naganawa et al. reported that there was an enhancement of the perivascular spaces observed 4 h after the administration of an intravenous GBCA injection, even in patients without renal dysfunction, and they speculated that the GBCA in the blood vessels might have permeated into the CSF space and the perivascular spaces [38]. However, there are no published studies outlining the exact dynamics of GBCAs in the brain parenchyma that lead to gadolinium accumulation, and the glymphatic system may be the major contributory factor to the accumulation and clearance of gadolinium in the brain tissue [37].

9.4.4 Accumulation in Other Parts of the Human Body

Gadolinium accumulation has not only been reported in the brain but also in other parts of the body such as in the bones, liver, and skin [39, 40]. It can occur regardless of renal function. Although it cannot be detected by MRI, the amounts of accumulation in these parts are reported to be greater than in the brain.

9.4.5 Effects on the Human Body

Until now, there is no evidence of brain toxicity that resulted from gadolinium accumulation. According to a previous population-based study, there was no association between GBCA administration and Parkinson's symptoms [41]. Thus, the possibility of developing severe symptoms due to gadolinium accumulation in the brain seems to be low, but concerns still remain regarding the possibility of complications that have not been detected yet. The clinical significance of gadolinium accumulation in other parts of the human body is also unknown. The EMA recommended the removal of linear GBCAs from the market in 2017 because of the gadolinium accumulation in the brain [42]. In Japan, it is recommended to use macrocyclic GBCAs as the primary choice and to use a linear GBCA when using a macrocyclic GBCA is not appropriate because of a history of adverse effects [43] On the other hand, the American College of Radiology and the US Food and Drug Administration (FDA) announced that they would not restrict the use of linear GBCAs [44].

9.5 GBCAs for Pregnant or Lactating Women

For pregnant or lactating women with renal dysfunction, the administration of GBCAs should be avoided. Important points to consider when using GBCAs for pregnant or lactating women without renal dysfunction are described below.

9.5.1 Safety During Pregnancy

Only when there is a very strong indication for the use of a contrast-enhanced MRI, the smallest possible dose of macrocyclic (= low risk) GBCAs may be administered to pregnant women [7]. In animal studies, it has been confirmed that GBCAs pass through the placenta, and gadolinium accumulation was observed in fetal organs; the accumulation levels of linear GBCAs (gadodiamide (Omniscan®)) were higher than those of macrocyclic GBCAs (gadoterate meglumine (Magnescope®)) [45, 46]. Once a GBCA has reached the fetal circulation via the umbilical vein, it is excreted into the amniotic fluid via the fetal kidneys. However, the fetus can swallow and reabsorb it; thus, the recirculation mechanism of chelated gadolinium can be established in the amniotic fluid. The persistence of chelated gadolinium in the fetal environment may increase the risk of the dechelation of Gd^{3+} ions [47]. In humans, the percentage of GBCAs administered to the mother that pass through the placenta and recirculates in the fetal environment is yet to be quantified. Further, a precise quantification of the half-life and stability of GBCAs in the human fetus are yet to be known. Perinatal exposure to GBCAs in mice, owing to maternal administration, affected the offspring's behavior when they reach adulthood, manifesting in symptoms such as anxiety-like behavior, disrupted motor coordination, impaired memory function, stimulated tactile sensitivity, and decreased muscle strength [46]. These results suggest that exposure to Gd^{3+} ions or that gadolinium accumulation occurring during postnatal development may lead to impaired brain development. In a study that was focused on humans, 26 pregnant women who inadvertently received GBCAs in the first trimester were observed, and no subsequent evidence of teratogenesis or mutagenesis was found [48]. In a population-based cohort study conducted in Canada that involved more than 1.4 million pregnant women, it was revealed that GBCA administration at any time during pregnancy was associated with a higher risk of stillbirth or neonatal death and the development of a broad set of rheumatological, inflammatory, or infiltrative skin conditions [49]. The influence that administering GBCAs to a pregnant woman is still controversial; however, restricting their use only to cases in which the potential benefits outweigh the potential risks to the fetus is important.

9.5.2 Safety During Lactation

Breast feeding may be continued normally after macrocyclic GBCAs are administered to the mother [7]. According to previous reports, only a low percentage (0.011–0.04%) of the maternal dose of gadopentetate dimeglumine (Magnevist®) was excreted into breast milk [50–53], and a much lower percentage was absorbed by the infant's gastrointestinal system [52]. There are no reports on adverse events occurring due to GBCAs in breast milk.

9.6 GBCAs for Children

The safety considerations associated with using contrast media in neonates are similar to those associated with their use in adults, but the reactions to these agents are not the same as the ones observed in adults. We use GBCAs only when the benefits outweigh the risks; furthermore, when using GBCAs, the dose must be adjusted according to a patient's age and body weight. The administration of high-risk GBCAs should be avoided in children [7], and macrocyclic GBCAs should be chosen. Adverse reactions to GBCAs in children are rare and are less common than in adults [54]. According to previous reports, no severe adverse reactions to GBCAs were observed among pediatric patients, and the rate of the occurrence of mild reactions was only 0.05–0.5% [55, 56]. Although developing NSF is extremely rare among the pediatric population, it can develop in some cases [57–59]. Therefore, similar to adults cases involving adults, it is important to evaluate the renal function before administering GBCAs to children; however, in addition, age-specific normal values of serum creatinine or eGFR must also be evaluated for children in order to choose the appropriate dose [7].

Gadolinium accumulation in the brain is also reported among the pediatric population [60–62] (Fig. 9.3). The effects of gadolinium accumulation on human health have not been documented to date; however, special care should be taken in cases involving pediatric patients because their remaining lifespans are longer compared to an adult's, which makes them more susceptible to long-term toxicity manifesting later on in the course of their lives [54].

9.7 Conclusion

Macrocyclic GBCAs are the primary choice because of their high stability, and linear GBCAs are used only when the use of macrocyclic GBCAs is not adequate. GBCAs should be administered in doses that are as small as possible. It is essential to check for risk factors of acute adverse reactions and to evaluate the renal function before using GBCAs. Further studies are needed to find out whether there are clinical problems associated with gadolinium accumula-

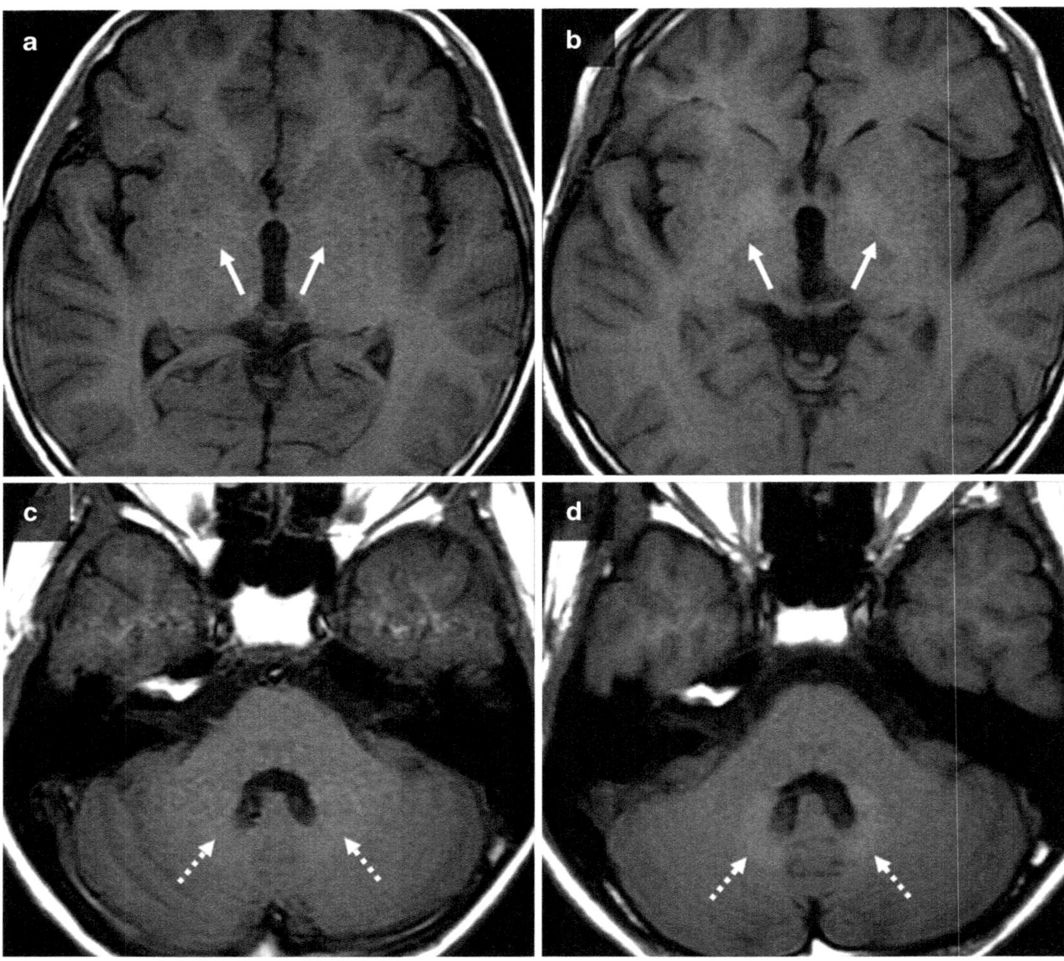

Fig. 9.3 T1-weighted images (T1WI) of a 15-year-old boy who received administrations of gadopentetate dimeglumine (Magnevist®) 12 times. (**a**, **c**) T1WI from his initial MRI (without the history of GBCA administration). (**b**, **d**) T1WI from his current MRI (with the history of 12 gadopentetate dimeglumine administrations). The globus pallidus (arrows) and dentate nucleus (dashed arrows) regions show a higher intensity in the images (**b**) and (**d**) than in (**a**) and (**c**). The signal increase of the dentate nucleus is more obvious than that of the globus pallidus

tion in various parts of the human body. The use of GBCAs in case of pregnant women or pediatric patients should be considered carefully.

References

1. Kanda T, Ishii K, Kawaguchi H, et al. High signal intensity in the dentate nucleus and globus pallidus on unenhanced T1-weighted MR images: relationship with increasing cumulative dose of a gadolinium-based contrast material. Radiology. 2014;270(3):834–41.
2. Errante Y, Cirimele V, Mallio CA, et al. Progressive increase of T1 signal intensity of the dentate nucleus on unenhanced magnetic resonance images is associated with cumulative doses of intravenously administered gadodiamide in patients with normal renal function, suggesting dechelation. Invest Radiol. 2014;49(10):685–90.
3. Adin ME, Kleinberg L, Vaidya D, et al. Hyperintense dentate nuclei on T1-weighted MRI: relation to repeat gadolinium administration. AJNR Am J Neuroradiol. 2015;36(10):1859–65.
4. McDonald RJ, McDonald JS, Kallmes DF, et al. Intracranial gadolinium deposition after contrast-enhanced MR imaging. Radiology. 2015;275(3):772–82.
5. Ramalho J, Castillo M, AlObaidy M, et al. High signal intensity in globus pallidus and dentate nucleus on unenhanced T1-weighted MR images: evaluation of two linear gadolinium-based contrast agents. Radiology. 2015;276(3):836–44.
6. Weberling LD, Kieslich PJ, Kickingereder P, et al. Increased signal intensity in the dentate nucleus on unenhanced T1-weighted images after gadobenate dimeglumine administration. Invest Radiol. 2015;50(11):743–8.
7. ESUR guidelines on contrast agents v10.0. 2018. http://www.esur-cm.org/index.php/en/.
8. Bellin MF, Van Der Molen AJ. Extracellular gadolinium-based contrast media: an overview. Eur J Radiol. 2008;66(2):160–7.
9. Frenzel T, Lengsfeld P, Schirmer H, et al. Stability of gadolinium-based magnetic resonance imaging contrast agents in human serum at 37 degrees C. Invest Radiol. 2008;43(12):817–28.
10. Prybylski JP, Semelka RC, Jay M. The stability of gadolinium-based contrast agents in human serum: a reanalysis of literature data and association with clinical outcomes. Magn Reson Imaging. 2017;38:145–51.
11. Tsushima Y. Safety information of gadolinium-based contrast agents: up to date. J Jpn Soc Pediatr Radiol. 2017;33(2):91–6.
12. Cochran ST. Anaphylactoid reactions to radiocontrast media. Curr Allergy Asthma Rep. 2005;5(1):28–31.
13. Katayama H, Yamaguchi K, Kozuka T, et al. Adverse reactions to ionic and nonionic contrast media. A report from the Japanese Committee on the Safety of Contrast Media. Radiology. 1990;175(3):621–8.
14. Prince MR, Zhang H, Zou Z, et al. Incidence of immediate gadolinium contrast media reactions. AJR Am J Roentgenol. 2011;196(2):W138–43.
15. Power S, Talbot N, Kucharczyk W, et al. Allergic-like reactions to the MR imaging contrast agent gadobutrol: a prospective study of 32991 consecutive injections. Radiology. 2016;281(1):72–7.
16. Tsushima Y, Awai K, Shinoda G, et al. Post-marketing surveillance of gadobutrol for contrast-enhanced magnetic resonance imaging in Japan. Jpn J Radiol. 2018;36(11):676–85.
17. Nagai H, Nishigori C. A delayed reaction to the magnetic resonance imaging contrast agent gadobutrol. J Allergy Clin Immunol Pract. 2017;5(3):850–1.
18. Marckmann P, Skov L, Rossen K, et al. Nephrogenic systemic fibrosis: suspected causative role of gadodiamide used for contrast-enhanced magnetic resonance imaging. J Am Soc Nephrol. 2006;17(9):2359–62.
19. Zou Z, Zhang HL, Roditi GH, et al. Nephrogenic systemic fibrosis: review of 370 biopsy-confirmed cases. JACC Cardiovasc Imaging. 2011;4(11):1206–16.
20. Kanda T, Fukusato T, Matsuda M, et al. Gadolinium-based contrast agent accumulates in the brain even in subjects without severe renal dysfunction: evaluation of autopsy brain specimens with inductively coupled plasma mass spectroscopy. Radiology. 2015;276(1):228–32.
21. Kanda T, Osawa M, Oba H, et al. High signal intensity in dentate nucleus on unenhanced T1-weighted MR images: association with linear versus macrocyclic gadolinium chelate administration. Radiology. 2015;275(3):803–9.
22. Radbruch A, Weberling LD, Kieslich PJ, et al. Gadolinium retention in the dentate nucleus and globus pallidus is dependent on the class of contrast agent. Radiology. 2015;275(3):783–91.
23. Radbruch A, Haase R, Kieslich PJ, et al. No signal intensity increase in the dentate nucleus on unenhanced T1-weighted MR images after more than 20 serial injections of macrocyclic gadolinium-based contrast agents. Radiology. 2017;282(3):699–707.
24. Yoo RE, Sohn CH, Kang KM, et al. Evaluation of gadolinium retention after serial administrations of a macrocyclic gadolinium-based contrast agent (gadobutrol): a single-institution experience with 189 patients. Invest Radiol. 2018;53(1):20–5.
25. Bjornerud A, Vatnehol SAS, Larsson C, et al. Signal enhancement of the dentate nucleus at unenhanced MR imaging after very high cumulative doses of the macrocyclic gadolinium-based contrast agent gadobutrol: an observational study. Radiology. 2017;285(2):434–44.
26. Khant ZA, Hirai T, Kadota Y, et al. T1 shortening in the cerebral cortex after multiple administrations of gadolinium-based contrast agents. Magn Reson Med Sci. 2017;16(1):84–6.
27. Zhang Y, Cao Y, Shih GL, et al. Extent of signal hyperintensity on unenhanced T1-weighted brain

MR images after more than 35 administrations of linear gadolinium-based contrast agents. Radiology. 2017;282(2):516–25.
28. Schmitt-Willich H. Stability of linear and macrocyclic gadolinium based contrast agents. Br J Radiol. 2007;80(955):581–2; author reply 4–5.
29. Schmitt-Willich H, Brehm M, Ewers CL, et al. Synthesis and physicochemical characterization of a new gadolinium chelate: the liver-specific magnetic resonance imaging contrast agent Gd-EOB-DTPA. Inorg Chem. 1999;38(6):1134–44.
30. Ichikawa S, Motosugi U, Omiya Y, et al. Contrast agent-induced high signal intensity in dentate nucleus on unenhanced T1-weighted images: comparison of gadodiamide and gadoxetic acid. Invest Radiol. 2017;52(7):389–95.
31. Kahn J, Posch H, Steffen IG, et al. Is there long-term signal intensity increase in the central nervous system on T1-weighted images after MR imaging with the hepatospecific contrast agent gadoxetic acid? A cross-sectional study in 91 patients. Radiology. 2017;282(3):708–16.
32. Radbruch A, Weberling LD, Kieslich PJ, et al. Intraindividual analysis of signal intensity changes in the dentate nucleus after consecutive serial applications of linear and macrocyclic gadolinium-based contrast agents. Invest Radiol. 2016;51(11):683–90.
33. Behzadi AH, Farooq Z, Zhao Y, et al. Dentate nucleus signal intensity decrease on T1-weighted MR images after switching from gadopentetate dimeglumine to gadobutrol. Radiology. 2018;287(3):816–23.
34. Smith AP, Marino M, Roberts J, et al. Clearance of gadolinium from the brain with no pathologic effect after repeated administration of gadodiamide in healthy rats: an analytical and histologic study. Radiology. 2017;282(3):743–51.
35. Daneman R, Prat A. The blood-brain barrier. Cold Spring Harb Perspect Biol. 2015;7(1):a020412.
36. Kanda T, Nakai Y, Oba H, et al. Gadolinium deposition in the brain. Magn Reson Imaging. 2016;34(10):1346–50.
37. Taoka T, Naganawa S. Gadolinium-based contrast media, cerebrospinal fluid and the glymphatic system: possible mechanisms for the deposition of gadolinium in the brain. Magn Reson Med Sci. 2018;17(2):111–9.
38. Naganawa S, Nakane T, Kawai H, et al. Gd-based contrast enhancement of the perivascular spaces in the basal ganglia. Magn Reson Med Sci. 2017;16(1):61–5.
39. Murata N, Murata K, Gonzalez-Cuyar LF, et al. Gadolinium tissue deposition in brain and bone. Magn Reson Imaging. 2016;34(10):1359–65.
40. Roberts DR, Lindhorst SM, Welsh CT, et al. High levels of gadolinium deposition in the skin of a patient with normal renal function. Invest Radiol. 2016;51(5):280–9.
41. Welk B, McArthur E, Morrow SA, et al. Association between gadolinium contrast exposure and the risk of parkinsonism. JAMA. 2016;316(1):96–8.
42. PRAC concludes assessment of gadolinium agents used in body scans and recommends regulatory actions, including suspension for some marketing authorisations. 2017. https://www.ema.europa.eu/en/news/prac-concludes-assessment-gadolinium-agents-used-body-scans-recommends-regulatory-actions-including.
43. Kanda T. The new restrictions on the use of linear gadolinium-based contrast agents in Japan. Magn Reson Med Sci. 2019;18(1):1–3.
44. FDA Drug Safety Communication: FDA warns that gadolinium-based contrast agents (GBCAs) are retained in the body; requires new class warnings. 2017. https://www.fda.gov/Drugs/DrugSafety/ucm589213.htm.
45. Erdene K, Nakajima T, Kameo S, et al. Organ retention of gadolinium in mother and pup mice: effect of pregnancy and type of gadolinium-based contrast agents. Jpn J Radiol. 2017;35(10):568–73.
46. Khairinisa MA, Takatsuru Y, Amano I, et al. The effect of perinatal gadolinium-based contrast agents on adult mice behavior. Invest radiol. 2018;53(2):110–8.
47. Pasquini L, Napolitano A, Visconti E, et al. Gadolinium-based contrast agent-related toxicities. CNS Drugs. 2018;32(3):229–40.
48. De Santis M, Straface G, Cavaliere AF, et al. Gadolinium periconceptional exposure: pregnancy and neonatal outcome. Acta Obstet Gynecol Scand. 2007;86(1):99–101.
49. Ray JG, Vermeulen MJ, Bharatha A, et al. Association between MRI exposure during pregnancy and fetal and childhood outcomes. JAMA. 2016;316(9):952–61.
50. Rofsky NM, Weinreb JC, Litt AW. Quantitative analysis of gadopentetate dimeglumine excreted in breast milk. J Magn Reson Imaging. 1993;3(1):131–2.
51. Schmiedl U, Maravilla KR, Gerlach R, et al. Excretion of gadopentetate dimeglumine in human breast milk. AJR Am J Roentgenol. 1990;154(6):1305–6.
52. Kubik-Huch RA, Gottstein-Aalame NM, Frenzel T, et al. Gadopentetate dimeglumine excretion into human breast milk during lactation. Radiology. 2000;216(2):555–8.
53. Webb JA, Thomsen HS, Morcos SK, Members of Contrast Media Safety Committee of European Society of Urogenital Radiology. The use of iodinated and gadolinium contrast media during pregnancy and lactation. Eur Radiol. 2005;15(6):1234–40.
54. Soares BP, Lequin MH, Huisman T. Safety of contrast material use in children. Magn Reson Imaging Clin N Am. 2017;25(4):779–85.
55. Davenport MS, Dillman JR, Cohan RH, et al. Effect of abrupt substitution of gadobenate dimeglumine for gadopentetate dimeglumine on rate of allergic-like reactions. Radiology. 2013;266(3):773–82.
56. Glutig K, Bhargava R, Hahn G, et al. Safety of gadobutrol in more than 1,000 pediatric patients: subanalysis of the GARDIAN study, a global multicenter prospective non-interventional study. Pediatr Radiol. 2016;46(9):1317–23.
57. Ozkur E, Kivanc Altunay I, Erdem Y, et al. Nephrogenic systemic fibrosis: in a child with primary hyperoxaluria. Clin Exp Dermatol. 2019;44(1):70–2.

58. Nardone B, Saddleton E, Laumann AE, et al. Pediatric nephrogenic systemic fibrosis is rarely reported: a RADAR report. Pediatr Radiol. 2014;44(2):173–80.
59. Weller A, Barber JL, Olsen OE. Gadolinium and nephrogenic systemic fibrosis: an update. Pediatr Nephrol. 2014;29(10):1927–37.
60. Flood TF, Stence NV, Maloney JA, et al. Pediatric brain: repeated exposure to linear gadolinium-based contrast material is associated with increased signal intensity at unenhanced T1-weighted MR imaging. Radiology. 2017;282(1):222–8.
61. Ichikawa S, Omiya Y, Onishi H, et al. Linear gadolinium-based contrast agent (gadodiamide and gadopentetate dimeglumine)-induced high signal intensity on unenhanced T1-weighted images in pediatric patients. J Magn Reson Imaging. 2019;49(4):1046–52. https://doi.org/10.1002/jmri.26311.
62. McDonald JS, McDonald RJ, Jentoft ME, et al. Intracranial gadolinium deposition following gadodiamide-enhanced magnetic resonance imaging in pediatric patients: a case-control study. JAMA Pediatr. 2017;171(7):705–7.

Basic Properties of Ultrasound Contrast Agents

10

Vito Cantisani, Christoph Frank Dietrich, Chandra Bortolotto, Shaun Ivan Muzic, Emanuele David, Yana Solskaya, and Fabrizio Calliada

10.1 Introduction

The acronym CEUS refers to contrast-enhanced ultrasound techniques in general [1–11]. Dynamic contrast-enhanced ultrasound (DCE-US) refers to quantitative time-intensity curve (TIC) analysis [11–13] using either bolus injection of microbubbles [13–16] or intravenous infusion with disruption-replenishment technique [17, 18].

Ultrasound contrast agents for transcutaneous ultrasound (TUS) have been developed to enhance Doppler signals. Later this technique was applied to contrast-specific imaging, and the CEUS was adopted to refer to this research and clinical technique.

In this chapter we describe the composition and basic properties of currently available ultrasound contrast agents (UCAs). The UCA application, specific imaging techniques and safety issues are also discussed.

10.2 Short History of UCA

The first experience with UCA has been reported in 1968 with short-living air bubbles. Gramiak and Shah reported clouds of air bubbles after arterial catheter injection of saline [19]. Unfortunately, the bubbles were unstable and the results were not achieved. It has taken many research years to develop the stable ultrasound contrast agents that are used till nowadays.

A different approach was used to produce more stable bubbles to reach the right heart including autologous blood injections [20]. Saline and also dextrose, indocyanine green, hydrogen peroxide and other iodine contrast agents coupled with air were used [21]. Neither the mentioned agents nor gelatine- or agarose-containing combinations [22], poly(D,L-lactide-*co*-glycolide) [23, 24] and poly(vinyl-alcohol) [25] stabilised the bubbles

V. Cantisani
Department of Radiological, Oncological and Anbathomo-Pathology Sciences, University of Rome La Sapienza, Rome, Italy
e-mail: vito.cantisani@uniroma1.it

C. F. Dietrich
Caritas-Krankenhaus, Wasserburg, Germany

Kliniken Hirslanden Beau Site, Salem und Permanence, Bern, Switzerland
e-mail: ChristophFrank.Dietrich@hirslanden.ch

C. Bortolotto (✉)
Radiology Department, Fondazione IRCCS Policlinico San Matteo, Pavia, Italy

S. I. Muzic · F. Calliada
Radiology Unit, University of Pavia, Pavia, Italy

E. David
Radiology Unit, Papardo Hospital, Messina, Italy

Y. Solskaya
P.Stradina Clinical University Hospital, Diagnosic Radiology Institute, Riga, Latvia

S. M. Erturk et al. (eds.), *Medical Imaging Contrast Agents: A Clinical Manual*,
https://doi.org/10.1007/978-3-030-79256-5_10

sufficiently to allow real-time imaging. Synthetic cyanoacrylate polymers with air bubbles were first produced under the marketing name of Sonovist® (Schering, Berlin, Germany) [26, 27]. After some minutes, the air bubbles were taken up by the reticuloendothelial system (RES) [26, 27].

The early developed experimental and commercially available UCA consisted of air or inert gas bubbles ranging from 1 to 10 μm in size encapsulated by a shell of different material. The shell is mainly responsible for the acoustic (viscoelastic) properties to allow stability and, therefore, durability [28], while the gas determines solubility and the acoustic properties. In addition, some UCAs are taken up by the RES (Kupffer cell and macrophages within and outside of the liver) including Levovist® and Sonazoid® and to lesser degree also other UCAs [29], whereas others are not. The later phases have been also termed as "post-vascular phase" [4, 30]. Since the lung capillaries are efficient filters, UCAs were differentiated if they pass such filters or not [31]. The so-called true blood pool agents including phospholipids and perfluorocarbons allow passage from the peripheral venous system via the pulmonary vascularity into the left heart and main arterial circulation contrast agents. The newly developed UCA defined by non-linear oscillations could be differentiated from tissue signals using specific software algorithms [32]. Albumin (protein)-shelled microbubbles were also developed. Optison® consists of a perfluoropropane gas covered by an albumin shell. The terms "first-, second-, third- and fourth-generation UCA" are sometimes misleading because the terms are not uniformly used.

In contrast to microbubbles, also nanobubbles with a size of 400–800 nm have been developed for treatment purposes. They allow less oscillation, but nanobubbles penetrate neoplastic tissue [28]. The accumulation of nanobubbles in neoplastic tissue allows targeting [33].

10.3 Ultrasound Contrast Agents (UCAs) [31, 34]

- Echovist® (approval 1991). Galactose-based microparticle. Indication: Shunt imaging in cardiology, hysterosalpingo-contrast sonography [34–36].
- Albunex® (approval 1995). Perflutren shell with air. Indication: Cardiology [21, 34, 37]. Disadvantage: Due to the air component, no real-time imaging was possible [34].
- Levovist® (approval 1995). Mix of galactose and palmitic acid as shell with air. Indication: Cardiology, liver imaging and imaging of vesicoureteral reflux [36]. Disadvantage: Due to the air component, no real-time imaging was possible [34].
- Optison® (approval 1997). Albumin shell with perflutren gas. Indication: Left ventricular opacification and endocardial border definition.
- SonoVue® or Lumason® (approval 2001). Phospholipid shell and sulphur hexafluoride gas. Indication: Left ventricular opacification and endocardial border definition, breast, liver, portal vein, extracranial carotid and peripheral arteries. Paediatric indications in the US. It is the most used.
- Definity® (approval 2001). Phospholipid shell and octofluoropropane gas. Indication: Enhancement of left ventricle endocardial border for its delineations in patients with suboptimal echocardiogram.
- Sonazoid® (approval 2007). Lipid shell with perfluorobutane gas. Indication: Liver, breast.
- Focal liver lesions and also for focal breast lesions in Japan.

10.4 UCA Imaging

Firstly UCAs change the reflection pattern with the increase of the backscattered signal [38]. In relation to the acoustic pressure (AP) applied, first linear resonation occurs. By increasing the AP, also non-linear resonation can be observed [4, 11, 18, 31, 39].

Therefore, the enhancement intensity of a focal lesion is compared with the surrounding reference tissue which can be subtracted, and the corresponding appearance is described as contrast enhancement pattern.

10.4.1 Contrast-Specific Imaging

The contrast imaging should provide high-resolution real-time imaging over a sufficient long period of time with B-mode information side by side or as an overlay to the UCA signal [18, 34].

Different techniques have been described depending on the manufacturer. Initially a low-pass filter was used to remove fundamental waves.

The next evolution generating higher spatial resolution was the use of phase inversion modes with the complete bandwidth of the transducer.

10.4.2 Stimulated Acoustic Emission

According to the definition, acoustic power (acoustic emission) is the transient elastic waves in a tissue that are caused by the release of stress energy from the system [40].

In B-mode high acoustic energy is used to avoid attenuation of such structure as cartilage or bones, but during the DCE-US, acoustic field is weak that increases the attenuating effect of additional structures [41].

Mechanical index (MI) is the ability of ultrasound beam to cause cavitation effects in the tissues and micromechanical damage and is proportional to the frequency of the beam—higher frequency, lower MI [42].

All microbubbles used in UCA are very sensitive to ultrasound energy that can destroy them easily. The typical range of acoustic power (MI), during the DCE-US examination, is <0.1 that shows the minimal or no microbubble destruction, but some differences in the MI value according to the manufactures' applications are allowed. Also, the excessive scanning in a single plane can cause the destruction of microbubbles [41]. Disruption is characterized with the gas diffusion from microbubble, and loss scattering property and UCA cannot be used effectively and even can mimic the false-positive wash-out of lesion.

Therefore, it is very important for the clinicians to find the optimal MI range without the destruction of microbubbles, for example, to avoid the "flash" phenomena, if seen—reduce the MI until the flashes of perfused parenchyma are not visualized [43]. Continuous scanning and recording help imprint the earliest UCA microbubbles' arrival, arterial enhancement and venous phase after 60 s with further storage of 30–60 s recordings for wash-out detection [41].

10.4.3 Artefacts

Reduced MI can lead to problems in depth penetration [44, 45].

The main artefact is the pseudo-enhancement of tissue due to the high concentration of microbubbles. Identifying non-physiologic nature of microbubble can help distinguish pseudo-enhancement from the true microbubble signal, as also image of microbubble can be compared with the tissue to detect bright target in both.

The increasing of non-linear coefficient ("bulk" coefficient) with the microbubbles can cause occurrence of non-linear propagation without low MI administration. That way hyperechoic bright targets may produce non-linear component echoes, caused by propagation, but not microbubble scattering.

To prevent the artefact during the examination, high UCA doses and presence of large vessel near the area of interest have to be avoided. Equipment application settings with the correct MI and penetration mode are as much important as the UCA dosage.

Artefact problem is very common in clinical practice in follow-up of liver tumours after ablation—bright hyperenhanced focus in treated area can show linear artefact and become evaluated as recurrent or residual tumour. Dynamic enhancement of arterial phase has to be evaluated: tumour is perfused in arterial phase, but non-linear artefacts attribute to increase enhancement in portal phase and even delayed phase.

As known, higher MI provides better penetration but increases the microbubble destruction, so the balance of the signal intensity and fixity of microbubbles is most important and hard during the CEUS examination. In the early phase, the dose of the contrast agent should be balanced with the enhancement intensity and the duration of the enhancement (sufficient concentration in late phase).

For example, CEUS circle of disaster can be described as the originally high MI, and after the UCA administration, the microbubble destruction may appear, with the following additional microbubble injection and increased attenuation → higher MI and as the result destruction of all microbubbles [41].

10.4.4 Heterogeneous Long Liver Enhancement [46]

Prolonged innocuous liver enhancement, after the bolus injection of microbubble contrast agents, appears as a heterogeneous enhancement in the liver during the performance of the CEUS examination, often beginning at around 2 min and lasting up to 5 h after contrast injection on both B-mode and contrast-specific modes. It is not destroyed by conventional B-mode imaging. The enhanced signals can also be observed in the portal and superior mesenteric veins, though not in the systemic circulation [46]. It is similar in appearance to the US finding of free portal venous gas.

10.5 Examination Technique

10.5.1 CEUS Phases

Herewith we summarize the expert opinions reported in the WFUMB (World Federation of Ultrasound in Medicine and Biology) position paper on how to perform CEUS [18]. CEUS allows real-time recording and evaluation of the wash-in and wash-out phases of the ultrasound contrast agent (UCA) over several minutes [18]. Owing to the specific supply of blood to the liver, three different phases have been defined: the arterial (AP), the portal venous (PVP) and the late (sinusoidal) phases (LP) [47, 48] (Fig. 10.1). Some contrast agents (such as Sonazoid™, BR14, BR38) are phagocytosed by cells of the mononuclear phagocyte system (reticulo-endothelium, e.g. Kupffer cells in the liver). Phagocytosis may start as early as the arterial phase and becomes pronounced in the late phase. This results in accelerated clearance of the agents from the vascular distribution volume [49]. These UCAs persist significantly longer in the liver parenchyma than purely vascular agents, so that a fourth phase, the post-vascular phase (also known as the Kupffer cell phase), can be defined. For these reasons, transit times and time-intensity curves (TIC) differ for purely blood pool versus reticuloendothelial UCAs. The latter should not be used to evaluate hepatic transit times, as they do not reflect the hepatic kinetics [18].

The main diagnostic features are [18]:

1. Vascular architecture (evaluated in the early wash-in phase) (Fig. 10.2)
2. Contrast enhancement of the lesion compared to the adjacent tissue (time course of wash-in and wash-out) (Fig. 10.3)

The combined evaluation of the above diagnostic features makes it possible to characterize focal liver lesions (FLL) in healthy parenchyma [50–53] as malignant or benign.

Similar characteristics apply to other organs [18, 54, 55].

10.5.1.1 Enhancement (Degree and Timing)

The contrast behaviour of a lesion depends if the liver is healthy or diseased (e.g. liver cirrhosis, fibrosis or steatosis). In fact, the different clinical conditions may affect the contrast behaviour of the lesion and liver parenchyma as well. Enhancement refers to the intensity of the signal relative to the adjacent parenchyma as isoenhancing, hyperenhancing and hypoenhancing.

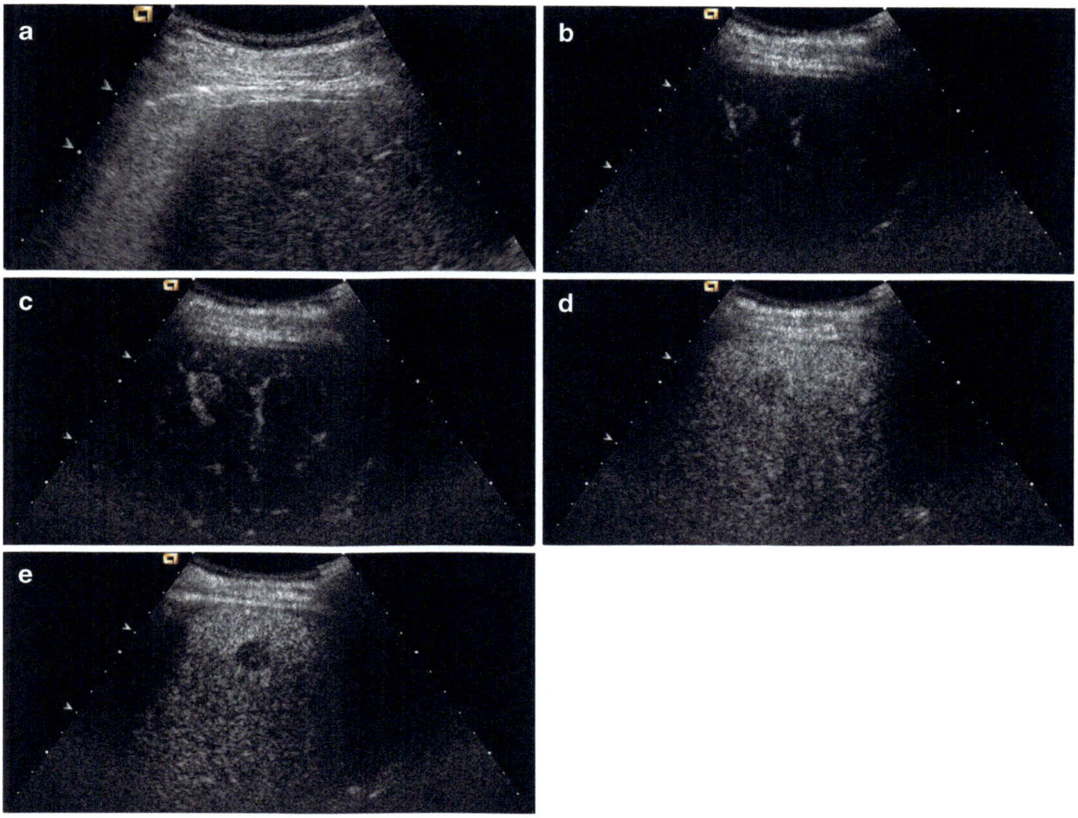

Fig. 10.1 CEUS phases. (**a**) B-mode ultrasound of a hepatic lesion appearing as scarcely recognizable nodule with a hypoechoic rim in the hepatic parenchyma. (**b**, **c**) CEUS shows homogeneous arterial contrast enhancement during arterial phase, seen at 13″ and 15″ (**d**) portal-venous phase; initial wash-out already evident at 3″ (**e**) late phase; complete wash-out at 3 min

Sustained enhancement refers to continuation of the same or greater intensity of enhancement in the lesion relative to the adjacent parenchyma over time. It applies to lesions that are iso- or hyperenhancing in the arterial phase. Complete absence of enhancement can be described as non-enhancing [4, 5, 56].

10.5.1.2 "Wash-In" and "Wash-Out"

"Wash-in", used for both qualitative and quantitative analyses, refers to the progressive enhancement within a region of interest from the arrival of microbubbles in the field of view, to "peak enhancement", and "wash-out" to the reduction in enhancement which follows peak enhancement [4, 5]. As explained above, the timing (early versus late onset, fast versus slow), degree (complete, incomplete) and pattern should be described in comparison to the surrounding "normal" parenchyma. The characteristic features of a TIC analysis are shown in [11, 57]. This model for quantification of tumour vascularization was applied in multicentric studies validating the UCA as a predictive marker [58, 59].

10.6 Indications for UCA

According to the WFUMB and EFSUMB (European Federation of Societies for Ultrasound in Medicine and Biology) guidelines, the main following indications in adults and paediatric patients can be summarized [18, 43, 54, 55, 60, 61]:

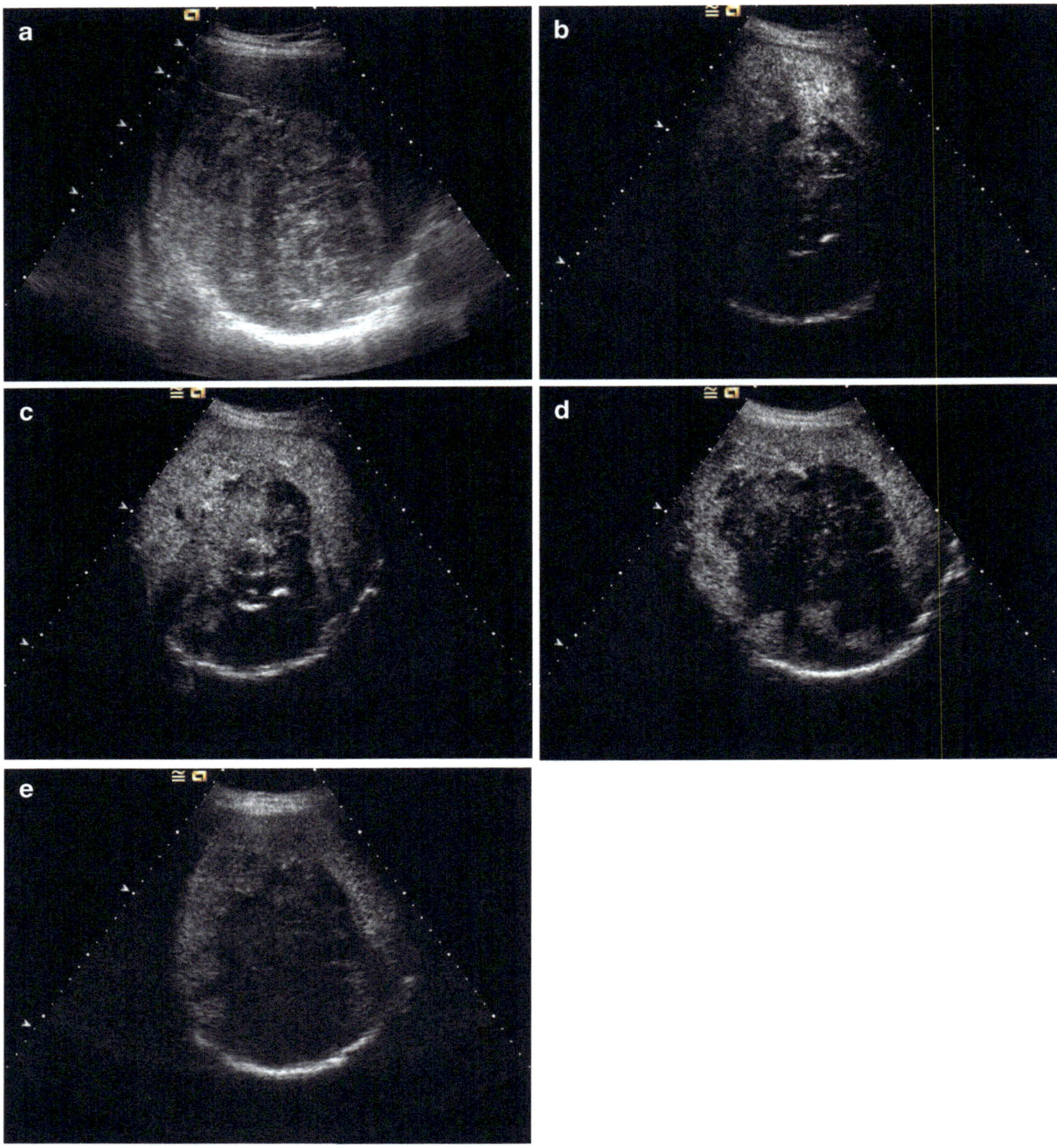

Fig. 10.2 Vascular architecture. (**a**) B-mode ultrasound of a hepatocellular adenoma shows a large lesion that is markedly inhomogeneous for its content of fat tissue, necrosis, haemorrhage and calcifications. (**b**, **c**) CEUS shows in the arterial phase deranged and dystrophic vessels especially in the very early arterial phase (**b**), while the portal and late phases show wash-out with an inhomogeneous pattern (**d**, **e**). The differential diagnosis of such a lesion with the sole use of CEUS imaging is difficult, as the diagnostic algorithm must be integrated with clinical and laboratory data

- Characterization of focal liver lesions in the noncirrhotic and cirrhotic liver
- Lesion(s) or suspected lesion(s) in patients with history of malignancy as an alternative to CT or MRI
- In patients with contraindicated contrast CT and MRI (renal failure)
- Inconclusive MRI/CT
- Inconclusive cytology/histology results
- Characterization of portal vein thrombosis

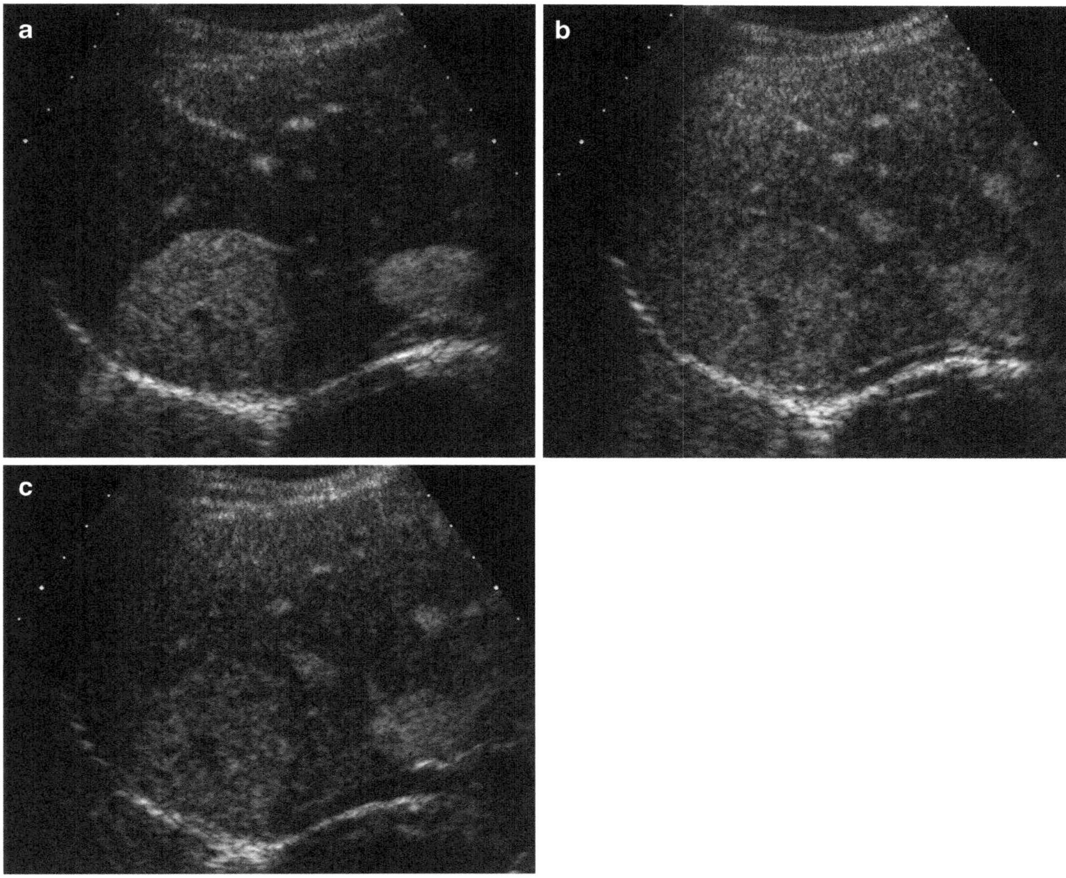

Fig. 10.3 Contrast enhancement of the lesion compared to the adjacent tissue. CEUS of a focal nodular hyperplasia shows a lesion with brisk, homogeneous enhancement in the arterial phase (**a**), with the portal (**b**) and late phase (**c**) showing mild sustained enhancement. The central scar is seen as a hypoechoic area within the lesion, becoming more evident in the portal venous phase than in the arterial phase

- Liver and kidney transplantation.
- CT/MRI contraindication
- Vascular studies such as carotid artery evaluation, aortic aneurysm pre- and post-treatment evaluation
- GI evaluation
- MSK diseases
- Pancreas lesion characterization
- Post-treatment evaluations
- Renal trauma
- Renal infarction and necrosis
- Renal artery stenosis
- Tumour (vascularity and visualization)
- Complicated infection diagnostics
- Complicated cysts
- Transplants

As contraindications have to be mentioned:

- History of allergic reaction or hypersensitivity
- Right-to-left shunts
- Systemic and pulmonary hypertension

10.6.1 CEUS-Guided Interventions

CEUS-guided interventions for practical considerations are performed very much like a standard US-guided procedure except that two injections of UCAs are used, one to plan the procedure and second to guide the actual intervention. In some cases, a continuous infusion may be the better choice, while in other cases, the procedure may be performed without a second contrast injection, if the perfusion conditions are adequately demonstrated with the first CEUS to allow for a standard ultrasound-guided procedure. CEUS-guided biopsy has been reported to increase the diagnostic accuracy rate by up to 10% either by directing the biopsy towards contrast-enhanced—and thus viable—tissue inside the tumour and thereby avoiding sampling of necrotic material or by identifying previously non-visualised lesions more accessible for biopsy [4, 39, 62–65]. Furthermore, CEUS may visualise active bleeding, hemobilia or segmental liver infarction.

CEUS is also helpful in performing and follow-up for radiofrequency ablation or cryotherapy for hepatic and renal masses [49, 66, 67]. CEUS allows evaluation of the extent of the ablated zone at the end of the procedure. If residual tumour is identified, the ablation can be extended after repositioning the needle to the residual tumour using CEUS guidance. On follow-up studies, CEUS is able to identify—immediately following treatment—small amounts of residual tumour, which can be too small or too soon to detect with CECT or CT/MRI [18, 68, 69].

10.6.2 Paediatric Patients and Newborns

The use of CEUS in children, first reported in 2002, has been addressed in an EFSUMB position statement discussing the current status of CEUS and its further development in children [61]. Currently sulphur hexafluoride gas microbubbles (SonoVue™/Lumason™, Bracco SpA, Milan) have been approved in the United States by the Food and Drug Administration (FDA) as Lumason™ for characterising focal liver lesions in children ["Lumason is indicated for use with ultrasound of the liver in adult and pediatric patients to characterize focal liver lesions"] and vesicoureteral reflux. In Europe, CEUS in children is mostly "off-label" use, except for a few indications including vesicoureteral reflux [70]. The same is true for many drugs, which are used off-label in paediatric practice, and the question of "off-label use" has been widely discussed [71, 72]. The recent approval of SonoVue™/Lumason™ for use in paediatrics in the United States is a welcome first step towards the acceptance of this technique in the non-ionising imaging of children [73].

10.6.3 Extravascular (Intracavitary)

Extravascular (intracavitary) CEUS (EV-CEUS) is used for imaging physiological and non-physiological body cavities. Physiological cavities include the peritoneal cavity, pleural cavity, biliary tract, gastrointestinal tract, urinary tract, etc., and pathological cavities include abscesses, cysts, diverticula, etc. [39, 74]. The UCA is given through a needle or catheter, for instance, at cholangiography or nephrostomy. However, UCAs can also be given orally or as an enema for imaging the upper and lower gastrointestinal tract [75, 76].

The following clinical applications of EV-CEUS have been described in case studies: percutaneous nephrostomy [77], biliary tract imaging via percutaneous transhepatic cholangiography and drainage (PTCD) [78], abscess drainage [79], swallow CEUS for imaging Zenker's diverticulum, voiding vesicoureteral reflux sonography [80, 81], salivary gland duct imaging [82], contrast-enhanced hysterosalpingo-sonography (CE-HyCoSy) [83], biliary tract imaging via endoscopic retrograde cholangiography (ERCP) [84] and fistula imaging [85].

The transducer used in extravascular CEUS is the same as that used in conventional US. SonoVue™ is currently the most often used UCA for VUR [86] though it is not licensed for other extravascular indications of CEUS. To date, no standard dosage of UCA has been established for extravascular CEUS. The reported range is 0.1–1 mL SonoVue™ (most commonly just a few drops) diluted in 50 mL or more of 0.9% saline. A higher content of SonoVue™ may be needed for high-frequency US probes [39].

Compared with X-ray contrast techniques, EV-CEUS does not require exposure to ionizing radiation and can be performed at the bedside.

10.7 Quantification

The term of quantification in contrast-enhanced ultrasound implies the kinetics of ultrasound contrast agent uptake by tissues in dynamic contrast-enhanced ultrasound (DCE-US). There are two dynamic contrast-enhanced ultrasound injection modes that provide estimation of parameters related to perfusion:

- Bolus injection
- Constant infusion

Bolus and infusion techniques provide the perfusion evaluation for different parameters in the tissues. It should be noticed that it is necessary to use the same administration method of UCA (quantification method) for the follow-up, to keep the identity of imaging settings.

Bolus injection is a standard mode for non-cardiac indications. During the ultrasound examination, contrast-specific sequences are used, and single intravenous injection of contrast agent is performed. Bubbles reach the target tissues, according to its localization: the first enhancement or "opacification" of arteries, heart, liver and other good vascularized organs happens in the first seconds after the intravenous bolus injection, while the enhancement of soft tissues, glands and lymph nodes starts some seconds later, because of the lower blood supply. Enhancement effect persists for 3–6 min. In cardiac patients, hemodynamic status and in case of inappropriate dosage of UCA time of enhancement can be reduced. ROI is used as region of interest, and TIC (time-intensity curve) describes the wash-in and wash-out of the contrast agent.

During the bolus injection, low mechanical index (MI) is performed at 10–20 frames/s for the enhancement period. The contrast agent wash-in and wash-out is described with the time-intensity curve (TIC) in the region of interest (ROI) that is displayed as function time. For additional evaluation, several ROI can be placed in the lesson or reference tissue [43].

In case of constant infusion, UCA is administered continuously with the specific pump or drip bag for 5–20 min, but time of infusion and amount of UCA depend on clinical application. Constant infusion is mostly used for cardiac indications, where the prolonged steady state with the disruption-replenishment analysis method is applied [43, 87].

In the beginning evaluation starts with the low MI, without disrupting the bubbles; then high MI is set for few frames to cause the disruption of the bubbles; and low MI is reverted back to visualize the fresh UCA arrival. Image sequences form the time-intensity curve (TIC) and measures the UCA rate of replenishment in the ROI.

Infusion using the pump or drip can be performed only using the Definity® UCA, but to perform the slow infusion injection with SonoVue®-specific rotating pump for vertical placement is required [43].

In the presence of liver malignancy or cirrhosis, hepatic shunting may occur. For that, hepatic vein transit time can be evaluated and measured as arrival time of microbubbles in hepatic veins, portal vein and hepatic arteries with the transit time calculated [43].

10.8 UCA Safety

As mentioned earlier, UCAs are safe with a very low incidence of side effects. As there are no cardio-, hepato-, or nephro-toxic effects, it is not necessary to perform laboratory checks to assess liver, renal or thyroid function before administration. The incidence of severe adverse events is lower than with current X-ray contrast agents and is comparable to those encountered with MR contrast agents. Life-threatening anaphylactic reactions in abdominal applications have been reported with a rate of 0.001%, with no death in a series of >23,000 abdominal patients [88]. Further studies have reproduced this very low adverse event rate [89, 90]. Nonetheless, investigators should be trained in resuscitation and have the appropriate facilities available to react in cases of adverse events [4, 5]. In particular, each centre should be prepared with a crash chart and ability to treat anaphylactic shock if it occurs.

Safety studies and reports by far more than 300,000 patients receiving SonoVue®, Optison® and Definity® demonstrated a very low adverse event rate [88, 90–94].

UCAs are extremely safe with low incidence of side effects [88] and no cardio-, hepato- or nephrotoxic effects. Therefore, it is not necessary to perform laboratory tests to assess liver or kidney function prior to their administration [18, 31].

10.9 Conclusions

Contrast-enhanced ultrasound (CEUS), performed with the intravenous injection of microbubble contrast agents, has expanded, as shown above, the horizon for ultrasound imaging by providing a technique capable of showing the vascular phase enhancement in dynamic real time for over 5 min, allowing the demonstration of blood flow at the microcirculatory or perfusion level in ultrasound. Its safe performance without any requirement for ionizing radiation and with no nephrotoxicity makes it a competitive and effective choice in many clinical arenas and certainly for children. In spite of many obvious benefits of CEUS, it is still not yet widely worldwide used outside of specialized secondary and tertiary institutions due to its labour-intensive nature, considerable learning curve for attainment of expertise at performance, and frequent lack of reimbursement. However, future developments and more diffuse use are advisable in this era of cost containment and radiation awareness.

References

1. Albrecht T, Blomley M, Bolondi L, Claudon M, Correas JM, Cosgrove D, Greiner L, et al. Guidelines for the use of contrast agents in ultrasound. January 2004. Ultraschall Med. 2004;25:249–56.
2. Claudon M, Cosgrove D, Albrecht T, Bolondi L, Bosio M, Calliada F, Correas JM, et al. Guidelines and good clinical practice recommendations for contrast enhanced ultrasound (CEUS)—update 2008. Ultraschall Med. 2008;29:28–44.
3. Piscaglia F, Nolsoe C, Dietrich CF, Cosgrove DO, Gilja OH, Bachmann NM, Albrecht T, et al. The EFSUMB Guidelines and Recommendations on the Clinical Practice of Contrast Enhanced Ultrasound (CEUS): update 2011 on non-hepatic applications. Ultraschall Med. 2012;33:33–59.
4. Claudon M, Dietrich CF, Choi BI, Cosgrove DO, Kudo M, Nolsoe CP, Piscaglia F, et al. Guidelines and good clinical practice recommendations for contrast enhanced ultrasound (CEUS) in the liver—update 2012: a WFUMB-EFSUMB initiative in cooperation with representatives of AFSUMB, AIUM, ASUM, FLAUS and ICUS. Ultraschall Med. 2013;34:11–29.
5. Claudon M, Dietrich CF, Choi BI, Cosgrove DO, Kudo M, Nolsoe CP, Piscaglia F, et al. Guidelines and good clinical practice recommendations for Contrast Enhanced Ultrasound (CEUS) in the liver—update 2012: a WFUMB-EFSUMB initiative in cooperation with representatives of AFSUMB, AIUM, ASUM, FLAUS and ICUS. Ultrasound Med Biol. 2013;39:187–210.
6. Dietrich CF, Ignee A, Trojan J, Fellbaum C, Schuessler G. Improved characterisation of histologically proven liver tumours by contrast enhanced ultrasonography during the portal venous and specific late phase of SHU 508A. Gut. 2004;53:401–5.
7. Dietrich CF, Schuessler G, Trojan J, Fellbaum C, Ignee A. Differentiation of focal nodular hyperplasia and hepatocellular adenoma by contrast-enhanced ultrasound. Br J Radiol. 2005;78:704–7.
8. Dietrich CF, Becker D. Signalverstärkte Lebersonographie zur verbesserten Detektion und Charakterisierung von Leberraumforderungen. Dt Aerzteblatt. 2002;24:7.
9. Dietrich CF. [3D real time contrast enhanced ultrasonography,a new technique]. Rofo. 2002;174:160–3.
10. Dietrich CFWD, Brunner V, Braden B, Zeuzem S, Caspary WF. Erste Erfahrungen mit einem neuen Signalverstärker bei der Untersuchung der Leber. Ultraschall Med. 1998;19.
11. Dietrich CF, Averkiou MA, Correas JM, Lassau N, Leen E, Piscaglia F. An EFSUMB introduction into Dynamic Contrast-Enhanced Ultrasound (DCE-US) for quantification of tumour perfusion. Ultraschall Med. 2012;33:344–51.
12. Ignee A, Jedrejczyk M, Schuessler G, Jakubowski W, Dietrich CF. Quantitative contrast enhanced ultrasound of the liver for time intensity curves-reliability and potential sources of errors. Eur J Radiol. 2010;73:153–8.
13. Lassau N, Cosgrove D, Armand JP. Early evaluation of targeted drugs using dynamic contrast-enhanced ultrasonography for personalized medicine. Future Oncol. 2012;8:1215–8.
14. Lassau N, Koscielny S, Chami L, Chebil M, Benatsou B, Roche A, Ducreux M, et al. Advanced hepatocellular carcinoma: early evaluation of response to beva-

cizumab therapy at dynamic contrast-enhanced US with quantification—preliminary results. Radiology. 2011;258:291–300.
15. Lassau N, Koscielny S, Albiges L, Chami L, Benatsou B, Chebil M, Roche A, et al. Metastatic renal cell carcinoma treated with sunitinib: early evaluation of treatment response using dynamic contrast-enhanced ultrasonography. Clin Cancer Res. 2010;16:1216–25.
16. Frampas E, Lassau N, Zappa M, Vullierme MP, Koscielny S, Vilgrain V. Advanced Hepatocellular Carcinoma: early evaluation of response to targeted therapy and prognostic value of Perfusion CT and Dynamic Contrast Enhanced-Ultrasound. Preliminary results. Eur J Radiol. 2013;82:e205–11.
17. Williams R, Hudson JM, Lloyd BA, Sureshkumar AR, Lueck G, Milot L, Atri M, et al. Dynamic microbubble contrast-enhanced US to measure tumor response to targeted therapy: a proposed clinical protocol with results from renal cell carcinoma patients receiving antiangiogenic therapy. Radiology. 2011;260:581–90.
18. Dietrich CF, Averkiou M, Nielsen MB, Barr RG, Burns PN, Calliada F, Cantisani V, et al. How to perform Contrast-Enhanced Ultrasound (CEUS). Ultrasound Int Open. 2018;4:E2–E15.
19. Gramiak R, Shah PM. Echocardiography of the aortic root. Invest Radiol. 1968;3:356–66.
20. Kremkau FW, Gramiak R, Carstensen EL, Shah PM, Kramer DH. Ultrasonic detection of cavitation at catheter tips. Am J Roentgenol Radium Ther Nucl Med. 1970;110:177–83.
21. Feinstein SB, Shah PM, Bing RJ, Meerbaum S, Corday E, Chang BL, Santillan G, et al. Microbubble dynamics visualized in the intact capillary circulation. J Am Coll Cardiol. 1984;4:595–600.
22. D'Arrigo JS, Mano Y. Bubble production in agarose gels subjected to different decompression schedules. Undersea Biomed Res. 1979;6:93–8.
23. Cui W, Bei J, Wang S, Zhi G, Zhao Y, Zhou X, Zhang H, et al. Preparation and evaluation of poly(L-lactide-co-glycolide) (PLGA) microbubbles as a contrast agent for myocardial contrast echocardiography. J Biomed Mater Res B Appl Biomater. 2005;73:171–8.
24. Eisenbrey JR, Hsu J, Wheatley MA. Plasma sterilization of poly lactic acid ultrasound contrast agents: surface modification and implications for drug delivery. Ultrasound Med Biol. 2009;35:1854–62.
25. Cavalieri F, El Hamassi A, Chiessi E, Paradossi G. Stable polymeric microballoons as multifunctional device for biomedical uses: synthesis and characterization. Langmuir. 2005;21:8758–64.
26. Forsberg F, Basude R, Liu JB, Alessandro J, Shi WT, Rawool NM, Goldberg BB, et al. Effect of filling gases on the backscatter from contrast microbubbles: theory and in vivo measurements. Ultrasound Med Biol. 1999;25:1203–11.
27. Fritzsch T, Schlief R. Future prospects for echo-enhancing agents. Clin Radiol. 1996;51(Suppl 1):56–8.
28. Paefgen V, Doleschel D, Kiessling F. Evolution of contrast agents for ultrasound imaging and ultrasound-mediated drug delivery. Front Pharmacol. 2015;6:197.
29. Chen CC, Borden MA. The role of poly(ethylene glycol) brush architecture in complement activation on targeted microbubble surfaces. Biomaterials. 2011;32:6579–87.
30. Yanagisawa K, Moriyasu F, Miyahara T, Yuki M, Iijima H. Phagocytosis of ultrasound contrast agent microbubbles by Kupffer cells. Ultrasound Med Biol. 2007;33:318–25.
31. Appis AW, Tracy MJ, Feinstein SB. Update on the safety and efficacy of commercial ultrasound contrast agents in cardiac applications. Echo Res Pract. 2015;2:R55–62.
32. Leong-Poi H, Song J, Rim SJ, Christiansen J, Kaul S, Lindner JR. Influence of microbubble shell properties on ultrasound signal: implications for low-power perfusion imaging. J Am Soc Echocardiogr. 2002;15:1269–76.
33. Yin T, Wang P, Zheng R, Zheng B, Cheng D, Zhang X, Shuai X. Nanobubbles for enhanced ultrasound imaging of tumors. Int J Nanomedicine. 2012;7:895–904.
34. Ignee A, Atkinson NS, Schuessler G, Dietrich CF. Ultrasound contrast agents. Endosc Ultrasound. 2016;5:355–62.
35. Uzuner N, Horner S, Pichler G, Svetina D, Niederkorn K. Right-to-left shunt assessed by contrast transcranial Doppler sonography: new insights. J Ultrasound Med. 2004;23:1475–82.
36. Cosgrove D. Echo enhancers and ultrasound imaging. Eur J Radiol. 1997;26:64–76.
37. Feinstein SB, Cheirif J, Ten Cate FJ, Silverman PR, Heidenreich PA, Dick C, Desir RM, et al. Safety and efficacy of a new transpulmonary ultrasound contrast agent: initial multicenter clinical results. J Am Coll Cardiol. 1990;16:316–24.
38. Calliada F, Campani R, Bottinelli O, Bozzini A, Sommaruga MG. Ultrasound contrast agents: basic principles. Eur J Radiol. 1998;27(Suppl 2):S157–60.
39. Piscaglia F, Nolsoe C, Dietrich CF, Cosgrove DO, Gilja OH, Bachmann Nielsen M, Albrecht T, et al. The EFSUMB Guidelines and Recommendations on the Clinical Practice of Contrast Enhanced Ultrasound (CEUS): update 2011 on non-hepatic applications. Ultraschall Med. 2012;33:33–59.
40. Cantisani V, Wilson SR. CEUS: where are we in 2015? Eur J Radiol. 2015;84(9):1621–2. https://doi.org/10.1016/j.ejrad.2015.05.028. Epub 2015 Jun 17.
41. Hagiwara Y, Saijo Y, Ando A, et al. Comparison of articular cartilage images assessed by high-frequency ultrasound microscope and scanning acoustic microscope. Int Orthop. 2012;36(1):185–90. https://doi.org/10.1007/s00264-011-1263-1.
42. Averkiou MA, Bruce MF, Powers JE, et al. Imaging methods for ultrasound contrast agents. Ultrasound Med Biol. 46(3):498–517. https://doi.org/10.1016/j.ultrasmedbio.2019.11.004.
43. Dietrich CF, Averkiou MA, Correas J-M, et al. An EFSUMB introduction into Dynamic Contrast-

Enhanced Ultrasound (DCE-US) for quantification of tumour perfusion. Ultraschall Med. 2012;33:344–51.
44. Dietrich CF, Ignee A, Greis C, Cui XW, Schreiber-Dietrich DG, Hocke M. Artifacts and pitfalls in contrast-enhanced ultrasound of the liver. Ultraschall Med. 2014;35:108–25; quiz 126–7.
45. Dietrich CF, Ignee A, Hocke M, Schreiber-Dietrich D, Greis C. Pitfalls and artefacts using contrast enhanced ultrasound. Z Gastroenterol. 2011;49:350–6.
46. Cui XW, Ignee A, Hocke M, Seitz K, Schrade G, Dietrich CF. Prolonged heterogeneous liver enhancement on contrast-enhanced ultrasound. Ultraschall Med. 2014;35:246–52.
47. Solbiati L, Tonolini M, Cova L, Goldberg SN. The role of contrast-enhanced ultrasound in the detection of focal liver leasions. Eur Radiol. 2001;11(Suppl 3):E15–26.
48. D'Onofrio M, Martone E, Faccioli N, Zamboni G, Malago R, Mucelli RP. Focal liver lesions: sinusoidal phase of CEUS. Abdom Imaging. 2006;31:529–36.
49. Dietrich CF, Lorentzen T, Appelbaum L, Buscarini E, Cantisani V, Correas JM, Cui XW, et al. EFSUMB Guidelines on Interventional Ultrasound (INVUS), part III—abdominal treatment procedures (long version). Ultraschall Med. 2016;37:E1–E32.
50. Strobel D, Seitz K, Blank W, Schuler A, Dietrich C, von Herbay A, Friedrich-Rust M, et al. Contrast-enhanced ultrasound for the characterization of focal liver lesions—diagnostic accuracy in clinical practice (DEGUM multicenter trial). Ultraschall Med. 2008;29:499–505.
51. Bernatik T, Seitz K, Blank W, Schuler A, Dietrich CF, Strobel D. Unclear focal liver lesions in contrast-enhanced ultrasonography—lessons to be learned from the DEGUM multicenter study for the characterization of liver tumors. Ultraschall Med. 2010;31:577–81.
52. Seitz K, Greis C, Schuler A, Bernatik T, Blank W, Dietrich CF, Strobel D. Frequency of tumor entities among liver tumors of unclear etiology initially detected by sonography in the noncirrhotic or cirrhotic livers of 1349 patients. Results of the DEGUM multicenter study. Ultraschall Med. 2011;32:598–603.
53. Strobel D, Bernatik T, Blank W, Schuler A, Greis C, Dietrich CF, Seitz K. Diagnostic accuracy of CEUS in the differential diagnosis of small (</= 20 mm) and subcentimetric (</= 10 mm) focal liver lesions in comparison with histology. Results of the DEGUM multicenter trial. Ultraschall Med. 2011;32:593–7.
54. Sidhu PS, Cantisani V, Dietrich CF, Gilja OH, Saftoiu A, Bartels E, Bertolotto M, et al. The EFSUMB guidelines and recommendations for the clinical practice of Contrast-Enhanced Ultrasound (CEUS) in non-hepatic applications: update 2017 (long version). Ultraschall Med. 2018;39:e2–e44.
55. Sidhu PS, Cantisani V, Dietrich CF, Gilja OH, Saftoiu A, Bartels E, Bertolotto M, et al. The EFSUMB guidelines and recommendations for the clinical practice of Contrast-Enhanced Ultrasound (CEUS) in non-hepatic applications: update 2017 (short version). Ultraschall Med. 2018;39:154–80.
56. Kudo M. Defect reperfusion imaging with Sonazoid(R): a breakthrough in hepatocellular carcinoma. Liver Cancer. 2016;5:1–7.
57. Dietrich CF, Greis C. [How to perform contrast enhanced ultrasound]. Dtsch Med Wochenschr. 2016;141:1019–24.
58. Lassau N, Bonastre J, Kind M, Vilgrain V, Lacroix J, Cuinet M, Taieb S, et al. Validation of dynamic contrast-enhanced ultrasound in predicting outcomes of antiangiogenic therapy for solid tumors: the French multicenter support for innovative and expensive techniques study. Invest Radiol. 2014;49:794–800.
59. O'Connor JP, Aboagye EO, Adams JE, Aerts HJ, Barrington SF, Beer AJ, Boellaard R, et al. Imaging biomarker roadmap for cancer studies. Nat Rev Clin Oncol. 2017;14:169–86.
60. Jenssen C, Gilja OH, Serra AL, Piscaglia F, Dietrich CF, Rudd L, Sidhu PS. European Federation of Societies for Ultrasound in Medicine and Biology (EFSUMB) policy document development strategy—clinical practice guidelines, position statements and technological reviews. Ultrasound Int Open. 2019;5:E2–E10.
61. Sidhu PS, Cantisani V, Deganello A, Dietrich CF, Duran C, Franke D, Harkanyi Z, et al. Role of Contrast-Enhanced Ultrasound (CEUS) in paediatric practice: an EFSUMB position statement. Ultraschall Med. 2017;38:33–43.
62. Wu W, Chen MH, Yin SS, Yan K, Fan ZH, Yang W, Dai Y, et al. The role of contrast-enhanced sonography of focal liver lesions before percutaneous biopsy. AJR Am J Roentgenol. 2006;187:752–61.
63. Bang N, Bachmann Nielsen M, Vejborg I, Mellon Mogensen A. Clinical report: contrast enhancement of tumor perfusion as a guidance for biopsy. Eur J Ultrasound. 2000;12:159–61.
64. Sparchez Z, Radu P, Zaharia T, Kacso G, Grigorescu I, Botis G, Badea R. Usefulness of contrast enhanced ultrasound guidance in percutaneous biopsies of liver tumors. J Gastrointestin Liver Dis. 2011;20:191–6.
65. Yoon SH, Lee KH, Kim SY, Kim YH, Kim JH, Lee SH, Kim TK. Real-time contrast-enhanced ultrasound-guided biopsy of focal hepatic lesions not localised on B-mode ultrasound. Eur Radiol. 2010;20:2047–56.
66. Lackey L 2nd, Peterson C, Barr RG. Contrast-enhanced ultrasound-guided radiofrequency ablation of renal tumors. Ultrasound Q. 2012;28:269–74.
67. Ignee A, Boerner N, Bruening A, Dirks K, von Herbay A, Jenssen C, Kubale R, et al. Duplex sonography of the mesenteric vessels—a critical evaluation of inter-observer variability. Z Gastroenterol. 2016;54:304–11.
68. Sanz E, Hevia V, Arias F, Fabuel JJ, Alvarez S, Rodriguez-Patron R, Gomez V, et al. Contrast-

enhanced ultrasound (CEUS): an excellent tool in the follow-up of small renal masses treated with cryoablation. Curr Urol Rep. 2015;16:469.
69. Meloni MF, Bertolotto M, Alberzoni C, Lazzaroni S, Filice C, Livraghi T, Ferraioli G. Follow-up after percutaneous radiofrequency ablation of renal cell carcinoma: contrast-enhanced sonography versus contrast-enhanced CT or MRI. AJR Am J Roentgenol. 2008;191:1233–8.
70. Schreiber-Dietrich DG, Cui XW, Piscaglia F, Gilja OH, Dietrich CF. Contrast enhanced ultrasound in pediatric patients: a real challenge. Z Gastroenterol. 2014;52:1178–84.
71. Dietrich CF, Maurer M, Riemer-Hommel P. Challenges for the German health care system—pharmaceuticals. Endheu. 2014;27:45–53.
72. Esposito F, Di Serafino M, Sgambati P, Mercogliano F, Tarantino L, Vallone G, Oresta P. Ultrasound contrast media in paediatric patients: is it an off-label use? Regulatory requirements and radiologist's liability. Radiol Med. 2012;117:148–59.
73. Chiorean L, Cui XW, Tannapfel A, Franke D, Stenzel M, Kosiak W, Schreiber-Dietrich D, et al. Benign liver tumors in pediatric patients—review with emphasis on imaging features. World J Gastroenterol. 2015;21:8541–61.
74. Ignee A, Schuessler G, Cui XW. Endocavernous contrast-enhanced ultrasound—different applications, literature review and future perspectives. Ultraschall Med. 2013;34:2–26.
75. Nylund K, Maconi G, Hollerweger A, Ripolles T, Pallotta N, Higginson A, Serra C, Dietrich CF, Sporea I, Saftoiu A, Dirks K, Hausken T, Calabrese E, Romanini L, Maaser C, Nuernberg D, Gilja OH. EFSUMB Recommendations and Guidelines for Gastrointestinal Ultrasound. Ultraschall Med. 2017;38(3):e1–15. English. https://doi.org/10.1055/s-0042-115853. Epub 2016 Sep 7. PMID: 27604052.
76. Nylund K, Maconi G, Hollerweger A, Ripolles T, Pallotta N, Higginson A, Serra C, Dietrich CF, Sporea I, Saftoiu A, Dirks K, Hausken T, Calabrese E, Romanini L, Maaser C, Nuernberg D, Gilja OH. EFSUMB Recommendations and Guidelines for Gastrointestinal Ultrasound. Ultraschall Med. 2017;38(3):273–84. English. https://doi.org/10.1055/s-0042-115410. Epub 2016 Sep 7. PMID: 27604051.
77. Cui XW, Ignee A, Maros T, Straub B, Wen JG, Dietrich CF. Feasibility and usefulness of intra-cavitary contrast-enhanced ultrasound in percutaneous nephrostomy. Ultrasound Med Biol. 2016;42:2180–8.
78. Ignee A, Cui X, Schuessler G, Dietrich CF. Percutaneous transhepatic cholangiography and drainage using extravascular contrast enhanced ultrasound. Z Gastroenterol. 2015;53:385–90.
79. Ignee A, Jenssen C, Cui XW, Schuessler G, Dietrich CF. Intracavitary contrast-enhanced ultrasound in abscess drainage—feasibility and clinical value. Scand J Gastroenterol. 2016;51:41–7.
80. Darge K. Voiding urosonography with US contrast agents for the diagnosis of vesicoureteric reflux in children. II. Comparison with radiological examinations. Pediatr Radiol. 2008;38:54–63; quiz 126–7.
81. Darge K. Voiding urosonography with ultrasound contrast agents for the diagnosis of vesicoureteric reflux in children. I. Procedure. Pediatr Radiol. 2008;38:40–53.
82. Zengel P, Siedek V, Berghaus A, Clevert DA. Intraductally applied contrast-enhanced ultrasound (IA-CEUS) for improved visualization of obstructive diseases of the salivary glands, primary results. Clin Hemorheol Microcirc. 2010;45:193–205.
83. Lanzani C, Savasi V, Leone FP, Ratti M, Ferrazzi E. Two-dimensional HyCoSy with contrast tuned imaging technology and a second-generation contrast media for the assessment of tubal patency in an infertility program. Fertil Steril. 2009;92:1158–61.
84. Zuber-Jerger I, Endlicher E, Scholmerich J, Klebl F. Endoscopic retrograde cholangiography with contrast ultrasonography. Endoscopy. 2008;40(Suppl 2):E202.
85. Chew SS, Yang JL, Newstead GL, Douglas PR. Anal fistula: Levovist-enhanced endoanal ultrasound: a pilot study. Dis Colon Rectum. 2003;46:377–84.
86. Rosch T, Meining A, Fruhmorgen S, Zillinger C, Schusdziarra V, Hellerhoff K, Classen M, et al. A prospective comparison of the diagnostic accuracy of ERCP, MRCP, CT, and EUS in biliary strictures. Gastrointest Endosc. 2002;55:870–6.
87. Tranquart F, Mercier L, Frinking P, et al. Perfusion quantification in Contrast-Enhanced Ultra-sound (CEUS)—ready for research projects and routine clinical use. Ultraschall Med. 2012;33:S31–8.
88. Piscaglia F, Bolondi L, Italian Society for Ultrasound in Medicine and Biology (SIUMB) Study Group on Ultrasound Contrast Agents. The safety of Sonovue in abdominal applications: retrospective analysis of 23188 investigations. Ultrasound Med Biol. 2006;32:1369–75.
89. Kusnetzky LL, Khalid A, Khumri TM, Moe TG, Jones PG, Main ML. Acute mortality in hospitalized patients undergoing echocardiography with and without an ultrasound contrast agent: results in 18,671 consecutive studies. J Am Coll Cardiol. 2008;51:1704–6.
90. Main ML, Ryan AC, Davis TE, Albano MP, Kusnetzky LL, Hibberd M. Acute mortality in hospitalized patients undergoing echocardiography with and without an ultrasound contrast agent (multicenter registry results in 4,300,966 consecutive patients). Am J Cardiol. 2008;102:1742–6.
91. Dolan MS, Gala SS, Dodla S, Abdelmoneim SS, Xie F, Cloutier D, Bierig M, et al. Safety and efficacy of commercially available ultrasound contrast agents for rest and stress echocardiography a multicenter experience. J Am Coll Cardiol. 2009;53:32–8.

92. Aggeli C, Giannopoulos G, Roussakis G, Christoforatou E, Marinos G, Toli C, Pitsavos C, et al. Safety of myocardial flash-contrast echocardiography in combination with dobutamine stress testing for the detection of ischaemia in 5250 studies. Heart. 2008;94:1571–7.
93. Szebeni J. Complement activation-related pseudoallergy: a new class of drug-induced acute immune toxicity. Toxicology. 2005;216:106–21.
94. Bokor D, Chambers JB, Rees PJ, Mant TG, Luzzani F, Spinazzi A. Clinical safety of SonoVue, a new contrast agent for ultrasound imaging, in healthy volunteers and in patients with chronic obstructive pulmonary disease. Invest Radiol. 2001;36:104–9.

Contrast Agents in Pregnancy and Breastfeeding

11

Bora Korkmazer

Abbreviations

ACLS	Advanced cardiovascular life support
ACOG	The American College of Obstetricians and Gynecologists
ACR	The American College of Radiology
CSF	Cerebrospinal fluid
CT	Computed tomography
ESUR	The European Society of Urogenital Radiology
FDA	The Food and Drug Administration
GBCA	Gadolinium-based contrast agent
HOCM	High-osmolar contrast media
HSG	Hysterosalpingography
IV	Intravenous
LOCM	Low-osmolar contrast media
MRI	Magnetic resonance imaging
PO	Per Os
SAR	Specific absorption rate
TSH	Thyroid-stimulating hormone
USCA	Ultrasound contrast agent

11.1 Introduction

Radiological imaging is an important key player which ultimately leads to determining the final diagnosis. In the last few decades due to the advancements in technology, emergence of new radiological modalities, and ease of access to imaging methods, there is an increasing trend especially in the use of noninvasive diagnostic radiological modalities. Pregnancy also does not constitute an exception in this trend, and utilization rates of all radiological examinations on pregnant women were demonstrated to increase 107% from 1997 to 2006 by a study conducted by Lazarus et al. [1]. The main share in this increment was attributed to CT examinations (approximately 25% per year), and the most common indications were trauma and suspected pulmonary embolism [1, 2]. Similar to the significant increase in radiological examinations in pregnant women, CT and MRI are being increasingly used in the evaluation of women during breastfeeding period [3].

Although ultrasonography is the first step radiological examination in pregnancy and lactation period, radiological modalities, which may require contrast material to increase the diagnostic yield, such as CT and MRI are also frequently used for definitive diagnosis when medically indicated. When the use of a contrast-enhanced modality is being considered in pregnancy or lactation, besides the ionizing radiation exposure

B. Korkmazer (✉)
Radiology, Istanbul University-Cerrahpasa
Cerrahpasa Medical Faculty, Istanbul, Turkey

S. M. Erturk et al. (eds.), *Medical Imaging Contrast Agents: A Clinical Manual*,
https://doi.org/10.1007/978-3-030-79256-5_11

and high magnetic field, the potential harmful effects related to contrast media should also be kept in mind.

In this chapter, the use of different types of contrast media during pregnancy and lactation, as well as the management of allergic reactions following contrast agent use during pregnancy and periprocedural counseling, are discussed in detail.

11.2 Iodinated Contrast Agents

When radiological examinations, which require iodinated contrast agents, are considered during pregnancy, the major concern is the exposure of fetus to ionizing radiation. Ionizing radiation exposure in the fetal period has the potential to cause stochastic effects that may result in carcinogenesis and deterministic effects such as malformation, growth retardation, mental retardation, and death. Despite these potential risks, CT remains an essential imaging modality especially in the emergency setting, and a significant increase was demonstrated by Lazarus et al. in the use of CT examinations during pregnancy in the last few decades [1, 4]. One of the most important sources of this trend is pulmonary CT angiography, which requires IV administration of iodinated contrast agents.

11.2.1 Types and FDA Categories

Iodinated contrast agents are derived from a triiodobenzoic acid which is a benzene ring covalently bonded to the three iodine atoms. Modifications of non-iodinated positions 1, 3, and 5 on the benzene ring lead to change in the physical, pharmacological, and chemical properties of the compound [5]. These agents are classified according to the chemical structures, iodine content, ionization in solution, viscosity, and osmolarity [6].

The first-generation iodinated contrast agents are high-osmolar ionic monomers with an osmolarity up to 7 or 8 times greater than blood (1400 mOsm/kg) and have been associated with a relative high risk of adverse reactions. Low-osmolar (600–800 mOsm/kg) nonionic compounds (second-generation) and iso-osmolar (290 mOsm/kg) nonionic dimer iodixanol (third-generation) have been developed to replace first-generation compounds for providing better safety [5, 6].

Except diatrizoate meglumine and diatrizoate meglumine sodium whose parenteral forms are listed as pregnancy category C drugs, iodinated contrast agents are classified as pregnancy category B drugs [7].

11.2.2 Transplacental Transfer and Biodistribution Within Fetus

The placenta allows the physiologic exchange of various substances between the maternal and fetal circulations by acting as a dynamic barrier that evolves over the course of pregnancy [3, 8]. This barrier mainly forms a single layer of chorionic epithelium between the fetal connective tissue and the placental villi surrounded by maternal blood [9].

Although there are several mechanisms of transplacental passage of nutrients, hormones, waste products, and drugs, passive diffusion is the main pathway by which drugs cross the placental barrier [9, 10]. In this transition process, the chorionic epithelium acts as other lipid membranes in the body, permitting the passage of fat-soluble molecules and low-molecular-weight water-soluble structures (<100 Da). Nonionic iodinated contrast agents currently used in radiological examinations are water-soluble, and their molecular weight ranges between 777 and 1550 Da. Therefore, the transplacental transition of these contrast agents with passive diffusion is limited when compared to small water-soluble molecules [9].

Contrast agents that enter the fetal systemic circulation by crossing the placental barrier are excreted from the fetal kidneys to the bladder and reach the amniotic fluid via the urine. By swallowing the amniotic fluid, a small amount of contrast material enters the fetal gastrointestinal tract. In addition, as an alternative way, it is thought that little amount of contrast material passes directly from the maternal blood to the amniotic fluid [9].

Experimental studies in animals and humans have shown transplacental passage of ionic contrast agents, especially following IV urography and cholecystography [7, 11, 12].

Iobitridol, a nonionic iodinated contrast medium, was shown to be below the quantification limits in the amniotic fluid (<0.1 mgI/mL) and fetal plasma (<0.2 mgI/mL) up to 24 h after administration of intravenous injection in gestating rabbits [13]. It was reported that only 0.003% of the injected dose of iohexol and iobitridol reached fetal blood in rabbits [13]. In addition, it has also been demonstrated that nonionic contrast agents may pass the human placenta and accumulate in various fetal tissues and body fluids such as gastrointestinal system, urine, and CSF [14–16].

11.2.3 Potential Harmful Effects

11.2.3.1 Mutagenicity and Teratogenicity

In vitro studies in cultured human lymphocytes using both bacterial (Ames) testing and sister chromatid exchange methods showed no mutagenic activity with three ionic iodinated agents [17]. Several in vitro systems and in vivo studies in animals with nonionic iodinated contrast media elicited no evidence of teratogenic or mutagenic potential [18–21]. There are no well-controlled studies regarding the teratogenic effects of iodinated contrast agents in pregnant women [22].

11.2.3.2 Effects on Fetal-Neonatal Thyroid Function

Thyroid function during fetal and neonatal period is crucial for neurological development and metabolism. Studies with both animals and humans reported that the maternal administration of pharmacologic quantities of iodine found in some medications may lead to neonatal thyroid dysfunction [23, 24]. Maternal administration of iodinated contrast agents may also impair fetal-neonatal thyroid function, and this is one of the most important potential harmful effects of iodinated contrast agents after transplacental passage [25].

The free iodide in the iodinated contrast media is thought to be the harmful component, and this forms either as a result of deiodination of the contrast agent or as a contamination product [26]. Free iodide as a contaminant is known to occur in both ionic and nonionic iodinated contrast media without significant difference between these groups [27]. The extent of deiodination that occurs is dependent partially on the duration that contrast media remains in the circulation [27].

Biologically effective load of free iodide is closely related to the status of thyroid maturation, and at a gestational age less than 36 weeks, thyroid follicular cells are unable to modify iodine uptake adequately by autoregulation [28]. This leads to inhibition of biosynthesis and secretion of thyroid hormones (Wolff-Chaikoff effect) as a consequence of high intracellular iodide concentration following iodine exposure [28, 29].

The adverse effects of iodinated contrast media on fetal thyroid function were firstly shown after amniofetography using liposoluble compounds with impaired TSH values in the neonatal period [30]. Similarly, neonatal hypothyroidism was shown following maternal HSG using liposoluble contrast agents in patients with infertility problems. The frequency of neonatal thyroid dysfunction after maternal ethiodized-oil HSG was higher (2.4%) when compared with the recall rate for the first congenital hypothyroidism screening (0.7%) in Tokyo, Japan [31]. Liposoluble iodinated contrast agents (e.g., Lipiodol) cross placental barrier more easily and are deposited in the vernix [32]. Due to their relatively poor excretion, they cause prolonged exposure of fetal thyroid to excessive iodine, thus leading to a more pronounced effect on fetal thyroid function [29]. These agents are no longer used in imaging during pregnancy [32].

Several studies in the literature demonstrated that maternal exposure to water-soluble nonionic iodinated contrast agents does not significantly affect neonatal thyroid function as indicated by normal neonatal TSH levels, because the total amount of free excess iodide present in fetal circulation is small and exposure of fetal thyroid is transient [25, 29, 32–34].

In the case of impaired maternal renal function, the elimination of contrast material from circulation is delayed, and therefore the detrimental effect of iodides on fetal thyroid may increase in maternal renal failure [33].

If the mother received iodinated contrast material during her pregnancy, the Contrast Media Safety Committee of the European Society of Urogenital Radiology recommends the evaluation of thyroid function of the newborn in the first week of life [9]. However, it is suggested that this approach should be reserved for premature infants and newborns whose mothers are exposed to other drugs during pregnancy [7].

11.2.4 Excretion of Iodinated Contrast Agents into Breast Milk

The drugs can gain entry to breast milk by two routes, through alveolar cells or intercellular clefts. In the first, the drug moves through multiple membranes and intracellular fluids to ultimately reach the alveolar lumen. The second way is an alternative route which provides a more direct passage through the intercellular clefts if they are of low molecular weight [35]. If a drug has high lipid solubility and high affinity for plasma and milk proteins, it is more likely to be concentrated in breast milk [9, 35]. In view of these general concepts, transition of iodinated contrast agents, which have high water solubility and minimal protein binding, into breast milk is limited [9].

Liposoluble cholecystographic agent, iopanoic acid; intrathecally administered nonionic water-soluble agent, metrizamide; and monomer ionic water-soluble contrast media for urography showed limited excretion into breast milk [36–38]. Nielsen et al. demonstrated that the amount of 24-h excretion into milk was approximately 0.5% of the weight-adjusted maternal dose for intravenously administered iohexol and metrizoate [39].

Only a very small portion of the iodinated contrast material, which enters the gut through breastfeeding, reaches into the bloodstream. The expected absorbed dose of contrast material by the breast-fed infant ends up being less than 0.05% of the recommended dose if the infant were to undergo a contrast-enhanced imaging study [4]. The likelihood of direct toxicity or allergic reaction following the use of iodinated contrast agents during lactation is very low [4, 9]. Consequently, iodinated contrast agents are considered safe for nursing mothers. However, preterm infants, who may have immature autoregulation mechanisms of thyroid axis, are at risk for transient hypothyroidism and require special consideration [3, 32].

Similar to all medicines and foodstuffs, the iodinated contrast agents may slightly alter the taste of milk for a short period of time [9, 32].

11.2.5 Current Recommendations for the Use of Iodinated Contrast Agents in Pregnancy

Different scientific societies have published recommendations suggesting that iodine-based contrast media may be given to pregnant or potentially pregnant patients if it is necessary to obtain additional diagnostic information that may affect the care of the fetus or woman (Table 11.1) [22, 40, 41].

The use of iodinated contrast agents may be wise if the contrast agent is likely to contribute to the definitive diagnosis and non-diagnostic CT examination is possibly to be repeated due to imaging limitations [2].

Since there are no available data indicating that exposure to iodinated contrast media may lead to any possible harm to the fetus, the ACR does not recommend routine screening for pregnancy prior to contrast media use [22].

To reduce the potential risks related to contrast media agents, different institutions have developed a series of steps for the use of contrast media. These steps mainly consist of intravenous or oral hydration, selection of the appropriate iodinated contrast agent (LOCM vs. HOCM),

Table 11.1 Professional society guidelines for iodinated contrast agent use in pregnancy and lactation

	ACR 2021 [22]	ESUR 2018 [40]	ACOG 2017 [41]
Iodinated contrast agents in pregnancy	"We do not recommend withholding the use of iodinated contrast agents in pregnant or potentially pregnant patients when it is needed for diagnostic purposes" "Given the current available data and routine evaluation of all newborns for congenital hypothyroidism by measurement of TSH levels at the time of their birth, no extra attention is felt to be necessary"	"In exceptional circumstances, when radiographic examination is essential, iodine-based contrast media may be given to the pregnant female" "Following administration of iodine-based contrast media to the mother during pregnancy, thyroid function should be checked in the neonate during the first week"	"Iodinated contrast should only be used if absolutely required to obtain additional diagnostic information that will affect the care of the fetus or woman during the pregnancy"
Iodinated contrast agents in lactation	"Because of the very small percentage of iodinated contrast medium that is excreted into the breast milk and absorbed by the infant's gut, we believe that the available data suggest that it is safe for the mother and infant to continue breast-feeding after receiving such an agent"	"Breast feeding may be continued normally when iodine-based contrast media is given to the mother"	"Breastfeeding can be continued without interruption after the use of iodinated contrast"

ACOG American Congress of Obstetricians and Gynecologists, *ACR* American College of Radiology, *ESUR* European Society of Urogenital Radiology

administration of the lowest possible iodinated contrast agent dose for diagnosis, and obtaining renal function tests within 3 months of the contrast agent administration [7].

Following maternal administration of iodinated contrast media during pregnancy, the newborn should be screened for hypothyroidism in the first week of life, which is already a standard practice in most regions of the world [2, 22, 40].

11.2.6 Current Recommendations for the Use of Iodinated Contrast Agents in Breastfeeding

Different scientific societies advise that breastfeeding can be continued without interruption after administration of intravenous iodinated contrast agents that have been shown to reach into the infant's bloodstream at very low levels (Table 11.1) [22, 40, 41].

Before deciding to temporarily stop breastfeeding after the intravenous administration of the contrast agent, the mother should be informed that even short-term cessation periods might lead to complete weaning and the decision must be left to the mother. If the mother decides to stop breastfeeding temporarily, this period should be between 12 and 24 h and during which time breast milk should be pumped and discarded. There is no value of breastfeeding cessation beyond 24 h, since contrast agent is undetectable in the maternal circulation after this period. It may also be advisable to use a breast pump for obtaining milk before contrast-enhanced examination to feed the infant during the period of cessation [2, 22].

11.3 Gadolinium-Based Contrast Agents (GBCAs)

Pregnancy and lactation are unique periods in which patients were differentiated from other patient groups in terms of diagnostic imaging considering the radiosensitivity of the fetus and maternal breast tissue. As a result, imaging algorithms in these periods are based on the use of ultrasound primarily and MRI as the second choice in order to minimize the risk of exposure to ionizing radiation [42, 43]. Despite the potential for tissue heating due to MR gradient changes and fetal ear damage secondary to acoustic noise, no damage to a developing human fetus caused by MRI has been documented [3, 44]. MRI is considered to be safe in any gestational age [45]; however, it should be performed only when benefits outweigh potential risks, and care should be taken regarding SAR limits [44].

Following the approval of the first gadolinium-based MRI contrast agent by the FDA in 1988, the use of MRI was significantly increased, and gadolinium-based contrast agents are administered in up to 35% of MRI examinations currently performed in clinical practice [43].

In addition to GBCAs, iron particulates and manganese-based agents are also used in contrast-enhanced MRI studies; however, none of them have provided large-scale alternative to gadolinium-based agents [46]. Manganese-based agents are no longer available due to their toxicity [7, 47].

11.3.1 Types and FDA Categories

The gadolinium ion is a known toxic rare earth metal and has a long biologic half-life; it should be administrated as a complex with a chelating ligand in humans [46, 47]. The chelate is a carrier molecule whose aim is to remain bound to gadolinium ion until it is excreted from circulation, thereby preventing intracellular uptake and deposition of free gadolinium in tissues [43]. GBCAs can be classified depending on their molecular structure (linear, macrocyclic) and also be subdivided according to their chemical preparation (ionic, nonionic) [7]. Since the gadolinium ion is trapped in a molecular cavity within the chelating agent, macrocyclic compounds (gadobutrol, gadoteridol, and gadoterate meglumine) tend to be more stable than linear compounds, allowing a lower rate of dissociation of the free gadolinium ion [46]. While nonionic linear contrast agents (gadodiamide and gadoversetamide) are the least chemically stable molecules in which gadolinium is prone to dissociate from the chelated form, the ionic linear chelate molecules (gadopentetate dimeglumine, gadobenate dimeglumine, and gadofosveset) have intermediate stability [7, 46].

GBCAs are classified as pregnancy category C drugs by the FDA, meaning that animal studies have demonstrated adverse effects on the fetus (at supraclinical and repeated doses); however, there have been no well-controlled studies in humans. Therefore, they should be administered only if the potential benefits outweigh the potential risks to the fetus [3, 7].

11.3.2 Transplacental Transfer and Biodistribution Within Fetus

GBCAs currently used in radiological examinations are water-soluble, and their molecular weight ranges between 558 and 1058 Da. Therefore, the transplacental transition of these contrast agents with passive diffusion is limited when compared to small water-soluble molecules [9].

Studies were conducted with different contrast agents in order to evaluate the placental transfer of radiological contrast agents on gravid rats, rhesus monkeys, and macaques [48–51]. Studies with gadopentetate dimeglumine, gadodiamide, and gadoteridol showed very low levels (approximately 170 times lower than those in the maternal plasma) of contrast material in the placenta, amniotic fluid, and fetal tissues after maternal injection. 0.01% of the injected dose of gadodiamide in the first 4 h following maternal injection showed fetal distribution in rats [51].

Although the highest amount of GBCAs were detected in the first 5 min after the injection, the progressive decrease in the presence of contrast material was shown in the measurements up to 45 h with trace amounts in fetal tissues after 24 h [48, 49, 51].

Following maternal injection, gadolinium concentrations increase in fetal kidneys, and the relative concentration is found to be the highest in fetal kidneys among all fetal tissues [48, 49, 51]. This is an indicator of fetal renal excretion of gadolinium and can be used for the exclusion of renal and bladder-related pathologies in pregnant women with reduced amniotic fluid [48]. Concentrations of gadolinium remain low in fetal liver, muscle, heart, brain, femur, and skin [48, 49].

Because the contrast medium remains in the circulation for a longer period of time in pregnant women with impaired renal function, the fetal dose may increase due to more contrast material passage through placenta [3]. Furthermore, contrast agents may return to the maternal circulation through the placenta and reduce the fetal dose, thus allowing the maternal excretion of the contrast agent [9, 52, 53].

The longer GBCAs remain in the amniotic fluid, the greater the potential for dissociation from the chelating ligand and, thus, the risk of causing harm to the fetus [45].

11.3.3 Potential Harmful Effects

11.3.3.1 Mutagenicity and Teratogenicity

Free gadolinium is known to be toxic and is administered only in a chelated form [41]. Currently, the vast majority of the information regarding the use of GBCAs during pregnancy has been derived from animal studies. In an animal study on rabbits, repeated and high doses (two to seven times higher than those used in humans for medical imaging) of intravenous gadolinium have been shown to be teratogenic, possibly due to prolonged duration in the circulation allows dissociation of gadolinium from the chelation agent [41, 43, 54]. On the contrary, no teratogenic effect or chromosomal damage was demonstrated in several animal studies following administration of GBCAs [55–57].

There is no well-controlled fetal toxicity studies regarding the use of gadolinium-based contrast media conducted in humans during pregnancy. However, no teratogenic effect was reported in a prospective cohort study on neonates inadvertently exposed to gadolinium derivatives in utero during the first trimester of pregnancy [58]. Neonatal anomalies were also not detected in the infants of two women who underwent contrast-enhanced MRI to diagnose Crohn's disease during pregnancy [59]. Two studies with contrast-enhanced MRI using GBCAs to assess normal placenta and placental pathologies in the second and third trimesters of pregnancy did not detect any fetal effects secondary to gadolinium exposure [60, 61].

A recent study by Ray et al. demonstrated no significantly higher risk for congenital anomalies, neoplasm, and vision or hearing loss among infants exposed to GBCAs during the first trimester of pregnancy; however, gadolinium MRI at any time during pregnancy was associated with an increased risk of a broad set of rheumatological, inflammatory, or infiltrative skin conditions and for stillbirth or neonatal death [62]. Although these findings raise a concern regarding the use of gadolinium-based agents during pregnancy, there are substantial limitations in the study. The control group included patients who did not undergo MRI during pregnancy, rather than patients who underwent MRI without GBCAs [22, 41]. Whether any of the children were exposed to GBCAs after birth was not investigated. And also the number of cases of connective tissue or skin disease similar to nephrogenic systemic fibrosis was considered too small for statistical analysis [22].

There are no available animal or human studies evaluating the safety of maternally administered superparamagnetic iron oxide contrast agents on the fetus or breast-fed baby; therefore if contrast-enhanced MR is to be performed, GBCAs should be preferred [41].

11.3.4 Excretion of Gadolinium-Based Contrast Agents into Milk

Similar to iodinated contrast agents, GBCAs are water-soluble and have low affinity to milk proteins. Therefore gadolinium-based contrast media are excreted into human breast milk at low levels [9, 43]. In a study including 20 breastfeeding women who were administered IV gadopentetate dimeglumine, the cumulative amount of gadolinium excreted in human breast milk during 24 h was 0.003 mmol, with the dose being less than 0.04% of the maternal intravenous dose administered for all cases [63]. In addition, less than 1% of the dose in breast milk is absorbed by the infant gastrointestinal tract into the bloodstream. As a result, the effective circulatory dose of infant is at least 10,000 times less than the dose of intravenously administered gadolinium-based contrast media for contrast-enhanced MRI with any indication in the neonatal period [43].

There are no available case reports in the literature regarding adverse events in infants attributable to GBCA containing breast milk.

GBCAs may cause a temporary alteration in the taste of breast milk [9, 32].

11.3.5 Current Recommendations for the Use of Gadolinium-Based Contrast Agents in Pregnancy

Various professional societies have issued guidelines regarding the use of GBCAs during pregnancy to assist healthcare providers (Table 11.2) [22, 40, 41]. The general consensus is that GBCAs can be administered in pregnant patients on a case-by-case basis if maternal and fetal benefits outweigh the potential risks of fetal gadolinium exposure.

If the decision is made to administer a GBCA to a pregnant woman, agents which tightly bind the gadolinium ion and have high stability constants (macrocyclic compounds) should be used at the lowest possible dose [2, 22, 40, 43].

Neonatal tests are not required following the maternal administration of GBCAs during pregnancy [40].

11.3.6 Current Recommendations for the Use of Gadolinium-Based Contrast Agents in Breastfeeding

The ACR and the ACOG advise that breastfeeding should not be interrupted after maternal administration of GBCAs. The ESUR also recommends that breastfeeding may be continued normally when macrocyclic GBCAs are given to the mother [22, 40, 41] (Table 11.2).

Table 11.2 Guidelines for GBCA use in pregnancy and lactation

	ACR 2021 [22]	ESUR 2018 [40]	ACOG 2017 [41]
GBCAs in pregnancy	"Each case should be reviewed carefully by members of the clinical and radiology service groups, and a GBCA should be administered only when there is a potential significant benefit to the patient or fetus that outweighs the possible but unknown risk of fetal exposure to free gadolinium ions"	"When there is a very strong indication for enhanced MR, the smallest possible dose of a macrocyclic gadolinium contrast agent may be given to the pregnant female" "Following administration of gadolinium-based agents to the mother during pregnancy, no neonatal tests are necessary"	"The use of gadolinium contrast with MRI should be limited; it may be used as a contrast agent in a pregnant woman only if it significantly improves diagnostic performance and is expected to improve fetal or maternal outcome"
GBCAs in lactation	"Because of the very small percentage of gadolinium-based contrast medium that is excreted into the breast milk and absorbed by the infant's gut, we believe that the available data suggest that it is safe for the mother and infant to continue breast-feeding after receiving such an agent"	"Breastfeeding may be continued normally when macrocyclic gadolinium-based contrast agents are given to the mother"	"Breastfeeding should not be interrupted after gadolinium administration"

ACOG American Congress of Obstetricians and Gynecologists, *ACR* American College of Radiology, *ESUR* European Society of Urogenital Radiology, *GBCA* gadolinium-based contrast agent

If the mother remains to be concerned about any possible adverse effects to the infant despite appropriate counseling, she may temporarily stop breastfeeding for 12–24 h after administration of the contrast agent, and breast milk should be pumped and discarded in this period [2, 22]. Similar to iodinated contrast agents, GBCAs have a plasma half-life of about 2 h and are completely cleared from the bloodstream within 24 h in patients with normal renal function [22].

11.4 Ultrasound Contrast Agents (USCAs)

The USCAs are composed of inert gas encapsulated by a protective shell and are used to demonstrate blood flow at the microcirculatory level by specialized imaging techniques [64, 65]. Following IV injection, they improve the visualization of blood flow with respect to the surrounding tissues mainly by increasing back-scattering intensity when compared to body fluids and other tissues [64].

Microbubble size and uniformity are of great importance because microbubbles with a diameter of smaller than 10 μm are not trapped within capillary structures and thus reducing the risk of microembolism [66]. There are only a few products approved for clinical use, and they all consist of gas-filled microbubbles with a mean diameter less than a red blood cell [64].

These contrast media are used mainly in cardiovascular applications and diagnosis of tumors. Although the characterization of the liver masses constitutes the main field of application, they have been shown to be effective in the diagnosis of many other solid organ pathologies over recent years [65]. These agents can also be used to evaluate the placenta, corpus luteum, and uteroplacental circulation [7, 66].

These agents are fundamentally intravascular and do not show any interstitial distribution as opposed to other contrast agents administered through IV route. Neither do these agents interact with the thyroid gland nor have renal excretion thus can be safely applied in case of acute or chronic renal failure [67, 68].

Although the biochemical structure of USCAs does not permit transplacental passage and none of the studies using these agents in pregnant patients show fetal or maternal side effects, ultrasound contrast media have not yet been approved for clinical use in pregnancy and lactation [7, 66, 69, 70]. The main concerns regarding the use of ultrasound contrast agents in pregnancy are lodging of contrast agent in the microcirculation, complement activation, and microhemorrhages as a result of cavitation [71].

Serious adverse reactions after administration of USCAs are reported to be approximately in 1/10,000 patients [72].

11.5 Gastrointestinal Contrast Agents

Barium agents are non-water-soluble contrast media which are preferred to visualize the gastrointestinal tract. The particles of barium sulfate suspension remain in the gastrointestinal lumen and are not absorbed from the gut due its extremely low solubility [73, 74].

Barium sulfate has not been formally assigned to a pregnancy category by the FDA. Although the radiological modalities using barium are not preferred in pregnancy due to the possible harmful effects of ionizing radiation to the fetus, almost all of barium studies performed during pregnancy have been done inadvertently in women who are yet unaware of their pregnancies [75, 76].

Studies conducted by Han et al. demonstrated no association between the use of barium sulfate for gastrointestinal imaging during pregnancy and adverse fetal outcomes [75, 76]. Results of these studies and poor absorption of barium sulfate from gastrointestinal system suggest that barium salts are unlikely to be of major concern in pregnancy [7, 75]. However, the effects of ionizing radiation in pregnancy constitute the main concern that prevents the frequent use of radiological modalities requiring barium agents.

The incidence of adverse effects and allergic reactions following barium sulfate administration in pregnant women is similar to the rest of the population and is rare [7]. The most common adverse effects related to barium contrast media are almost always mild with symptoms such as nausea, vomiting, abdominal cramps, and discomfort. Allergic-like reactions secondary to enteric barium are very rare with frequencies of mild reactions, and moderate-severe reactions are reported to be 1/750,000 examinations and 1/2,500,000 exposures, respectively [22].

11.6 Management of Adverse Reactions Following Contrast Agent Use During Pregnancy

Adverse reactions following IV administration of low-osmolarity iodinated or gadolinium-based contrast agents are estimated to have an incidence of less than 1% [77]. In the literature, there is no evidence that pregnancy increases the risk of allergic reactions to contrast agents, and the factors that increase the risk of adverse reactions to IV contrast agents in pregnancy are similar to those in non-pregnant patients. These factors include a history of prior allergic reaction (especially following the administration of contrast media), asthma, bronchospasm, atopy, significant cardiac or renal disease, and anxiety [78, 79].

11.6.1 Premedication in Patients with Prior Allergic-Like Reactions to Iodinated or Gadolinium-Based Contrast Agents

During pregnancy, anaphylaxis can lead to destructive consequences such as hypoxic-ischemic encephalopathy and persistent central nervous system damage or death [80], and the risk of damage to the fetus is higher than that of the mother [22]. Therefore, the ACR recommends that otherwise-indicated premedication to reduce the risk of contrast media reaction should not be withheld because the patient is pregnant and a standard PO or IV regimen might be employed [22].

Diphenhydramine (FDA pregnancy category B) and corticosteroids (FDA pregnancy category C) are commonly used for prophylaxis in patients at risk for allergic-like contrast reactions to contrast media [22]. Although prednisone and dexamethasone cross the placenta, most of these agents are metabolized within the placenta before reaching the fetus and therefore are not associated with teratogenicity in humans. However, cases of sporadic fetal adrenal suppression have been reported. When methylprednisolone is used before 10 weeks of gestation, it carries a potential risk for development of cleft lip in the fetus [22]. Both referring clinicians and pregnant patients receiving premedication prior to the administration of contrast agents should be counseled appropriately and should indicate that they understand the potential risks and benefits of the medications being used, as well as alternative diagnostic options [22].

11.6.2 Treatment

If a pregnant patient has been considered to have a reaction to the contrast agent, it should be classified as mild, moderate, or severe according to the ACR guidelines [78]. It is important to know that various potential symptoms of anaphylactic reactions unique to pregnancy may be seen such as intense pruritus in the vulva and vagina, low back pain, and uterine cramps [80]. Fetal distress and preterm labor should also be considered as severe reactions [78, 80].

The management of an acute reaction in a pregnant patient is similar to that of a non-pregnant patient, except for a few modifications [78].

During the evaluation and treatment of the reactions to the contrast agents, IV access should be provided, and the vital signs should be monitored for at least 30 min or as long as necessary to ensure clinical stability and improvement of symptoms. The patient should be monitored with pulse oximetry, and oxygen should be given by mask if indicated [78].

Diphenhydramine is the preferred medication for mild to moderate reactions [7].

When interfering with acute anaphylactoid reaction in a pregnant patient, ACLS guidelines should be followed [78]. In addition, the mother should be placed in the left lateral decubitus position, supine with a leftward tilt using a wedge, or supine with manual left uterine displacement for increasing the venous return to the heart by reducing the compression of the inferior vena cava [22, 78]. In the third trimester of pregnancy, continuous external fetal heart rate monitoring should also be initiated to aid in guiding resuscitation efforts due to potential fetal viability [78].

11.7 Periprocedural Counseling

With increasing use of radiological modalities in the evaluation of pregnant and lactating patients in recent years, misperceptions regarding diagnostic radiation and contrast agents often cause unwarranted concerns among patients and clinicians. Consequently these concerns might lead to delays in diagnosis and treatment or even unnecessary termination of pregnancy [2, 54].

Surveys among practitioners have revealed substantial deficiencies in knowledge regarding the safety of diagnostic radiation and contrast agent use during pregnancy [2].

For any radiological examination in pregnancy and lactation, the referring physician and radiologist should take into account the risks and benefits of the proposed contrast-enhanced study and potential imaging alternatives that may provide better diagnostic information. When used appropriately in pregnancy and lactation, benefits derived from contrast-enhanced CT and MR imaging often outweigh the risks [2, 3].

Radiologists should have up-to-date knowledge regarding the effects of radiation and contrast agents during pregnancy and lactation [3]. Radiologists should inform patients appropriately and provide a realistic understanding of the risks associated with imaging modality during pregnancy and lactation [2].

Appropriate counseling services for pregnant women who were exposed to diagnostic radiation and contrast agents during pregnancy can help reduce concerns and prevent unnecessary pregnancy termination [3, 75, 81].

A medical physicist might be consulted post-procedurally to provide accurate dose estimations in order to help the patient in understanding the risks associated with diagnostic radiation exposure especially following studies performed in women who are yet unaware of their pregnancies.

Written informed consent regarding the use of any radiological imaging modality in pregnancy should be obtained before performing the examination. It provides information about the risks and benefits of relevant radiological examination to pregnant patients or relatives of the patient but also allows the clinicians to address the patient's questions and concerns. Informed consent should be prepared in a simple manner and, if appropriate, confirmed by asking the patient to explain the risks and benefits in her own words [2].

References

1. Lazarus E, DeBenedectis C, North D, Spencer PK, Mayo-Smith WW. Utilization of imaging in pregnant patients: 10-year review of 5270 examinations in 3285 patients—1997–2006. Radiology. 2009;251:517–24.
2. Tirada N, Dreizin D, Khati NJ, Akin EA, Zeman RK. Imaging pregnant and lactating patients. Radiographics. 2015;35:1751–65.
3. Tremblay E, Thérasse E, Thomassin-Naggara I, Trop I. Quality initiatives: guidelines for use of medical imaging during pregnancy and lactation. Radiographics. 2012;32:897–911.
4. Wang PI, Chong ST, Kielar AZ, Kelly AM, Knoepp UD, Mazza MB, Goodsitt MM. Imaging of pregnant and lactating patients: part 1, evidence-based review and recommendations. Am J Roentgenol. 2012;198:778–84.
5. Spampinato MV, Abid A, Matheus MG. Current radiographic iodinated contrast agents. Magn Reson Imaging Clin N Am. 2017;25:697–704.
6. Singh J, Daftary A. Iodinated contrast media and their adverse reactions. J Nucl Med Technol. 2008;36:69–74; quiz 76–7.
7. Puac P, Rodríguez A, Vallejo C, Zamora CA, Castillo M. Safety of contrast material use during pregnancy and lactation. Magn Reson Imaging Clin N Am. 2017;25:787–97.
8. Ross Michael H, Kaye Gordon I, Wojciech P. Histology a text and atlas. 4th ed. Baltimore: Susan Katz; 2003.
9. Webb JAW, Thomsen HS, Morcos SK, Members of Contrast Media Safety Committee of European Society of Urogenital Radiology (ESUR). The use of

iodinated and gadolinium contrast media during pregnancy and lactation. Eur Radiol. 2005;15:1234–40.
10. Bourget P, Roulot C, Fernandez H. Models for placental transfer studies of drugs. Clin Pharmacokinet. 1995;28:161–80.
11. David RR, Alexander DS, Wilkins L. Placental transfer of an organic radiopaque medium resulting in a prolonged elevation of the protein-bound iodine. J Pediatr. 1961;59:223–6.
12. Dean PB. Fetal uptake of an intravascular radiologic contrast medium. RöFo. 1977;127:267–70.
13. Bourrinet P, Dencausse A, Havard P, Violas X, Bonnemain B. Transplacental passage and milk excretion of iobitridol. Invest Radiol. 1995;30:156–8.
14. Kato H, Kanematsu M, Orii KE, Morimoto M, Kato Z, Kondo N. Apparition of iodinated contrast agents in twin neonatal gastrointestinal tracts after maternal contrast-enhanced computed tomography. Jpn J Radiol. 2011;29:521–3.
15. Moon AJ, Katzberg RW, Sherman MP. Transplacental passage of iohexol. J Pediatr. 2000;136:548–9.
16. Vanhaesebrouck P, Verstraete AG, De Praeter C, Smets K, Zecic A, Craen M. Transplacental passage of a nonionic contrast agent. Eur J Pediatr. 2005;164:408–10.
17. Nelson JA, Livingston GK, Moon RG. Mutagenic evaluation of radiographic contrast media. Invest Radiol. 1982;17:183–5.
18. Ralston WH, Robbins MS, James P. Reproductive, developmental, and genetic toxicology of ioversol. Invest Radiol. 1989;24(Suppl 1):S16–22.
19. Donandieu AM, Idee JM, Doucet D, Legros A, Penati S, Nain-Dit-Ducret M, Marmion F, Bonnemain B. Toxicologic profile of iobitridol, a new nonionic low-osmolality contrast medium. Acta Radiol Suppl. 1996;400:17–24.
20. Fujikawa K, Sakaguchi Y, Harada S, Holtz E, Smith JA, Svendsen O. Reproductive toxicity of iodixanol, a new non-ionic, iso-tonic contrast medium in rats and rabbits. J Toxicol Sci. 1995;20(Suppl 1):107–15.
21. Morisetti A, Tirone P, Luzzani F, de Haën C. Toxicological safety assessment of iomeprol, a new X-ray contrast agent. Eur J Radiol. 1994;18(Suppl 1):S21–31.
22. American College of Radiology Manual on contrast media. https://www.acr.org/Clinical-Resources/Contrast-Manual. Accessed: 26 June 2021.
23. Robuschi G, Montermini M, Alboni A, Borciani E, Cersosimo G, Negrotti L, Gnudi A, Safran M, Braverman LE, Roti E. Cord blood iodothyronine and thyrotropin concentrations in newborns of mothers exposed to povidone iodine in the last trimester. J Endocrinol Invest. 1987;10:183–6.
24. Theodoropoulos T, Braverman LE, Vagenakis AG. Iodide-induced hypothyroidism: a potential hazard during perinatal life. Science. 1979;205:502–3.
25. Kochi MH, Kaloudis EV, Ahmed W, Moore WH. Effect of in utero exposure of iodinated intravenous contrast on neonatal thyroid function. J Comput Assist Tomogr. 2012;36:165–9.
26. van der Molen AJ, Thomsen HS, Morcos SK, Contrast Media Safety Committee, European Society of Urogenital Radiology (ESUR). Effect of iodinated contrast media on thyroid function in adults. Eur Radiol. 2004;14:902–7.
27. Laurie AJ, Lyon SG, Lasser EC. Contrast material iodides: potential effects on radioactive iodine thyroid uptake. J Nucl Med. 1992;33:237–8.
28. Dembinski J, Arpe V, Kroll M, Hieronimi G, Bartmann P. Thyroid function in very low birthweight infants after intravenous administration of the iodinated contrast medium iopromide. Arch Dis Child Fetal Neonatal Ed. 2000;82:F215–7.
29. Atwell TD, Lteif AN, Brown DL, McCann M, Townsend JE, LeRoy AJ. Neonatal thyroid function after administration of iv iodinated contrast agent to 21 pregnant patients. Am J Roentgenol. 2008;191:268–71.
30. Rodesch F, Camus M, Ermans AM, Dodion J, Delange F. Adverse effect of amniofetography on fetal thyroid function. Am J Obstet Gynecol. 1976;126:723–6.
31. Satoh M, Aso K, Katagiri Y. Thyroid dysfunction in neonates born to mothers who have undergone hysterosalpingography involving an oil-soluble iodinated contrast medium. Horm Res Paediatr. 2015;84:370–5.
32. Bourjeily G, Chalhoub M, Phornphutkul C, Alleyne TC, Woodfield CA, Chen KK. Neonatal thyroid function: effect of a single exposure to iodinated contrast medium in utero. Radiology. 2010;256:744–50.
33. Rajaram S, Exley CE, Fairlie F, Matthews S. Effect of antenatal iodinated contrast agent on neonatal thyroid function. Br J Radiol. 2012;85:e238–42.
34. Chauvet P, Terral D, Colombier M, Mulliez A, Suarez C, Brunhes A, Gallot D. Iodinated contrast in pregnant women and neonatal thyroid function. Gynecol Obstet Fertil. 2016;44:685–9.
35. Wilson JT, Brown RD, Cherek DR, Dailey JW, Hilman B, Jobe PC, Manno BR, Manno JE, Redetzki HM, Stewart JJ. Drug excretion in human breast milk 1,2. Clin Pharmacokinet. 1980;5:1–66.
36. FitzJohn TP, Williams DG, Laker MF, Owen JP. Intravenous urography during lactation. Br J Radiol. 1982;55:603–5.
37. Holmdahl KH. Cholecystography during lactation. Acta Radiol. 1956;45:305–7.
38. Ilett KF, Hackett LP, Paterson JW, McCormick CC. Excretion of metrizamide in milk. Br J Radiol. 1981;54:537–8.
39. Nielsen ST, Matheson I, Rasmussen JN, Skinnemoen K, Andrew E, Hafsahl G. Excretion of iohexol and metrizoate in human breast milk. Acta Radiol. 1987;28:523–6.
40. ESUR. ESUR guidelines on contrast media. 2019. http://www.esur-cm.org/index.php/c-miscellaneous-2#C_5. Accessed 19 May 2019.
41. The American College of Obstetricians and Gynecologists' Commitee on Obstetric Practice Commitee Opinion No.723. Guidelines for diagnostic imaging during pregnancy and lactation. Obstet Gynecol. 2017;130(4):e210–6.

42. Patel SJ, Reede DL, Katz DS, Subramaniam R, Amorosa JK. Imaging the pregnant patient for nonobstetric conditions: algorithms and radiation dose considerations. Radiographics. 2007;27:1705–22.
43. Fraum TJ, Ludwig DR, Bashir MR, Fowler KJ. Gadolinium-based contrast agents: a comprehensive risk assessment. J Magn Reson Imaging. 2017;46:338–53.
44. Bulas D, Egloff A. Benefits and risks of MRI in pregnancy. Semin Perinatol. 2013;37:301–4.
45. Kanal E, Barkovich AJ, Bell C, et al. ACR guidance document on MR safe practices: 2013. J Magn Reson Imaging. 2013;37:501–30.
46. Czeyda-Pommersheim F, Martin DR, Costello JR, Kalb B. Contrast agents for MR imaging. Magn Reson Imaging Clin N Am. 2017;25:705–11.
47. Lin S-P, Brown JJ. MR contrast agents: physical and pharmacologic basics. J Magn Reson Imaging. 2007;25:884–99.
48. Novak Z, Thurmond AS, Ross PL, Jones MK, Thornburg KL, Katzberg RW. Gadolinium-DTPA transplacental transfer and distribution in fetal tissue in rabbits. Invest Radiol. 1993;28:828–30.
49. Oh KY, Roberts VHJ, Schabel MC, Grove KL, Woods M, Frias AE. Gadolinium chelate contrast material in pregnancy: fetal biodistribution in the nonhuman primate. Radiology. 2015;276:110–8.
50. Panigel M, Wolf G, Zeleznick A. Magnetic resonance imaging of the placenta in rhesus monkeys, Macaca mulatta. J Med Primatol. 1988;17:3–18.
51. Okazaki O, Murayama N, Masubuchi N, Nomura H, Hakusui H. Placental transfer and milk secretion of gadodiamide injection in rats. Arzneimittelforschung. 1996;46:83–6.
52. Etling N, Gehin-Fouque F, Vielh JP, Gautray JP. The iodine content of amniotic fluid and placental transfer of iodinated drugs. Obstet Gynecol. 1979;53:376–80.
53. Garcia-Bournissen F, Shrim A, Koren G. Safety of gadolinium during pregnancy. Can Fam Physician. 2006;52:309–10.
54. Chen MM, Coakley FV, Kaimal A, Laros RK. Guidelines for computed tomography and magnetic resonance imaging use during pregnancy and lactation. Obstet Gynecol. 2008;112:333–40.
55. Rofsky NM, Pizzarello DJ, Weinreb JC, Ambrosino MM, Rosenberg C. Effect on fetal mouse development of exposure to MR imaging and gadopentetate dimeglumine. J Magn Reson Imaging. 1994;4:805–7.
56. Soltys RA. Summary of preclinical safety evaluation of gadoteridol injection. Invest Radiol. 1992;27(Suppl 1):S7–11.
57. Morisetti A, Bussi S, Tirone P, de Haën C. Toxicological safety evaluation of gadobenate dimeglumine 0.5 M solution for injection (MultiHance), a new magnetic resonance imaging contrast medium. J Comput Assist Tomogr. 1999;23(Suppl 1):S207–17.
58. De Santis M, Straface G, Cavaliere AF, Carducci B, Caruso A. Gadolinium periconceptional exposure: pregnancy and neonatal outcome. Acta Obstet Gynecol Scand. 2007;86:99–101.
59. Shoenut JP, Semelka RC, Silverman R, Yaffe CS, Micflikier AB. MRI in the diagnosis of Crohn's disease in two pregnant women. J Clin Gastroenterol. 1993;17:244–7.
60. Marcos HB, Semelka RC, Worawattanakul S. Normal placenta: gadolinium-enhanced dynamic MR imaging. Radiology. 1997;205:493–6.
61. Tanaka YO, Sohda S, Shigemitsu S, Niitsu M, Itai Y. High temporal resolution dynamic contrast MRI in a high risk group for placenta accreta. Magn Reson Imaging. 2001;19:635–42.
62. Ray JG, Vermeulen MJ, Bharatha A, Montanera WJ, Park AL. Association between MRI exposure during pregnancy and fetal and childhood outcomes. JAMA. 2016;316:952.
63. Kubik-Huch RA, Gottstein-Aalame NM, Frenzel T, Seifert B, Puchert E, Wittek S, Debatin JF. Gadopentetate dimeglumine excretion into human breast milk during lactation. Radiology. 2000;216:555–8.
64. Jakobsen J, Oyen R, Thomsen HS, Morcos SK, Members of Contrast Media Safety Committee of European Society of Urogenital Radiology (ESUR). Safety of ultrasound contrast agents. Eur Radiol. 2005;15:941–5.
65. Sawhney S, Wilson SR. Can ultrasound with contrast enhancement replace nonenhanced computed tomography scans in patients with contraindication to computed tomography contrast agents? Ultrasound Q. 2017;33:125–32.
66. Ordén M-R, Gudmundsson S, Kirkinen P. Intravascular ultrasound contrast agent: an aid in imaging intervillous blood flow? Placenta. 1999;20:235–40.
67. Miele V, Piccolo CL, Galluzzo M, Ianniello S, Sessa B, Trinci M. Contrast-enhanced ultrasound (CEUS) in blunt abdominal trauma. Br J Radiol. 2016;89:20150823.
68. Pinto F, Miele V, Scaglione M, Pinto A. The use of contrast-enhanced ultrasound in blunt abdominal trauma: advantages and limitations. Acta Radiol. 2014;55:776–84.
69. Schmiedl UP, Komarniski K, Winter TC, Luna JA, Cyr DR, Ruppenthal G, Schlief R. Assessment of fetal and placental blood flow in primates using contrast enhanced ultrasonography. J Ultrasound Med. 1998;17:75–80; discussion 81–2.
70. Ordén MR, Leinonen M, Kirkinen P. Contrast-enhanced ultrasonography of uteroplacental circulation does not evoke harmful CTG changes or perinatal events. Fetal Diagn Ther. 2000;15:139–45.
71. Roberts VHJ, Lo JO, Salati JA, Lewandowski KS, Lindner JR, Morgan TK, Frias AE. Quantitative assessment of placental perfusion by contrast-enhanced ultrasound in macaques and human subjects. Am J Obstet Gynecol. 2016;214:369.e1–8.
72. Piscaglia F, Bolondi L, Italian Society for Ultrasound in Medicine and Biology (SIUMB) Study Group on Ultrasound Contrast Agents. The safety of Sonovue®

in abdominal applications: retrospective analysis of 23188 investigations. Ultrasound Med Biol. 2006;32:1369–75.
73. Morcos SK. Barium preparations: safety issues. In: Contrast media. Berlin Heidelberg: Springer; 2009. p. 223–6.
74. Aspelin P, Bellin MF, Jakobsen JÅ, Webb JAW. Classification and terminology. In: Contrast media. Berlin Heidelberg: Springer; 2009. p. 3–9.
75. Han BH, Lee KS, Han JY, Choi JS, Ahn HK, Ryu HM, Yang JH, Han HW, Nava-Ocampo AA. Pregnancy outcome after 1st-trimester inadvertent exposure to barium sulphate as a contrast media for upper gastrointestinal tract radiography. J Obstet Gynaecol (Lahore). 2011;31:586–8.
76. Han BH, Han JY, Choi JS, Ahn HK, Nava-Ocampo AA. Conventional barium enema in early pregnancy. J Obstet Gynaecol (Lahore). 2010;30:559–62.
77. Boyd B, Zamora CA, Castillo M. Managing adverse reactions to contrast agents. Magn Reson Imaging Clin N Am. 2017;25:737–42.
78. Sikka A, Bisla JK, Rajan PV, Chalfoux LA, Goodhartz LA, Miller FH, Yaghmai V, Horowitz JM. How to manage allergic reactions to contrast agent in pregnant patients. Am J Roentgenol. 2016;206:247–52.
79. Beckett KR, Moriarity AK, Langer JM. Safe use of contrast media: what the radiologist needs to know. Radiographics. 2015;35:1738–50.
80. Simons FER, Schatz M. Anaphylaxis during pregnancy. J Allergy Clin Immunol. 2012;130:597–606.
81. Brent RL. Saving lives and changing family histories: appropriate counseling of pregnant women and men and women of reproductive age, concerning the risk of diagnostic radiation exposures during and before pregnancy. Am J Obstet Gynecol. 2009;200:4–24.

Contrast-Enhanced CT Scanning of the Liver and Pancreas

12

Shintaro Ichikawa

12.1 Introduction

Liver cancer is the third leading cause of cancer-related deaths, with 841,100 newly diagnosed patients and 781,000 deaths per year worldwide [1]. Hepatocellular carcinoma (HCC) is the predominant primary liver cancer in many countries, and HCC-related mortality continues to increase [2–4]. The computed tomography (CT) characteristics of HCC are well described, and a diagnostic algorithm for HCC (Liver Reporting and Data System (LI-RADS®)), which is based on contrast-enhanced CT, has been established [5].

Pancreatic adenocarcinoma is the most common solid pancreatic tumor and still has a poor prognosis. Pancreatic cancer is newly diagnosed in 458,900 patients and causes 433,200 deaths per year worldwide [1]. Despite the poor prognosis of pancreatic adenocarcinoma, surgical resection represents the only potentially curative treatment. Therefore, careful patient selection based on accurate disease staging is of prime importance.

Dynamic CT is a widely used and well-established technique for the evaluation of hepatic and pancreatic disease. It shows high diagnostic performance; however, if it is not properly used, it cannot be effective. Thus, this chapter focuses on the optimal protocol for hepatic and pancreatic dynamic CT and its important characteristics.

12.2 Contrast-Enhanced CT of the Liver

12.2.1 Why Dynamic CT?

We can often detect focal liver lesions using non-contrast-enhanced CT (NE-CT). Do we need dynamic CT in such cases? The answer is yes because we cannot make qualitative diagnoses without using dynamic CT. For example, Figs. 12.1a, 12.2a, and 12.3a show low attenuation lesions on NE-CT in three different patients. We can detect them using NE-CT but cannot differentiate between even benign and malignant lesions. However, we can diagnose these lesions easily by referring to arterial phase (AP) images (Figs. 12.1b, 12.2b, 12.3b). The AP is the most important phase in dynamic CT. Typical imaging findings of HCC, hemangioma, and metastatic tumor from colorectal adenocarcinoma are shown Figs. 12.1, 12.2, and 12.3.

While in cases with liver steatosis or cirrhosis, it may be difficult to detect focal liver lesions on NE-CT. Diffuse steatosis reduces liver attenuation. Liver cirrhosis causes parenchymal heterogeneity due to regeneration nodules or fatty infiltration. In those cases, focal liver lesions may not be visible on NE-CT, because the contrast

S. Ichikawa (✉)
Department of Radiology, Hamamatsu University School of Medicine, Hamamatsu, Japan
e-mail: shintaro@hama-med.ac.jp

S. M. Erturk et al. (eds.), *Medical Imaging Contrast Agents: A Clinical Manual*,
https://doi.org/10.1007/978-3-030-79256-5_12

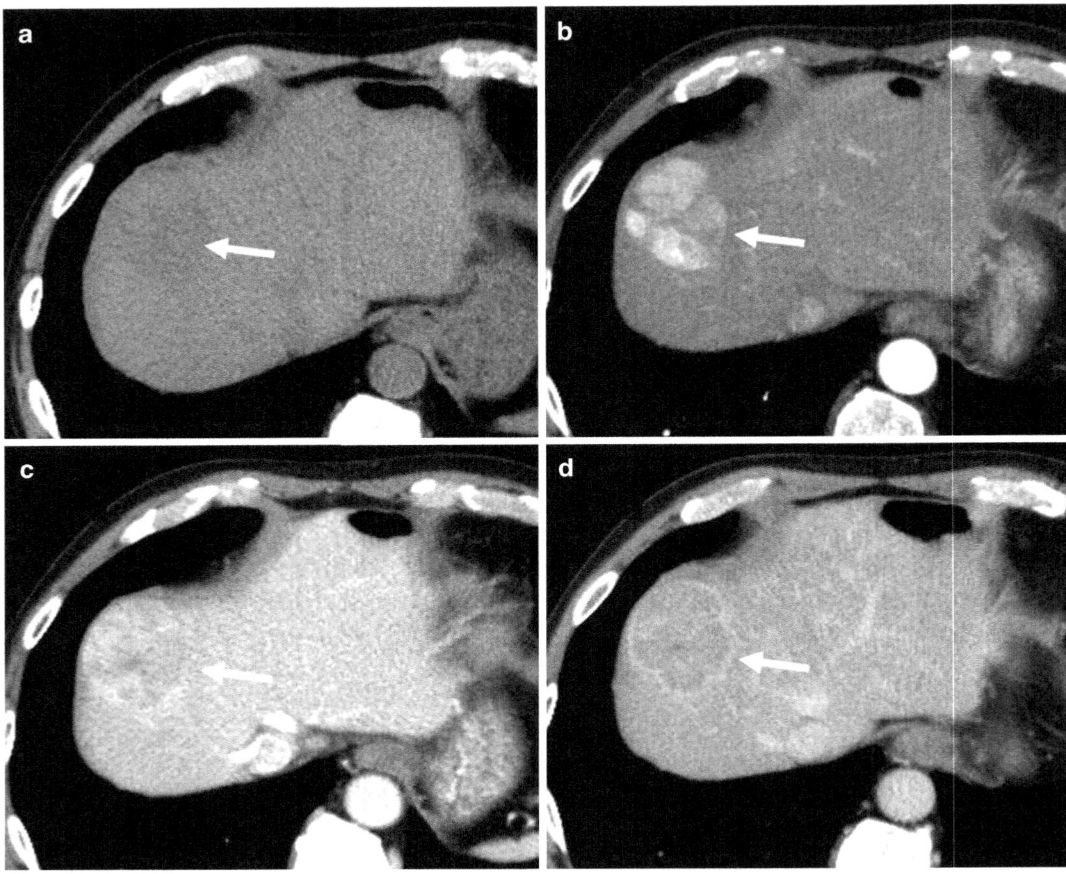

Fig. 12.1 Dynamic CT of a 64-year-old man with HCC secondary to chronic hepatitis C. (**a**) NE-CT, (**b**) AP, (**c**) PVP, and (**d**) DP. NE-CT shows a low attenuation lesion in segment 8 (**a**) (arrow). The lesion shows non-rim APHE in AP (**b**) and non-peripheral washout and enhancing capsule in PVP and DP (**c**, **d**) which are typical findings of hypervascular HCC (arrow). It shows non-peripheral washout and enhancing capsule in the PVP and DP (**c**, **d**) (arrow). Non-peripheral washout and enhancing capsule are clearer in DP than PVP in this case. *CT* computed tomography, *NE* non-contrast-enhanced, *AP* arterial phase, *PVP* portal venous phase, *DP* delayed phase, *HCC* hepatocellular carcinoma, *APHE* arterial phase hyperenhancement

between lesions and surrounding liver parenchyma becomes too low (Fig. 12.4a). However, AP images are useful in detecting liver lesions even in such cases (Fig. 12.4b). The conspicuity of liver lesions depends on the difference in attenuation between lesions and the surrounding liver parenchyma.

12.2.2 Recommended Protocol

The liver has a unique blood supply that comprises the hepatic artery and portal vein (PV). It is essential to understand the dual blood supply to the liver when we think of dynamic CT. Of the normal liver parenchyma, 70–80% is supplied by the PV, and the remaining 20–30% is supplied by the hepatic artery; therefore, the normal liver parenchyma is enhanced maximally in the portal venous phase (PVP) and enhanced weakly in AP. An appropriate dynamic CT protocol consists of NE-CT, AP, PVP, and delayed phase (DP). These phases are defined based on the time after intravenous administration of iodine-based contrast medium (CM). According to LI-RADS® v2018, a multidetector CT with ≥8 detector rows

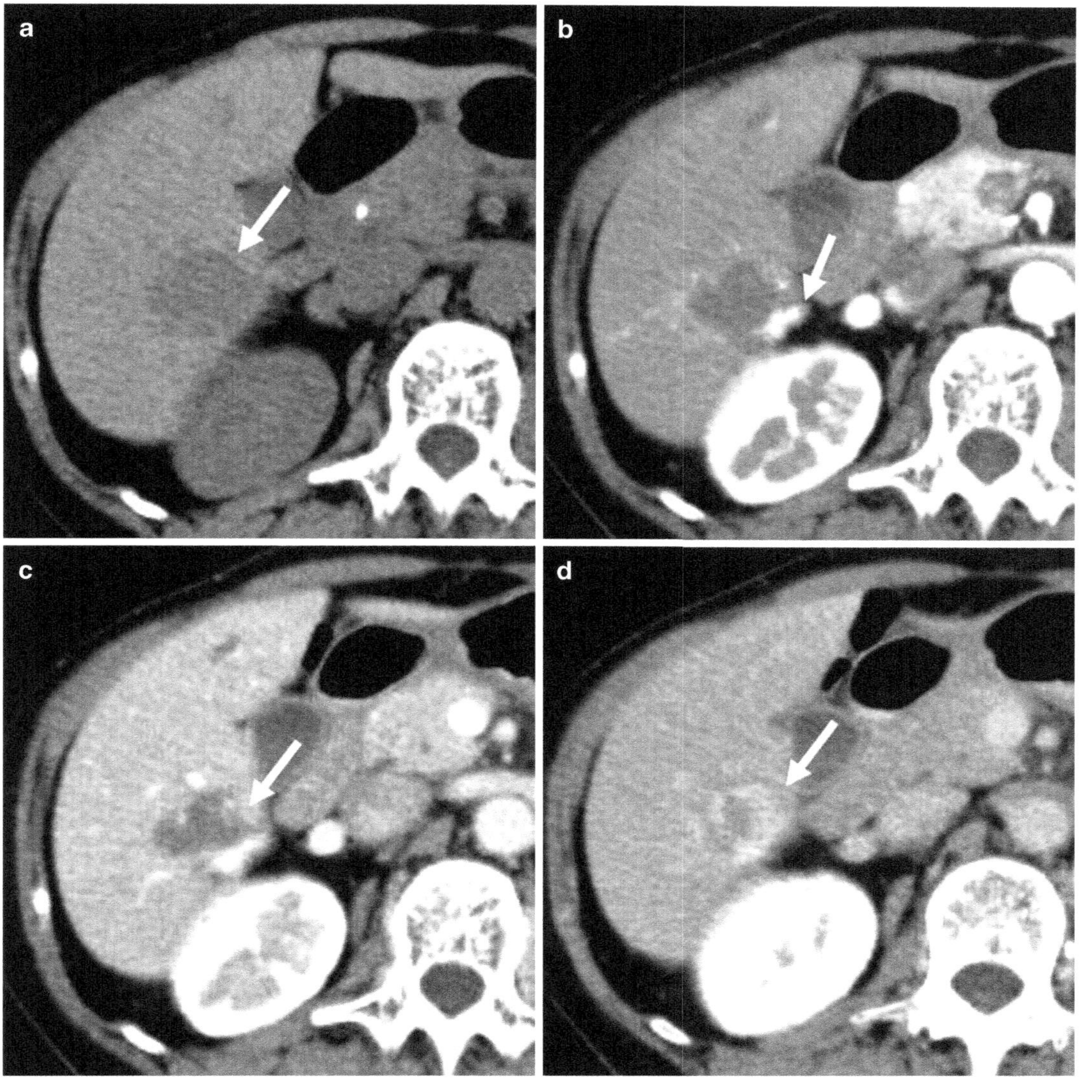

Fig. 12.2 Dynamic CT of a 45-year-old woman with hepatic hemangioma. (**a**) NE-CT, (**b**) AP, (**c**) PVP, and (**d**) DP. NE-CT shows a low attenuation lesion in segment 6 (**a**) (arrow). The lesion shows a discontinuous, nodular, peripheral enhancement in the AP (**b**) and irregular fill-in pattern in the PVP and DP (**c**, **d**), which are typical findings of hepatic hemangioma (arrow). *CT* computed tomography, *NE* non-contrast-enhanced, *AP* arterial phase, *PVP* portal venous phase, *DP* delayed phase

is recommended [5]. Details of each phase are as follows.

12.2.2.1 NE-CT

Images obtained before the administration of CM. It is useful for detecting calcifications, fat, hemorrhage, and post-treatment change, including lipiodol deposition, in focal liver lesions.

12.2.2.2 AP (Late AP Is Strongly Preferred)

Images obtained 35–40 s after administration of CM. The optimal timing of AP is when the hepatic artery and branches and PV are enhanced, but the hepatic vein is not yet enhanced by antegrade flow (Fig. 12.5a) [5]. If only the hepatic artery is enhanced, the scan timing is too early

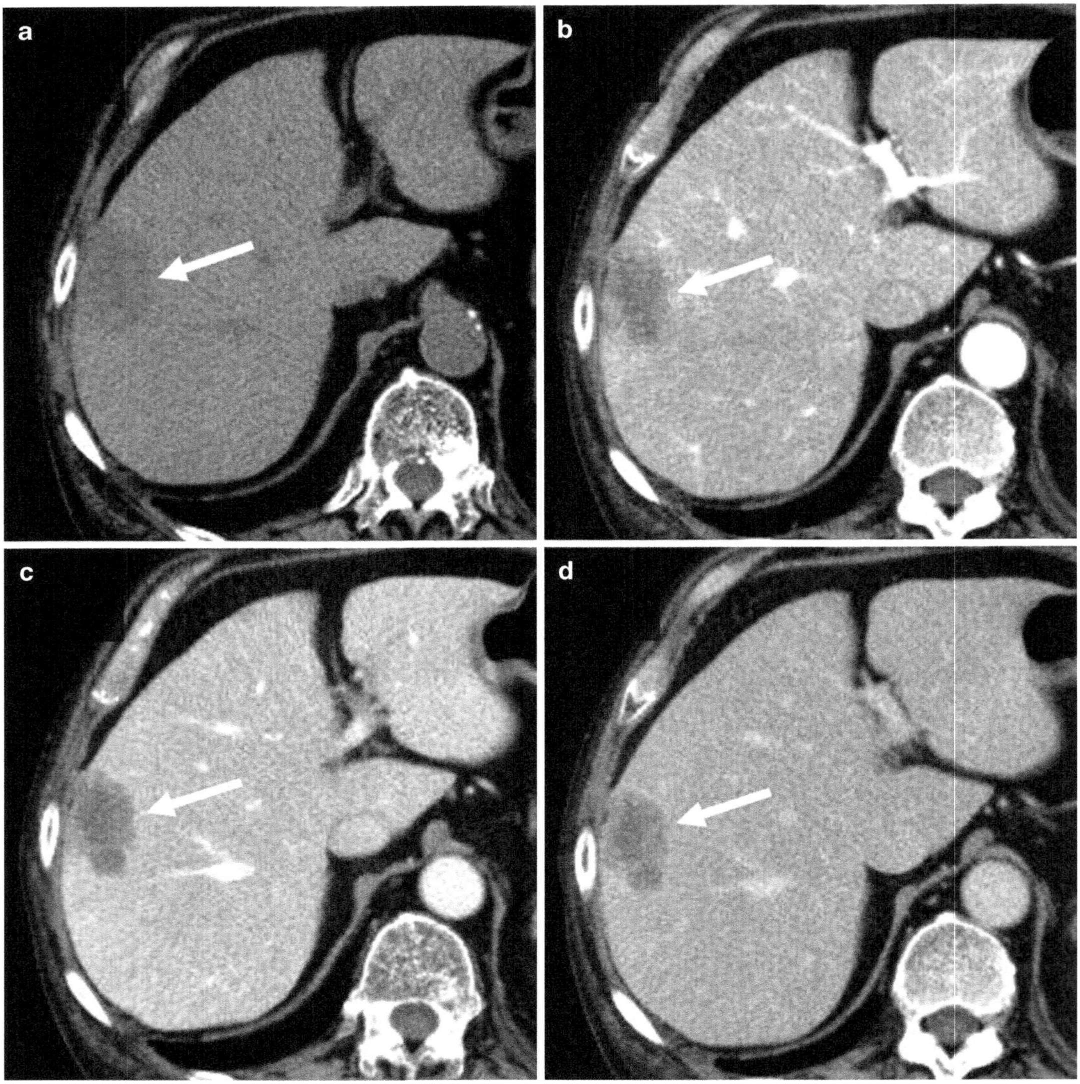

Fig. 12.3 Dynamic CT of a 76-year-old man with liver metastasis from sigmoid colon cancer. (**a**) NE-CT, (**b**) AP, (**c**) PVP, and (**d**) DP. NE-CT shows a low attenuation lesion in segment 8/5 (**a**) (arrow). The lesion shows a hypovascular pattern with ill-defined margin in the AP (**b**) and peripheral enhancement in the PVP and DP (**b**, **c**), which are the typical findings of liver metastasis from colorectal adenocarcinoma (arrow). *CT* computed tomography, *NE* non-contrast-enhanced, *AP* arterial phase, *PVP* portal venous phase, *DP* delayed phase

(early AP) (Fig. 12.5b). If the hepatic vein is already enhanced, the scan timing is too late (Fig. 12.5c). HCC is most strongly enhanced in this phase because it receives 100% of its blood supply from the hepatic artery. Non-rim arterial phase hyperenhancement (APHE) is the most important major imaging feature in LI-RADS®; therefore, obtaining optimal AP images is crucial for the diagnosis of HCC. Non-rim APHE is defined as non-rim-like enhancement in AP unequivocally greater in whole or in part than in the liver (Figs. 12.1b and 12.4b). The enhanced part must have higher attenuation than the liver parenchyma [5].

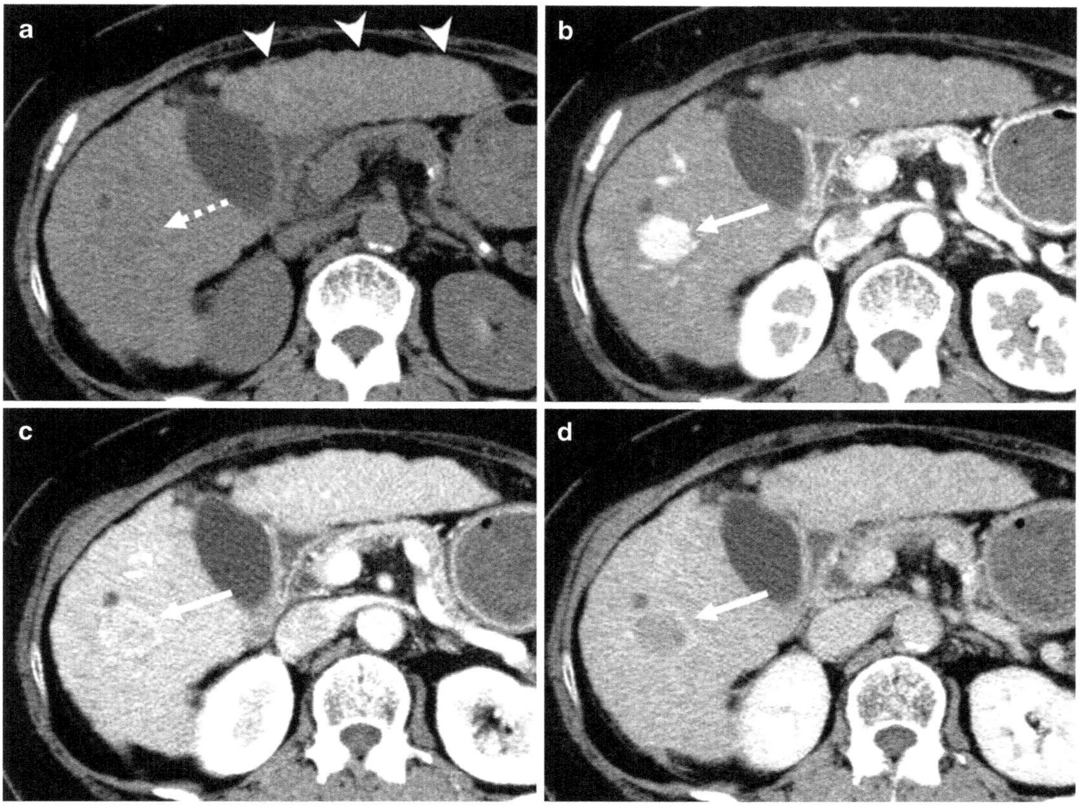

Fig. 12.4 Dynamic CT of a 60-year-old woman with HCC secondary to alcoholic hepatitis. (**a**) NE-CT, (**b**) AP, (**c**) PVP, and (**d**) DP. The liver surface shows a nodular pattern that corresponds to liver cirrhosis (arrowheads). The contrast between the liver parenchyma and intrahepatic blood vessels is low on NE-CT, indicating a fatty liver (**a**). It is difficult to detect the mass in segment 5 on NE-CT (dotted arrow) (**a**). However, the lesion shows non-rim APHE in the AP (**b**) and non-peripheral washout and enhancing capsule in the PVP and DP (**c**, **d**), which are typical findings of hypervascular HCC (arrow). It shows non-peripheral washout and enhancing capsule in PVP and DP (**c**, **d**) (arrow). Non-peripheral washout is clearer in the DP than in the PVP. *CT* computed tomography, *NE* non-contrast-enhanced, *AP* arterial phase, *PVP* portal venous phase, *DP* delayed phase, *HCC* hepatocellular carcinoma, *APHE* arterial phase hyperenhancement

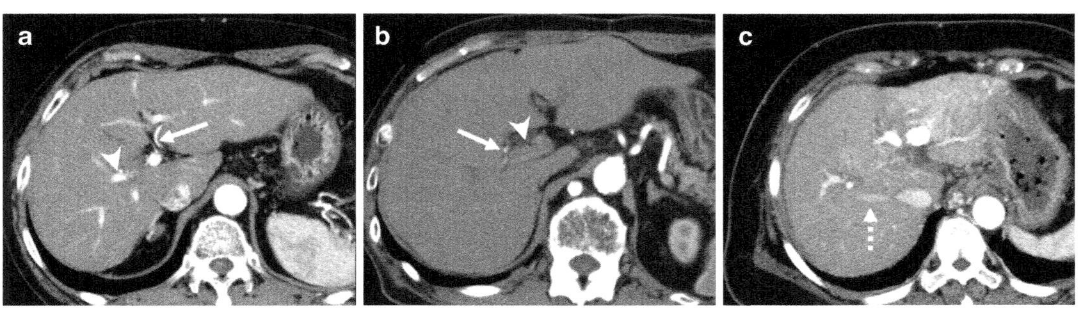

Fig. 12.5 Scan timing of the AP. (**a**) Optimal, (**b**) too early, and (**c**) too late. The optimal timing of the AP is when the hepatic artery and branches (arrow) and portal vein (arrowhead) are enhanced, but the hepatic vein is not yet enhanced by antegrade flow (**a**). If only the hepatic artery is enhanced (arrow), the scan timing is too early (**b**). If the hepatic vein is already enhanced (dotted arrow), the scan timing is too late (**c**). *AP* arterial phase

12.2.2.3 PVP

Images obtained 55–70 s after administration of CM. The time range is characterized by full enhancement of the PV, and the hepatic vein is enhanced by antegrade flow [5]. The liver parenchyma usually shows peak enhancement in this phase. Non-peripheral washout and enhancing capsule, which are major imaging features in LI-RADS®, should be evaluated in this phase or following DP. Non-peripheral washout is defined as a non-peripheral visually assessed temporal reduction in enhancement in whole or in part relative to the surrounding liver parenchyma in the PVP or DP (Figs. 12.1c, d and 12.4d). It can apply to any enhancing observation in AP, even if there is no APHE [5]. The enhancing capsule is defined as a smooth, uniform, and sharp border around most or all of an observation, unequivocally thicker or more conspicuous than fibrotic tissue around background nodules, and visible as an enhancing rim in PVP or DP (Figs. 12.1c, d and 12.4c, d) [5]. Moreover, hypovascular liver tumors are best seen in this phase because the surrounding liver parenchyma is well enhanced.

12.2.2.4 DP

Images obtained 150–200 s after administration of CM. In this phase, the PV, hepatic vein, and liver parenchyma are enhanced but less than in PVP [5]. As mentioned above, non-peripheral washout and enhancing capsule are evaluated in PVP or DP. Non-peripheral washout is observed more often in DP than PVP. Moreover, focal liver lesions that have abandoned fibrotic tissue, like intrahepatic cholangiocarcinoma, hold the contrast much longer than normal parenchyma; therefore, they may show delayed enhancement in this phase.

Early AP and multiplanar reconstructions (MPR) are considered as optional images. Early AP is defined as the phase where only the hepatic artery and its branches are enhanced, but the PV and hepatic vein are not yet enhanced. It is useful for pre-treatment planning for hepatic tumors. It is essential to assess the anatomy of the hepatic artery in detail before hepatectomy or interventional radiology. Three-dimensional images of the arterial vasculature, such as the maximum intensity projection (MIP) and volume rendering (VR), can be reconstructed from early AP images. It is easy to understand the spatial relationship between arterial branches and liver parenchyma or portal/hepatic veins. Anatomical variation of the hepatic artery can also be depicted clearly. However, van den Hoven et al. reported that early AP images did not significantly improve detection of small intra- and extra-hepatic branches [6]. Therefore, further studies are needed in order to clarify whether early AP is truly necessary. MPR is the process of converting data from a certain plane, usually axial, into other planes such as coronal, sagittal, or oblique. It has significant applications in the diagnosis of focal liver lesions in the hepatic dome. Since modern multidetector-row CT scanners can obtain isovoxel data, it is easy to create high-quality MPR images routinely.

12.2.3 Recommended Injection Method of CM

Dynamic CT images are affected by several factors, including iodine dose, iodine concentration, injection duration, and saline flush [7]. It is important to know how these factors affect contrast enhancement and scan timing in order to obtain optimal dynamic CT images. The recommended injection method of CM includes 600 mgI/kg iodine dose with a standard tube voltage (120 kVp) CT, CM with a low iodine concentration, and fixed injection duration (30 s) protocol. The details are described below.

12.2.3.1 Iodine Dose

The iodine dose of CM should be tailored according to the patients' body weight to obtain optimal contrast between the focal liver lesion and liver parenchyma [7, 8]. According to a multicenter prospective study in 77 general hospitals in Japan, the recommended iodine doses of CM for AP and PVP are 567–647 mgI/kg and 572 mgI/kg, respectively, for investigating hypervascular HCC [8]. Therefore, in general, 600 mgI/kg has been chosen in daily practice in Japan. Recently, there have been several published studies that showed by using low tube voltage (80 or 100 kVp) CT with iterative reconstruction, the iodine dose of CM can be reduced by 17–50% compared to standard tube voltage (120 kVp) CT [9–13].

12.2.3.2 Iodine Concentration

Commercially available intravenous iodine-based CM has various concentrations (240–370 mgI/mL). When the iodine dose is tailored according to the patients' body weight, using CM with a low iodine concentration requires a larger amount of CM. The volume of CM left in dead space does not contribute to the enhancement of the aorta or hypervascular focal liver lesions, such as HCCs. Dead space here refers to the intravenous space between the brachial vein and superior vena cava, which would be approximately 10–30 mL. When CM with a high iodine concentration is used, the total amount of iodine in the dead space is higher. Furthermore, the injection rate would be lower when using CM with a high iodine concentration because as described below, a fixed injection duration is recommended. It is known that the higher the injection rate, the higher the aortic peak enhancement [7, 14]. On the other hand, it has been reported that there were no significant differences in the peak enhancement values of the PV and liver parenchyma between high and low iodine concentrations when using same iodine dose [15]. Therefore, CM with a low iodine concentration might be recommended over CM with a high iodine concentration when using the same iodine dose to detect hypervascular HCC on AP. However, in case of patients with a high body weight, the total iodine dose of CM with a low iodine concentration can be insufficient. Therefore, the iodine concentration should be decided based on the patients' body weight and availability in each institution.

12.2.3.3 Injection Duration

Injection duration is defined as the time from the beginning to the completion of the injection [7]. The scan delay after the beginning of CM administration for each phase, especially AP, varies in each patient; therefore it is impossible to determine the optimal fixed scan delays that can be applied in all patients because there are several uncontrollable patient-based factors such as body weight, cardiac output, and circulation time [15]. The bolus tracking method is one of the solutions to this problem. It is a computer-assisted technique that automatically initiates a scan triggered by the contrast enhancement, namely, if the contrast enhancement reaches the predicted threshold in a previously set region-of-interest [16]. The usefulness of the bolus tracking method is well-known [17]; however, it has some disadvantages, including a slightly complicated method and additional radiation exposure (although a very small dose). In contrast, a fixed injection duration protocol is a quite simple and useful method. It can minimize patient-dependent factors in scan delays and achieve optimal scan timing for each phase among most patients [7, 15]. The fixed injection duration protocol depends on the fact that the peak enhancement time of the abdominal aorta (pET-Ao) observed on the time-density curve is defined by the injection duration. The mean time delay from the completion of the CM injection to pET-Ao was approximately 10 s [15, 18]. The mean delays with any fixed injection duration from the completion of CM injection to the peak enhancement time of the PV (pET-PV) and the liver parenchyma (pET-liver) are also constant (approximately 20 and 30 s, respectively) [15]. The peak enhancement time for hypervascular HCC (pET-HCC) might occur approximately 5 s after pET-Ao because hypervascular HCC receives arterial blood supply from the hepatic artery following the abdominal aorta [15]. The recommended fixed injection duration has been established as 30 s in a practical dynamic CT protocol of the liver. Therefore, each peak enhancement time can be calculated as follows:

$$\mathrm{pET-Ao} = 30 + 10 = 40\,\mathrm{s}$$

$$\mathrm{pET-HCC} = 30 + 15 = 45\,\mathrm{s}$$

$$\mathrm{pET-PV} = 30 + 20 = 50\,\mathrm{s}$$

$$\mathrm{pET-liver} = 30 + 30 = 60\,\mathrm{s}$$

A fixed injection duration protocol is advantageous over a fixed injection rate protocol because the scan timing can be more easily standardized, and the iodine administration rate can be adjusted based on the patient size [7].

12.2.3.4 Saline Flush

A saline flush pushes the previously injected CM that remains in the dead space, including the injection tube and venous space, into the central blood volume. Therefore, it can improve contrast enhancement and the efficiency of CM use and is particularly beneficial when the total volume of CM is small [7]. However, it takes more time to prepare because a saline flush requires a dual-syringe power injector for the injection of CM and saline, so it is not essential for dynamic CT of the liver. If you apply this technique, 20–30 mL of saline flush is enough.

12.2.4 Scan Timing of CT

Scan timing is important in order to obtain the optimal moment of maximal contrast differences between focal liver lesion and surrounding liver parenchyma. As described above, when 30 s is used as the fixed injection duration, pET-Ao, pET-HCC, pET-PV, and pET-liver are calculated to be at 40, 45, 50, and 60 s, respectively. In AP, the timing of pET-HCC (45 s) should be placed in the scan center because hypervascular HCC shows maximal enhancement and it is easy to detect APHE at this point. You must adapt your protocol to the type of CT scanner because the scan duration varies depending on the CT scanner. For example, if the scan duration for each phase is 10 s, you start at 40 s after the beginning of the injection of CM. If the scan duration for each phase is 4 s, you start at 43 s after the beginning of the injection of CM.

Theoretically, the timing of pET-liver (60 s) should be placed in the scan center for PVP because liver parenchyma shows maximal enhancement and it is easy to detect washout of HCC at this point. Thus, if the scan duration for each phase is 10 s, you start at 55 s after the beginning of the injection of CM. However, it is not undesirable to be too early for PVP, because it is necessary to load the liver with CM, and it takes time for CM to reach the liver parenchyma from the PV. Therefore, you can start at 55–70 s after the beginning of the injection of CM regardless of the CT scanner. DP needs to be obtained at a sufficiently late timing; therefore, in general, 150–200 s after the beginning of the injection of CM is chosen regardless of the CT scanner.

12.3 Contrast-Enhanced CT of the Pancreas

12.3.1 Why Dynamic CT?

The most common solid pancreatic lesion is pancreatic adenocarcinoma followed by neuroendocrine neoplasms. It is often difficult to detect them using NE-CT (Figs. 12.6a, 12.7a, and 12.8a); therefore, dynamic CT is essential for the diagnosis of solid pancreatic lesions. Dynamic CT is useful for distinguishing these tumors because typical dynamic CT findings are completely different, namely, pancreatic adenocarcinoma is hypovascular (Fig. 12.6b), and neuroendocrine neoplasms are hypervascular (Fig. 12.7b). Moreover, preoperative evaluation on dynamic CT is quite important because only surgical resection has the potential to be curative for pancreatic adenocarcinoma. The principal goal of preoperative evaluation of dynamic CT is to identify patients with potentially resectable disease and avoid surgical exploration in those with unresectable disease.

12.3.2 Recommended Protocol

High-resolution dynamic CT is the established technique for evaluating pancreatic tumors. The protocol for dynamic CT of the pancreas is similar to that of the liver.

12.3.2.1 NE-CT

Images obtained before the administration of CM. It is useful for detecting calcifications, fat, and hemorrhage. Calcifications on the background pancreatic parenchyma are particularly important because it is essential for the diagnosis of chronic pancreatitis.

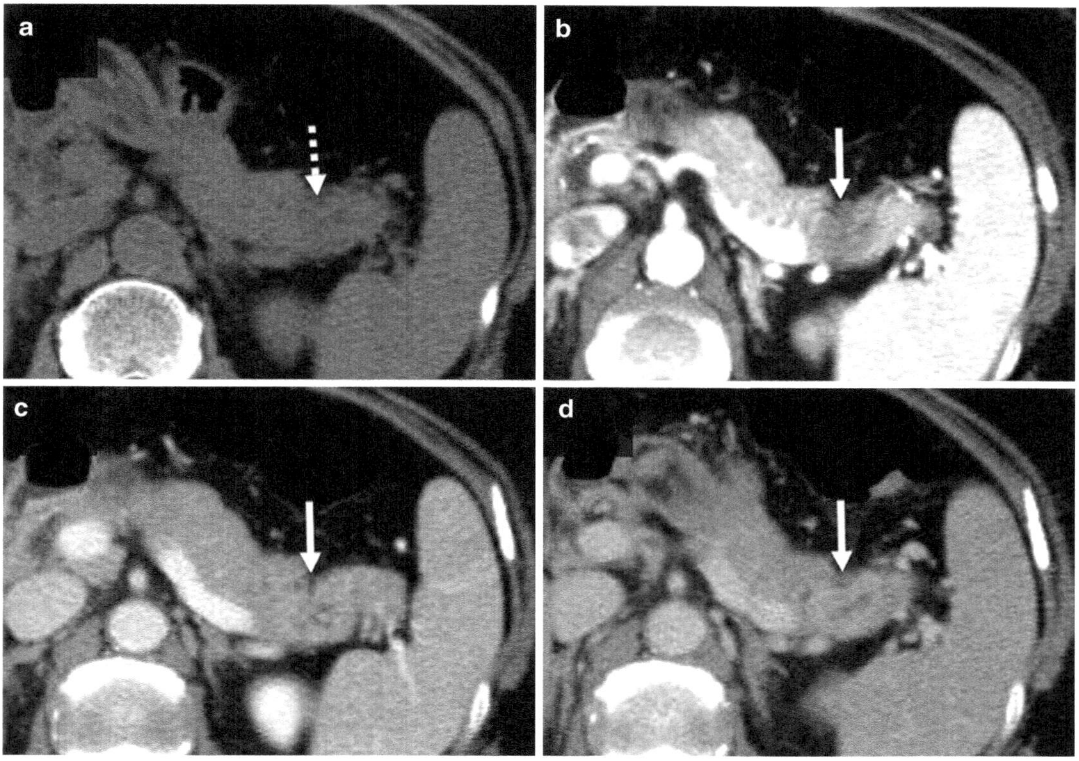

Fig. 12.6 Dynamic CT of a 61-year-old woman with pancreatic adenocarcinoma. (**a**) NE-CT, (**b**) PPP, (**c**) PVP, and (**d**) DP. It is difficult to detect the mass in the tail of the pancreas on NE-CT (dotted arrow) (**a**). The lesion shows a hypovascular pattern with an ill-defined margin in the PPP (**b**) and delayed enhancement in the PVP to DP (**c**, **d**), which are typical findings of pancreatic adenocarcinoma (arrow). This is a resectable case because no CA, SMA, CHA, SMV, or PV invasion is observed. *CT* computed tomography, *NE* non-contrast-enhanced, *PPP* pancreatic parenchymal phase, *PVP* portal venous phase, *DP* delayed phase

12.3.2.2 Late AP or Pancreatic Parenchymal Phase (PPP) (Almost the Same)

Images obtained 40–45 s after the administration of CM. Pancreatic parenchyma shows maximum enhancement in this phase [19, 20], allowing optimal visualization of the tumor, because maximum contrast is obtained between the hypovascular tumor and surrounding pancreatic parenchyma in this phase. This phase is also useful for evaluating tumor spread to the peripancreatic arteries because they are markedly enhanced.

12.3.2.3 PVP

Images obtained 55–70 s after administration of CM. This phase is optimal for detecting metastatic disease in the liver and for assessing the PV. In PPP, the PV is not sufficiently enhanced; therefore, it is not appropriate for evaluating PV invasion and should be evaluated in PVP. The poorly enhanced PV may be confused with pancreatic head masses in PPP; in such cases PVP is required. Moreover, the contrast of lymph nodes and other abdominal organs is good in this phase; therefore, PVP is suitable for the evaluation of the whole abdomen.

12.3.2.4 DP

Images obtained 240–300 s after administration of CM. Pancreatic adenocarcinoma has abandoned fibrotic tissue; therefore, it holds the contrast much longer than normal parenchyma and may show delayed enhancement in this phase (Figs. 12.7d and 12.8d). Some pancreatic adenocarcinomas are isoattenuated in PPP and PVP and show delayed enhancement in DP (Fig. 12.8) [21, 22].

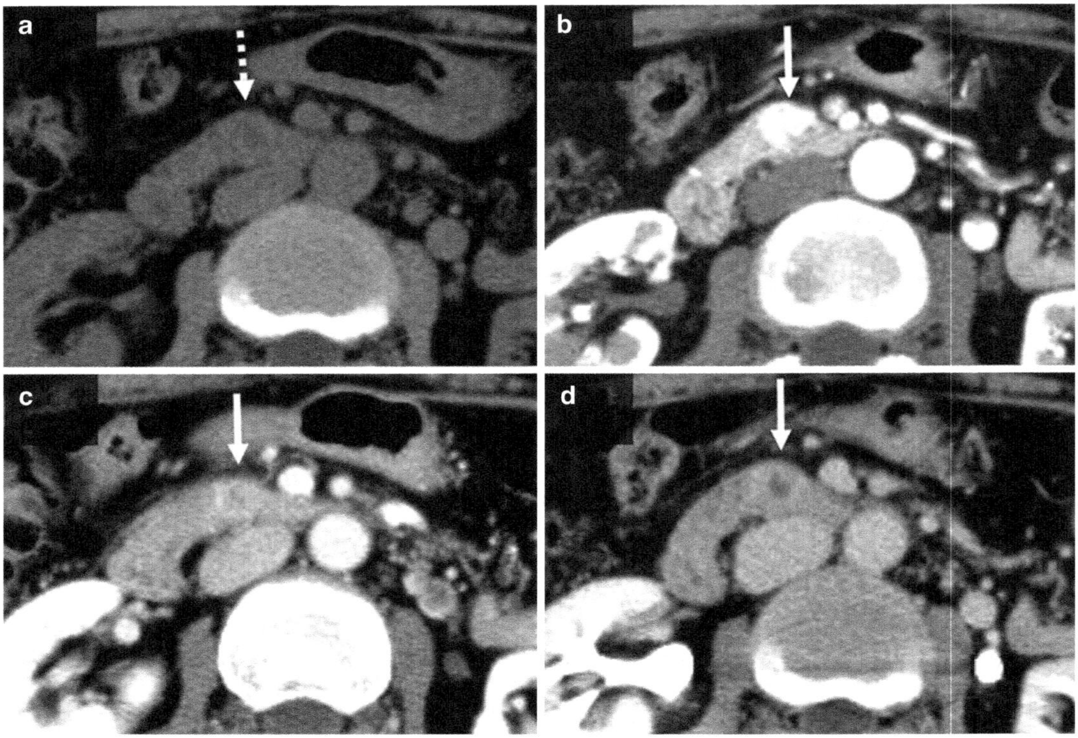

Fig. 12.7 Dynamic CT of a 59-year-old woman with pancreatic neuroendocrine neoplasm. (**a**) NE-CT, (**b**) PPP, (**c**) PVP, and (**d**) DP. It is difficult to detect the mass in the head of the pancreas on NE-CT (dotted arrow) (**a**). The lesion shows avid enhancement with a well-defined margin in the PPP (**b**), which is the typical finding of pancreatic neuroendocrine neoplasm (arrow). This mass shows slightly higher attenuation than that of the pancreas parenchyma in the PVP and DP in this case (**c, d**). *CT* computed tomography, *NE* non-contrast-enhanced, *PPP* pancreatic parenchymal phase, *PVP* portal venous phase, *DP* delayed phase

Thin slice images (Figs. 12.9a, c and 12.10b) and MPR images (Fig. 12.9b) are necessary to allow full assessment of the circumferential and longitudinal vascular contact, changes in vessel caliber, and presence of contour deformity secondary to the tumor, which may not be appreciated on normal axial images alone. Early AP is considered an optional image. It is useful for preoperative planning for pancreatic tumor because it is essential to assess the anatomy of peripancreatic arteries in detail before surgery.

12.3.3 Recommended Injection Method of CM

The recommended injection method of CM includes a 600 mgI/kg iodine dose with a standard tube voltage (120 kVp) CT and fixed injection duration (30 s) protocol. For the pancreas, CM theory has not been studied as in detail as for the liver; however, dynamic CT should be performed according to the liver protocol. See I-3 and I-4 in detail.

12.3.4 Assessment of Tumor Spread

Staging of pancreatic adenocarcinoma is based on the tumor size, location within the pancreas, involvement of the surrounding vessels, and presence of metastatic lesions. The commonly used staging systems in the USA are those proposed by the American Joint Committee on Cancer and the National Comprehensive Cancer Network (NCCN). The NCCN guidelines define a staging

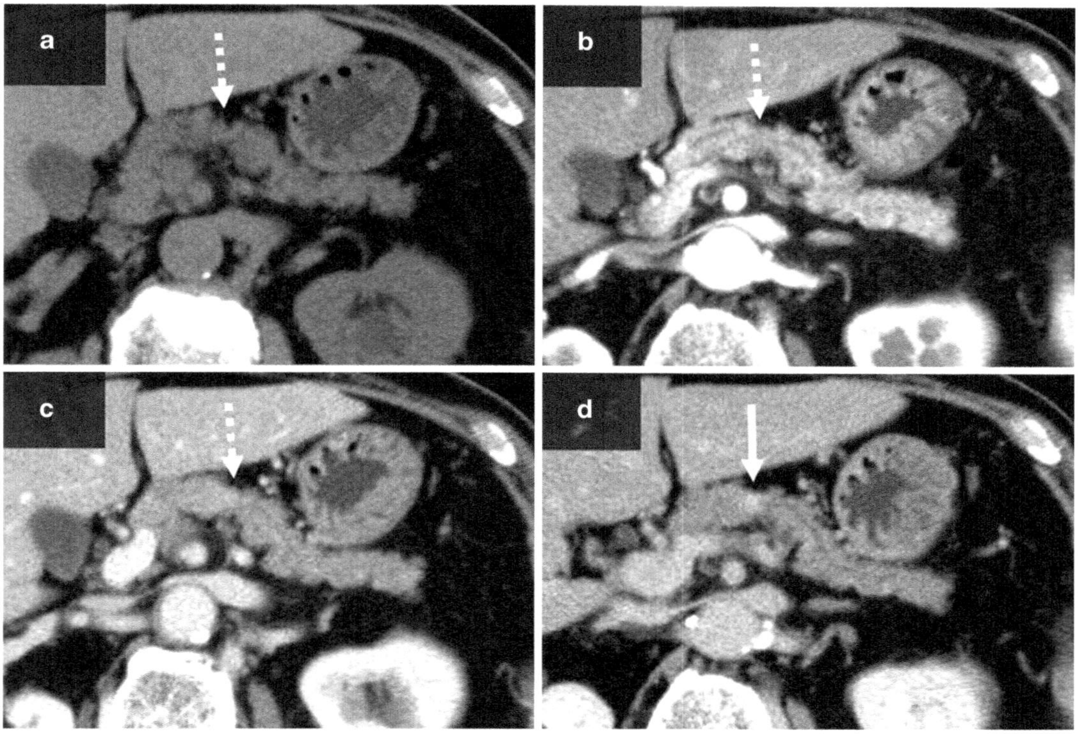

Fig. 12.8 Dynamic CT of a 70-year-old man with pancreatic adenocarcinoma. (**a**) NE-CT, (**b**) PPP, (**c**) PVP, and (**d**) DP. It is difficult to detect the mass in the body of the pancreas on NE-CT, PPP, and PVP (dotted arrow) (**a**–**c**). The lesion shows a delayed enhancement in the DP (arrow) (**d**). Some pancreatic adenocarcinomas can be detected only in the DP, such as in this case. This is a resectable case because no CA, SMA, CHA, SMV, or PV invasion is observed. *CT* computed tomography, *NE* non-contrast-enhanced, *PPP* pancreatic parenchymal phase, *PVP* portal venous phase, *DP* delayed phase

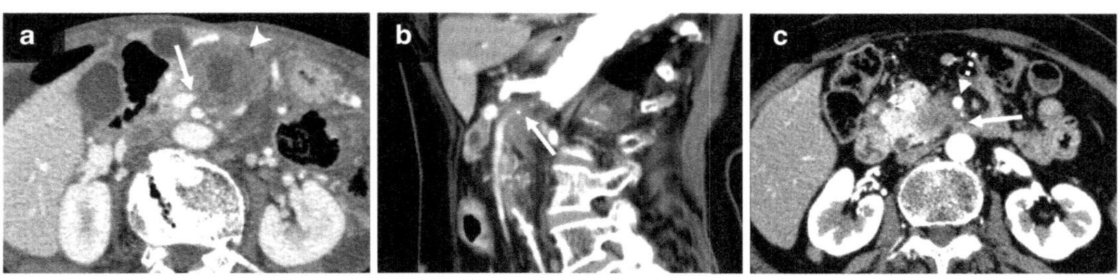

Fig. 12.9 Tumor involvement of the surrounding tissues. (**a**) Thin slice (1-mm thickness) PVP image of a 79-year-old woman with pancreatic adenocarcinoma. The contour of the SMV shows a change in the caliber (arrow) due to the contact of the tumor (arrowhead) ("tear drop" deformity). It is considered a sign of PV invasion and this case is unresectable. (**b**) Sagittal PPP image of a 90-year-old woman with pancreatic adenocarcinoma. This case shows direct abutment of the SMA and severe stenosis. It is considered a sign of SMA invasion, and this case is unresectable. (**c**) Thin slice (1-mm thickness) PPP image of a 76-year-old woman with pancreatic adenocarcinoma. The hypovascular mass is in the head of the pancreas (arrowhead). The peripancreatic retroperitoneal space and fat space around the SMA are replaced with irregular soft tissue (arrow). This finding indicates extrapancreatic neural plexus invasion. The SMA is marked with a dotted arrow. *PVP* portal venous phase, *SMV* superior mesenteric vein, *PPP* pancreatic parenchymal phase, *SMA* superior mesenteric artery

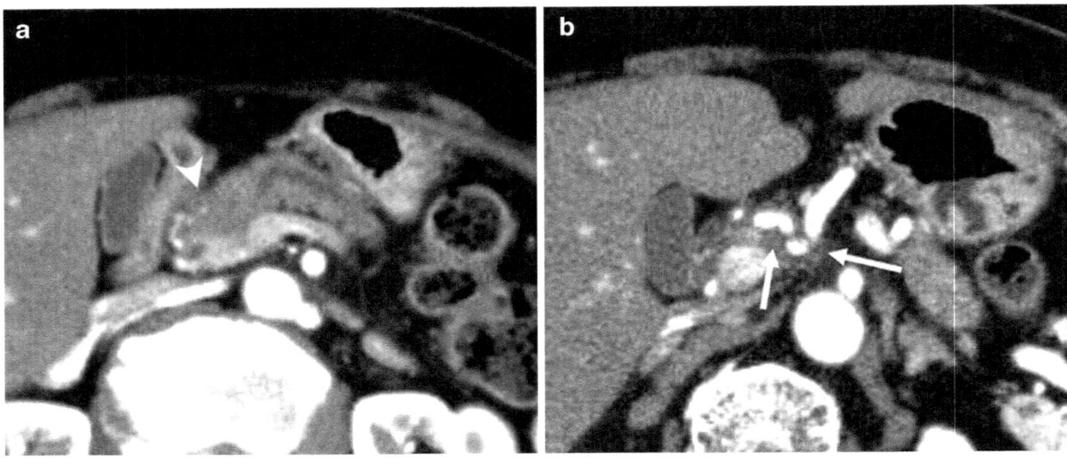

Fig. 12.10 PPP of a 64-year-old woman with borderline resectable pancreatic adenocarcinoma. (**a**) Normal slice thickness image (5 mm), (**b**) thin slice image (1-mm thickness). The hypovascular mass is in the head of the pancreas (arrowhead) (**a**). CHA is surrounded by irregular soft tissue (arrows) (**b**). This finding indicates CHA invasion; therefore, this case is borderline resectable. *PPP* pancreatic parenchymal phase, *CHA* common hepatic artery

system based on tumor extent and offer treatment recommendations accordingly [23]. In the absence of metastatic disease, pancreatic cancer cases are classified into three main categories—resectable, borderline resectable, and unresectable. The disease category selection depends on the tumor location within the pancreas and the arterial (celiac axis (CA), superior mesenteric artery (SMA), and common hepatic artery (CHA)) or venous (superior mesenteric vein (SMV) and PV) involvement [24]. More than 180° of tumor-vessel contact is highly specific for tumor invasion of the vessels [25]. Irregularity of the vessel contour, including a "tear drop" deformity or change in caliber, is also considered a sign of vascular invasion, regardless of the degree of contact between the tumor and vessel (Fig. 12.9a) [25]. Resectable cases show clear fat planes around the CA, SMA, and CHA and no SMV or PV distortion (Figs. 12.6 and 12.8). Unresectable cases show direct abutment of the SMA/CA exceeding 180° (Fig. 12.9b) or unreconstructive SMV/PV due to tumor involvement or occlusion (Fig. 12.9a). Other than that, they are classified as borderline resectable cases (Fig. 12.10).

Extrapancreatic nerve plexus invasion is another important factor to be assessed. It is one of the most important prognostic factors in patients with pancreatic adenocarcinoma in the head of the pancreas [26]. Cancer cells possibly spread and metastasize through the perineural space, leading to recurrence after surgery. Therefore, preoperative imaging diagnosis of extrapancreatic nerve plexus invasion from pancreatic adenocarcinoma in the head of the pancreas is clinically important for predicting the prognosis and deciding surgical strategy, including extended resection with removal of the adjacent major vessels. The CT findings of extrapancreatic neural plexus invasion are as follows: (1) replacement fat space in the peripancreatic retroperitoneal space with irregular soft tissue, (2) disappearance of the fat space around SMA/SMV/CA, and (3) narrowing or disappearance of the fat space behind the splenic vein (Fig. 12.9c) [27, 28].

12.4 Conclusion

Dynamic CT is a very useful noninvasive diagnostic method for evaluating hepatic and pancreatic tumors; however, if appropriate conditions are not used, it will not be sufficiently effective.

CM theory has been well established for the liver, making it important to understand and practice. The recommended injection method of CM includes 600 mgI/kg iodine dose with standard tube voltage (120 kVp) CT, CM with a low iodine concentration, and fixed injection duration (30 s) protocol. For the pancreas, CM theory has not been studied as in detail as that for the liver; however, dynamic CT should be performed according to the liver protocol.

References

1. Ferlay J, Colombet M, Soerjomataram I, et al. Estimating the global cancer incidence and mortality in 2018: GLOBOCAN sources and methods. Int J Cancer. 2019;144(8):1941–53.
2. Beal EW, Tumin D, Kabir A, et al. Trends in the mortality of hepatocellular carcinoma in the United States. J Gastrointest Surg. 2017;21(12):2033–8.
3. Zhu RX, Seto WK, Lai CL, Yuen MF. Epidemiology of hepatocellular carcinoma in the Asia-Pacific region. Gut Liver. 2016;10(3):332–9.
4. Ascione A, Fontanella L, Imparato M, Rinaldi L, De Luca M. Mortality from cirrhosis and hepatocellular carcinoma in Western Europe over the last 40 years. Liver Int. 2017;37(8):1193–201.
5. American College of Radiology. CT/MRI LI-RADS® v2018. 2018. https://www.acr.org/Clinical-Resources/Reporting-and-Data-Systems/LI-RADS/CT-MRI-LI-RADS-v2018.
6. van den Hoven AF, Braat MN, Prince JF, et al. Liver CT for vascular mapping during radioembolisation workup: comparison of an early and late arterial phase protocol. Eur Radiol. 2017;27(1):61–9.
7. Bae KT. Intravenous contrast medium administration and scan timing at CT: considerations and approaches. Radiology. 2010;256(1):32–61.
8. Ichikawa T, Okada M, Kondo H, et al. Recommended iodine dose for multiphasic contrast-enhanced mutidetector-row computed tomography imaging of liver for assessing hypervascular hepatocellular carcinoma: multicenter prospective study in 77 general hospitals in Japan. Acad Radiol. 2013;20(9):1130–6.
9. Taguchi N, Oda S, Utsunomiya D, et al. Using 80 kVp on a 320-row scanner for hepatic multiphasic CT reduces the contrast dose by 50 % in patients at risk for contrast-induced nephropathy. Eur Radiol. 2017;27(2):812–20.
10. Iyama Y, Nakaura T, Yokoyama K, et al. Impact of knowledge-based iterative model reconstruction in abdominal dynamic CT with low tube voltage and low contrast dose. AJR Am J Roentgenol. 2016;206(4):687–93.
11. Nakaura T, Nagayama Y, Kidoh M, et al. Low contrast dose protocol involving a 100 kVp tube voltage for hypervascular hepatocellular carcinoma in patients with renal dysfunction. Jpn J Radiol. 2015;33(9):566–76.
12. Nakamoto A, Yamamoto K, Sakane M, et al. Reduction of the radiation dose and the amount of contrast material in hepatic dynamic CT using low tube voltage and adaptive iterative dose reduction 3-dimensional. Medicine (Baltimore). 2018;97(34):e11857.
13. Noda Y, Kanematsu M, Goshima S, et al. Reducing iodine load in hepatic CT for patients with chronic liver disease with a combination of low-tube-voltage and adaptive statistical iterative reconstruction. Eur J Radiol. 2015;84(1):11–8.
14. Han JK, Choi BI, Kim AY, Kim SJ. Contrast media in abdominal computed tomography: optimization of delivery methods. Korean J Radiol. 2001;2(1):28–36.
15. Ichikawa T, Erturk SM, Araki T. Multiphasic contrast-enhanced multidetector-row CT of liver: contrast-enhancement theory and practical scan protocol with a combination of fixed injection duration and patients' body-weight-tailored dose of contrast material. Eur J Radiol. 2006;58(2):165–76.
16. Mehnert F, Pereira PL, Trubenbach J, Kopp AF, Claussen CD. Biphasic spiral CT of the liver: automatic bolus tracking or time delay? Eur Radiol. 2001;11(3):427–31.
17. Sween S, Samar C, Binu SM. Triple-phase MDCT of liver: scan protocol modification to obtain optimal vascular and lesional contrast. Indian J Radiol Imaging. 2018;28(3):315–9.
18. Leggett RW, Williams LR. A proposed blood circulation model for Reference Man. Health Phys. 1995;69(2):187–201.
19. Tang A, Billiard JS, Chagnon DO, et al. Optimal pancreatic phase delay with 64-detector CT scanner and bolus-tracking technique. Acad Radiol. 2014;21(8):977–85.
20. Yanaga Y, Awai K, Nakayama Y, et al. Pancreas: patient body weight tailored contrast material injection protocol versus fixed dose protocol at dynamic CT. Radiology. 2007;245(2):475–82.
21. Scialpi M, Cagini L, Pierotti L, et al. Detection of small (</= 2 cm) pancreatic adenocarcinoma and surrounding parenchyma: correlations between enhancement patterns at triphasic MDCT and histologic features. BMC Gastroenterol. 2014;14:16.
22. Yamada Y, Mori H, Matsumoto S, Kiyosue H, Hori Y, Hongo N. Pancreatic adenocarcinoma versus chronic pancreatitis: differentiation with triple-phase helical CT. Abdom Imaging. 2010;35(2):163–71.
23. National Comprehensive Cancer Network®. NCCN Clinical Practice Guidelines in Oncology (NCCN Guidelines®). Pancreatic Adenocarcinoma. NCCN Guidelines version 2.2018. 2018. https://www.nccn.org/professionals/physician_gls/default.aspx.
24. Garces-Descovich A, Beker K, Jaramillo-Cardoso A, James Moser A, Mortele KJ. Applicability of current

NCCN Guidelines for pancreatic adenocarcinoma resectability: analysis and pitfalls. Abdom Radiol (NY). 2018;43(2):314–22.
25. Al-Hawary MM, Francis IR, Chari ST, et al. Pancreatic ductal adenocarcinoma radiology reporting template: consensus statement of the Society of Abdominal Radiology and the American Pancreatic Association. Radiology. 2014;270(1):248–60.
26. Shimada K, Nara S, Esaki M, Sakamoto Y, Kosuge T, Hiraoka N. Intrapancreatic nerve invasion as a predictor for recurrence after pancreaticoduodenectomy in patients with invasive ductal carcinoma of the pancreas. Pancreas. 2011;40(3):464–8.
27. Zuo HD, Tang W, Zhang XM, Zhao QH, Xiao B. CT and MR imaging patterns for pancreatic carcinoma invading the extrapancreatic neural plexus (Part II): imaging of pancreatic carcinoma nerve invasion. World J Radiol. 2012;4(1):13–20.
28. Mochizuki K, Gabata T, Kozaka K, et al. MDCT findings of extrapancreatic nerve plexus invasion by pancreas head carcinoma: correlation with en bloc pathological specimens and diagnostic accuracy. Eur Radiol. 2010;20(7):1757–67.

Contrast-Enhanced Magnetic Resonance Imaging of the Liver and Pancreas

13

Tomoaki Ichikawa

13.1 Liver

13.1.1 Selection of Contrast Material for Contrast-Enhanced Magnetic Resonance Imaging (CE-MRI) of the Liver

Detection and characterization of hepatic lesions using CE-MRI require multiphasic acquisition that includes the hepatic arterial-dominant (HAP), portal venous (PVP), and delayed (DP) phases, and gadolinium ethoxybenzyl diethylenetriamine pentaacetic acid (Gd-EOB-DTPA; gadoxetic acid) is commonly utilized as the contrast material for image acquisition. Conventional acquisition utilizing extracellular gadolinium-based contrast material (ECCM-MRI) allows assessment of lesion hemodynamics, but more detailed information requires acquisition of additional imaging during the hepatocyte phase (HP), which reflects absorption of the contrast medium into the hepatic cells. Acquisition of EOB-MRI, obtained using Gd-EOB-DTPA for contrast, includes imaging of all four phases and has permitted the highest detection of lesions in comparison among findings using various imaging modalities. EOB-MRI reflects the degree of contrast material taken up by hepatic cells and the associated iso, hypo-, or hyperintensity of signal of lesions.

However, gadolinium-based contrast material is contraindicated in some patients, such as those with severe renal dysfunction or allergic reaction, and in these cases, superparamagnetic iron oxide (SPIO) may be substituted for ECCM and Gd-EOB-DTPA for image acquisition.

13.1.2 Acquisition of CE-MRI with ECCM or Gd-EOB-DTPA

Acquisition of MRI utilizing Gd-EOB-DTPA in both ECCM-MRI and EOB-MRI usually employs three-dimensional (3D), fat-suppressed, gradient-echo T1-weighted (3D-FSGRE T1W) sequences because these sequences demonstrate excellent spatial and contrast resolution. Evaluation of hepatic lesions requires multiphasic acquisition that includes the hepatic arterial-dominant (HAP), portal venous (PVP), and delayed (DP) phases, followed by acquisition of hepatocyte-phase imaging. For ECCM-MRI, 0.2 mL/kg of ECCM is injected at 2 to 3 mL/s followed by saline flush, and for EOB-MRI, 0.1 mL/kg of Gd-EOB-DTPA is injected at a rate of about 1 mL/s followed by saline flush. Faster injection of such a small amount of contrast material in EOB-MRI may produce severe artifacts in HAP images [1]

T. Ichikawa (✉)
Department of Diagnostic Radiology and Nuclear Medicine, Gunma University Graduate School of Medicine, Maebashi, Gunma, Japan

S. M. Erturk et al. (eds.), *Medical Imaging Contrast Agents: A Clinical Manual*,
https://doi.org/10.1007/978-3-030-79256-5_13

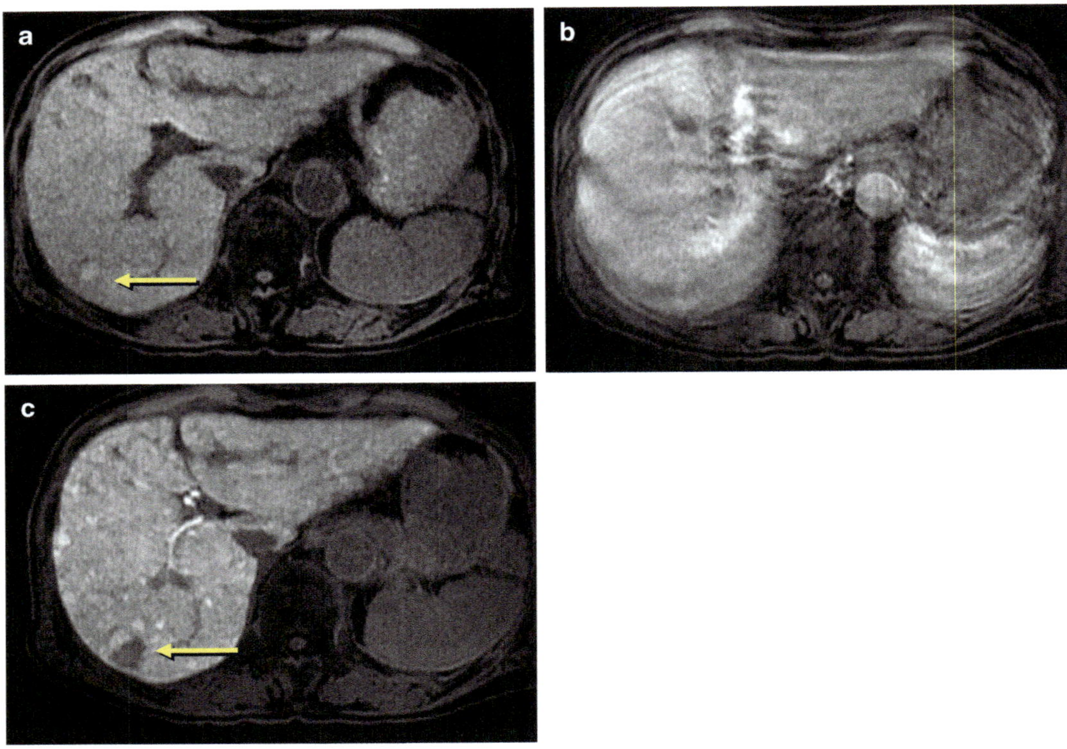

Fig. 13.1 A 79-year-old man with a partially dedifferentiated hepatocellular carcinoma (HCC) from an early hypovascular HCC (yellow arrows). Magnetic resonance images obtained with Gd-EOB-DTPA (EOB-MRI): (**a**) unenhanced phase, (**b**) hepatic arterial-dominant phase (HAP), and (**c**) hepatocyte phase (HP). A nodular lesion showing (**a**) partial hyperintensity in an unenhanced image and (**b**) partial hypointensity in an image obtained during hepatocyte phase (**c**) is noted at the inferoposterior segment of the right lobe of the liver. The area of hypointensity in (**c**) suggests the partially dedifferentiated component of the HCC, and the presence of early contrast enhancement may be presumed in the area in (**a**). Note that transient severe image artifacts in (**a**) alone prevent evaluation of early contrast enhancement

(Fig. 13.1), but diluting the injected dose of Gd-EOB-DTPA may avoid this effect [2]. Any method of bolus tracking can be used for HAP imaging with either ECCM- or EOB-MRI. It is important to set the scan timing of the center of the k-space to initiate HAP imaging 15–20 s after the contrast material reaches the aorta, as determined by the bolus tracking [3]. PVP images are then obtained about 70 s after the initiation of injection of the contrast material and DP images, about 3 min after injection is begun. Acquisition of HP images with EOB-MRI is begun 15–20 min after the start of the injection of Gd-EOB-DTPA [4].

13.1.3 EOB-MRI

13.1.3.1 Principle of Hepatic Uptake of Gd-EOB-DTPA in EOB-MRI

In EOB-MRI, Gd-EOB-DTPA is conveyed through the sinusoidal membranes of hepatocytes by the transport protein, organic anion transporter polypeptide 1B3 (OATP1B3) [5, 6], and it is excreted into the bile by another transporter, multidrug resistance protein 2 (MRP2) [7]. Decreased expression of OATP1B3 in some kinds of hepatic lesions provides excellent image contrast between lesions and adjacent normal liver parenchyma in hepatocyte-phase images [5]. The expression pattern of MRP2 may have some influence on image contrast, but it is the expression of OATP1B3 by hepatic lesions that is considered the primary determiner of enhancement patterns in HP images [5–7].

Kitao's team elegantly demonstrated a stepwise decrease in transporter expression in multistep hepatocarcinogenesis [8]. Similarly, our immunohistochemical analysis [9] demonstrated decreased expression of OATP1B3 in 92% of early (hypovascular) hepatocellular carcinomas (e-HCC) from the normal expression in all dysplastic nodules (DN). In addition, we observed excellent correlation between OATP1B3 expression in both DN and e-HCC and the intensity of signal in HP images, noting iso-/high signal intensity in all DN and in e-HCC demonstrating normal OATP1B3 expression and hypointensity in most e-HCC demonstrating decreased or no expression. Thus, the expression of OATP1B3 serves as a major determiner of the hypointensity of e-HCC in HP images. We have noted similar association as well between hypointensity and conventional (hypervascular) hepatocellular carcinoma (c-HCC) which ordinarily demonstrates no OATP1B3 expression.

13.1.3.2 Characteristics of Hemodynamics and Image Contrast in EOB-MRI

Theoretically, approximately half of Gd-EOB-DTPA is hepatocyte-specific, taken into the hepatocytes and finally excreted into the biliary tract, and the other half works outside the liver cells (extracellular) and is excreted via the kidney (ECCM). Therefore, both CE-MRI obtained with conventional acquisition utilizing extracellular gadolinium-based contrast material (ECCM-MRI) and that of EOB allow assessment of the arterial hemodynamics of lesions in hepatic arterial-dominant-phase images. However, the hepatocytic uptake of Gd-EOB-DTPA in EOB-MRI permits subsequent acquisition of HP images [4, 10].

Time-intensity measurement indicates that Gd-EOB-DTPA uptake into hepatocytes begins from 1.5 min after its injection [10], with hepatocyte-specific contrast enhancement visually identifiable from around 3 min that becomes dominant in images obtained 4–5 min after injection. Thus, the degree of hepatocyte-specific contrast enhancement is the chief determiner of visual image contrast, and extracellular contrast enhancement cannot be assessed on images obtained after 5 min (Fig. 13.2). So, the delayed phase of EOB-MRI differs from that with ECCM-MRI. In EOB-MRI, acquisition of delayed-phase images 3 min after the injection of Gd-EOB-DTPA may not allow sufficient time to acquire diagnostically optimal images that clearly depict lesion characteristics that are readily apparent in delayed-phase images of ECCM-MRI. As examples, delayed-phase images of ECCM-MRI can show the washout that is characteristic of c-HCC, the pooling of contrast material typical of hemangioma, or delayed enhancement commonly manifested in cholangiocarcinoma.

Generally, hepatic-phase images should be obtained 20 min after injection of GD-EOB-DTPA, but personal experience has shown that 10–15 min may be adequate for imaging in a healthy liver. It is helpful to know that the ratio of contrast between the signal intensity of the liver and that of the spleen (LSCR) in HP images aids visual estimation of optimal image contrast, that is, visually assessing whether hepatocytic uptake of Gd-EOB-DTPA is sufficient to demonstrate hepatic lesions in HP images. Based on our results [11], LSCR of at least 1.5 represents sufficient contrast to detect lesions in HP images (Fig. 13.3), but LSCR below 1.5 may not offer adequate contrast to identify all lesions (Fig. 13.4). LSCR is frequently below 1.5 in images of patients with cirrhotic liver, so that contrast is insufficient to classify the degree of liver failure as Child-Pugh A, B, or C. This lack of contrast has been noted at 10 min after injection of Gd-EOB-DTPA in 23% of patients with diagnosed Child-Pugh A disease, 59% with Child-Pugh B, and 100% with Child-Pugh C and at 20 min after injection in 9% with Child-Pugh A disease, 38% with Child-Pugh B, and 75% with Child-Pugh C. One disadvantage with EOB-MRI is the prolongation of examination time to accommodate acquisition of HP images 20 min after the injection of contrast material. The shortening of overall imaging duration of EOB-MRI has been reported with the acquisition of T2-

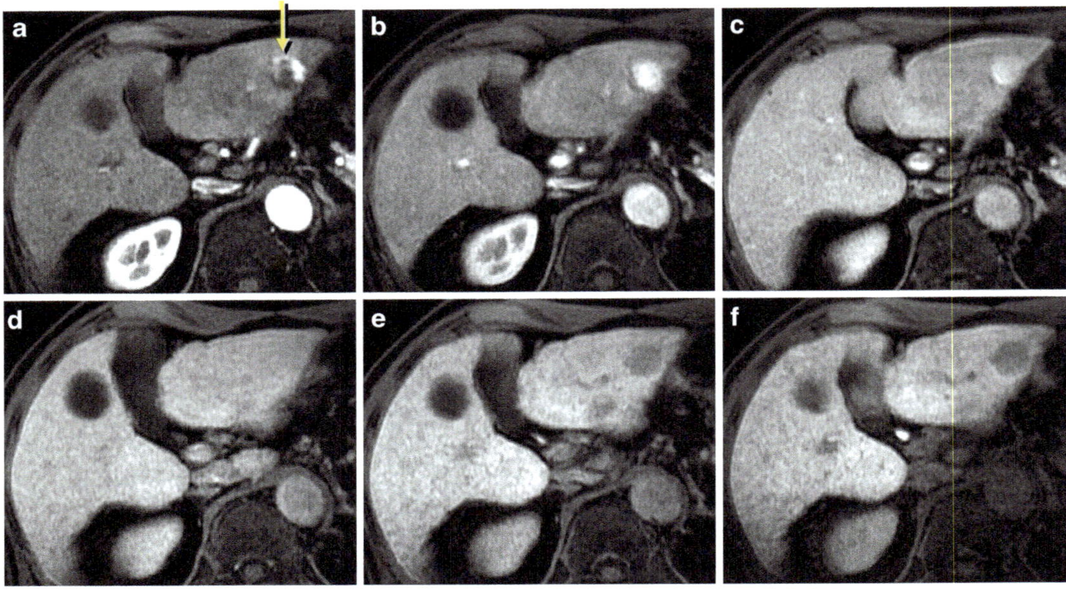

Fig. 13.2 An 81-year-old woman with a typical hepatic hemangioma (yellow arrow). Magnetic resonance images obtained with Gd-EOB-DTPA (EOB-MRI): (**a**) 20 s after injection of contrast material (hepatic arterial-dominant phase [HAP]), (**b**) 2 min after injection (portal venous phase [PVP]), (**c**) 3 min after injection (delayed phase [DP]), and (**d**) 5 min, (**e**) 10 min, and (**f**) 20 min after injection (hepatocyte phase [HP]). A nodular lesion is observed at the lateral segment of the left lobe of the liver. The nodule shows (**a**) peripheral, nodular early contrast enhancement in the HAP image and (**b**) and (**c**) centripetal extracellular contrast enhancement throughout the nodule in (**b**) PVP and (**c**) DP phases, typical findings of hepatic hemangioma. However, the nodule (**d**) becomes unclear 5 min after injection of Gd-EOB-DTPA and demonstrates hypointensity compared with the peripheral hepatic parenchyma in images obtained (**e**) 10 min and (**f**) 20 min after contrast injection due to the predominance of hepatocyte-specific contrast enhancement

or diffusion-weighted MR images (T2WI or DWI) between delayed and hepatocyte phases [12], and using this technique, we have observed no significant changes in enhancement of images obtained before and after either T2WI or DWI acquisition that affect lesion detection [13] (Fig. 13.5).

13.1.3.3 Clinical Application of EOB-MRI

Conventional (Hypervascular) Hepatocellular Carcinoma (c-HCC)

Detection of c-HCC is most common in the hepatic arterial-dominant phase. Previous studies have mentioned similar detectability of c-HCC using classic ECCM-MRI and multiphasic contrast-enhanced multidetector CT (CE-MDCT), but findings of each of these modalities have been inferior to results obtained using a combination of CT during arterial portography (CTAP) and CT during hepatic arteriography (CTHA) [14–16]. Furthermore, recent investigations have emphasized the greater sensitivity of EOB-MRI to that of the CTAP-CTHA combination to detect c-HCC, especially lesions smaller than 2 cm [17]. Hepatocyte-phase images of EOB-MRI have been particularly useful in the detection, differentiation, and diagnosis of HCC (Fig. 13.6). Di Martino and associates [18] found that the addition of HP imaging to the dynamic phases of EOB-MRI significantly improved sensitivity and specificity in the detection of c-HCC, whereas without the additional HP imaging, sensitivity and specificity were comparable between EOB-MRI and CE-MDCT.

Conventional hepatocellular carcinoma typically shows no expression of OATP1B3 and appears as hypointensity in HP images. However, in the current study, we observed increased expression of OATP1B3 and entire or partial iso-/hyperintensity on HP images in approximately 10% of c-HCC [19, 20]. Although the precise

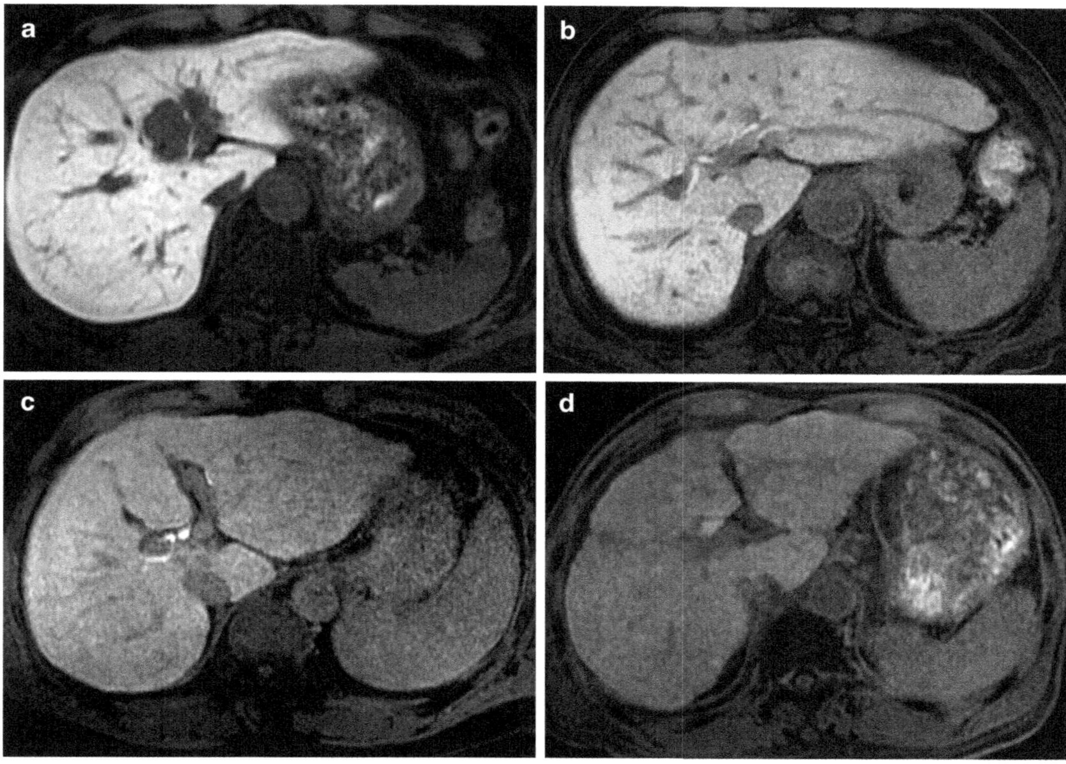

Fig. 13.3 Effects of hepatic function for hepatocyte-specific contrast enhancement on hepatocyte phase (HP). Magnetic resonance images obtained with Gd-EOB-DTPA (EOB-MRI). HP images obtained of patients with (**a**) normal liver and (**b**) cirrhotic liver classified as (**b**) Child-Pugh A, (**c**) Child-Pugh B, and (**d**) Child-Pugh C. Visual contrast of the liver to the spleen (LS) is considered (**a**) excellent and (**b**) good (**b**). Quantitatively, the ratio of the contrast in signal intensity between the liver and the spleen (LSCR) is 1.5 or more. (**c and d**) Visual LS contrast gradually diminishes in proportion to liver function, and LSCR is below 1.5

mechanism of the increased expression of OATP1B3 in c-HCC remains uncertain, this phenomenon may be important because most c-HCC that demonstrate iso-/hyperintensity on HP images are moderately as opposed to well or poorly differentiated (Fig. 13.7) and may show better clinical outcome [19, 20].

Early (Hypovascular) Hepatocellular Carcinoma (e-HCC)

Clinical Background and Diagnostic Significance in the Detection and Differentiation of e-HCC and Dysplastic Nodules

Early detection of HCC is important to improve prognosis [21]. Treatment in its early stages results in a lower rate of recurrence, longer time to recurrence, and higher 5-year survival rate than those of more advanced disease.

HCC develops by multi-step carcinogenesis from low- to high-grade DN to early HCC to progressed disease [22, 23]. However, precise detection of early HCC and its accurate differentiation from DN are extremely difficult with conventional diagnostic modalities, such as multiphasic contrast-enhanced CT or dynamic MRI with extracellular gadolinium contrast agents. The very similar pathological features, including the hemodynamic condition of early HCC, with those seen in DN and sometimes even surrounding liver parenchyma contribute to this difficulty [24].

A distinct pathological definition of early HCC has been established only recently by a group of 34 pathologists and 2 clinicians from 13 countries [25,

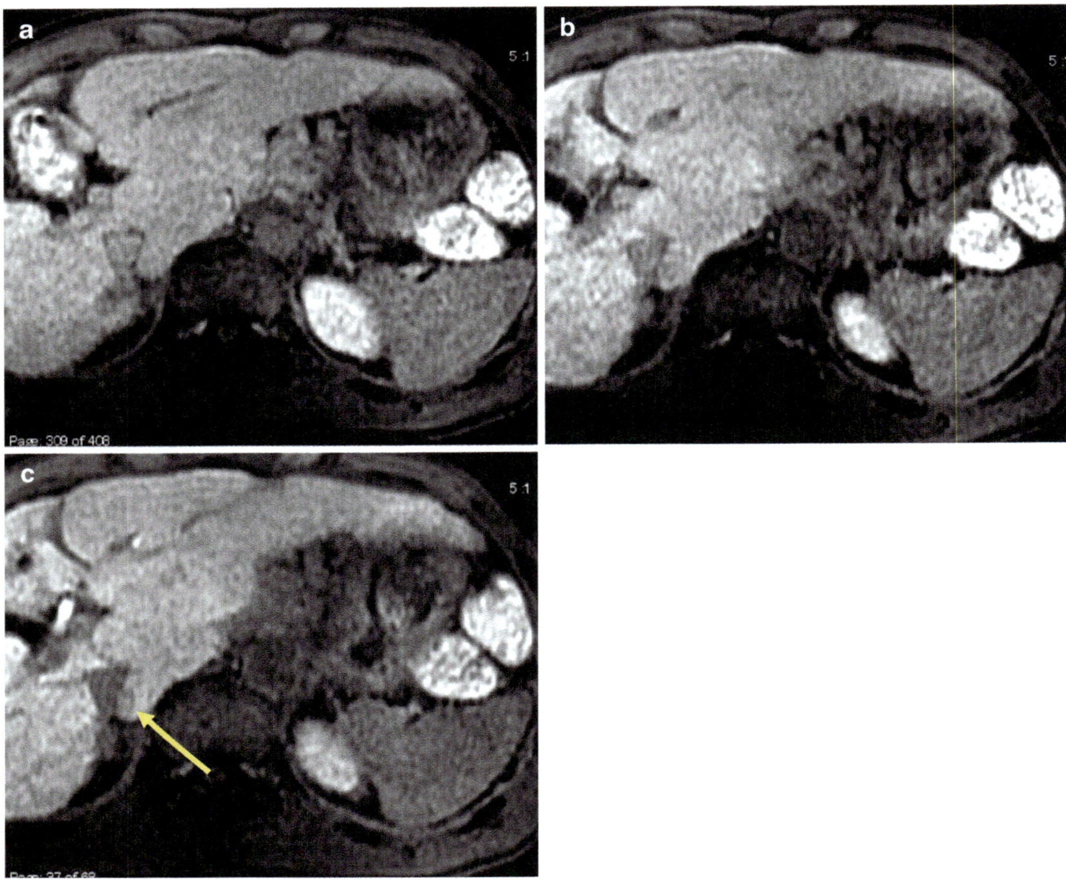

Fig. 13.4 A 70-year-old man with a conventional hepatocellular carcinoma (HCC) (yellow arrow). Magnetic resonance images obtained with Gd-EOB-DTPA (EOB-MRI): (**a**) 5 min, (**b**) 10 min, and (**c**) 20 min after injection of contrast material (hepatocyte phase [HP]). Visual contrast between the liver and the spleen (LS) is considered (**a**) nondiagnostic 5 min after Gd-EOB-DTPA injection and (**b**) poor 10 min after injection. Quantitatively, the ratio of contrast between signal intensity in the liver and that in the spleen (LSCR) is below 1.5, 1.11 in (**a**) and 1.23 in (**b**). (**c**) Visual LS contrast is improved 20 min after the administration of Gd-EOB-DTPA, and the LSCR is more than 1.5 (1.59). Finally, the HCC just adjacent to the inferior vena cava can be detected as hypointensity compared with the peripheral hepatic parenchyma only on (**c**)

26]. The International Consensus Group for Hepatocellular Neoplasia (ICGHN) set forth very specific criteria that characterize the pathology of early HCC and its differentiation from DN that take into account the diagnostic ability of each imaging modality to detect early HCC [25, 27]. After efforts by many others over decades to describe adequately diagnostic features of this disease process, the ICGHN has produced the first reliable and reproducible guide for the sometimes very daunting task of assessing HCC at all its stages.

The important role of EOB-MRI has recently come into focus among various imaging modalities, and its excellent depiction of e-HCC lesions in HP images is expected. Early reports of multicenter phase III studies have predicted that the lack of uptake of Gd-EOB-DTPA by e-HCC as well as most c-HCC may demonstrate hypointensity on HP images [28]. Moreover, no other imaging technique has permitted accurate differentiation between e-HCC and DN on HP images [17].

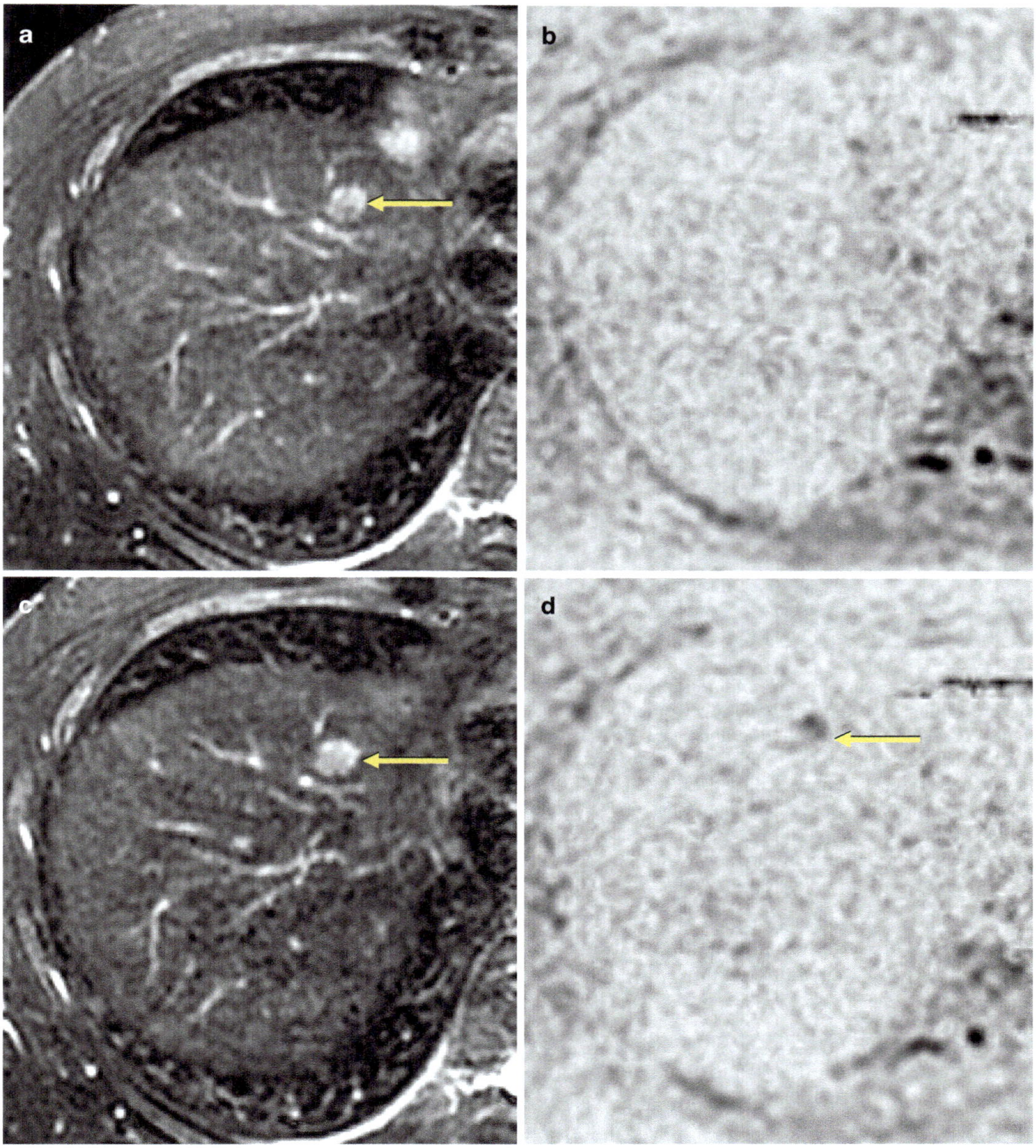

Fig. 13.5 A 68-year-old man with a conventional hepatocellular carcinoma (HCC) (yellow arrows). (**a**) Precontrast T2-weighted, (**b**) diffusion-weighted, (**c**) postcontrast T2-weighted, and (**d**) diffusion-weighted magnetic resonance (MR) images. (**a**, **c**) T2-weighted MR images demonstrate hyperintensity of HCC at the medial segment of the left lobe of the liver. Delineation of the tumor is clearer in the postcontrast image (**c**) than the image acquired before contrast administration (**a**). (**b**, **d**) In diffusion-weighted MR images, (**b**) prior to contrast administration, the tumor cannot be detected and (**d**) appears only after administration of Gd-EOB-DTPA because the signal intensity of the peripheral hepatic parenchyma decreases on the postcontrast MR images

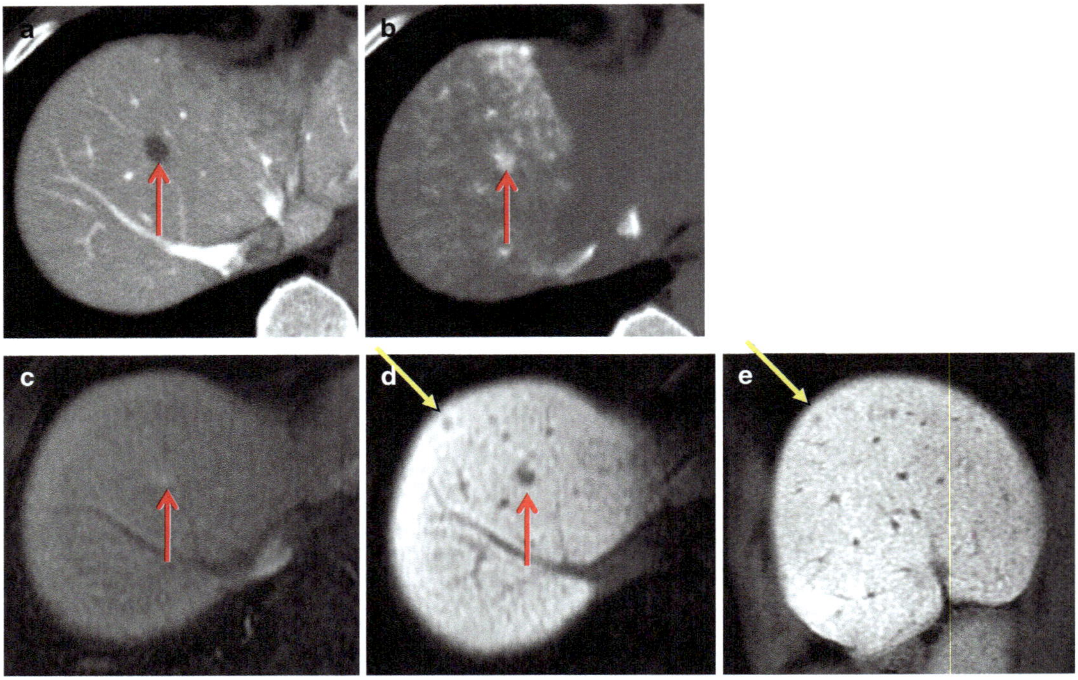

Fig. 13.6 A 58-year-old man with multiple conventional hepatocellular carcinomas (HCC). (**a**) Computed tomography (CT) during arterioportography (CTAP), (**b**) CT during hepatic arteriography (CTHA), (**c–e**) magnetic resonance images obtained with Gd-EOB-DTPA (EOB-MRI) in (**c**) hepatic arterial-dominant phase (HAP), and (**d**) and (**e**) hepatocyte phase (HP) (axial (**d**), sagittal (**e**)). A nodule is seen at the anterosuperior segment of the right lobe of the liver. The nodule shows (**a**) lack of portal flow in CTAP, (**b**) and (**c**) early contrast enhancement (arterial flow) in CTHA and HAP phase of EOB-MRI, and (**d**) hypointensity in axial image of hepatocyte phase in EOB-MRI, typical findings of conventional HCC (red arrows). (**d, e**) An additional small HCC was revealed at the anterosuperior segment of the right lobe of the liver during surgery (yellow arrows)

Comparison of Detection and Differentiation of e-HCC Among EOB-MRI and Other Imaging Modalities

Differentiating early HCC from high-grade DN can be extremely delicate and even impossible for some nodules, especially in the analysis and diagnosis of biopsy specimens. We therefore undertook the evaluation of the entire surgically resected hepatocellular nodules diagnosed according to the criteria set forth by the ICGHN [17]. We found hypointensity on HP images of EOB-MRI to be the most important imaging feature for both the detection of e-HCC and its differentiation from DN (Figs. 13.8 and 13.9); only one e-HCC lesion showed isointensity compared with the surrounding liver parenchyma. EOB-MRI demonstrated excellent sensitivity (97%) and specificity (100%) in differentiating e-HCC and DN.

Other imaging modalities, including contrast-enhanced CT, unenhanced MRI, CTAP, and CTHA, highlighted different features for the detection of e-HCC and its differentiation from DN, but the sensitivities of these features were fat-containing appearance determined by hypoattenuation on unenhanced CT (42%) or combined with in- and opposed-phase T1-weighted MR images (T1WI) (52%) (Fig. 13.8b, c) and portal flow decrease to any degree (hypoattenuation) on CTAP (42%).

Thus, only hypointensity on HP images of EOB-MRI demonstrated near-perfect sensitivity and specificity for evaluating e-HCC.

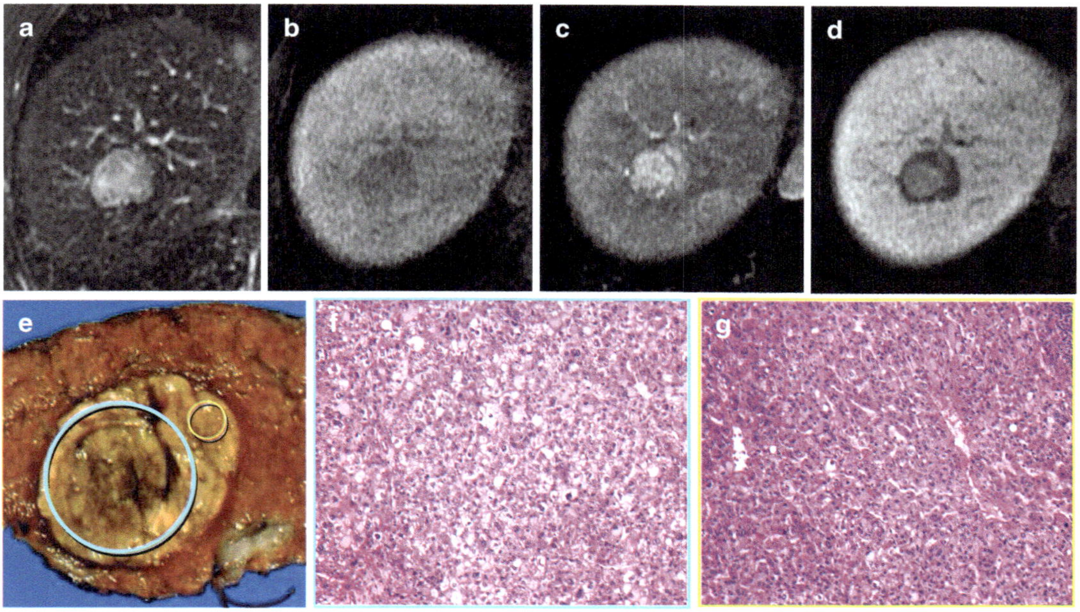

Fig. 13.7 A 62-year-old man with conventional hepatocellular carcinoma (HCC). Magnetic resonance images obtained with Gd-EOB-DTPA (EOB-MRI): (**a**) T2-weighted, (**b**) unenhanced, (**c**) hepatic arterial-dominant phase (HAP), and (**d**) hepatocyte phase (HP). (**e**) Macroscopic and (**f**, **g**) microscopic pathological specimens. A nodule at the anterosuperior segment of the right lobe of the liver shows (**a**) hyperintensity in T2-weighted image and (**c**) early contrast enhancement in HAP, typical findings of conventional HCC. (**d**) The nodule shows partial uptake of Gd-EOB-DTPA. Pathologically, the area showing the uptake of Gd-EOB-DTPA (**e**) looks slightly greenish in macroscopic specimen (so-called green hepatoma; blue circle) and corresponds with (**f**) the moderately differentiated component of a microscopic specimen, whereas (**e**) the area lacking uptake of Gd-EOB-DTPA in the macroscopic specimen (yellow circle) corresponds with (**g**) the well-differentiated component of the other microscopic specimen

Current Consensus for the Diagnosis of e-HCC with EOB-MRI

Sano and colleagues [17] have reported excellent sensitivity (97%) and specificity (100%) in HP imaging, and Golfieri's team [29] has reported its accuracy (95–100%) in the detection of e-HCC and the differentiation of e-HCC from DN. It might therefore be reasonable to assume from their results, based on the correlation of imaging and pathologic findings and clinical follow-up for nodules showing hypointensity on HP images, that most hypovascular early-stage hepatocellular nodules that demonstrate hypointensity on HP images comprise a greater proportion of early HCC and lower proportion of high-grade DN and should therefore be treated clinically as malignancy. This understanding has been researched and developed in Eastern and Western countries [30, 31], and a review paper by authors in Western country has reported the utility of EOB-MRI for differentiating e-HCC from DN, observing the hypointensity of most HCC, including early disease, and the predominant absence of hypointensity on HP images of dysplastic nodules [32].

Hepatic Metastasis

The excellent detectability of hepatic metastases by HP imaging compared with various other imaging methods has been noted [33, 34]. Muhi and associates [34] confirmed similar findings for HP detection of hepatic metastases from colorectal cancers, observing the highest mean sensitivity (95%) and mean positive predictive value (98%) with HP imaging, followed by SPIO-MRI (80%, 96%), ultrasonography (US) (73%, 84%), and CE-MDCT (63%, 96%). In addition, their group clarified the superior sensitivity (92%) and specificity (100%) of HP imaging to detect

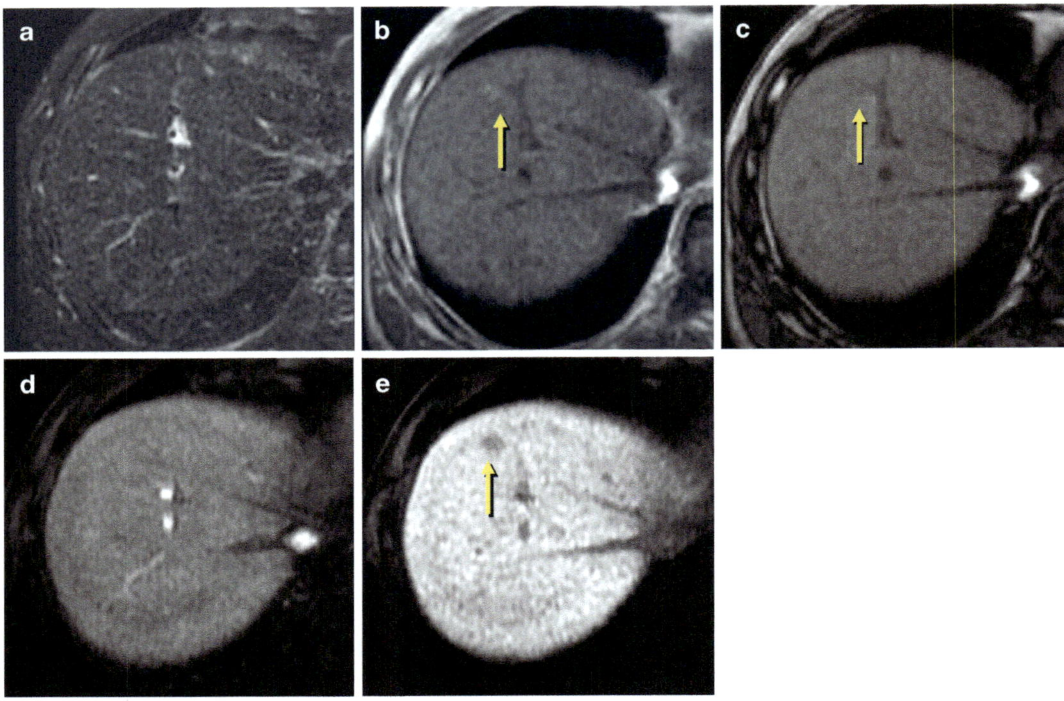

Fig. 13.8 A 70-year-old man with early (hypovascular) hepatocellular carcinoma (HCC) (yellow allows). Magnetic resonance images obtained with Gd-EOB-DTPA (EOB-MRI): (**a**) T2-weighted, (**b**) in-phase and (**c**) opposed-phase T1-weighted, (**d**) hepatic arterial-dominant phase (HAP), and (**e**) hepatocyte phase (HP). (**a**) A nodule at the anterosuperior segment of the right lobe of the liver cannot be detected on T2-weighted image. (**b**) Slightly high signal intensity in in-phase T1-weighted image and (**c**) decreased signal in opposed-phase T1 imaging suggest the presence of a fat component within the nodule. The nodule shows (**d**) no early contrast enhancement in HAP and (e) hypointensity in hepatocyte phase. These MR imaging findings are typical for early HCC

hepatic metastases of 10 mm or less. They observed sensitivity and specificity of 63 and 96% with SPIO-MRI, 41 and 90% with US, and 26 and 93% with CE-MDCT (Fig. 13.10). Thus, the widespread recognition of EOB-MRI as the strongest tool for the assessment of the liver suggests that it should be adopted in place of classic ECCM-MRI as the standard method for the acquisition of CE-MRI.

Hemangioma

As noted, 5 min or more after Gd-EOB-DTPA injection, hepatocyte-specific contrast enhancement becomes dominant and prevents assessment of extracellular enhancement. As a result, DP images of EOB-MRI are defined as those obtained 3 min after the injection of contrast material (Fig. 13.2). However, it should be noted that 3 min may not be sufficient to permit display of the centripetal delayed contrast enhancement characteristically observed in typical hemangiomas with ECCM-MRI, and it can never be identified on images obtained more than 5 min after Gd-EOB-DTPA injection. This is especially true in so-called slow-flow hemangiomas [35] (Fig. 13.11). Therefore, the diagnosis of hemangiomas and differentiation of hepatic metastases require comprehensive analysis of MRI findings. Particular attention should be paid to marked hyperintensity on T2WI and peripheral, nodular early contrast enhancement in HAP images. Compared to findings in hemangiomas, hepatic metastases have been reported to demonstrate lower hyperintensity on T2WI and ring-like, early contrast enhancement on HAP [36].

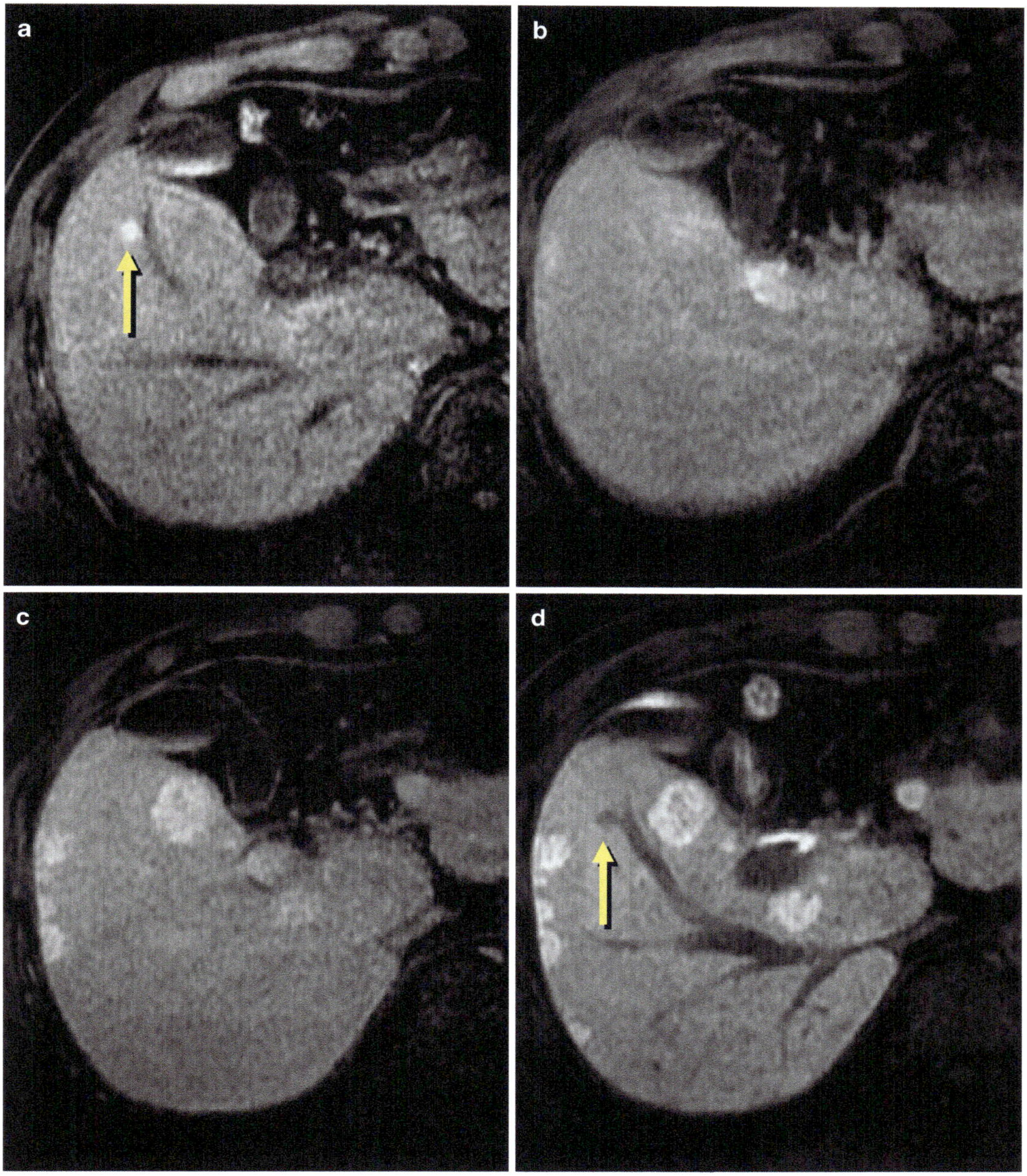

Fig. 13.9 A 63-year-old man with conventional hepatocellular carcinoma (HCC) (yellow arrows) and multiple dysplastic nodules (DN). Magnetic resonance images obtained with Gd-EOB-DTPA (EOB-MRI): (**a**) hepatic arterial-dominant phase (HAP), (**b**) 2 min after contrast injection (portal venous phase [PVP]), (**c**) 3 min after contrast injection (delayed phase [DP]), and (**d**) 20 min after injection (hepatocyte phase [HP]). Conventional HCC at the anteroinferior segment of the right lobe of the liver shows (**a**) early contrast enhancement in HAP and (**d**) hypointensity in hepatocyte phase. Multiple hypovascular nodules demonstrated throughout the liver were proven dysplastic (DN) at surgery. Unlike early HCC, all DN show hyperintensity in (**c**) delayed phase and (**d**) hepatocyte phase because of the uptake of Gd-EOB-DTPA

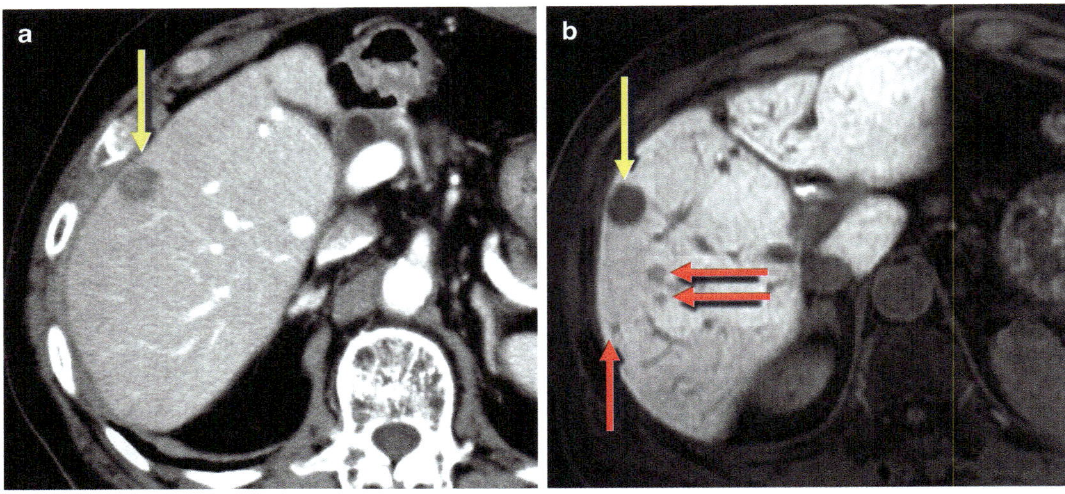

Fig. 13.10 A 66-year-old woman with multiple hepatic metastases from sigmoid colon cancer (yellow allows). (**a**) Portal venous phase (PVP) of contrast-enhanced computed tomography (CT) and (**b**) hepatocyte phase (HP) of magnetic resonance image obtained with Gd-EOB-DTPA (EOB-MRI) obtained 20 min contrast injection. (**a**, **b**) CT and MRI images demonstrate metastasis of 2-cm size (yellow arrows). (**b**) Three additional small metastases are apparent in HP of EOB-MRI (red arrows). Thus, HP imaging with EOB-MRI is superior to contrast-enhanced CT to detect small hepatic metastases smaller than 1 cm

Pseudolesion (Arterioportal Shunt; AP Shunt)

In patients with cirrhotic liver, the hypervascularity of AP shunt on HAP images with CE-MDCT and ECCM-MRI can mimic findings of c-HCC. Their similar shapes may make it difficult to distinguish the two [37–39] (Fig. 13.12). The lack of washout of AP shunt on DP images obtained with CE-MDCT/MRI is the most important image finding to distinguish it from c-HCC, which usually shows washout [37, 38]. However, c-HCC, especially of small size, does not always demonstrate washout. Theoretically, EOB-MRI is useful to distinguish AP shunt from c-HCC because lesion hemodynamics do not influence the static images of hepatocyte phase. In HP images, most AP shunt shows isointensity with the surrounding liver parenchyma and is thus invisible, whereas c-HCC generally shows hypointensity. Our investigation showed that 13% (4/32) of AP shunt demonstrated hypointensity on HP images and was difficult to distinguish from c-HCC [39]. Thus, it should be emphasized that hypervascular lesions should be carefully assessed using multi-imaging diagnostic criteria even if they show hypointensity on HP images.

13.2 Pancreas

13.2.1 CE-MRI of the Pancreas

The detection and characterization of pancreatic lesions, similarly to those of hepatic lesions, also require multiphasic acquisition that consists of pancreatic parenchymal (PPP), portal venous (PVP), and delayed (DP) phases. ECCM is generally used for CE-MRI of the pancreas. The technical details, including the dose of ECCM, scan timing for each phase, and sequence parameters for ECCM-MRI of the pancreas, are the same as those outlined above for ECCM-MRI of the liver. However, in pancreatic imaging, PPP acquisition replaces the HAP scanning of the liver, and PPP scanning is initiated 25–30 s after the contrast material reaches the aorta as determined by bolus tracking, which is 5–10 s later than HAP scanning of the liver. Pancreatic lesions demonstrate very similar contrast enhancement patterns with ECCM-MRI to those with CE-MDCT.

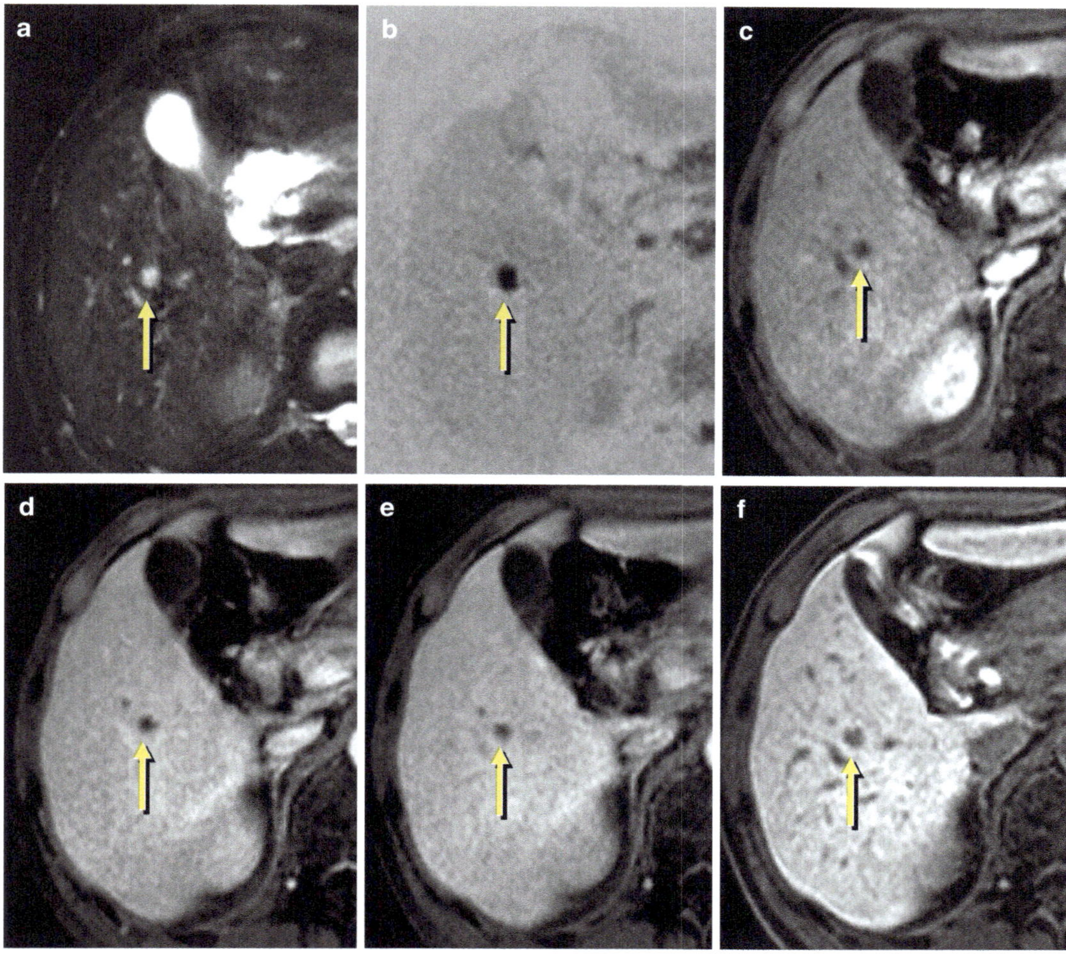

Fig. 13.11 A 46-year-old woman with an atypical (slow-flow) hemangioma (yellow allows). (**a**) T2-weighted magnetic resonance image (MRI). (**b**) diffusion-weighted MRI. (**c**, **f**) Magnetic resonance images obtained with Gd-EOB-DTPA (EOB-MRI): (**c**) hepatic arterial-dominant phase (HAP), (**d**) 2 min after contrast injection (portal venous phase [PVP]), (**e**) 3 min after contrast injection (delayed phase [DP]), and (**f**) 20 min after contrast injection (hepatocyte phase [HP]). A nodule showing marked hyperintensity in (**a**) T2-weighted and (**b**) diffusion-weighted images at the anteroinferior segment of the right lobe of the liver shows neither early nor delayed contrast enhancement in (**c**) HAP, (**d**) PVP, and (**e**) DP and finally (**f**) demonstrates hypointensity in hepatocyte phase. Based on these imaging findings, it is difficult to distinguish the nodule from hepatic metastasis

13.2.2 Application of EOB-MRI to Assess Pancreatic Lesions (Especially Invasive Ductal Adenocarcinoma)

Of the pancreatic neoplasms, invasive ductal adenocarcinoma of the pancreas (pancreatic cancer) is the most common and is the fourth leading cause of cancer death in the United States. Several recent studies have reported the value of ECCM-MRI for preoperative assessment of pancreatic cancer and have suggested that it is almost equivalent to CE-MDCT, though older reports describe the superiority of ECCM-MRI to CE-MDCT [40–43]. In addition, comparable diagnostic performance in the assessment of tumor resectability is reported between ECCM-MRI with the addition of MR cholangiopancreatography and imaging with CE-MDCT [44]. As noted, the detectability of

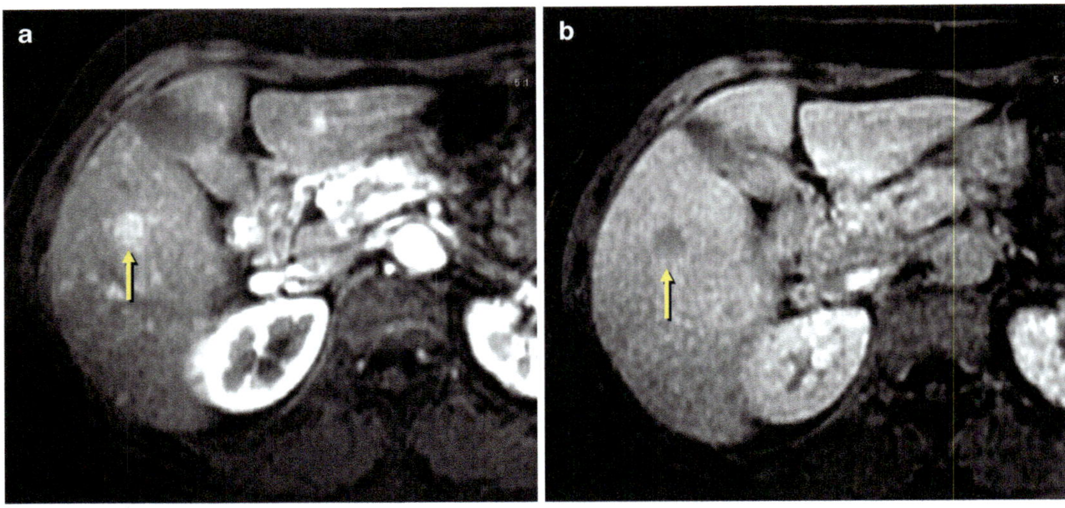

Fig. 13.12 A 74-year-old man with a hypervascular pseudolesion (arterioportal shunt) (yellow allows). Magnetic resonance images obtained with Gd-EOB-DTPA (EOB-MRI): (**a**) hepatic arterial-dominant phase (HAP) and (**b**) 20 min after injection of contrast material (hepatocyte phase, HP). A round lesion at the anteroinferior segment of the right lobe of the liver shows (**a**) early contrast enhancement in HAP and (**b**) hypointensity in HP, findings that mimic those of conventional HCC. Please note that the obscure margin of the hypointense lesion in hepatocyte phase may help distinguish this lesion from conventional HCC

hepatic metastases with HP images of EOB-MRI is significantly higher than that with CE-MDCT and the highest among all imaging modalities [33, 34]. Approximately 20% of patients with pancreatic cancer demonstrate hepatic metastases, and the presence of even one such lesion rules out surgical treatment. Accurate diagnosis is therefore extremely important in preoperative assessment. Thus, clinical management for pancreatic cancers might seem best to rely on Gd-EOB-DTPA rather than ECCM as the first choice for CE-MRI of the pancreas [45, 46].

In terms of differences in enhancement effects between ECCM and Gd-EOB-DTPA, the T1-relaxivity of Gd-EOB-DTPA measured in human blood at 1.5-T is approximately twice that of standard ECCM, such as gadopentetate dimeglumine (Gd-DTPA), at a quarter of the dose (0.025 mmol/kg for Gd-EOB-DTPA versus 0.1 mmol/kg for Gd-DTPA) [47, 48]. Therefore, the enhancement effect of Gd-EOB-DTPA in solid organs and vessels during arterial phase would be about half that of Gd-DTPA. As a result, the degree of contrast enhancement with Gd-EOB-DTPA should be significantly lower than in ECCM-MRI [47]. However, it may be hypothesized that less contrast material may be required for 3D-FSGRE T1W sequences, commonly employed for EOB-MRI of the liver and the pancreas, because the pancreas naturally shows sufficient hyperintensity on unenhanced images [49, 50] to obtain sufficient tumor conspicuity. In our investigation [46], we observed no significant differences between EOB-MRI and CE-MDCT in the detection of pancreatic cancers based on analyses of areas under the receiver operating characteristic curves, sensitivity, specificity, and positive/negative predictive values, whereas sensitivity in the detection of hepatic metastases was significantly higher with EOB-MRI than CE-MDCT (Fig. 13.13).

Overall, we choose EOB-MRI rather than ECCM-MRI at our institution for the preoperative evaluation of pancreatic cancer, particularly valuing the excellent demonstration of hepatic metastases in HP images.

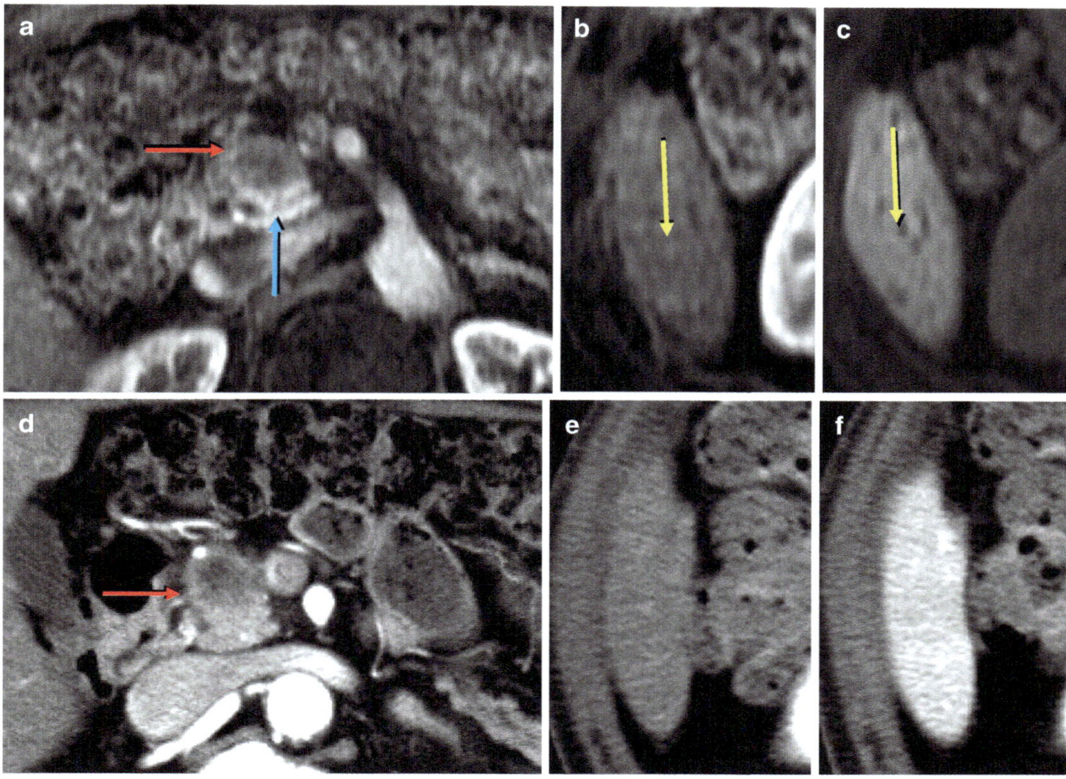

Fig. 13.13 A 72-year-old man with pancreatic cancer at the head of the pancreas (red arrow) and hepatic metastasis (yellow allows). (**a–c**) Magnetic resonance images obtained with Gd-EOB-DTPA (EOB-MRI): (**a**) and (**b**) hepatic arterial-dominant phase (HAP) and (**c**) 20 min injection of contrast material (hepatocyte phase [HP]). (**d, e**) Contrast-enhanced images of multidetector computed tomography (CE-MDCT): (**d**) hepatic arterial-dominant phase (HAP) and (**e**) 2 min after injection of contrast material (portal venous phase (PVP]). (**a, d**) A hypovascular lesion (red arrows) is clearly demonstrated at the head of the pancreas. (**a**) Please note the sufficient image contrast between the hypointense lesion and well-enhanced hyperintense normal parenchyma of the head of the pancreas (blue arrow). A nodular lesion showing (**b**) early contrast enhancement in HAP and (**c**) clear demonstration of hypointensity in hepatocyte phase of MRI was accurately diagnosed preoperatively as hepatic metastasis. However, this lesion is not apparent in the HAP (**e**) and PVP (**f**) image of MDCT. Finally, pathological evaluation of surgical specimens proved the lesion at the head of the pancreas was indeed pancreatic cancer and the hepatic nodule was hepatic metastasis

13.2.3 Acquisition of Magnetic Resonance Cholangiopancreatography (MRCP) with Hepatocyte-Specific Contrast Material

All types of hepatocyte-specific contrast materials, exemplified by Gd-EOB-DTPA, are finally excreted into the bile duct. Both manganese dipyridoxyl diphosphate (Mn-DPDP) and Gd-EOB-DTPA begin to appear in the bile duct 10 min after contrast injection, and gadobenate dimeglumine (Gd-BOPTA) begins to appear 20 min after injection [51, 52]. Contrast-enhanced T1-weighted magnetic resonance cholangiopancreatography (CE-MRCP) images can be obtained after pancreatic imaging with EOB-MRI because the excreted Gd-EOB-DTPA produces a strong T1-shortening effect in the bile duct. CE-MRCP may provide valuable additional information to that of conventional MRCP images obtained with heavily T2-weighted MR sequences (c-MRCP), which have been widely used. CE-MRCP imaging acquired with

Mn-DPDP that employs 3D-FSGRE T1W sequences to improve resolution has more accurately demonstrated anatomic variants of the intrahepatic bile ducts than findings reported with c-MRCP [51]. It has also been emphasized that CE-MRCP can provide information regarding function that cannot be evaluated using c-MRCP images. Examples include information regarding biliary excretion that may be particularly useful in identifying the site of bile leakage as a complication after surgery or elucidation of stenosis/obstruction of the biliary tree [53].

However, CE-MRCP can render the contrast of c-MRCP images nondiagnostic. Acquisition of c-MRCP after the administration of contrast material results in a strong T2-shortening effect as hepatocyte-specific contrast material is excreted, so care should be taken to acquire c-MRCP images before its appearance in the bile duct.

References

1. Zech CJ, et al. Vascular enhancement in early dynamic liver MR imaging in an animal model: comparison of two injection regimen and two different doses Gd-EOB-DTPA with standard Gd-DTPA. Invest Radiol. 2009;44:305–10.
2. Motosugi U, Ichikawa T, Sou H, Sano K, Ichikawa S, Tominaga L, Araki T. Dilution method of gadolinium ethoxybenzyl diethylenetriaminepentaacetic acid (Gd-EOB-DTPA)-enhanced magnetic resonance imaging (MRI). J Magn Reson Imaging. 2009;30:849–54.
3. Kagawa Y, et al. Optimal scanning protocol of arterial dominant phase for hypervascular hepatocellular carcinoma with gadolinium-ethoxybenyldiethylenetriamine pentaacetic acid-enhanced MR. J Magn Reson Imaging. 2011;33:864–72.
4. Reimer P, Rummeny EJ, Shamsi K, Balzer T, Daldrup HE, Tombach B, Hesse T, Berns T, Peters PE. Phase II clinical evaluation of Gd-EOB-DTPA: dose, safety aspects, and pulse sequence. Radiology. 1996;199:177–83.
5. Kitao A, Zen Y, Matsui O, et al. Hepatocellular carcinoma: signal intensity at gadoxetic acid-enhanced MR imaging—correlation with molecular transporters and histopathologic features. Radiology. 2010;256(3):817–26.
6. Narita M, Hatano E, Arizono S, et al. Expression of OATP1B3 determines uptake of Gd-EOB-DTPA in hepatocellular carcinoma. J Gastroenterol. 2009;44(7):793–8.
7. Tsuboyama T, Onishi H, Kim T, et al. Hepatocellular carcinoma: hepatocyte-selective enhancement at gadoxetic acid-enhanced MR imaging—correlation with expression of sinusoidal and canalicular transporters and bile accumulation. Radiology. 2010;255(3):824–33.
8. Kitao A, Matsui O, Yoneda N, et al. The uptake transporter OATP8 expression decreases during multistep hepatocarcinogenesis: correlation with gadoxetic acid enhanced MR imaging. Eur Radiol. 2011;21(10):2056–66.
9. Ichikawa T, Sano K, Morisaka H. Diagnosis of pathologically early HCC with EOB-MRI: experiences and current consensus. Liver Cancer. 2014;3(2):97–107.
10. Vogl TJ, Kümmel S, Hammerstingl R, Schellenbeck M, Schumacher G, Balzer T, Schwarz W, Müller PK, Bechstein WO, Mack MG, Söllner O, Felix R. Liver tumors: comparison of MR imaging with Gd-EOB-DTPA and Gd-DTPA. Radiology. 1996;200:59–67.
11. Motosugi U, Ichikawa T, Sou H, Sano K, Tominaga L, Kitamura T, Araki T. Liver parenchymal enhancement of hepatocyte-phase images in Gd-EOB-DTPA enhanced MR imaging: which biological markers of the liver function affect the enhancement? J Magn Reson Imaging. 2009;30(5):1042–6.
12. Kim YK, et al. Detection and characterization of focal hepatic tumors: a comparison of T2-weighted MR images before and after the administration of gadxetic acid. J Magn Reson Imaging. 2009;30:437–43.
13. Motosugi U, Ichikawa T, Tominaga L, Sou H, Sano K, Ichikawa S, Araki T. Delay before the hepatocyte phase of Gd-EOB-DTPA-enhanced MR imaging: is it possible to shorten the examination time? Eur Radiol. 2009;19(11):2623–9.
14. Hori M, et al. Sensitivity in detection of hypervascular hepatocellular carcinoma by helical CT with intra-arterial injection of contrast medium, and by helical CT and MR imaging with intravenous injection of contrast medium. Acta Radiol. 1998;39:144–51.
15. Jang HJ, et al. Hepatocellular carcinoma: are combined CT during arterial portography and CT gepatic angiography in addition to triple-phase helical CT all necessary for preoperative evaluation? Radiology. 2000;215:473–380.
16. Kanematsu M, et al. Detection of hepatocellular carcinoma in patients with cirrhosis: MR imaging versus angiographically assisted helical CT. AJR. 1997;169:1507–15.
17. Sano K, Ichikawa T, Motosugi U, Sou H, Muhi A, Matsuda M, Nakano M, Sakamoto M, Nakazawa T, Asakawa M, Fujii H, Kitamura T, Enomoto N, Araki T. Imaging study of early hepatocellular carcinoma: usefulness of gadoxetic acid-enhanced MR imaging. Radiology. 2011;261(3):834–44.
18. Martino D, et al. Hepatocellular carcinoma in cirrhotic patients: prospective comparison of US CT and MR imaging. Eur Radiol. 2013;23:887–96.
19. Kitao A, Matsui O, Yoneda N, et al. Hypervascular hepatocellular carcinoma: correlation between bio-

logic features and signal intensity on gadoxetic acid enhanced MR images. Radiology. 2012;265:780–9.
20. Kim JY, Kim MJ, Kim KA, Jeong HT, Park YN. Hyperintense HCC on hepatobiliary phase images of gadoxetic acid-enhanced MRI: correlation with clinical and pathological features. Eur J Radiol. 2012;81:3877–82.
21. Kudo M. Early hepatocellular carcinoma: definition and diagnosis. Liver Cancer. 2013;2:69–72.
22. Kudo M. Multistep human hepatocarcinogenesis: correlation of imaging with pathology. J Gastroenterol. 2009;44(Suppl 19):112–8.
23. Kitao A, Zen Y, Matsui O, Gabata T, Nakanuma Y. Hepatocarcinogenesis: multistep changes of drainage vessels at CT during arterial portography and hepatic arteriography—radiologic-pathologic correlation. Radiology. 2009;252:605–14.
24. Sakamoto M, Hirohashi S, Shimosato Y. Early stages of multistep hepatocarcinogenesis: adenomatous hyperplasia and early hepatocellular carcinoma. Hum Pathol. 1991;22:172–8.
25. International Working Party. Terminology of nodular hepatocellular lesions. Hepatology. 1995;22:983–93.
26. Desmet VJ. East-West pathology agreement on precancerous liver lesions and early hepatocellular carcinoma. Hepatology. 2009;49:355–7.
27. The International Consensus Group for Hepatocellular Neoplasia. Pathologic diagnosis of early hepatocellular carcinoma: a report of the international consensus group for hepatocellular neoplasia. Hepatology. 2009;49:658–64.
28. Ichikawa T, Saito K, Yoshioka N, Tanimoto A, Gokan T, Takehara Y, Kamura T, Gabata T, Murakami T, Ito K, Hirohashi S, Nishie A, Saito Y, Onaya H, Kuwatsuru R, Morimoto A, Ueda K, Kurauchi M, Breuer J. Detection and characterization of focal liver lesions: a Japanese phase III, multicenter comparison between gadoxetic acid disodium-enhanced magnetic resonance imaging and contrast-enhanced computed tomography predominantly in patients with hepatocellular carcinoma and chronic liver disease. Invest Radiol. 2010;45(3):133–41.
29. Golfieri R, et al. Focak lesions in the cirrhotic liver: their pivotal role in gadoxetic acid-enhanced MRI and recognition by the Western guidelines. Dig Dis. 2014;32:696–704.
30. Kudo M. Natural course of hypovascular nodule, which shows low intense on hepatobiliary phase Gd-EOBDTPA. Kantansuigazo. 2012;14:369–70.
31. Van Beers BE, Pastor CM, Hussain HK. Primovist, Eovist: what to expect? J Hepatol. 2012;57:421–9.
32. Lee JM, Zech CJ, Bolondi L, Jonas E, Kim MJ, Matsui O, Merkle EM, Sakamoto M, Choi BI. Consensus report of the 4th international forum for gadoliniumethoxybenzyl-diethylenetriamine pentaacetic acid magnetic resonance imaging. J Hepatol. 2011;12:403–15.
33. Kim YK, Lee YH, Kwak HS, Kim CS, Han YM. Detection of liver metastases: gadoxetic acid enhanced three-dimensional MR imaging versus ferucarbotran-enhanced MR imaging. Eur J Radiol. 2010;73:131–6.
34. Muhi A, Ichikawa T, Motosugi U, Sou H, Nakajima H, Sano K, Sano M, Kato S, Kitamura T, Fatima Z, Fukushima K, Iino H, Mori Y, Fujii H, Araki T. Diagnosis of colorectal hepatic metastases: comparison of contrast-enhanced CT, contrast-enhanced US, superparamagnetic iron oxide-enhanced MRI, and gadoxetic acid-enhanced MRI. J Magn Reson Imaging. 2011;34:326–35.
35. Jang HJ, Kim TK, Lim HK, et al. Hepatic hemangioma: atypical appearances on CT, MR imaging, and sonography. AJR. 2003;180:135–41.
36. Motosugi U, Ichikawa T, Onohara K, Sou H, Sano K, Muhi A, Araki T. Distinguishing hepatic metastasis from hemangioma using gadoxetic acid-enhanced magnetic resonance imaging. Invest Radiol. 2011;46:359–65.
37. Kim TK, et al. Nontumorous arterioportal shunt mimicking hypervascular tumor in cirrhotic liver: two-phase spiral CT findings. Radiology. 1998;208:597–603.
38. Ahn JH, et al. Nontumorous arterioportal shunt in the liver: CT and MRI findings considering mechanisms and fate. Eur Radiol. 2010;20:385–94.
39. Motosugi U, Ichikawa T, Sou H, Sano K, Tominaga L, Muhi A, Araki T. Distinguishing hypervascular pseudolesions of the liver from hypervascular hepatocellular carcinomas with gadoxetic acid-enhanced MR imaging. Radiology. 2010;256(1):151–8.
40. Sheridan MB, Ward J, Guthrie JA, et al. Dynamic contrast-enhanced MR imaging and dual-phase helical CT in the preoperative assessment of suspected pancreatic cancer: a comparative study with receiver operating characteristic analysis. AJR. 1999;173:583–90.
41. Sironi S, De Cobelli F, Zerbi A, Balzano G, Di Carlo V, DelMaschio A. Pancreatic carcinoma: MR assessment of tumor invasion of the peripancreatic vessels. J Comput Assist Tomogr. 1995;19:739–44.
42. Spencer JA, Ward J, Guthrie JA, Guillou PJ, Robinson PJ. Assessment of resectability of pancreatic cancer with dynamic contrast enhanced MR imaging: technique, surgical correlation and patient outcome. Eur Radiol. 1998;8:23–9.
43. Erturk SM, Ichikawa T, Sou H, et al. Pancreatic adenocarcinoma: MDCT versus MRI in the detection and assessment of locoregional extension. J Comput Assist Tomogr. 2006;30:583–90.
44. Park HS, Lee JM, Choi HK, Hong SH, Han JK, Choi BI. Preoperative evaluation of pancreatic cancer: comparison of gadolinium enhanced dynamic MRI with MR cholangiopancreatography versus MDCT. J Magn Reson Imaging. 2009;30:586–95.
45. Koelblinger C, et al. Gadolinium dimeglumine enhanced 3.0-T MR imaging versus multiphasic 64-detector row CT: prospective evaluation in patients suspected of having pancreatic cancer. Radiology. 2011;259:757–66.
46. Motosugi U, Ichikawa T, Morisaka H, Sou H, Muhi A, Kimura K, Sano K, Araki T. Detection of pancreatic carcinoma and liver metastases with gadoxetic acid-enhanced MR imaging: comparison with

contrast-enhanced multi-detector row CT. Radiology. 2011;260(2):446–53.
47. Tamada T, Ito K, Sone T, et al. Dynamic contrast-enhanced magnetic resonance imaging of abdominal solid organ and major vessel: comparison of enhancement effect between Gd-EOB-DTPA and Gd-DTPA. J Magn Reson Imaging. 2009;29:636–40.
48. Rohrer M, Bauer H, Mintorovitch J, Requardt M, Weinmann HJ. Comparison of magnetic properties of MRI contrast media solutions at different magnetic field strengths. Invest Radiol. 2005;40:715–24.
49. Ichikawa T, Peterson MS, Federle MP, et al. Islet cell tumor of the pancreas: biphasic CT versus MR imaging in tumor detection. Radiology. 2000;216:163–71.
50. Kim YK, Kim CS, Han YM. Role of fat suppressed t1-weighted magnetic resonance imaging in predicting severity and prognosis of acute pancreatitis: an intraindividual comparison with multidetector computed tomography. J Comput Assist Tomogr. 2009;33:651–6.
51. Fayad LM, Holland GA, Bergin D, et al. Functional magnetic resonance cholangiography (fMRC) of the gallbladder and biliary tree with contrast-enhanced magnetic resonance cholangiography. J Magn Reson Imaging. 2003;18:449–60.
52. Dahlstrom N, Persson A, Albiin N, Smedby O, Brismar TB. Contrast-enhanced magnetic resonance cholangiography with Gd-BOPTA and GdEOB-DTPA in healthy subjects. Acta Radiol. 2007;48:362–8.
53. Hoeffel C, Azizi L, Lewin M, et al. Normal and pathologic features of the postoperative biliary tract at 3D MR cholangiopancreatography and MR imaging. RadioGraphics. 2006;26:1603–20.

CT and MR Enterography and Enteroclysis

14

Sehnaz Evrimler and Oktay Algin

14.1 Small Bowel Imaging Methods

Several imaging methods have been developed for small bowel imaging. The purpose of these methods is to diagnose small bowel diseases such as inflammatory bowel disease, obscure gastrointestinal tract bleeding, intestinal malabsorption syndromes, and intestinal neoplasm precisely and confidentially. Small bowel follow-through and enteroclysis were the first small bowel imaging methods and were followed by multidetector-row CT and magnetic resonance imaging (MRI) with technological developments. Enterography examinations are based on CT or MRI after drinking a large amount of oral contrast agent (OCA). The enteroclysis term is used for imaging after administration of OCA via nasojejunal intubation [1]. Capsule endoscopy is used for mucosal assessment and may be preferred in gastrointestinal (GI) bleeding cases of which conventional endoscopy is negative [2]. Early Crohn's disease and neoplasms which have only mucosal findings may be detected by only capsule endoscopy. On the other hand, extra-intestinal findings cannot be evaluated by this method. The complications of this technique are the retention and aspiration of the capsule. It is not recommended for patients with a stricture. CTE or MRE imaging should be performed before capsule endoscopy to avoid small bowel obstruction associated with capsule retention [3].

The most important factor in bowel imaging is luminal distension, because intraluminal lesions may be concealed in a collapsed bowel. Also, inadequate distension can cause misinterpretation for abnormal wall thickening. Optimal luminal distension may be obtained by fluoroscopic enteroclysis, but extraluminal findings cannot be evaluated. Also, it is a time-consuming method that is less tolerable for patients. CT enteroclysis can demonstrate extraluminal findings with optimal luminal distension but still shows less tolerability [1, 4–6]. Thus, MRE and CTE examinations exhibiting similar diagnostic performance with better tolerability were developed [7, 8]. CTE is a faster and easily achievable method, while MRE is a radiation-free technique with higher contrast resolution [1, 9–11]. Ingestion of a large amount of OCA is a prerequisite for both CTE and MRE to obtain adequate luminal distension. OCAs also decrease MRI susceptibility artifacts secondary to intraluminal air via luminal distension in colonic segments [12]. Lots of oral contrast agents (OCAs) have been studied for enterography examinations in

S. Evrimler (✉)
Department of Radiology, Suleyman Demirel University, Faculty of Medicine, Isparta, Turkey
e-mail: sehnazevrimler@sdu.edu.tr

O. Algin
Department of Radiology, Yidirim Beyazit University, Faculty of Medicine, Ankara, Turkey

National MR Research Center, UMRAM, Bilkent University, Ankara, Turkey
e-mail: oktay.algin@umram.bilkent.edu.tr

S. M. Erturk et al. (eds.), *Medical Imaging Contrast Agents: A Clinical Manual*,
https://doi.org/10.1007/978-3-030-79256-5_14

literature. Hyperosmolar agents are more preferred [13]. Ingestion of OCAs over 45–60 min is recommended [14]. The optimal volume is not strictly determined, but volume below 1-L liquid will probably be inadequate for luminal distension [15]. On the other hand, there is also a study suggesting that acceptable quality can be achieved with 450 mL [4]. Also, there is not a certain decision about whether OCA should be drunk in split aliquots or continuously. In a condition of stoma or bowel resection, plugging and earlier scanning may be recommended [5].

Comparison of CTE with small bowel follow-through and conventional enteroclysis [9, 16]:

1. Extraluminal and luminal pathologies can be evaluated in a single examination.
2. Overlapping of loops is not a limitation, and all small bowel segments can be visualized.
3. Multiplanar images can be reconstructed.
4. It improves diagnostic performance, cost-efficiency, and patient tolerance.
5. Motility cannot be evaluated.
6. Sinus and fistula patency may be missed.

Comparison of CTE with MRE

The superiorities of CTE [9, 16]:

1. Higher spatial and temporal resolution
2. Faster imaging which can be performed in single breath-hold
3. Cost-efficiency
4. The ability of luminal navigation

The superiorities of MRE [9, 16]:

1. Higher contrast resolution
2. Better fistula detection
3. A safer intravenous contrast agent
4. Radiation-free method

14.2 CT Enterography and Enteroclysis

14.2.1 CT Enterography (CTE)

In 1996, Raptopoulos et al. described CTE for the first time. Patients drank 1600 mL 2% flavored barium suspension as an OCA in 1–2 h, and abdomino pelvic images were obtained 50 s after intravenous (IV) contrast material injection (enteric phase) in the prone position [17]. There have been new technological advancements in CTE imaging since that day such as shortening the imaging time to within one breath-hold and enabling multiplanar reformatted imaging with improved spatial resolution. Neutral OCAs with IV contrast material administration have been more preferred for CTE because they exhibit low intraluminal density, which improves detection of inflammation and neoplasm compared to positive OCAs [18]. Although routine CTE images are obtained in the enteric phase, multi-phase imaging can be performed for the assessment of vascular pathologies and GI bleeding. CTE is superior to MRE in the detection of GI bleeding. Biphasic (arterial-portal venous phase) or triphasic (arterial-enteric-delayed phase) imaging can demonstrate negative capsule endoscopy obscure GI bleeding with progressive accumulation of iodinated contrast in the small bowel lumen. Vascular pathologies such as arteriovenous malformation may be observed as arterial enhancement accompanied by early draining veins. Meckel's diverticulum may be the cause of GI bleeding in young patients and can be demonstrated on CTE images [6, 9, 19, 20].

Small bowel imaging methods are mostly used for Crohn's disease which is a chronic disease, usually seen in young adults, and requires follow-up imaging for evaluating treatment response. Therefore, it is crucial to minimize radiation dose [3]. CTE may be considered for imaging the first diagnosis of Crohn's disease, but MRE is more preferred for follow-up imaging or evaluation of complicated cases. Automatic exposure is recommended to lower the radiation dose. According to studies in literature, CT dose index volume (CTDI-vol) ranges between 11 and 15 mGy for CTE [9, 21, 22].

The attenuation of tissues differs according to photon energies. Dual-energy (DE) CT technique separates high-energy X-ray photons from low-energy X-ray photons. DECT can make iodine quantification which is a quantitative marker for perfusion [23–25]. CTDI-vol of DE CTE was measured 9.89 mGy in a study which is lower than routine CTE [24].

14.2.2 CT Enteroclysis (CTEc)

CT enteroclysis (CTEc) is based on CT imaging of the small bowel after administration of oral contrast via the nasojejunal tube. The disadvantages of small bowel follow-through are overlapping of intestinal loops and the inability for direct evaluation of intestinal wall and extraluminal structures [7–9]. CTEc obviates these disadvantages with the contribution of cross-sectional modality features such as multiplanar imaging and three-dimensional (3-D) reconstructions [3, 10–13]. This method is also superior to small bowel follow-through for detection of level and cause of obstruction in high-grade and long-standing small bowel obstruction cases. Fluoroscopic nasojejunal intubation is needed for CTEc which is an invasive procedure impairing patient tolerance and increasing radiation exposure. Therefore, the radiation dose of CTEc is higher than CTE. Luminal distension provided by CTEc is generally better or similar when compared with CTE, especially in the jejunum. However, the image or distention quality of CTE is generally good enough to evaluate Crohn's disease involvement which predominantly affects the ileum [26–30].

14.2.3 CT Enterography and CT Enteroclysis Imaging Protocol

Patient preparation and imaging protocol recommendations for MRE and MREc are as follows [5, 28, 31–34]:

Patient Preparation Avoid solid foods and liquids for 4–6 h before the imaging. Water is allowed. There is no consensus for bowel cleansing with laxatives the day before, but can be recommended for colonic imaging.

Oral Contrast Agent Ingestion of 1–2 L of neutral oral contrast over 45–60 min is recommended. If patients have a stoma, it should be plugged.

Ten milligrams of IV metoclopramide may be administered 60 min before scanning for stimulating gastric emptying and increasing peristalsis to facilitate small bowel distension. It should be avoided in patients with Parkinsonism, pheochromocytoma, insulinoma, diabetes mellitus, and depression.

MDCT Sixteen-slice CT scanners are the minimum, and 64-slice CT scanners are the optimal scanners required for CTE/CTEc examinations.

Spasmolytic Agent It is optional to use a spasmolytic agent, but 20 mg of IV hyoscine butylbromide just before scanning is recommended as the first-line agent, and 1 mg of IV glucagon may be used as a second-line agent.

Scanning Scanning should be performed from the diaphragm to the perineum either in a supine or prone position. Some authors suggest that the prone position provides better distension, but the supine position is more comfortable and tolerable for patients.

Scan Acquisition Automatic exposure control is recommended. The tube current should be kept as low as possible. Tube voltage should be between 80 and 120 kV for inflammatory bowel disease and 80 and 140 kV for GI bleeding according to patient body habitus.

It is advised to record cumulative radiation dose for repeating CT examinations such as inflammatory bowel disease imaging.

Slice Thickness Multiplanar reformatted images are obtained. Therefore slice thickness should be 3 mm or less to avoid stair-step artifacts in coronal reformatted images, and overlap should be at least 30–40% for slice thickness of 3 mm (2 mm reconstruction interval). The overlap is not necessary for a slice thickness of 1 mm.

Scan Timing It is recommended to perform the enteric phase (50 s) or portal venous phase (70 s) for inflammatory bowel disease. Arterial (20–25 s) and portal venous phase imaging are recommended for the detection of GI bleeding.

Intravenous Contrast Material Recommended pump injection rate is 3–5 mL/s via an 18-guage cannula, iodine content is 300–370 mg/mL, and iodine dose is 1.5 mL/kg.

CTEc The same protocol with CTE is applied, and the only difference is the administration of OCA via 8–10 F nasojejunal tube at a rate of 80–120 mL/min with an automated pump. The volume should be decided by monitoring on CT.

14.2.4 Oral Contrast Agents: CT Enterography and Enteroclysis

In the mid-1980s negative OCAs such as air and carbon dioxide that darken the bowel lumen, causing < −200 HU [35–37], and neutral OCAs such as water or corn oil emulsions [38] that cause similar density with water and show grey density in the lumen were studied in CT imaging.

The success of CTE depends on the luminal distension provided by the OCA. Therefore, the importance of drinking the OCA for the success of the examination should be explained, and patients should be encouraged to drink all of the mixture as much as they can [9].

14.2.4.1 Neutral Oral Contrast Agents

Neutral OCAs have a lower density than the intestinal wall, thus enabling better assessment of mural-mucosal contrast enhancement and mesenteric vasculature. Major neutral OCAs used in daily practice are water, milk, polyethylene glycol (PEG), water with methylcellulose, lactulose, and 0.1% barium solution with sorbitol (Volumen; Bracco, Milan, Italy) [29, 38–43]. Neutral OCAs facilitate bowel wall visualization, luminal distension, and assessment of vascular structures [42]. On the other hand, they may conceal suspected perforation or make it difficult to differentiate between complete and incomplete obstruction [38, 44, 45].

PEG, water, methylcellulose, mannitol, and low-concentration barium with sorbitol have been studied as OCA for CTE in literature. Patients drink 1350–2000 mL OCA mixture in 45–75 min by dividing the mixture into 2–4 aliquots. In general, 75% of mixtures are drunk in the first 10–15 min [18, 29, 42, 43]. Better distension is obtained in ileal loops than jejunal loops [14, 18, 29, 42, 43].

Volumen consists of a low amount of barium which causes intraluminal attenuation of 20–40 HU. This amount of attenuation is not high enough to obscure wall enhancement. In addition, it enables the differentiation of adjacent cystic lesions and fluid collections with a higher density than water. There is not a specific contraindication for Volumen, but it carries the same risks with other barium consisting agents [42]. Nine hundred to one thousand milliliters of Volumen is recommended to be ingested in 20–30 min and last 200 mL just before scanning. Volumen is not the first choice for acute appendicitis, because positive OCAs enable better visualization of the appendix [42, 46].

Studies are suggesting that there is no significant difference between milk and Volumen [41] and milk is superior to water [47].

Lactulose was found to be the most successful OCA in a study comparing water, Metamucil, PEG (GoLYTELY Braintree Laboratories, MA), and lactulose (Euro-LAC; Euro-Pharm, Montreal, Canada) for luminal distension. Lactulose has a better taste than the others [48]. Lactulose is a synthetic non-digestible sugar. There are pharmaceutical products containing 667 mg/mL (250 mL Osmolak, Biofarma) or 670 mg/mL (250 mL Duphalac, Solvay) of lactulose. Ingestion of 1.5 L of lactulose in 60 min, divided into three aliquots, and immediate scanning afterward is recommended. It is contraindicated for acute abdominal pain, fever, vomiting, and galactose intolerance. Diarrhea is a relative contraindication. The side effects are diarrhea, nausea, vomiting, and abdominal pain [48].

Metamucil contains psyllium husk, a soluble fiber supplement, and a bulk-producing laxative. Therefore, it is not advised for stricture-associated Crohn patients who eat a low-fiber diet It is recommended to drink 2 L of Metamucil solution in 80 min, divided into four aliquots, each consisting of two packages (12 g/package) and scan 20 min after finishing the last one. Another ingestion direction for psyllium solution is to drink

1000 mL of solution, prepared in eight cups each consisting of one teaspoon of psyllium [49]. Abdominal distension, abdominal cramp, and bloating are side effects of Metamucil [48].

PEG is an osmotic laxative. PEG was found successful for luminal distension. It can cause diarrhea, abdominal distension, excess gas, and bloating [43, 48]. Although it provides better results than milk and water, it is less tolerable [39]. The price of Metamucil and lactulose is similar, whereas PEG is more expensive in our country [48].

Mannitol is a type of sugar alcohol. One thousand milliliters of mannitol solution is prepared by mixing 125 mL 20% mannitol (Mannitol 20% w/v Osmitrol, Baxter Healthcare, Old Toongabbie, NSW, Australia) with 875 mL water (2.5% concentration). Mannitol is a more cost-efficient agent that demonstrates similar distension and tolerability with Volumen [50]. Mannitol is also observed to be superior to psyllium fiber [49]. Mannitol has an osmotic effect which can cause diarrhea, but there is no significant difference for adverse effects between mannitol and Metamucil [49, 51].

14.2.4.2 Positive Oral Contrast Agents

Positive OCAs provide opacification in both small and large bowel loops, which improves visibility of both intraluminal and extraluminal pathologies. However, they obscure the mural enhancement by decreasing the contrast difference between the bowel wall and lumen [11]. They should also be omitted in CT angiography of GI bleeding cases, because of the same reason. Negative OCAs have some limitations: (1) it is difficult to differentiate distended bowel from adjacent cystic lesions, abscess, and fluid collections; (2) perforation can be missed; and (3) enteric fistula and postoperative anastomosis leak may not be demonstrated clearly and missed [38, 44, 45]. In such cases, water-soluble positive OCAs are preferred to overcome these limitations. Positive OCAs are beneficial for demonstrating intraluminal tumors and polyps on unenhanced scans. Positive OCA ingestion is also useful for identifying the grade of small bowel obstruction (SBO) and differentiation of complete or incomplete SBO. They can be preferred in partial obstruction cases. The amount of OCA differs according to the grade and level of obstruction. A smaller amount (100–200 mL) of water-soluble positive OCA in higher concentration is preferred for high-grade or proximal-level obstruction. On the other hand, a larger amount of OCA-water mixture (400–600 mL) in lower concentration (1:2) is preferred for low-grade or distal-level obstruction. A high-grade obstruction causes dilution of the OCA which is advised for high concentration OCAs [30].

Diatrizoate meglumine (Gastrografin, Bracco Diagnostics; Gastroview, Covidien) (Gastrografin; Schering, Berlin, Germany), a dilute high-osmolar contrast media (HOCM), is used as an oral contrast agent in CT imaging. It is a well-tolerated, water-soluble positive OCA with high osmolarity and low absorption that can provide luminal distension. Even less amount of Gastrografin ingestion would cause distension as a result of intestinal secretion caused by duodenal receptors because of the high osmolarity. This also results in the dilution of the contrast [30]. Also, the obscuring of the intestinal wall is less with Gastrografin than other high-density OCAs such as iodinated contrast material or barium sulfate suspension. Water-soluble iodinated contrast agents can be safely used in perforation-suspected cases [52]. The most specific finding is the detection of extraluminal positive OCA [53]. Small bowel follow-through with Gastrografin may have a therapeutic effect on adhesive SBO [54]. However, inappropriate dilution of HOCM can cause electrolyte imbalance in neonates and small children with low plasma volume. Aspiration pneumonia is another adverse effect that can rarely occur. Water-soluble iodinated contrast agents can cause an anaphylactic reaction [55].

Dilute iodine-based low-osmolar contrast media (LOCM) can substitute HOCM for enteric use with a lower risk of adverse effects. Iodine-based oral contrast agents should be diluted to avoid streak artifact on CT. Dilute ioversol 320 (Optiray 320, Mallinckrodt) is a commercially available dilute iodine-based OCA. It can be administered to pediatric patients with flavored additives because it has no taste. Water-soluble iodinated OCA can be mixed with water or juice. Iohexol and ioversol are more favorable than diatrizoate meglumine [55].

14.3 MR Enterography and Enteroclysis

14.3.1 MR Enterography

MRE is a radiation-free, reproducible, multiphasic imaging method that enables the assessment of both jejunal and ileal loops according to the timing of image acquisition. Contraindications of MRE are the same with MR imaging which are metal implants, pacemakers, cochlear implants, claustrophobia, etc. Colonic segments may also be evaluated with late images without the need for rectal contrast administration [56]. Collapsed bowel segments show higher attenuation than distended segments. This can cause misinterpretation for contrast enhancement. Additional inflammation findings should be investigated in such cases. Multiphasic imaging enables an image of the distension of the contracted segment and differentiates contraction from the stricture. Dynamic contrast-enhanced sequences can be used for vascular and enteric evaluation. This also enables quantitative assessment of contrast enhancement. MRE is also functional imaging with cine imaging sequences. In addition, it can be preferred in patients that iodinated contrast material is contraindicated [18, 57].

The essential factors for an optimal MRE examination are adequate luminal distension, full anatomic coverage of intestinal loops and perineum, rapid sequences to evaluate anatomy, fluid-sensitive sequences for detection of a mural and mesenteric edema, and contrast-enhanced sequences for assessment of mucosal-mural enhancement in inflammatory bowel disease. Diffusion-weighted imaging (DWI), cine imaging, and magnetization transfer imaging (MTI) are optional [57]. If gadolinium is contraindicated, T2-weighted (T2-W) images and DWI are recommended for the assessment of inflammation.

14.3.2 MR Enteroclysis (MREc)

This method is the combination of conventional enteroclysis and MRI. It has the advantages of cross-sectional imaging with less radiation exposure and provides better bowel distension, especially in jejunal segments, in comparison with MRE. Thus, it is a superior technique for the detection of mucosal and intraluminal pathologies and fistula. MREc may be better in the assessment of early, superficial mucosal involvement of Crohn's disease than MRE. It may also be used for low-grade small bowel obstruction cases. On the other hand, because of being an interventional procedure, it impairs patient tolerance and is generally not preferred for imaging of inflammatory bowel disease [57–59].

14.3.3 MRI Protocol of MRE and MREc

Patient preparation and imaging protocol recommendations for MRE and MREc are as follows [5, 33, 34, 57, 60]:

Patient Preparation Avoid solid foods and liquids for 4–6 h before the imaging. Water is allowed. There is no consensus for bowel cleansing with laxatives the day before, but it may alleviate artifacts and also be beneficial for colonic imaging.

Ingestion of 1–2 L of biphasic OCA over 45–60 min is recommended. If patients have a stoma, it should be plugged.

Supine or prone position may be preferred. The supine position is more comfortable for the patient. Prone position may decrease motility artifacts secondary to reduced peristalsis, also decrease bowel loop interposition, and shorten acquisition time secondary to reduced anterior-posterior dimension.

Hardware Both phased array coils at 1.5 and 3 T are acceptable.

Spasmolytic Agent Administration of 20 mg IV hyoscine butylbromide as the first-line agent before motion artifact-susceptible sequences (postcontrast T1-weighted images) in either a single dose or a split dose, half before the examination, and half before IV contrast injection is recommended. One milligram of IV glucagon is the second-line agent.

Intravenous Contrast (Gadolinium) Injection 0.1–0.2 mmol/kg with an infusion rate of 2 mL/s.

Field of View All small and large bowel segments should be included. The perineum should be exhibited to detect perianal fistulas.

14.3.3.1 MRI Sequences (Table 14.1)

Rapid sequences: These are fast sequences which are not susceptible to motion artifacts and used for evaluating the anatomy and wall thickness:

1. Axial and coronal balanced steady-state free precession (BSSFP) gradient-echo sequences without fat saturation
2. Axial and coronal single-shot fast-spin echo (SSFSE) T2-W sequences without fat saturation

Fluid-sensitive sequence: An axial or coronal FSE T2-W sequence with fat saturation (FS).

It is used for identifying mural and mesenteric edema.

The maximal slice thickness is 5 mm.

Non-enhanced coronal T1-weighted (T1-W) sequence with fat saturation followed by contrast-enhanced coronal and axial T1-W sequences with fat saturation in enteric (45 s) or portal venous (70 s) phase. The maximal slice thickness is 3 mm.

Optional Sequences

Cine motility: Decreased or absent motility may be a sign of inflammation and stricture. For this purpose, BSSFP sequences (e.g., true-ISP, FIESTA, BTFE) are used.

DWI (free-breathing technique, range of lower *b* values; 0–50, upper *b* values: 600–900 s/mm^2, with a maximal thickness of 5 mm): Diffusion-weighted imaging may substitute for contrast-enhanced sequences in patients that IV contrast material cannot be used. Diffusion restriction correlates well with inflammation. Read-out segmented EPI DWI technique may be useful for the elimination of artifacts.

Table 14.1 Sequences used in MR enterography and enteroclysis

Plane	Generic	Siemens	Philips	General electric	Max slice thickness	Respiration	Evaluation
Coronal	BSSFP	TrueFISP	BTFE	FIESTA	7-10 mm	Free-breathing, Breath-holds	Surveillance scan Cine imaging
Coronal and axial	T2-W Half Fourier SS TSE with FS	HASTE FS	SSH T2 FS	SS FSE FS	5 mm	Respiratory triggering, navigation	Mural and mesenteric edema
Coronal and axial precontrast, axial postcontrast	T1-W Ultrafast 3-D gradient echo with FS	T1-W-VIBE FS 3-D	THRIVE FS 3-D	LAVA FS 3-D	3 mm	Breath-holds	Precontrast for baseline imaging and intraluminal content Postcontrast for inflammation, neoplasm, vascular structures

Notes = *T1-W* T1-weighted, *T2-W* T2-weighted, *3-D* Three-dimensional, *BSSFP* balanced steady-state free precession, *TrueFISP* true fast imaging using steady-state free precession, *BTFE* balanced turbo field echo, *FIESTA* fast imaging employing steady-state acquisition, *HASTE* half-Fourier axial single-shot fast spin-echo, *SS/SSH* single shot, *FSE* fast spin echo, *FS* fat-saturated, *VIBE* volumetric interpolated breath-hold examination, *THRIVE* T1-W high-resolution isotropic volume examination, *LAVA* liver acquisition with volume acceleration

Magnetization transfer imaging (MTI) is not recommended for a routine examination. It measures magnetization transfer ratio (MTR) which is found to identify the amount of tissue collagen and fibrosis in animal models.

MREc Nasojejunal tube is placed at the duodenojejunal flexure on the fluoroscopy table. Biphasic OCA is administered via 8–10 F nasojejunal tube at an infusion rate of 75–120 mL/min until it reaches the terminal ileum, and then the rate is increased to 200 mL/min to decrease motion artifact by reflex atony in the MR unit.

MRE is more preferred than CTE in the pediatric patient group owing to the lack of ionizing radiation exposure. If MRE and/or ultrasound cannot identify the pathology, CTE may be performed. CTE is performed only in the portal phase. Same MRE sequences with adult patients are used in pediatric patients. Instructions for patient preparation are applied according to the age of the patient. Administration of spasmolytic is optional. Older children tolerate spasmolytic and bowel cleanse diets better. The volume of OCA, spasmolytic agent, and IV contrast agent depends on the weight of the patient. Recommendations for pediatric patient preparation [5, 61]:

Children aged between 6 and 9 years should avoid food for 2–4 h, and fluid restriction is not recommended. Children aged over 9 years should avoid food for 4–6 h, and fluid restriction is not recommended.

The supine position is more comfortable for children. They are also told to empty their bladder before imaging to avoid bowel compression.

Immediate OCA ingestion is required in MRE examination; therefore scanning is not routinely performed under sedation. Also, children older than 5 years old usually don't need sedation. If sedation is required, then MREc is performed under general anesthesia. It is essential to empty the stomach after imaging, before extubation to prevent aspiration.

The optimal volume of OCA is 20–25 mL/kg. The OCA is ingested in three doses, for patients weighing less than 50 kg; first 10 mL/kg 60 min before scanning, then 5 mL/kg 30 min before scanning, and last 5 mL/kg just before scanning. Pediatric patients weighing equal to or more than 50 kg may drink equal doses of 450 mL at time intervals mentioned above, up to the total volume of 1350 mL.

Spasmolytic agent: Intravenous 0.5 mg/kg hyoscine butylbromide or 0.5 mg (<24.9 kg) and 1 mg (>24.9 kg) at slow infusion rate of 1 mL/s with IV saline is recommended. Glucagon is preferred in the case of hyoscine butylbromide contraindication. Intravenous administration of 0.25 mg in pediatric patients <20 kg or 0.5 mg in pediatric patients ≥20 kg is recommended. Glucagon may cause rebound hypoglycemia, and therefore drinking fruit juice after examination may be beneficial.

An intravenous contrast agent (gadolinium): 0.1 mmol/kg to a maximum of 5 mmol and a dose of 5 mL.

Balanced steady-state free precession (BSSFP) sequences are very fast sequences with a high signal-to-noise ratio (SNR), lacking intraluminal flow artifacts that allow free-breathing imaging with excellent delineation of bowel and extra-intestinal anatomy. On the other hand, these sequences are more prone to susceptibility artifacts secondary to intraluminal air and post-operative metallic material, especially at a 3 T magnetic field. They are also not appropriate for assessment of bowel wall because it causes black edge artifact which exaggerates bowel wall thickness. Coronal free-breathing BSSFP can be used as surveillance imaging to ensure the arrival of oral contrast in the terminal ileum. BSSFP acquisition allows the evaluation of extra-intestinal findings such as mesenteric fibrofatty tissue, vascular structures, and lymph nodes. Chemical shift artifacts may be useful for the detection of intramural fat. Coronal BSSFP images also allow cine imaging with breath-holds or free-breathing at a slice thickness of 4–7 mm and two images/s for 10–20 s. It is used for differentiation between contraction and stenosis/bowel wall thickening. Post-spasmolytic axial BSSFP acquisition with free-breathing/breath-holds/respiratory triggering is optional [61, 62].

Fat-saturated (FS) T2-W single-shot fast spin-echo (SSFSE) with respiratory triggering or navigation in axial and coronal planes is performed after IV spasmolytic administration. FS T2-W acquisitions are fluid-sensitive, enabling assessment of mural and mesenteric edema, also fistula, sinus tract, and abscess. SSFSE is more prone to motion artifacts and has lower SNR compared with BSSFP, thus performed after spasmolytic administration. Short inversion time recovery sequences (STIR) may be preferred for fat suppression instead of chemical fat suppression in MR imaging of patients with metallic clips or prostheses causing susceptibility artifacts secondary to field inhomogeneity [61, 62].

Coronal fat-saturated ultrafast 3-D T1-W gradient echo images with breath-holds are performed before and after IV contrast agent administration. Precontrast images demonstrate a baseline signal of the bowel wall and intraluminal content. Postcontrast images are acquired at 45 s in the coronal plane and at 70 s in the axial plane [61, 62].

DWI is a fat-saturated echo-planar imaging sequence in axial plane performed with free-breathing and 3–8 b values of 0–800 s/mm^2. Apparent diffusion coefficient (ADC) maps are formed for quantitative analysis of diffusion restriction. DWI has become a fundamental sequence for detection of the primary tumor and metastases in abdominal MR imaging. The major role of DWI in small bowel imaging is the detection of active inflammation. In addition, it improves the delineation of lymph nodes, fistula, and abscesses. DWI is also considered as an alternative for intravenous contrast administration in the detection of inflammatory bowel disease (IBD) [61, 62].

14.3.4 Oral Contrast Agents: MR Enterography and Enteroclysis

The ideal OCA should provide adequate, homogeneous bowel distension and be commercially available, inexpensive, and lack serious side effects. Adequate luminal distension is important for the evaluation of intestinal wall thickness and enhancement. Normal bowel wall may look thickened and enhancing in a collapsed segment. Therefore a non-absorbable solution is needed for providing luminal distension, especially in the terminal ileum while examining for inflammatory bowel disease. Patients are supposed to drink approximately 1.5–2 L of solution over a 40–60 min period divided into three aliquots to be ingested every 20 min. It is recommended to drink additional water just before the exam to provide distension of the stomach and proximal small bowel segments. Patients with bowel resection history or stoma may drink less OCA. Late imaging may be performed, or rectal enema may be used for colonic evaluation [57, 62].

OCAs used in MRE are categorized in three groups according to their signal intensity characteristics on T1-W and T2-W images: (1) negative OCAs, (2) positive OCAs, and (3) biphasic OCAs (Table 14.2) [63].

14.3.4.1 Negative Oral Contrast Agents

This group includes superparamagnetic particles [small particle iron oxide (SPIO), ferumoxsil (GastroMARK), perfluorooctyl bromide, and oral magnetic particles], fruit juices (e.g., blueberry, pineapple, grape, acai) with very high manganese concentration, barium sulfate at high concentration, and room temperature air [12, 63, 64].

They show low intraluminal signal intensity on both T1-W and T2-W images, as a result of increasing magnetic field inhomogeneity. These agents can be utilized for improving the visibility of mesenteric fat tissue, peri-intestinal hyperintense lesions such as cysts, inter-loop abscesses, and fluid collections on T2-W images. Also, they facilitate bowel wall enhancement assessment or enhancing intraluminal lesion visibility on postcontrast T1-W images. Low signal intensity in the bowel lumen facilitates the visibility of the biliary system in MR cholangio pancreatography (MRCP) [65]. They are not routinely used regarding high cost and unavailability [12, 63, 64, 66].

Table 14.2 Classification of oral contrast agents used in MR enterography

MR enterography oral contrast agents	T1-W	T2-W	Examples
Negative			SPIO Ferumoxsil Perfluorooctyl bromide Fruit juices with very high manganese concentration
Positive			Gadolinium High-fat milk Ferric ammonium citrate Iron phytate Manganese chloride Fruit juices with high manganese concentration
Biphasic	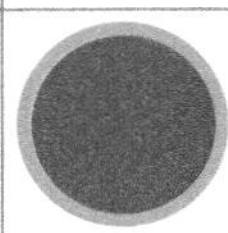		Water Methylcellulose Lactulose Mannitol Locust bean gum sorbitol Low-dose barium sulfate-sorbitol suspension Polyethylene glycol

14.3.4.2 Positive Oral Contrast Agents

This group includes gadolinium, high-fat milk, ferric ammonium citrate, iron phytate, and manganese chloride, fruit juices (blueberry, pineapple, grapefruit) owing to the high manganese concentration, and lipids with short T1 values (e.g., mineral oils, emulsions, and sucrose polyesters) [12, 63, 64].

They demonstrate high intraluminal signal intensity on both T1-W and T2-W images, as a result of a decrease in T1 relaxation time, while T2 relaxation time remains unaffected. This obscures the evaluation of mural and mucosal enhancement, because of both lumen and wall yielding high intensity on postcontrast T1-W images. Another disadvantage of this group is the motion artifact that can occur secondary to high intraluminal signal intensity on T1-W images. These agents are also not preferred in routine practice [12, 63, 64, 67].

Gadolinium in 1 mmol/L concentration may be used as positive OCA. It is contraindicated in ileus suspected cases and dehydrated patients [65]. A fistula between the rectum and adjacent organs may be hindered by perirectal fluid intensity on T2-W images. In such conditions, rectal administration of 0.5 mL of gadolinium in 500 mL of sterile saline (1:1000) via a rubber Foley catheter placed to gravity may facilitate the demonstration of the rectovesical or rectovaginal fistula by extraluminal extravasation of the contrast on fat-saturated T1-W images [63].

14.3.4.3 Biphasic Oral Contrast Agents

This group includes water, methylcellulose, lactulose, mannitol (2.5%), mannitol (2.5%) with locust bean gum (0.2%), sorbitol (2%), 0.1% low-dose barium-sulfate/sorbitol suspension (Volumen, EZ-E-M, Westbury, NY), and polyethylene glycol (PEG) [12, 63, 64].

They demonstrate low intraluminal signal intensity on T1-W and high signal intensity on T2-W images [12]. This facilitates mucosal and mural enhancement on postcontrast T1-W images and visibility of intraluminal and mural pathologies on T2-W images. They are the most preferred OCAs for MRE in daily routine practice, because of their availability and MRI characteristics. Tolerability, luminal distension, availability, and the cost of the agent should be considered while deciding which OCA to use in MRE. Water is well tolerated but absorbed quickly and generally cannot provide adequate distension, especially in distal segments. Therefore other agents are recommended for MRE. There is no consensus for which OCA should be preferred [12, 56, 66, 67].

Water is the cheapest, safest, and most tolerable OCA, but it is also the most rapidly reabsorbed agent that causes inadequacy in bowel distension [65]. Some compounds, highly osmolar agents such as polyethylene glycol, mannitol, sorbitol, or non-osmotic agents forming hydrogels such as locust bean gum, methylcellulose, and psyllium seed husk are added to reduce the reabsorption of water [15, 33].

Volumen contains 0.1% w/v barium sulfate, 1.4% sorbitol, and gum resins. Sorbitol and gum resins reduce the reabsorption of water by increasing the intraluminal osmolality. Barium-containing OCAs should be avoided in perforation suspected cases, within 1 week after endoscopic polypectomy, and before bowel operation [65]. It is recommended to drink 1 L of Volumen in 30–45 min before imaging.

Metamucil (Proctor & Gamble, Cincinnati, OH) contains psyllium seed husk [68]. Psyllium seed husk shows a laxative effect in low doses, whereas anti-diarrheal effect in high doses. Active portion, highly branched arabinoxylan consisting of copolymers of two pentose sugars, unlike found in cereal grains is not extensively fermented by colonic bacteria [69]. Nausea, diarrhea, and bloating are expected side effects that may also be observed with other biphasic OCAs. However, highly concentrated psyllium may cause small bowel obstruction. It is recommended to mix 500 mL of 1.6 g/kg psyllium in 2 L of water and ingest it every 30 min for 2 h [68].

Sorbitol, sugar, and hyperosmolar agent mostly reache the colon and ferment to lactulose, short-chain fatty acids, and gases, but unlike mannitol, explosive gas formation is not observed with sorbitol [70, 71]. It has a laxative effect in high doses and shows similar side effects with other biphasic OCAs. It is preferred owing to the lower price, availability, and adequate bowel distension. Sorbitol may be used on its own or with other agents such as barium sulfate and locust bean gum. Five hundred milliliters 3% sorbitol is recommended to be drunk every 15 min for 45 min [68].

Mannitol is another sugar alcohol with high osmolarity which reduces the reabsorption of water. The recommended administration protocol of 3% mannitol is a total 1500 mL solution ingested in 1 h, 500 mL 1 h before scanning, 500 mL 30 min before scanning, and 500 mL just before scanning for patients weighing more than 50 kg. Patients weighing less than 50 kg are recommended to drink 10 mL/kg 1 h before scanning, 5 mL/kg 30 min before scanning, and 5 mL/kg just before scanning [72]. Mannitol also may be used in combination with locust bean gum, a tasteless, insoluble fiber derived from carob seeds. Mannitol has a sweet taste, but it can cause moderate-severe diarrhea within 1 h after administration, whereas locust bean gum does not cause diarrhea [73].

PEG and sugar alcohol beverages and low-concentration barium solutions exhibit similar or better performance than methylcellulose for bowel distension, but PEG and sugar alcohol beverages are more favorable owing to their flavored taste. Breeza® (Beekley Corp., Bristol) is a sugar alcohol beverage that contains sorbitol, mannitol, and xanthan gum with lemon-lime flavor. PEG solution (MiraLAX) and Volumen are suggested to be administered with the addition of sugar-free fruit-flavored crystals for pediatric patients [74].

PEG is a polyether compound that has many different uses. It can be used as a laxative or oral contrast agent in medicine. It may provide better bowel distension than mannitol, lactulose, methylcellulose, and low-density barium but tastes worse [43, 64]. It is recommended to drink 1.5–2 L of PEG in 1 h in three aliquots of 500 mL; first in 15 min, second in 25 min, and last one 15 min before scanning [39].

Methylcellulose is a bulk-forming laxative, commercially available in powder form. Ten milligrams (two teaspoons) are homogenized in 650 mL of hot water with a mixer. Cold water and/or other biphasic OCAs such as lactulose and Volumen are added to the solution to obtain a 1–1.5 L mixture. Methylcellulose and water are the biphasic OCAs that have the least side effects [43, 64, 75].

Four different volumes (450, 900, 1350, and 1800 mL) of 2.5% mannitol with 0.2% locust bean gum, Volumen containing 2% sorbitol, Volumen containing 1.4% sorbitol, and water were compared with small bowel distension in a study. Better distension was achieved with OCAs containing sugar alcohol than water. Four hundred fifty milliliters of 2% sorbitol containing Volumen could provide adequate distension, but a high concentration of sorbitol may cause diarrhea. Adequate duodenal distension was obtained by 900 mL. Better jejunal and ileal distension was achieved by 1350 mL [76].

14.4 Imaging Findings of Small Bowel Diseases

14.4.1 Inflammatory Bowel Disease

Differential diagnosis of small bowel diseases is made by evaluating the localization, length, thickness, enhancement pattern of the affected bowel segment, and extra-intestinal findings [9, 11]. Enterography examinations are generally performed for diagnosis or follow-up imaging of Crohn's disease. Therefore we will emphasize the imaging findings of Crohn's disease more in this chapter.

CTE is suggested to be performed for older patients (>35 years old), patients with acute symptoms or suspicion of complex intra-abdominal penetrating disease which can require intervention or suspected perforation, and patients who have a contraindication for MRI or gadolinium [77]. CTE is superior to MRE in the detection of intramural and extraluminal air in ischemia and perforation cases, respectively [9, 11]. MRE is preferred in young adults and pediatric group, especially for follow-up imaging. Perianal fistula and extra-intestinal findings may be demonstrated better with MRE. It can be used in pregnant patients without IV contrast administration. MRE is recommended for patients who have iodinated contrast allergy [77].

The terminal ileum is the predominantly affected segment in Crohn's disease. Bowel segments are affected in a skipped pattern. CTE/CTEc and MRE/MREC examinations show a very good correlation with endoscopic findings. There is an imaging classification for Crohn's disease which exhibits a good correlation with clinical and laboratory findings. There are four types of Crohn's disease, which are active inflammatory, fistulizing/penetrating/perforating, fibrostenotic, and reparative/regenerative [78]. The enterography examination findings of Crohn's disease are as follows [9, 77]:

1. Small bowel wall thickening (more than 3 mm) and enhancement
2. Mesenteric vascular engorgement: "comb sign"
3. Mural and mesenteric edema
4. Mesenteric lymphadenopathy and fibrofatty proliferation
5. Transmural ulceration and complications such as sinus tract-fistula-abscess
6. Strictures with upstream dilatation
7. Extra-intestinal manifestations

14.4.1.1 The Role of MRE in the Diagnosis of Crohn's Disease

Asymmetric mural enhancement is pathognomonic for Crohn's disease, whereas symmetric enhancement is non-specific. The differentiation between active disease, fibrostenotic disease, and penetrating disease can be achieved according to the enhancement pattern. Target appearance created by stratified mural enhancement owing to early mucosal and serosal enhancement (high mucosal signal intensity-low submucosal signal intensity-high serosal signal intensity) on postcontrast images and high mural signal intensity on T2-W images which is a sign of intramural edema is an indicator of active disease (Fig. 14.1). Intramural fat is a sign of chronicity (Fig. 14.2). Mucosal enhancement correlates well with disease activity [11]. Mesenteric vascular engorgement creating "comb sign" is another finding for active inflammation. Mesenteric fibrofatty proliferation may be observed in both active and chronic phases [11, 79]. The findings of the fibrostenotic disease are mural iso-/hypo-intensity on T2-W images and lacking early mucosal enhancement on T1-W images. Progressive mural enhancement may be observed secondary to fibrosis. The treatment approach, whether to choose medical or surgical

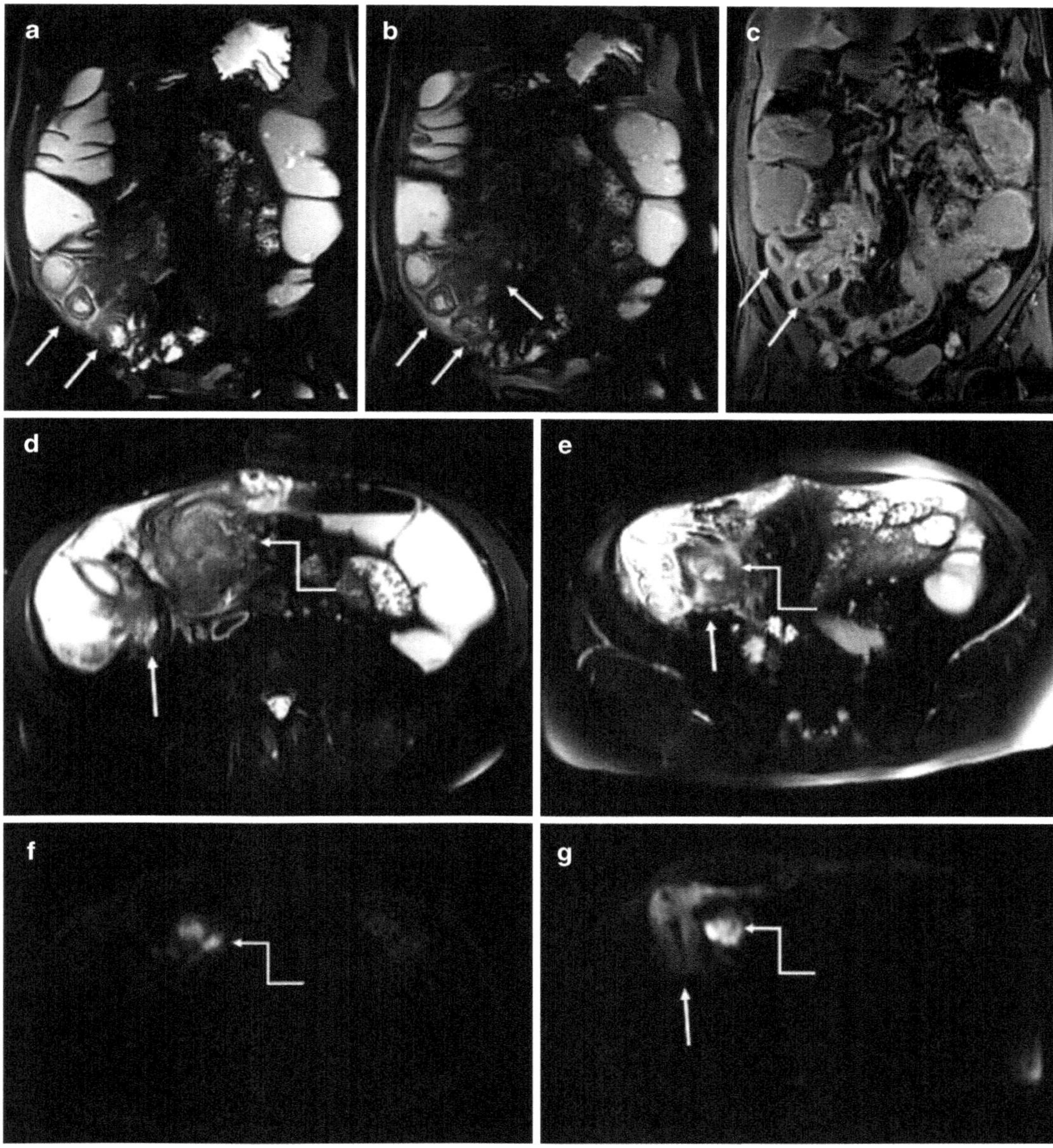

Fig. 14.1 MRE images of a 65-year-old male patient with Crohn's disease. On coronal FS T2-W (**a**, **b**), post-contrast T1-W (**c**), and axial FS T2-W (**d**, **e**) images; mural thickening, edema (*arrows* in **a** and **b**), and contrast enhancement (*arrows* in **c**) in distal ileum segments, accompanied with abscess, and mesenteric edema (*curved arrows* in **d** and **e**), restricted diffusion in these segments (*arrow* in **g**) and abscess in pericecal area (*curved arrows* in **f** and **g**) on b800 images of DWI

treatment, depends on the type of stricture; therefore distinction of either inflammatory, fibrotic, or combined form should be made. Acute inflammation within stricture is treated with medical therapy. Fibrosis-associated strictures require surgery. Surgical interventions are recommended to be applied in elective situations; otherwise, complication rates increase in case of emergent operations. Also, asymmetry, modularity, and soft tissue extension to mesen-

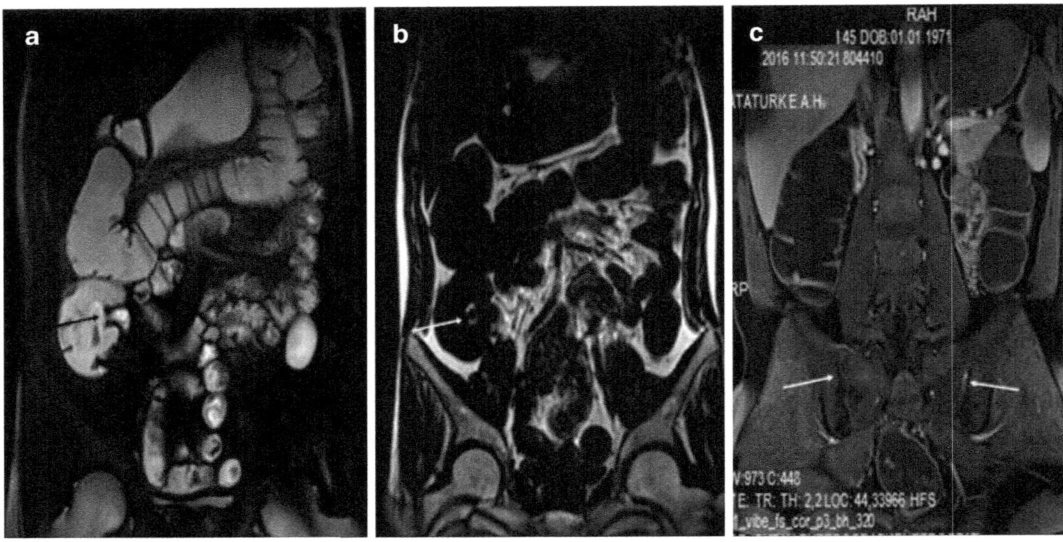

Fig. 14.2 Coronal plane FS T2-W (**a**), Dixon-fat (**b**), and postcontrast FS T1-W (**c**) images of a 45-year-old male with Crohn's disease, ileocecal valve involvement (*arrows* in **a** and **b**), bilateral active sacroiliitis (*arrows* in **c**), and intramural fat accumulation on Dixon-fat images related to chronic Crohn's disease (*arrow* in **b**)

tery are warning signs of neoplasm [59]. It is essential to perform CTE or MRE for detection of stricture before capsule endoscopy because it can induce small bowel obstruction [24, 25]. Radiology reports should include the localization, length of the involved bowel segment, and stricture type. The length and diameter of the upstream dilated bowel segment should also be identified [5, 77].

In penetrating disease, transmural inflammation exhibits extramural extension resulting in sinus tract, fistula, abscess formation, and even perforation. However, perianal fistulas are not accepted in this group. Sinus tracts may be within the bowel wall or blind end in mesentery/fascia. Fistulas occur between epithelial structures such as enteroenteric, enterocolic, enterocutaneous, enterovesical, etc. Kinked or tethered loops which form an "asterisk" shape are findings of the enteroenteric fistula which is a sign of penetrating disease. They present as hyperintense tracts on T2-W images and demonstrate contrast enhancement. Inter-loop abscess which is a fluid collection with peripheral rim enhancement may accompany (Fig. 14.3) [77].

Inflammation correlates well with diffusion restriction on DWI (Fig. 14.1). Cine MR imaging is used for motility assessment of the small bowel. Inflamed segments show decreased or absent motility. Strictures can be differentiated from a contraction by cine imaging. Fibrosis exhibits low mural signal intensity on MT pulse secondary to collagen content [80]. MT imaging may aid in the differentiation between acute and fibrotic strictures [64].

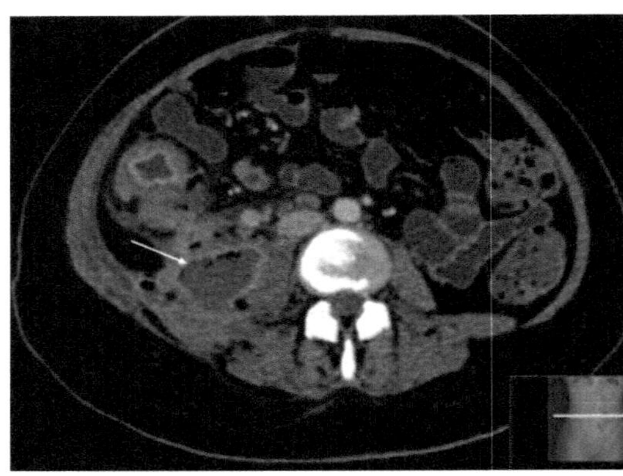

Fig. 14.3 Axial contrast-enhanced CT image of a 21-year-old female with Crohn's disease, abscesses, and inflammation around the right psoas muscle and pericecal area

Secondary involvement of the appendix can cause appendicitis in Crohn's disease. Mesenteric vein thrombosis and small bowel varices may also occur; therefore it is important to be able to evaluate vascular structures. Extra-intestinal manifestations of the disease are sacroiliitis, spondyloarthritis, primary sclerosing cholangitis, and avascular necrosis [77]. MRI would be a good choice for the assessment of these findings. FOV in MRE examination can be enlarged according to the suspected finding.

MRE can also aid in the evaluation of Crohn's disease severity and activity. Therefore, it can be used for monitoring treatment response [57]. MRE radiologic reports should also state the presence or lack of active inflammation in follow-up imaging. Complete or partial response to medical therapy may be observed. After alleviation of active inflammation, residual sequel findings may present. These are asymmetric mural fat deposits, pseudo-sacculations, scarring, and mural thickness without active inflammation findings [77].

Ulcerative colitis starts from the rectum and tends to involve all colonic segments continuously. Colonoscopy is more sensitive for diagnosis and grading of ulcerative colitis than CTE or MRE. Large bowel wall thickening, engorgement of vasa recta, and inflammatory pseudopolyps are common findings of both colonic involvements of Crohn's disease and ulcerative colitis. If the disease involves the entire colon and arrives at the terminal ileum level, it may cause backwash ileitis.

On the other hand, Crohn's disease involves predominantly the small bowel, and colitis occurs in a skipped pattern. Extra-intestinal manifestations tend to occur in Crohn's disease [9, 81].

Infectious bowel diseases can be misinterpreted as inflammatory bowel diseases. Especially, tuberculosis usually affects the cecum and terminal ileum, mimicking Crohn's disease. Tuberculosis may manifest with mural thickening accompanied by necrotic or calcified lymphadenopathies, peritonitis, and pulmonary findings. Transverse or star-shaped ulcers may be observed in tuberculosis. On the other hand, ulcers in Crohn's disease are in longitudinal shape [81, 82].

Chronic radiation enteritis may present with mural thickening, contrast enhancement, and luminal narrowing in a long segment of the distal ileum, accompanied by mesenteric stranding. These findings resemble inflammatory bowel disease. However, a focal abnormal bowel loop observed in the prior radiation therapy field leads to the diagnosis of radiation enteritis [83].

14.4.2 Small Bowel Neoplasms

Small bowel neoplasms account for <5% of gastrointestinal tumors [84]. The most common malignant small bowel tumors are adenocarcinoma, carcinoid tumor, lymphoma, and gastrointestinal stromal tumor in descending order. Hamartomatous polyps associated with Peutz-Jeghers syndrome and hyperplastic polyps are benign small bowel tumors. CTE is more sensitive than MRE for the detection of small bowel tumors owing to higher spatial resolution and less susceptibility to motion artifacts. Small bowel tumors are usually detected incidentally or in patients with occult gastrointestinal bleeding, iron deficiency anemia, weight loss, abdominal pain, luminal obstruction, jaundice, or obstruction [9, 11]. Small bowel tumors can present as a focal intraluminal mass, irregular transition, small bowel obstruction, intussusception, asymmetric mural thickening, and enhancement. Adenocarcinomas are usually located in the proximal small bowel, especially close to the ampulla. Gastrointestinal stromal tumors usually present as a pedunculated exoenteric mass and are located in the ileum or jejunum. Although they are usually homogeneous, large tumors can show necrosis. Lymphoma should be considered in the differential diagnosis of an exoenteric mass with lymphadenopathy or aneurysmal ulceration and asymmetric long segment circumferential wall thickening with dilatation. Mucosal/mural polypoid rapidly enhancing lesions and mural thickening combined with carpet-like appearance suggest carcinoid tumors. Carcinoid tumors are generally located in ileal segments. Mesenteric carcinoid metastases or liver metastases can occur. Mesenteric root clustering with desmoplastic reaction and eccentric calcifications suggest mesenteric carcinoid metastases. Hepatic metastases are usually hypervascular and show necrosis [9, 11, 81].

14.4.3 Coeliac Disease

Coeliac disease is a malabsorption syndrome caused by loss of villi and hyperplasia of crypts resulting in intraluminal excess fluid accumulation. Luminal dilatation, atrophy of jejunal folds, the reversal of jejunal and ileal fold pattern, temporary small bowel intussusception, duodenitis, mural edema, and intramural fat may be observed on CTE/CTEc and MRE/MREc (Fig. 14.4). Lymphadenopathy and celiac-associated T-cell lymphoma can accompany these findings. Dilution of barium, flocculation, and the slow passage of barium may be observed on small bowel follow-through and CTE/CTEc [85–89].

14.4.4 Intestinal Malformations

Meckel diverticulum is the most common (2–3%) congenital malformation of the gastrointestinal system. Intestinal atresia, stenosis, malrotation, duplications, and Nutcracker syndrome (superior mesenteric artery syndrome) are the other intestinal malformations. Meckel diverticulum is a blind-ending omphalomesenteric duct remnant, localized at the antimesenteric side of the distal ileum, 100 cm (30–90 cm in infants) proximal to the ileocecal valve. Complications of Meckel's diverticulum are hemorrhage, obstruction, intussusception, diverticulitis, enterolithiasis, and neoplasm [90–92].

14.4.5 Small Bowel Ischemia

Small bowel or mesenteric ischemia can be in acute or chronic form. Acute mesenteric ischemia is generally caused by mesenteric arterial or venous occlusion. Arterial thromboembolism is more common. The other causes are systemic hypotension, trauma, vasculitis, small bowel obstruction, strangulation, abdominal inflammatory conditions (pancreatitis, diverticulitis, etc.), and drugs (digitalis, amphetamine, cocaine). Chemotherapy and radiation therapy can result in vasculitis-associated enteropathy. Chronic mesenteric ischemia causes are atherosclerosis of the mesenteric artery and chronic radiation enteritis. Chronic mesenteric ischemia becomes symptomatic unless sufficient collaterals develop. CT-based images allow the evaluation of both vascular and nonvascular structures. Neutral OCAs are preferred for the accurate assessment

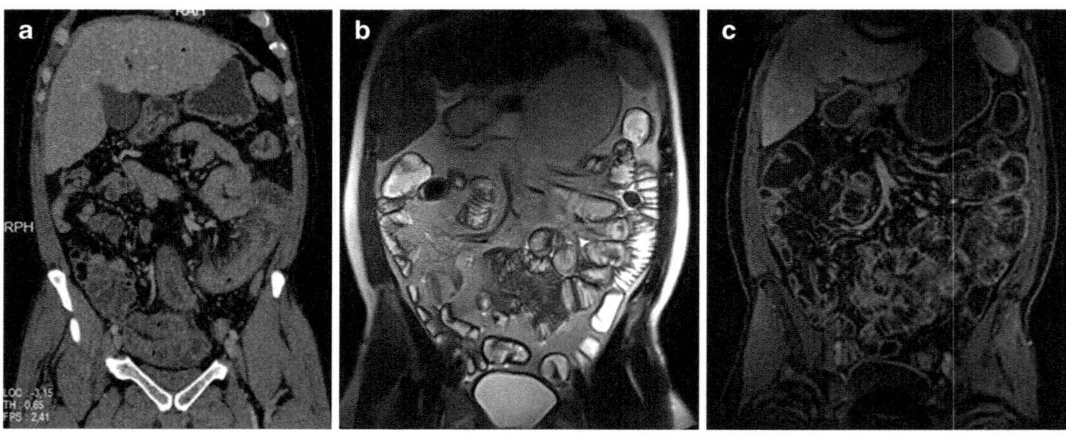

Fig. 14.4 Coronal CT (**a**), T2-W (**b**) and postcontrast FS T1-W (**c**) MR enterography images with biphasic oral contrast agent of a young male with celiac disease, flattening and loss of duodenal and jejunal folds, and in contrary prominent hypertrophic folds in the ileum

of bowel wall enhancement. Positive OCAs can obscure mural enhancement and also impair vascular assessment. Positive OCAs may be preferred in cases with IV contrast contraindication or suspected bowel obstruction. Both unenhanced and contrast-enhanced imagings are performed. Mural hemorrhage is demonstrated on non-contrast images with high attenuation. Biphasic imaging enables the assessment of the arterial and venous systems. CT findings of acute mesenteric ischemia are vascular occlusion or narrowing, bowel wall thickening, intramural gas (pneumatosis intestinalis), gas in portal vein/ mesenteric vein and branches, engorgement of mesenteric vasculature and abnormal prolonged enhancement secondary to stasis, and luminal dilatation secondary to decreased peristalsis. The most specific sign of mesenteric ischemia is the loss of contrast enhancement of the intestinal wall. Mural thickening with submucosal edema or hemorrhage may exhibit target sign [93, 94].

References

1. Markova I, Kluchova K, Zboril R, Mashlan M, Herman M. Small bowel imaging-still a radiologic approach. Biomed Pap Med Fac Univ Palacky Olomouc Czech Repub. 2010;154(2):123–32.
2. Maglinte DD, Sandrasegaran K, Chiorean M, Dewitt J, McHenry L, Lappas JC. Radiologic investigations complement and add diagnostic information to capsule endoscopy of small-bowel diseases. Am J Roentgenol. 2007;189(2):306–12.
3. Brenner DJ, Hall EJ. Computed tomography—an increasing source of radiation exposure. N Engl J Med. 2007;357(22):2277–84.
4. Kinner S, Kuehle CA, Herbig S, Haag S, Ladd SC, Barkhausen J, et al. MRI of the small bowel: can sufficient bowel distension be achieved with small volumes of oral contrast? Eur Radiol. 2008;18(11):2542–8.
5. Taylor S, Avni F, Cronin C, Hoeffel C, Kim S, Laghi A, et al. The first joint ESGAR/ESPR consensus statement on the technical performance of cross-sectional small bowel and colonic imaging. Eur Radiol. 2017;27(6):2570–82.
6. Yoon W, Jeong YY, Shin SS, Lim HS, Song SG, Jang NG, et al. Acute massive gastrointestinal bleeding: detection and localization with arterial phase multi–detector row helical CT. Radiology. 2006;239(1):160–7.
7. Horsthuis K, Bipat S, Bennink RJ, Stoker J. Inflammatory bowel disease diagnosed with US, MR, scintigraphy, and CT: meta-analysis of prospective studies. Radiology. 2008;247(1):64–79.
8. Siddiki HA, Fidler JL, Fletcher JG, Burton SS, Huprich JE, Hough DM, et al. Prospective comparison of state-of-the-art MR enterography and CT enterography in small-bowel Crohn's disease. Am J Roentgenol. 2009;193(1):113–21.
9. Ilangovan R, Burling D, George A, Gupta A, Marshall M, Taylor S. CT enterography: review of technique and practical tips. Br J Radiol. 2012;85(1015):876–86.
10. Paparo F, Garlaschi A, Biscaldi E, Bacigalupo L, Cevasco L, Rollandi GA. Computed tomography of the bowel: a prospective comparison study between four techniques. Eur J Radiol. 2013;82(1):e1–e10.
11. Paulsen SR, Huprich JE, Fletcher JG, Booya F, Young BM, Fidler JL, et al. CT enterography as a diagnostic tool in evaluating small bowel disorders: review of clinical experience with over 700 cases. Radiographics. 2006;26(3):641–57.
12. Kayhan A, Oommen J, Dahi F, Oto A. Magnetic resonance enterography in Crohn's disease: standard and advanced techniques. World J Radiol. 2010;2(4):113.
13. Borthne AS, Abdelnoor M, Storaas T, Pierre-Jerome C, Kløw N-E. Osmolarity: a decisive parameter of bowel agents in intestinal magnetic resonance imaging. Eur Radiol. 2006;16(6):1331.
14. Kuehle CA, Ajaj W, Ladd SC, Massing S, Barkhausen J, Lauenstein TC. Hydro-MRI of the small bowel: effect of contrast volume, timing of contrast administration, and data acquisition on bowel distention. Am J Roentgenol. 2006;187(4):W375–W85.
15. Ajaj W, Goehde SC, Schneemann H, Ruehm SG, Debatin JF, Lauenstein TC. Dose optimization of mannitol solution for small bowel distension in MRI. J Magn Reson Imaging. 2004;20(4):648–53.
16. Vogel J, da Luz Moreira A, Baker M, Hammel J, Einstein D, Stocchi L, et al. CT enterography for Crohn's disease: accurate preoperative diagnostic imaging. Dis Colon Rectum. 2007;50(11):1761–9.
17. Raptopoulos V, Schwartz R, McNicholas M, Movson J, Pearlman J, Joffe N. Multiplanar helical CT enterography in patients with Crohn's disease. AJR Am J Roentgenol. 1997;169(6):1545–50.
18. Fletcher JG. CT enterography technique: theme and variations. Abdom Imaging. 2009;34(3):283–8.
19. Huprich JE, Fletcher JG, Alexander JA, Fidler JL, Burton SS, McCullough CH. Obscure gastrointestinal bleeding: evaluation with 64-section multiphase CT enterography—initial experience. Radiology. 2008;246(2):562–71.
20. Scheffel H, Pfammatter T, Wildi S, Bauerfeind P, Marincek B, Alkadhi H. Acute gastrointestinal bleeding: detection of source and etiology with multi-detector-row CT. Eur Radiol. 2007;17(6):1555–65.
21. Siddiki H, Fletcher J, Bruining D. Performance of lower-dose CT enterography for detection of inflammatory Crohn's disease. RSNA abstact, Chicago, IL. 2007. p. 254.
22. Sodickson A, Baeyens PF, Andriole KP, Prevedello LM, Nawfel RD, Hanson R, et al. Recurrent CT,

cumulative radiation exposure, and associated radiation-induced cancer risks from CT of adults. Radiology. 2009;251(1):175–84.
23. Fulwadhva UP, Wortman JR, Sodickson AD. Use of dual-energy CT and iodine maps in evaluation of bowel disease. Radiographics. 2016;36(2):393–406.
24. Kim YS, Kim SH, Ryu HS, Han JK. Iodine quantification on spectral detector-based dual-energy CT enterography: correlation with Crohn's disease activity index and external validation. Korean J Radiol. 2018;19(6):1077–88.
25. Marin D, Boll DT, Mileto A, Nelson RC. State of the art: dual-energy CT of the abdomen. Radiology. 2014;271(2):327–42.
26. Boudiaf M, Jaff A, Soyer P, Bouhnik Y, Hamzi L, Rymer R. Small-bowel diseases: prospective evaluation of multi–detector row helical CT enteroclysis in 107 consecutive patients. Radiology. 2004;233(2):338–44.
27. Mazzeo S, Caramella D, Belcari A, Melai L, Cappelli C, Fontana F, et al. Multidetector CT of the small bowel: evaluation after oral hyperhydration with isotonic solution. Radiol Med. 2005;109(5–6):516–26.
28. Minordi LM, Vecchioli A, Mirk P, Bonomo L. CT enterography with polyethylene glycol solution vs CT enteroclysis in small bowel disease. Br J Radiol. 2011;84(998):112–9.
29. Wold PB, Fletcher JG, Johnson CD, Sandborn WJ. Assessment of small bowel Crohn disease: noninvasive peroral CT enterography compared with other imaging methods and endoscopy—feasibility study. Radiology. 2003;229(1):275–81.
30. Hong SS, Kim AY, Kwon SB, Kim PN, Lee M-G, Ha HK. Three-dimensional CT enterography using oral gastrografin in patients with small bowel obstruction: comparison with axial CT images or fluoroscopic findings. Abdom Imaging. 2010;35(5):556–62.
31. Schindera ST, Nelson RC, DeLong DM, Jaffe TA, Merkle EM, Paulson EK, et al. Multi–detector row CT of the small bowel: peak enhancement temporal window—initial experience. Radiology. 2007;243(2):438–44.
32. Vandenbroucke F, Mortele K, Tatli S, Pelsser V, Erturk S, De Mey J, et al. Noninvasive multidetector computed tomography enterography in patients with small-bowel Crohn's disease: is a 40-second delay better than 70 seconds? Acta Radiol. 2007;48(10):1052–60.
33. Ajaj W, Lauenstein TC, Langhorst J, Kuehle C, Goyen M, Zoepf T, et al. Small bowel hydro-MR imaging for optimized ileocecal distension in Crohn's disease: should an additional rectal enema filling be performed? J Magn Reson Imaging. 2005;22(1):92–100.
34. Friedrich C, Fajfar A, Pawlik M, Hoffstetter P, Rennert J, Agha A, et al. Magnetic resonance enterography with and without biphasic contrast agent enema compared to conventional ileocolonoscopy in patients with Crohn's disease. Inflamm Bowel Dis. 2012;18(10):1842–8.
35. Balthazar EJ, Megibow A, Hulnick D, Naidich D. Carcinoma of the colon: detection and preoperative staging by CT. Am J Roentgenol. 1988;150(2):301–6.
36. Megibow A, Bosniak M, Ho A, Beller U, Hulnick D, Beckman E. Accuracy of CT in detection of persistent or recurrent ovarian carcinoma: correlation with second-look laparotomy. Radiology. 1988;166(2):341–5.
37. Megibow AJ, Zerhouni EA, Hulnick DH, Beranbaum ER, Balthazar EJ. Air insufflation of the colon as an adjunct to computed tomography of the pelvis. J Comput Assist Tomogr. 1984;8(4):797–800.
38. Thompson SE, Raptopoulos V, Sheiman RL, McNicholas MM, Prassopoulos P. Abdominal helical CT: milk as a low-attenuation oral contrast agent. Radiology. 1999;211(3):870–5.
39. D'Ippolito G, Braga FA, Resende MC, Bretas EAS, Nunes TF, de Queiroz Rosas G, et al. Computed tomography enterography: a comparison of different neutral oral contrast agents. Radiol Bras. 2012;45(3):139–43.
40. Hebert J, Taylor A, Winter T, Reichelderfer M, Weichert J. Low-attenuation oral GI contrast agents in abdominal-pelvic computed tomography. Abdom Imaging. 2006;31(1):48–53.
41. Koo CW, Shah-Patel LR, Baer JW, Frager DH. Cost-effectiveness and patient tolerance of low-attenuation oral contrast material: milk versus VoLumen. Am J Roentgenol. 2008;190(5):1307–13.
42. Megibow AJ, Babb JS, Hecht EM, Cho JJ, Houston C, Boruch MM, et al. Evaluation of bowel distention and bowel wall appearance by using neutral oral contrast agent for multi–detector row CT. Radiology. 2006;238(1):87–95.
43. Young BM, Fletcher JG, Booya F, Paulsen S, Fidler J, Johnson CD, et al. Head-to-head comparison of oral contrast agents for cross-sectional enterography: small bowel distention, timing, and side effects. J Comput Assist Tomogr. 2008;32(1):32–8.
44. Rieber A, Aschoff A, Nüssle K, Wruk D, Tomczak R, Reinshagen M, et al. MRI in the diagnosis of small bowel disease: use of positive and negative oral contrast media in combination with enteroclysis. Eur Radiol. 2000;10(9):1377–82.
45. Winter TC, Ager JD, Nghiem HV, Hill RS, Harrison SD, Freeny PC. Upper gastrointestinal tract and abdomen: water as an orally administered contrast agent for helical CT. Radiology. 1996;201(2):365–70.
46. Jacobs JE, Birnbaum BA, Macari M, Megibow AJ, Israel G, Maki DD, et al. Acute appendicitis: comparison of helical CT diagnosis—focused technique with oral contrast material versus nonfocused technique with oral and intravenous contrast material. Radiology. 2001;220(3):683–90.
47. Lim BK, Bux SI, Rahmat K, Lam SY, Liew YW. Evaluation of bowel distension and mural visualisation using neutral oral contrast agents for multidetector-row computed tomography. Singap Med J. 2012;53(11):732.

48. Leduc F, De A, Rebello R, Muhn N, Ioannidis G. A comparative study of four oral contrast agents for small bowel distension with computed tomography enterography. Can Assoc Radiol J. 2015;66(2):140–4.
49. Wong J, Roger M, Moore H. Performance of two neutral oral contrast agents in CT enterography. J Med Imaging Radiat Oncol. 2015;59(1):34–8.
50. Wong J, Moore H, Roger M, McKee C. CT enterography: mannitol versus VoLumen. J Med Imaging Radiat Oncol. 2016;60(5):593–8.
51. Lauenstein TC, Schneemann H, Vogt FM, Herborn CU, Ruhm SG, Debatin JF. Optimization of oral contrast agents for MR imaging of the small bowel. Radiology. 2003;228(1):279–83.
52. Maniatis V, Chryssikopoulos H, Roussakis A, Kalamara C, Kavadias S, Papadopoulos A, et al. Perforation of the alimentary tract: evaluation with computed tomography. Abdom Imaging. 2000;25(4):373–9.
53. Brochwicz-Lewinski M, Paterson-Brown S, Murchison J. Small bowel obstruction—the water-soluble follow-through revisited. Clin Radiol. 2003;58(5):393–7.
54. Borthne A, Dormagen J, Gjesdal K, Storaas T, Lygren I, Geitung J. Bowel MR imaging with oral Gastrografin: an experimental study with healthy volunteers. Eur Radiol. 2003;13(1):100–6.
55. Callahan MJ, Talmadge JM, MacDougall R, Buonomo C, Taylor GA. The use of enteric contrast media for diagnostic CT, MRI, and ultrasound in infants and children: a practical approach. Am J Roentgenol. 2016;206(5):973–9.
56. Algin O, Evrimler S, Ozmen E, Metin MR, Ocakoglu G, Ersoy O, et al. A novel biphasic oral contrast solution for enterographic studies. J Comput Assist Tomogr. 2013;37(1):65–74.
57. Grand DJ, Guglielmo FF, Al-Hawary MM. MR enterography in Crohn's disease: current consensus on optimal imaging technique and future advances from the SAR Crohn's disease-focused panel. Abdom Imaging. 2015;40(5):953–64.
58. Cappabianca S, Granata V, Di Grezia G, Mandato Y, Reginelli A, Di Mizio V, et al. The role of nasoenteric intubation in the MR study of patients with Crohn's disease: our experience and literature review. Radiol Med. 2011;116(3):389–406.
59. Masselli G, Casciani E, Polettini E, Gualdi G. Comparison of MR enteroclysis with MR enterography and conventional enteroclysis in patients with Crohn's disease. Eur Radiol. 2008;18(3):438–47.
60. Dave-Verma H, Moore S, Singh A, Martins N, Zawacki J. Computed tomographic enterography and enteroclysis: pearls and pitfalls. Curr Probl Diagn Radiol. 2008;37(6):279–87.
61. Greer M-LC. How we do it: MR enterography. Pediatr Radiol. 2016;46(6):818–28.
62. Santillan CS. MR imaging techniques of the bowel. Magn Reson Imaging Clin. 2014;22(1):1–11.
63. Gupta MK, Khatri G, Bailey A, Pinho DF, Costa D, Pedrosa I. Endoluminal contrast for abdomen and pelvis magnetic resonance imaging. Abdom Radiol. 2016;41(7):1378–98.
64. Tolan DJ, Greenhalgh R, Zealley IA, Halligan S, Taylor SA. MR enterographic manifestations of small bowel Crohn disease. Radiographics. 2010;30(2):367–84.
65. Elsayed NM, Alsalem SA, Almugbel SAA, Alsuhaimi MM. Effectiveness of natural oral contrast agents in magnetic resonance imaging of the bowel. Egypt J Radiol Nucl Med. 2015;46(2):287–92.
66. Fidler JL, Guimaraes L, Einstein DM. MR imaging of the small bowel. Radiographics. 2009;29(6):1811–25.
67. Leyendecker JR, Bloomfeld RS, DiSantis DJ, Waters GS, Mott R, Bechtold RE. MR enterography in the management of patients with Crohn disease. Radiographics. 2009;29(6):1827–46.
68. Saini S, Colak E, Anthwal S, Vlachou P, Raikhlin A, Kirpalani A. Comparison of 3% sorbitol vs psyllium fibre as oral contrast agents in MR enterography. Br J Radiol. 2014;87(1042):20140100.
69. Marlett JA, Fischer MH. The active fraction of psyllium seed husk. Proc Nutr Soc. 2003;62(1):207–9.
70. Wang Y-M, van Eys J. Nutritional significance of fructose and sugar alcohols. Annu Rev Nutr. 1981;1(1):437–75.
71. La Brooy S, Fendick C, Avgerinos A, Williams C, Misiewicz J. Potentially explosive colonic concentrations of hydrogen after bowel preparation with mannitol. Lancet. 1981;317(8221):634–6.
72. Koplay M, Guneyli S, Cebeci H, Korkmaz H, Emiroglu H, Sekmenli T, et al. Magnetic resonance enterography with oral mannitol solution: diagnostic efficacy and image quality in Crohn disease. Diagn Interv Imaging. 2017;98(12):893–9.
73. Deeab DA, Dick E, Sergot AA, Sundblon L, Gedroyc W. Magnetic resonance imaging of the small bowel. Radiography. 2011;17(1):67–71.
74. Gottumukkala RV, LaPointe A, Sargent D, Gee MS. Comparison of three oral contrast preparations for magnetic resonance enterography in pediatric patients with known or suspected Crohn disease: a prospective randomized trial. Pediatr Radiol. 2019;49(7):889–96.
75. Evrimler S, Algin O. MR enterography with oral contrast agent composed of methylcellulose, low-dose barium sulfate, sorbitol, and lactulose: assessment of diagnostic performance, reliability, image quality, and patient tolerance. Clin Imaging. 2016;40(3):523–30.
76. Bharucha AE, Fidler JL, Huprich JE, Ratuapli SK, Holmes DR, Riederer SJ, et al. A prospective randomized controlled study of erythromycin on gastric and small intestinal distention: implications for MR enterography. Eur J Radiol. 2014;83(11):2001–6.
77. Bruining DH, Zimmermann EM, Loftus EV Jr, Sandborn WJ, Sauer CG, Strong SA, et al. Consensus recommendations for evaluation, interpretation, and utilization of computed tomography and magnetic resonance enterography in patients with small bowel Crohn's disease. Gastroenterology. 2018;154(4):1172–94.
78. Maglinte DD, Gourtsoyiannis N, Rex D, Howard TJ, Kelvin FM. Classification of small bowel Crohn's

subtypes based on multimodality imaging. Radiol Clin. 2003;41(2):285–303.
79. Koh D, Miao Y, Chinn R, Amin Z, Zeegen R, Westaby D, et al. MR imaging evaluation of the activity of Crohn's disease. Am J Roentgenol. 2001;177(6):1325–32.
80. Adler J, Swanson SD, Schmiedlin-Ren P, Higgins PD, Golembeski CP, Polydorides AD, et al. Magnetization transfer helps detect intestinal fibrosis in an animal model of Crohn disease. Radiology. 2011;259(1):127–35.
81. Algin O, Evrimler S, Arslan H. Advances in radiologic evaluation of small bowel diseases. J Comput Assist Tomogr. 2013;37(6):862–71.
82. Kapoor V. Abdominal tuberculosis. Postgrad Med J. 1998;74(874):459–67.
83. Algin O, Turkbey B, Ozmen E, Algin E. Magnetic resonance enterography findings of chronic radiation enteritis. Cancer Imaging. 2011;11(1):189.
84. Buckley JA, Fishman EK. CT evaluation of small bowel neoplasms: spectrum of disease. Radiographics. 1998;18(2):379–92.
85. Masselli G, Picarelli A, Di Tola M, Libanori V, Donato G, Polettini E, et al. Celiac disease: evaluation with dynamic contrast-enhanced MR imaging. Radiology. 2010;256(3):783–90.
86. Rubio-Tapia A, Kyle RA, Kaplan EL, Johnson DR, Page W, Erdtmann F, et al. Increased prevalence and mortality in undiagnosed celiac disease. Gastroenterology. 2009;137(1):88–93.
87. Scholz FJ, Afnan J, Behr SC. CT findings in adult celiac disease. Radiographics. 2011;31(4):977–92.
88. Tomei E, Diacinti D, Stagnitti A, Marini M, Laghi A, Passariello R, et al. MR enterography: relationship between intestinal fold pattern and the clinical presentation of adult celiac disease. J Magn Reson Imaging. 2012;36(1):183–7.
89. Amzallag-Bellenger E, Oudjit A, Ruiz A, Cadiot G, Soyer PA, Hoeffel CC. Effectiveness of MR enterography for the assessment of small-bowel diseases beyond Crohn disease. Radiographics. 2012;32(5):1423–44.
90. Levy AD, Hobbs CM. From the archives of the AFIP: Meckel diverticulum: radiologic features with pathologic correlation. Radiographics. 2004;24(2):565–87.
91. Schreyer A, Stroszczynski C. Radiological imaging of the small bowel. Dig Dis. 2011;29(Suppl 1):22–6.
92. Sozen S, Tuna Ö. A rare case of perforated Meckel's diverticulum presenting as a gastrointestinal stromal tumor. Arch Iran Med. 2012;15(5):325.
93. Furukawa A, Kanasaki S, Kono N, Wakamiya M, Tanaka T, Takahashi M, et al. CT diagnosis of acute mesenteric ischemia from various causes. Am J Roentgenol. 2009;192(2):408–16.
94. Rha SE, Ha HK, Lee S-H, Kim J-H, Kim J-K, Kim JH, et al. CT and MR imaging findings of bowel ischemia from various primary causes. Radiographics. 2000;20(1):29–42.

CT and MR Angiography in the Chest and Abdomen

15

Ilkay S. Idilman

15.1 Introduction

Cross-sectional imaging techniques have a widely accepted usage in varied vascular pathologies. Most of the diagnostic interventional procedures are replaced by computed tomography (CT) and magnetic resonance imaging (MRI), especially in the chest and abdomen. In this chapter, a summary of the techniques used in vascular imaging with CT and MRI in the chest and abdomen and an emphasis on clinical usage was aimed.

15.2 Computed Tomography Angiography (CTA)

CTA was developed in conjunction with the evolution of spiral CT that allows the acquisition of volumetric CT datasets in one breath-hold [1]. Short scan times made visualization of vascular structures possible with the usage of contrast material. By the 2000s, CTA become an alternative for conventional angiography for the diagnosis of many vascular diseases with superiority of CTA such as demonstration of the vessel wall, perivascular tissue, and end-organ parenchyma [2].

All CTA images are obtained after iodine-based contrast material injection which has the ability for absorption of x-rays that increase the absolute CT attenuation of the vessels [3, 4]. The goal of injection strategies is to achieve an adequate iodine concentration within the vasculature of interest [3]. In contrast with parenchymal opacification which is directly related to the total amount of administrated contrast material, arterial enhancement primarily depends on the amount of contrast material delivered per unit of time and injection duration [3]. In this connection, arterial opacification can be increased by increasing the iodine concentration of the contrast medium, increasing the injection flow rate (mL/s), or increasing injection duration time [3].

The iodine concentration of the contrast material is one of the important issues in CT angiography. The relationship between enhancement and iodine concentration is approximately 25–30 Hounsfield units (HU) per milligram (mg) of iodine per milliliter (mL) at 120 peak kilovoltage (kV) despite it differs at different CT scanners [5]. Therefore, contrast material preparations with a high iodine concentration preferably higher than 350 mg/mL are ideal for CT angiography protocols [6]. Besides, iodine delivery rate (IDR) that is formulized as [Contrast material iodine concentration (mg/mL)/1000] × flow rate (mL/s) can be used to standardize the rate of iodine delivery among different iodine concentrations [7] and it was shown that IDR of 1.5–2 g/s provides adequate arterial opacification in CTA protocols [8, 9].

I. S. Idilman (✉)
Hacettepe University, Ankara, Turkey

S. M. Erturk et al. (eds.), *Medical Imaging Contrast Agents: A Clinical Manual*,
https://doi.org/10.1007/978-3-030-79256-5_15

Changing iodine concentration of the contrast material has the same effect on arterial enhancement as changing the injection flow rate [3]. Increasing injection flow rate ends up with faster accumulation of contrast media in the aorta and increases peak aortic enhancement [6]. However, it was shown that increasing injection flow rates over 8 mL/s has no additional benefit as a result of pooling in the central venous system and reflux into the inferior vena cava [10]. An injection rate of 4–5 mL/s is efficacious for arterial opacification. The injection duration time is also important for arterial opacification as it increases cumulatively with the injection duration and a minimum of 10 s for injection duration is recommended for CTA [3, 6]. Saline flush is also recommended to push the tail of the contrast medium which would remain unused otherwise [5]. It is also useful for the reduction of streak artifact from dense contrast medium in the brachiocephalic vein and superior vena cava, especially in the chest CTAs.

The degree of CT contrast enhancement is also related to the level of x-ray energy besides the amount of iodine within the system [5]. X-ray output energy at low tube voltages is closer to the iodine k edge of 33 keV. By the way, selection of low tube voltage results in stronger contrast enhancement per iodine concentration. The use of low voltages such as 80 and 100 kVp has potential benefits like reduction of contrast material amount and radiation dose. However, tube current is increased by automatic exposure control (AEC) to maintain diagnostic image quality in many modern scanners and lowers estimated radiation dose reduction. The larger focal spot that is used for higher tube current causes a reduction in spatial resolution [11]. Exaggerated blooming artifact caused by metallic stents and calcified plaques is another limitation in usage of lower tube voltage [12].

On the other hand, there are other factors affecting arterial opacification that cannot be controlled such as cardiac output and physiologic or pathologic situations causing arterial filling delays. Cardiac output is inversely related to arterial opacification. Decreased cardiac output means delayed arrival of contrast material with stronger peak arterial enhancement and persistent enhancement in the vessels and highly perfused organs [5, 6]. It is also evident in patients with hypovolemic shock and systemic hypotension [5]. Age is another factor that is related to a delayed contrast enhancement according to the reduction of cardiac output with age [5]. Arrangement of injection rate and volume according to the patient's body weight reduces the effect of cardiac output on arterial enhancement [3]. It should also be considered that large-capacity vessels including aneurysm or ectasia or diseased vessels fill slower [12].

There are two methods, bolus tracking, and test bolus to designate the optimal arterial enhancement of the interested vessel. Bolus tracking is the most commonly used one without added contrast material administration and time. This technique is performed by placing a round of interest (ROI) on the interested vessel by acquiring a selected reference level in the topogram on a non-contrast image. The enhancement of ROI is monitored thereafter the contrast material administration after a fixed time delay. When the ROI reaches a specified level, such as 100–150 HU, scanning begins after a delay that allows peak arterial enhancement that is approximately 8 s. Test bolus method is performed by administration of a small amount of contrast material before a full bolus for diagnostic CT. Following this test bolus injection, multiple sequential images are acquired generally at the starting level of the diagnostic scan. The time to peak contrast enhancement is determined from the time-enhancement curve obtained by measuring enhancement within an ROI placed over the interested vessel.

A novel imaging technique, dual energy CT (DECT) that acquires two CT datasets at differing x-ray energy spectra has promising advancements in CTA [13]. The differences in photon absorption of different materials such as calcification, metallic materials, and contrast at various energy levels provide discrimination between them. There are two main DECT scanners; source-based DECT such as dual-source dual-energy (DSDE) and single-source dual-energy (SSDE) and detector-based DECT using dual layer of detectors. DECT improves arterial opacification of the vessel despite poor iodine concentration within it by reconstruction images at low keV levels. DECT is also useful to obtain virtual non-contrast images that can replace true non-contrast image acquisition. Therefore, it is useful for establishing real contrast extravasation and endoleaks and dose reduction. Artifacts caused by extensive vascular calcifications and metallic devices within the vessel can also be reduced by post-processing techniques in DECT. It is also possible to assess organ perfusion by using iodine map imaging.

Motion artifacts may be problematic especially in patients with high heart rates. It is obvious in the aortic root and may be misunderstood as a subtle aortic lesion. ECG-gating techniques are useful for reducing motion artifacts without need for administration of beta-blockers. It can be performed as prospective gating, retrospective gating, or high-pitch gated mode according to the available scanner. The image acquisition window is determined by the percent of R-R interval. The optimum phase for image acquisition for patients with a heart rate less than 75 beats per minute is a diastolic acquisition window of approximately 70–80%. A systolic phase acquisition (30–40%) is preferred in patients with higher heart rates [6].

The clinical indication is important to generate the optimal acquisition protocol in CTA. It is useful to obtain a non-contrast image first as it will give valuable information about the pathology. Hyperattenuating signs at non-contrast images are described for different pathologies that help the diagnosis including acute vascular occlusion, arterial dissection, and aortic rupture [14]. It is also useful in patients with clinical suspicion of active hemorrhage. The knowledge of factors affecting vascular opacification shows that there is no optimal contrast injection protocol for body CTA. Fleischmann et al. suggested a CTA protocol for a scanner with 64 channels and automated tube current modulation; a scan time of 10 s; injection duration of 18 s; scan timing of 8 s after the contrast arrival arranged with bolus triggering and injection rate according to the patient weight that is 4 mL/s for a 55 kg or a leaner patient and increasing 0.5 mL for every 10 kg of body weight with a pitch generally below 1 and usage of high-concentration contrast medium [12].

15.3 Magnetic Resonance Angiography (MRA)

MRA uses imaging techniques that discriminate flowing spins in blood from the surrounding stationary tissue. It was firstly described as a vascular imaging method without the need for a contrast medium based on gradient echo sequences called non-contrast MRA. Contrast-enhanced MRA (CE-MRA) is another technique in which gadolinium-based contrast agents (GBCA) are used that shortens longitudinal relaxation (T1) of the blood. The main advantage of both techniques is they do not expose the patient to ionizing radiation that enables repeated acquisitions, especially in children.

CE-MRA with the use of GBCA improves image quality by increasing SNR and reducing flow and motion artifacts [15]. The basic principle of CE-MRA is intravenous administration of a bolus of contrast medium and imaging the first passage of the contrast through the vessel of interest [16]. In accordance with this principle, it is important to maximize the signal enhancing effect of contrast medium in the interested vessel and minimize the signal of the surrounding tissue and unwanted vessels [17]. It is desired to reduce T1 value of blood to 50 ms or below to differ especially from fat which has the shortest T1 value in the surrounding tissues with approximately T1 value of 170–230 ms depending on field strength [17]. The concentration of contrast media in the first pass should be enough for this purpose and estimated by the injection rate divided by the cardiac output. Increasing injection rate increases concentration of GBCA and SNR till T2* effect reduces signal that occurs at an injection rate greater than 5 mL/s. Besides, increasing injection rate results in higher doses of contrast administration which is intolerable. Injection duration is also important for the totally administrated GBCA volume. The duration of injection should match the acquisition time of the MR pulse sequence. Choosing techniques using shorter acquisition time provides shorter duration of injection and leads to the use of lower GBCA with no need to change injection rate [17]. Rapid changes in the GBCA concentration create ringing artifacts and should also be avoided. It is generally recommended to use 2–3 mL/s as an injection rate for CE-MRAs.

The GBCA dose for CE-MRA changes across different institutions, indications, and available software and hardware. The dose can be arranged according to the weight of the patient between 0.1 and 0.4 mmol/kg (typically 0.2 mmol/kg) or 20–30 mL per patient for a single station and larger field of view [15]. Extending coverage should require increasing the contrast dose to 0.3 mmol/kg or 40–45 mL. Higher doses are also needed for venous evaluation because of dilution of the contrast agent or pathologies such as large aneurysms or dissections as it takes more contrast agents to fill the aneurysm or false lumen [18, 19].

It is important to inform the patient about the examination as performing the acquisition during patient breath-holding is necessary in many MRA applications in chest and abdomen. Relaxation also decreases cardiac output and increases arterial Gd concentration. A 20- or 22-gauge catheter is optimal for contrast administration and arms elevation is recommended. Hand or power injection can be performed for contrast material administration. It is mandatory to use saline flush after the contrast injection which is important for the delivery of the entire contrast and flushes the arm veins [15].

Spoiled-gradient-echo pulse sequence with short TE and TR is the standard pulse sequence for CE-MRA with different names according to the vendor as FLASH (Siemens), T1-FFE (Philips), or SPGR (GE). It is important to minimize TR for short acquisition times and increased saturation that result in signal reduction in the background tissue and TE for minimizing signal from T2 and magnetic susceptibility effects of the contrast medium. Two-dimensional or 3D acquisitions can be performed for CE-MRA. However, 3D sequences are generally preferred as they have higher spatial resolution with high signal-to-noise (SNR) values and thin slices that improves the quality of multiplanar reformatting (MPR) and maximum intensity projections (MIP). Flip angle values between 30° and 40° are preferred to improve saturation of the background. It is recommended to use lower flip angles such as 15°–25° in case of imaging systemic veins to maximize signal in later phases because of dilution of contrast agent [15].

Timing is the most crucial aspect of CE-MRA as scan acquisition should be in accordance with the peak contrast agent concentration in the interested vessel. Besides, central lines of k-space should be acquired at the time of highest concentration of contrast in the vessel as center of k-space primarily contributes to the contrast in an image. Timing can be organized in three ways; test bolus, automatic triggering, and MR fluoroscopy technique [15, 17]. A small bolus, approximately 2 mL of contrast administration and 20 mL saline infusion, and acquiring fast gradient echo images through the vessel of interest at fixed time intervals is used in the test bolus technique. Time to peak enhancement can be calculated by visual assessment or signal intensity measurements and image acquisition time can be planned by considering the injection duration of larger amount of contrast medium. Automatic triggering is an approach that uses a pulse sequence which automatically detects contrast arrival in the selected vessel and image acquisition is triggered when the signal intensity is above the selected threshold value. MR fluoroscopy is another way that uses rapid imaging techniques to watch contrast arrival to the interested vessel. The operator then triggers image acquisition.

There are different acquisition modes for CE-MRA and the two common ones are single phase and time-resolved MRA. The single phase mode describes acquiring vascular images at a single point of time, whereas time-resolved contrast-enhanced MRA techniques acquire multiple 3D datasets in a short time and provide consecutive dynamic angiography. Multiple phases such as arterial or venous can be obtained with no need to predetermine the timing of contrast agent in this technique. K-space is divided into several zones and the central part of k-space is reacquired more frequently than the other zones that result in updating contrast information rapidly in this technique [17]. This technique is useful for evaluating arteriovenous malformations and vascular anomalies [17].

Most GBCA are extracellular agents as they leak out of capillaries because of their small size. There are also different MRI contrast agents referred to as blood pool contrast agents that are large or bind large serum molecules reversibly and stay within the intravascular compartment. These agents enter venous circulation after the first pass in the arterial circulation and both arterial and venous vessels can be screened with a longer period of time which is named steady-state imaging [20]. Gadofosveset trisodium is one of them which was the only blood pool agent to receive United States Food and Drug Administration (FDA) approval and therefore the most widely used one. This agent reversibly binds to albumin with a serum half-time of 29 min that allows vascular imaging up to 1 h. Thakor et al. suggested a dosage of gadofosveset trisodium as 10 mL for patients with a weight of 70 kg and above and 0.12 mL/kg for smaller patients [20]. They also offered a 50:50 dilution of gadofosveset trisodium with saline for all cases; as undiluted gadofosveset trisodium causes irritation on injection [20].

Ferumoxytol is another one that is an ultrasmall superparamagnetic iron oxide (USPIO) coated with dextran that decreases its immunogenicity. The agent's serum half-life is 15 h and dilution of this agent generally as 1 part ferumoxytol to 4 parts sterile saline is also recommended [21]. The dosage can be organized as 1–4 mg/kg with an injection rate of 2 mL/s and the following saline flush [21, 22]. This agent can be safely used in patients with end-stage renal disease. Rapid bolus administration of this agent was reported to have adverse serious events including death which led to discontinuing of first-pass bolus imaging by many centers. Monitoring the patient's blood pressure, heart rate, and oxygen saturation for 30 min duration after administration of this agent is also recommended [21]. MRA with blood pool agents has potential benefits in thoracic and abdominal vascular imaging [20].

Non-contrast MRA options are generally reserved for patients with renal failure to avoid nephrogenic systemic fibrosis. The techniques depend on the motion of blood in or through the image plane. There are different ways to demonstrate vessels without contrast with MRI; flow independent ones including balanced steady-state free precession (bSSFP), non-subtractive inflow dependent including time of flight (TOF), inflow dependent inversion recovery (IFDIR) and Quiescent interval slice-selective (QISS), subtractive 3D MRA including cardiac gated 3D fast spin echo, flow sensitive dephasing (FSD) and arterial spin labeling (ASL), phase contrast (PC) including 2D, 3D, and 4D PC; and velocity-selective 3D MRA [23]. bSSFP sequence with cardiac gating is commonly used in thoracic and abdominal vascular imaging. The main problem with this sequence is off resonance artifact which is commonly seen in higher magnetic fields.

CTA and MRA provide large data sets which are difficult to review by using standard axial images. MPR means non-axial 2D images which may be in coronal, sagittal, oblique, or curved planes [24]. MIP displays only the highest attenuation value from the source image that is helpful especially to show contrast material-filled structures such as CTA and MRA. MIPs help to see longer segments of the vessel and are useful in rapid evaluation of vascular stenosis or occlusion. Overestimation of stenosis caused by a calcified plaque in CTA is the limitation of the technique and source images should be evaluated for confirmation [25]. It is also prone to artifacts in CE-MRA especially when the background signal is greater than the vascular structures or there are overlapping vessels [15]. Volume rendering (VR) is another post-processing method that is useful in displaying especially complex anatomy.

15.3.1 Pulmonary Arteries

The main indication for imaging pulmonary arteries is acute pulmonary embolism (PE). Chronic PE and pulmonary arteriovenous malformations are other indications for the evaluation of pulmonary arteries. In these specific

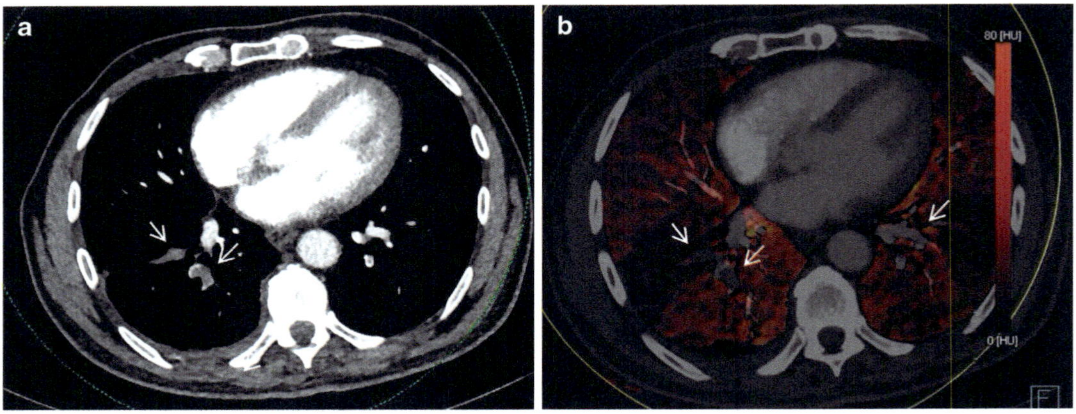

Fig. 15.1 A 67-year-old man with suspected acute pulmonary embolism. Axial dual energy CT image (**a**) and overlay image (**b**) demonstrate bilateral thrombus (arrows) at different levels with perfusion defects

indications, CTA is the modality of choice. The goal of pulmonary CTA is to provide optimum contrast material in the pulmonary arteries with minimal contrast in the superior vena cava which results in streak artifact [26, 27]. Test bolus or an ROI placed in the pulmonary trunk or main pulmonary artery should be used for optimizing contrast bolus timing. It is also important to minimize acquisition time to reduce motion artifacts. Inspiration immediately prior to the scan or Valsalva maneuver may lead to changes in intrathoracic pressure and cause inadequate or inhomogeneous intravascular contrast and careful instructions should be given to the patient [28]. Both cranio-caudal and caudo-cranial directions can be used with the most commonly preferred one is caudo-cranial as the final phase of the imaging is less disturbing in the upper portions of the lung and beam hardening artifact caused by the inflow of high contrast can be avoided [28]. Contrast material injection parameters are also important as injection with high flow rates (4–6 mL/s) and using high-concentration contrast material (370–400 mg of iodine/mL) result in better visualization of small and peripheral vessels [29]. Techniques reducing radiation dose and contrast material have come into prominence recently for pulmonary CTA. It is shown that reducing tube voltage from 120 to 100 kV results in reduction of both radiation exposure and contrast material requirement by 33% [30]. DECT has advanced in PE imaging. Beyond the luminal assessment, dual energy perfusion maps created by DECT show iodine-perfused lung tissues and by the way acts like scintigraphy and show hypoperfused areas (Fig. 15.1).

Pulmonary CTA is also useful for showing chronic pulmonary thromboembolic pulmonary hypertension (CTEPH) and pulmonary arteriovenous malformations (PAVMs) [31]. The CTA findings of CTEPH are vascular findings such as occlusion or narrowing of the pulmonary artery with eccentric or mural thrombus, webs or tortuous vessels, and a smaller pulmonary artery relative to the adjacent bronchus. Dilatation of the central pulmonary arteries and mosaic perfusion are other findings in CTEPH. PAVMs are direct communications between pulmonary arteries and veins. The imaging findings of PAVMs are enhancing nodular focus or ground-glass opacity with a feeding pulmonary artery and a draining pulmonary vein. CTA is also useful to demonstrate enlargement of bronchial or non-bronchial systemic arteries caused by variable pathologies such as CTEPH, chronic inflammatory diseases of lung parenchyma or airways, and malignity [32]. The main clinical importance of these vessels is rupture which leads to hemoptysis and CTA also plays a crucial role in mapping of these vessels prior to endovascular treatment in selected patients [32].

Assessment of pulmonary vessels can be performed with MRA especially in young or pregnant patients to avoid radiation exposure. The main MRA of pulmonary vessels is CE-MRA with 3D acquisition within a single breath-hold [33]. Large venous access such as antecubital vein is needed for high Gadolinium injection rates such as 5 mL/s to reduce venous contamination. Contrast doses of Gadolinium are 0.1–0.2 mmol/kg followed by 20 mL saline. Blood pool agents such as Gadomer-17, Gadofosveset trisodium, and ferumoxytol can be used especially in patients that cannot hold their breath [34]. Ferumoxytol can also be used in patients with contraindication to gadolinium. Imaging parameters of MRA are TR = 2.5–3 ms, TE = 1–1.5 ms, α = 30°–40°, FOV = 460 mm, matrix = 40 × 192 × 256 and parallel imaging factor $R = 2$ [35]. Central elliptic phase encoding with optimal scan timing ensures maximum SNR and separation of arterial and venous phases [33].

Capillary level tissue perfusion can be shown with perfusion MRI that has lower spatial but higher temporal resolution compared with MRA. A dynamic time-resolved MRA sequence with subtraction of post-contrast images from pre-contrast ones is used with a lower contrast material such as 0.005 mL/kg. Imaging parameters of dynamic contrast-enhanced perfusion MRI are TR = 2–2.5 ms, TE = 0.8–1 ms, α = 30–40°, FOV = 460 mm, and matrix = 32 × 96 × 128 [33]. Perfusion images allow demonstration of perfusion defects and their anatomical location and typically seen as wedge-shaped segmental or sub-segmental defects in acute PE, wedge-shaped or mottled defects in CTEPH, and diffuse defects in pulmonary hypertension [33]. Pulmonary blood flow (PBF), pulmonary blood volume (PBV), and mean transit time (MTT) can be quantified with post-processing.

Non-contrast-enhanced MRA and perfusion imaging can be an option in patients with risk for nephrogenic systemic fibrosis, pregnant patients, and pediatric population. Double inversion recovery fast spin echo (DIR FSE) imaging is useful in the evaluation of pulmonary embolism and slow flow or pulmonary clot is seen as high signal intensity relative to the flowing blood which is low signal intensity. 3D bSSFP sequence is another option in which clot or lesions can be identified in contrast with bright blood caused by long T2 (Fig. 15.2). In the ECG-gated 3D partial Fourier Fast spin echo (FSE) technique, arteries appear dark in systole due to fast flow and high in diastole due to relatively slow flow. Veins have some signal in both phases due to slow flow. Subtraction of systolic from diastolic images enables demonstration of the arterial system. ASL and TOF-MRA can be used in the chest. PC MRA has potential benefits in the evaluation of pulmonary vascular resistance and turbulent flow in the pulmonary arteries [36, 37]. Time-resolved imaging of the lungs during free breathing with Fourier decomposition (FD) analysis can be used for imaging of lung perfusion with no need to contrast material.

15.3.2 Thoracic Veins

Imaging studies of the veins in the chest such as pulmonary veins and central veins of the thorax can also be performed with both CT and MR. The indications for imaging of pulmonary veins include pulmonary venous anomalies and RF ablation planning in cases with atrial fibrillation. General purposes to evaluate a systemic vein are stenosis or thrombosis. Pulmonary venous anomalies including total and partial anomalous pulmonary venous return, pulmonary vein stenosis, pulmonary varix, and pulmonary vein atresia can be detected with both CT and MR [38]. Image acquisition time for CE-MRA should be timed for enhancement in the left atrium for imaging of pulmonary vein and as early equilibrium phase for systemic vein evaluation [39]. Direct MR venography can also be performed by administration of dilute GBCA directly into the peripheral veins during 3D image acquisition [15]. Non-contrast MRA can be useful in patients with gadolinium allergy or risk for nephrogenic systemic fibrosis [39].

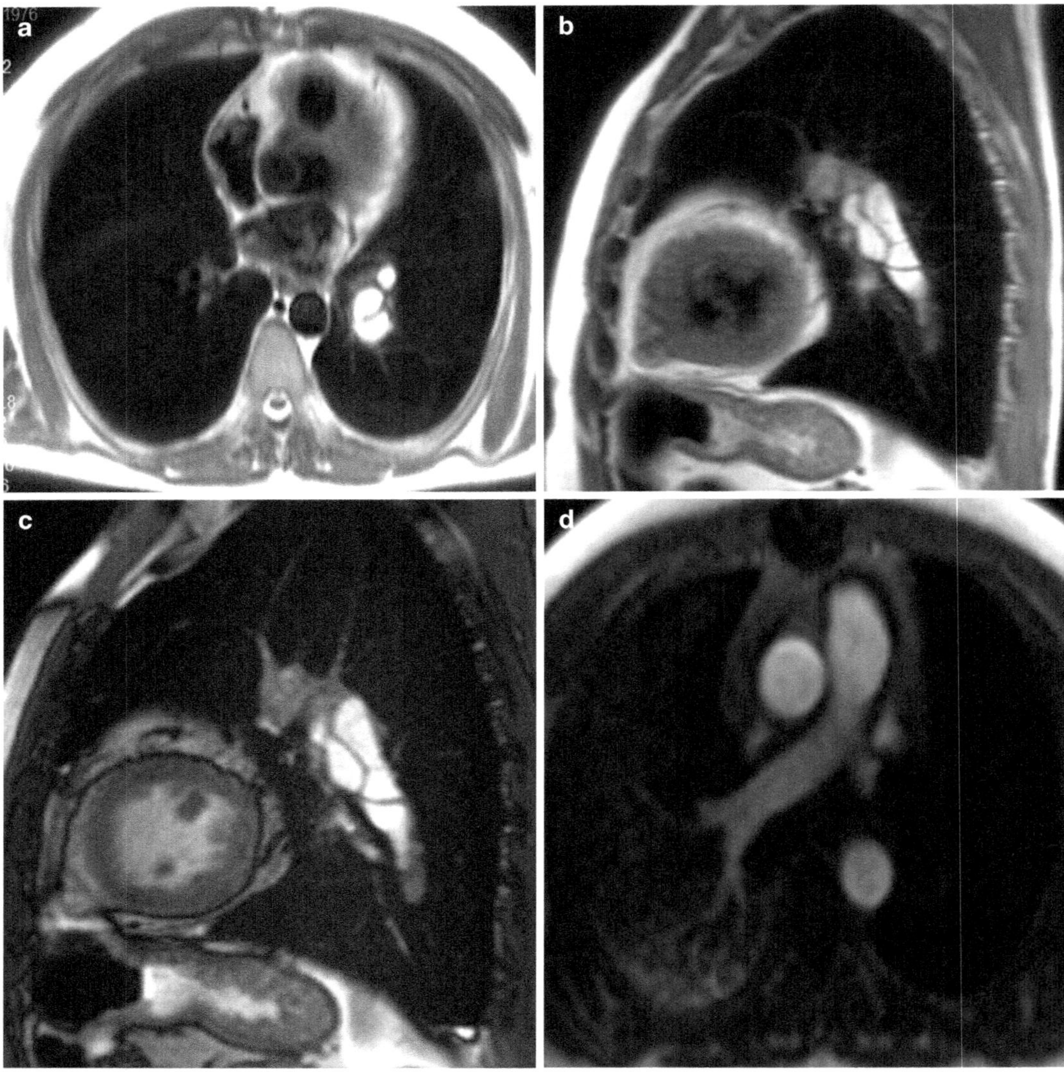

Fig. 15.2 A 43-year-old man with suspected pulmonary embolism. Axial (**a**) and sagittal (**b**) HASTE and sagittal True-FISP images (**c**) demonstrate hyper-intense filling defects in the left pulmonary artery. CE-MRA (**d**) also demonstrates the filling defect with hypoperfusion in the left lung. The patient was operated and the diagnosis was hydatid disease

15.3.3 Aorta

There are different pathologies affecting aorta with variable clinical scenarios. In emergency settings, CTA is generally the preferred modality to evaluate acute aortic traumatic injuries including aortic intimal flap, pseudoaneurysm, aortic thrombus, adventitial hematoma, aortic transection and acute aortic syndrome including aortic dissection (AD), intramural hematoma (IMH), penetrating atherosclerotic ulcer (PAU), and ruptured/leaking aneurysm [40] (Fig. 15.3). CTA has also an important role in the follow-up evaluation of surgical or endovascular treatment of these pathologies [41].

Oral contrast material is not indicated as it hinders the evaluation of aortoduodenal or aorto-enteric fistula. A non-enhanced scan with a sec-

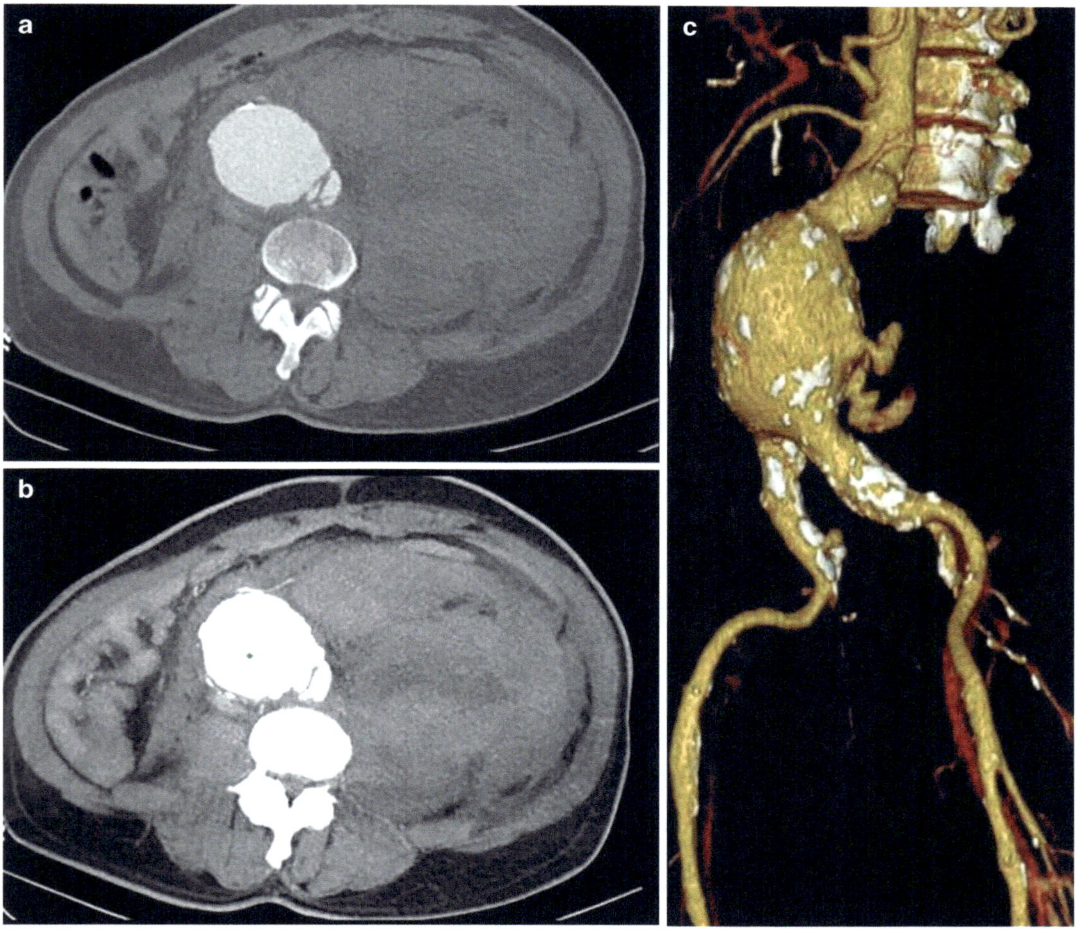

Fig. 15.3 A 60-year-old man presented with acute abdominal pain. Axial (**a**), MIP (**b**), and VR (**c**) CTA images demonstrate ruptured abdominal aortic aneurysm. With courtesy of Dr. Mehmet Ruhi Onur

tion thickness of 3–5 mm is needed to demonstrate an IMH which is thought to be an aortic dissection with an early thrombosed false lumen. This scan is also important to demonstrate hyperattenuating signs generally indicating clots in many diseases as discussed before [14]. In preoperative planning for endovascular stent graft repair (EVAR), this scan helps in the delineation of calcified plaques. In postoperative evaluation, it is useful to detect high-density surgical materials [42, 43]. The addition of a delayed non-enhanced scan in the eventuality of an abnormal CTA is another option. DECT enables the reconstruction of virtual non-contrast images with no need to acquire a separate non-contrast CT.

CTA of the aorta should cover the entire aorta from thoracic inlet to groin with a section thickness of 1 mm after intravenous administration of preferably high iodine concentration. ECG-gating is mandatory for the thoracic portion to reduce motion and pulsation artifacts that mimic dissection or subtle abnormalities. Tube current modulation that delivers full radiation in the diastole phase and limits in the other cardiac phases can be an option to reduce radiation dose in retrospective gating [44]. In prospective gating step and shoot, acquisition can be used for dose reduction if available and reported to reduce dose up to 75% [45]. Preferring lower kV values would reduce radiation dose in small patients.

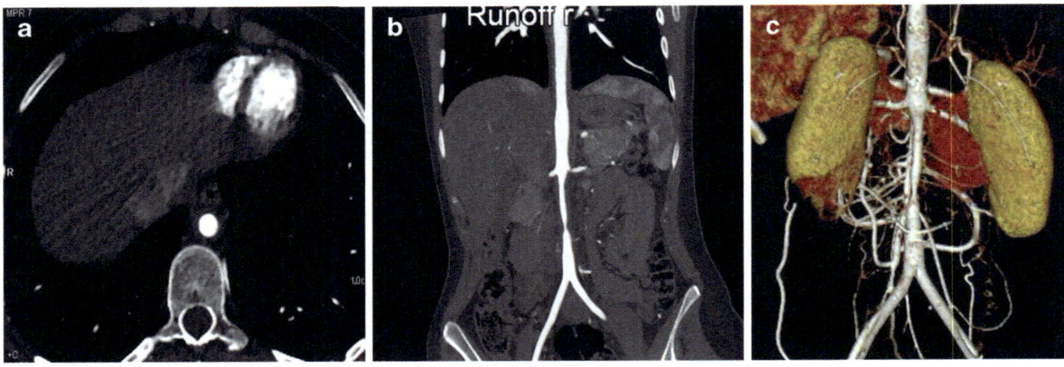

Fig. 15.4 A 21-year-old woman with suspicion of vasculitis was evaluated with CTA. On the axial image (**a**), diffuse wall thickening of the aorta is seen. On MIP (**b**) and VR (**c**) image, a diffuse narrowing of the infrarenal aorta is seen. With courtesy of Dr. Tuncay Hazirolan

Delayed phase imaging with 70 s delay is essential for detection of active bleeding and follow-up study of patients with EVAR to evaluate the size of the aneurysm and endoleak [46, 47]. A split bolus injection technique that acquires arterial and delayed phase images in one acquisition by injecting two sequential contrast material bolus, separated by a time delay of approximately 35 s has the potential to reduce radiation dose [48]. Image post-processing can help visualization of subtle and complex lesions and treatment planning [40] (Fig. 15.4).

Aorta MRA can be helpful in assessing the overall size, shape, and extend of aortic aneurysm. MRA has advances in the evaluation of AD such as determination of slow flow or thrombus in the false lumen [49]. MRA and MRI have also the capability to show IMH and PAU [50]. Aorta MRA is the preferred modality in patients with suspected aortic infections [51]. MRA enables to evaluate the site of narrowing, involvement of branch vessels, and the extent of collateral vessels in aortic coarctation [52]. It is also possible to measure velocities and by the way stenosis degree with PC MRI techniques.

SSFP is the main sequence to evaluate structural and functional characteristics of aortic valve and thoracic aorta and useful in the demonstration of aneurysms, AD, and aortic root structure [53]. ECG-gated cine sequences enable to evaluate flow disturbances within the aorta and by the way qualitatively analysis of aortic stenosis and regurgitation [54]. For quantitative evaluation of blood flow characteristics, PC MRI can be used. In this sequence selected peak velocity encoding (VENC) is important and should be 250 cm/s for the initial selection in patients with a suspicion of aortic stenosis [55]. To evaluate vessel wall and slow flow or static blood within the lumen such as false lumen in AD, DIR FSE is a useful sequence. It is also good for imaging of surrounding structures. CE-MRA demonstrates lumen and less prone to flow-related artifacts than bSSFP. ECG-gating sagittal oblique “candy-cane” CE-MRA is useful in the evaluation of aortic root motion [56]. Non-contrast-enhanced MRA can be performed with bSSFP with ECG-gating and respiratory navigation for thoracic aorta or 3D half-Fourier fast spin echo sequences [53]. In patients with clinical suspicion of large vessel vasculitis or aortic infection, it is important to add pre- and post-contrast T1 weighted 3D spoiled GRE sequence with a fat selective pre-pulse to demonstrate arterial enhancement [51, 57].

Bicuspid aortic valve (BAV) is the most common congenital cardiovascular malformation that can be associated with aortic stenosis, aortic regurgitation, and infective endocarditis [53]. In this clinical scenario, high-resolution cine SSFP is useful for the demonstration of BAV morphology and physiology, whereas PC MRI has roles in the evaluation of valvular stenosis and insufficiency. Spin Echo MR Images are good for anatomic evaluation of aortic coarctation and PC MRI helps understanding the severity of the disease as mild cases can be managed medically. It is also useful for preoperative planning and post-surgical follow-up. MRI is also helpful in the characterization of the plaques and evaluation of plaques that are vulnerable to thrombosis or embolization [58]. In the setting of acute aortic syndrome, MRA is not the preferred study. However, it is useful in the differentiation of intramural hematomas from mural thrombi [59]. Demonstration of flow dynamics is helpful in the differentiation of true and false lumen in AD. First-pass and steady-state imaging with blood pool agents were shown to demonstrate correct detection or exclusion of significant stenosis of abdominal aortic vessels [60].

15.3.4 Abdominopelvic Veins

Imaging of abdominal and pelvic venous structures is also feasible with CT and MR venography. The main indications for imaging veins are congenital anomalies, venous thrombosis, and May-Thurner syndrome. CT venography is the preferred modality in the evaluation of acute traumatic injuries and potential IVC complications [61] (Fig. 15.5). It should be noted that in the equilibrium phase of gadolinium distribution which is the optimal phase for venous imaging, the vascular signal is reduced and flip angle should be decreased [15]. MR venography with time-resolved imaging has benefits in the physiologic assessment of the direction of the flow within the veins and helps evaluation of pelvic venous insufficiency [62, 63].

15.3.5 Mesenteric Vessels

Demonstration of mesenteric vasculature and different pathologies involving them such as stenosis, occlusion, dissection, arteriovenous malformations, vasculitis, aneurysm, pseudoaneurysm, and bleeding is possible with CTA. In the suspicious of acute mesenteric ischemia (AMI) and gastrointestinal hemorrhage, CTA is the preferred imaging modality. CTA is also useful in the evaluation of hepatic, pancreatic, and splenic circulation in patients with tumor or evaluation of liver transplant living donors and recipients and complications after liver transplantation [64]. CTA protocol may differ according to the indication.

It is important to cover entire of the intestine by obtaining images from the dome of the liver to the perineum for evaluation of mesenteric

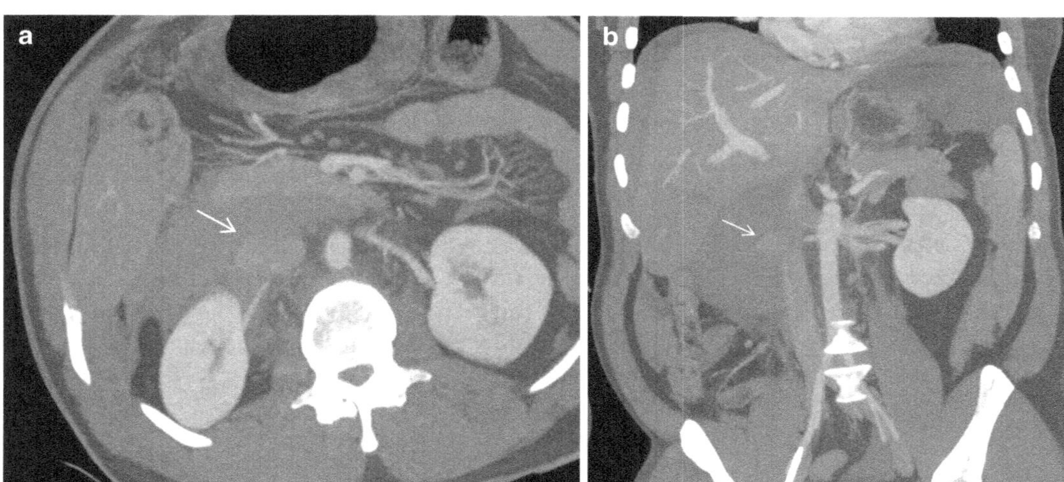

Fig. 15.5 A 43-year-old man with penetrating injury to inferior vena cava. Axial (**a**) and coronal (**b**) MIP images show contrast extravasation from the anterolateral aspect of IVC (arrows)

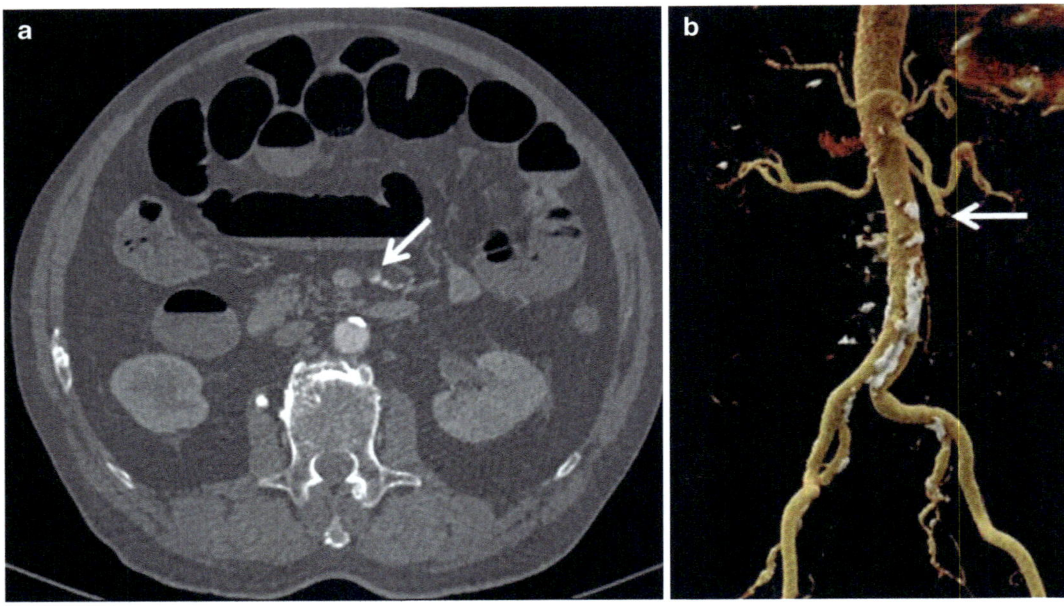

Fig. 15.6 A 78-year-old man admitted to the emergency department with a complaint of abdominal pain. Axial CTA image (**a**) shows clot in the SMA. VR image (**b**) demonstrate embolic occlusion of SMA

ischemia [65]. Non-enhanced images are necessary as well as arterial and venous phase images obtained after administration of 100–150 mL nonionic iodinated contrast material at a rate of 2.5–4 mL/s [65]. Multiplanar image reformations are helpful such as sagittal and coronal images and MIP and VR to show the interruption of the vessel with an embolus (Fig. 15.6) [65, 66]. Positive oral contrast material administration is not recommended as it obscures assessment of bowel wall enhancement in mesenteric ischemia and luminal contrast extravasation in gastrointestinal bleeding. It is also recommended to obtain three phase images—non-enhanced, arterial, and venous phase—and a rapid contrast material injection of 4–5 mL/s in order to maximize identification of contrast extravasation in gastrointestinal bleeding [67]. Non-enhanced images are helpful in the detection of high-attenuating lesions that may simulate disease and sentinel blood clots. The arterial phase is helpful in the demonstration of vascular anatomy and luminal extravasation in arterial source of bleeding with the use of MIP images and three-dimensional volume renderings [67] (Figs. 15.7 and 15.8). The portal venous phase is useful in the detection of luminal extravasation and venous source of bleeding. DECT also has advances in the evaluation of gastrointestinal bleeding. VNC images can be used instead of non-enhanced ones and by the way using DECT reduces radiation dose. Iodine maps and monochromatic images have potential benefits of increased detection of contrast material extravasation [68].

3D CE-MRA is the main imaging modality for mesenteric vasculature with MRA. With the usage of modern scanners and parallel imaging techniques, small vessels and branches can be visualized with this technique with a lower resolution than CTA [69, 70]. The images can be obtained in one breath-hold and repeated to obtain venous phase images after administration of 0.1 mmol/kg gadolinium with an injection rate of 1–2 mL/s [71]. Time-resolved MRA techniques provide morphologic and hemodynamic flow information about mesenteric vasculature with a significant reduction in acquisition times [70, 72]. Cardiac-triggered respiratory gating 3D SSFP sequences can be used for mesenteric noncontrast MRA in patients with risk for nephrogenic systemic fibrosis. QISS MRA which is a 2D bSSFP pulse sequence can be used for noncontrast arterial and venous imaging of the abdomen [73]. MRA can be useful in close follow-up

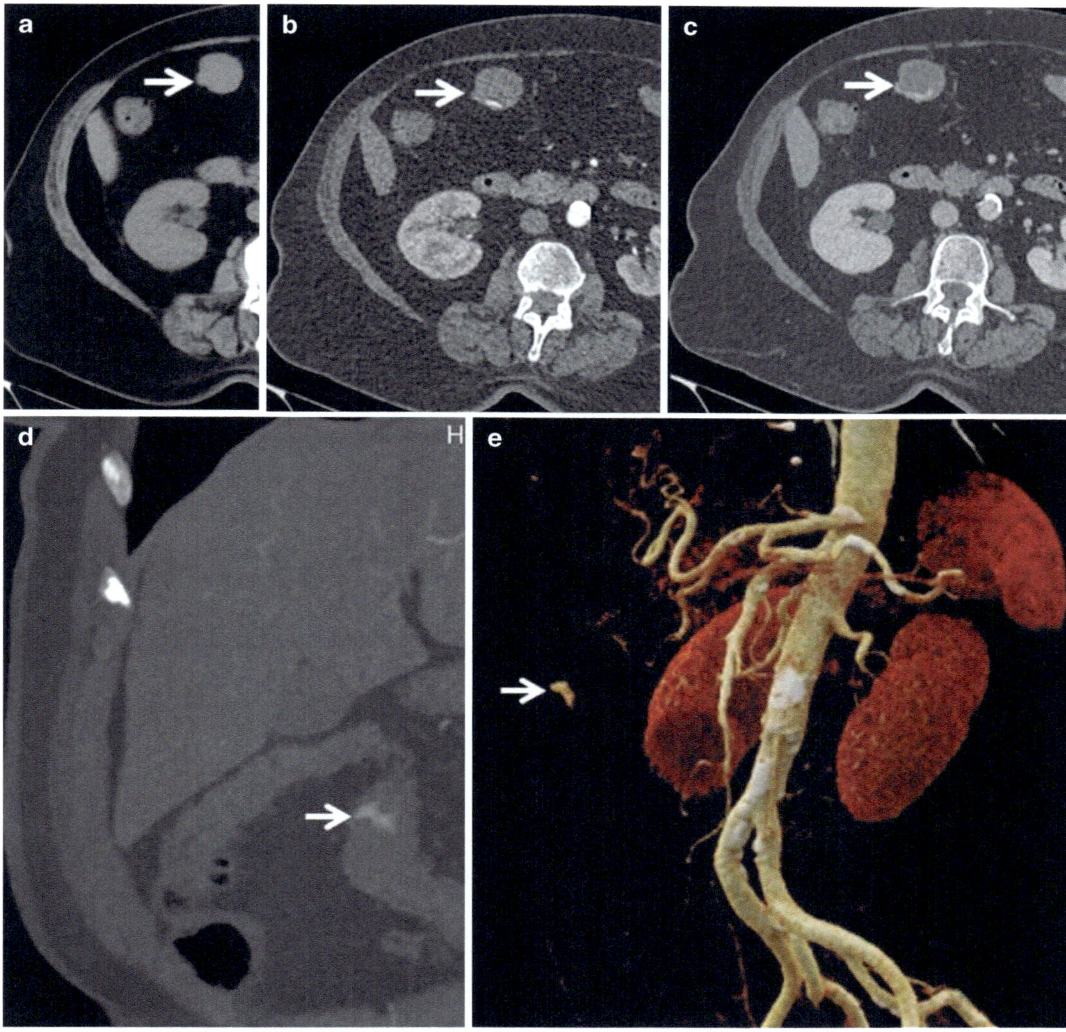

Fig. 15.7 A 76-year-old woman with complaints of hematochezia underwent CTA. Axial non-enhanced (**a**), arterial (**b**), and venous (**c**) phase coronal MIP (**d**), and VR (**e**) images demonstrate active extravasation from a diverticula in the transverse colon

of flow-related aneurysms caused by stenosis of celiac or superior mesenteric artery stenosis and recanalization after embolization [74, 75]. MRA with blood pool agents can be used for the assessment of median arcuate ligament syndrome [20].

15.3.6 Renal Vessels

The main indications for demonstration of renal vasculature are suspected renovascular hypertension and potential donors and recipients for renal transplantation. CTA is commonly used for these indications. Renal arterial flow is approximately 25% of cardiac output with a predominantly distribution to the renal cortex which leads to an initial cortical angionephrogram effect after contrast material delivery [76]. This effect lasts up to 80 s after injection and then medullary enhancement increases due to glomerular filtration. Between 120 and 180 s, a uniform nephrogram occurs and afterward excretory phase begins with calyceal excretion of contrast material [77]. The main renal vein opacification

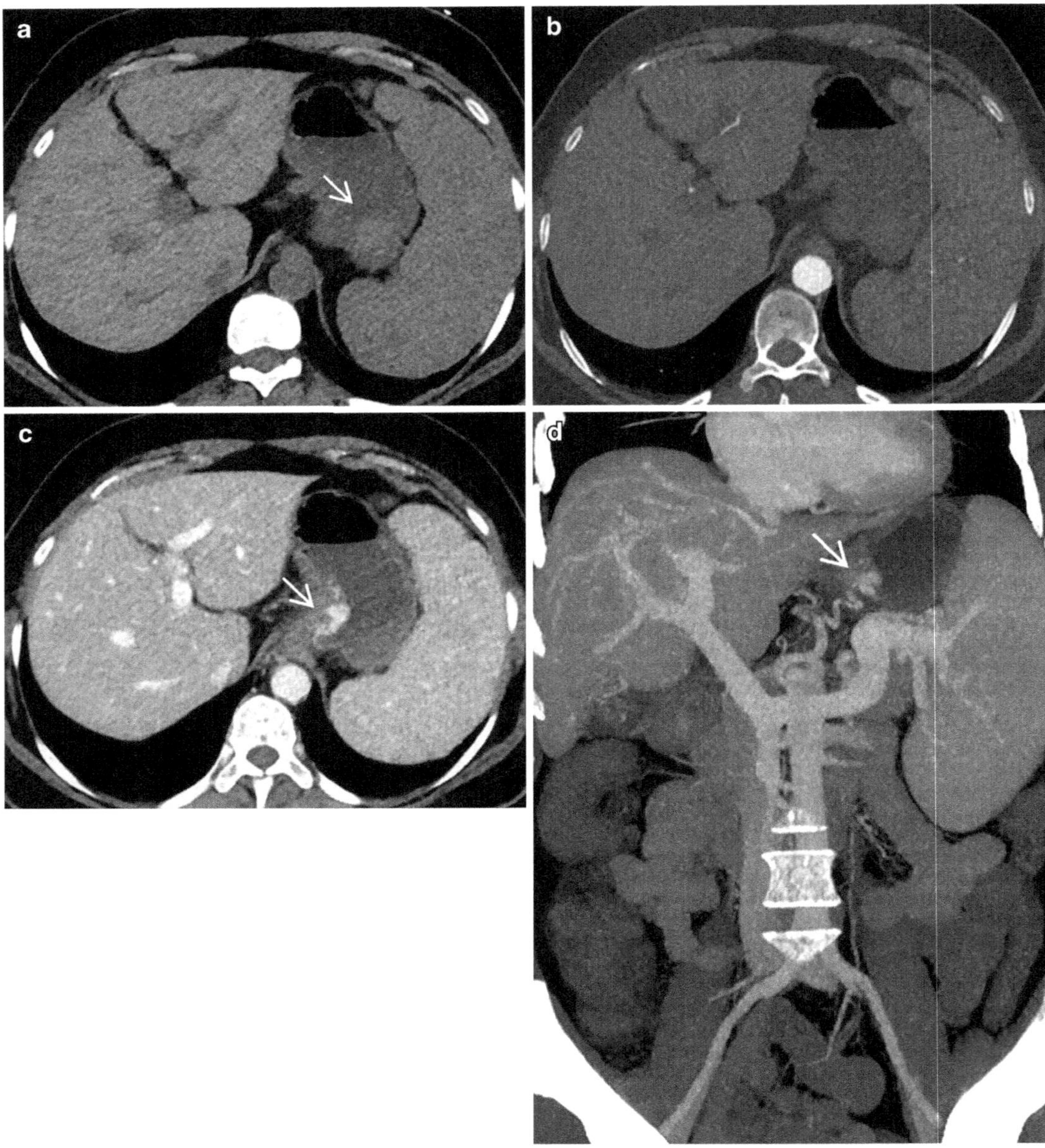

Fig. 15.8 A 50-year-old woman with a history of portal hypertension applied to the emergency department with hematemesis. A CTA was performed. On axial non-contrast image (**a**), a clot is seen in the stomach (arrow). On arterial phase, axial image (**b**) no contrast extravasation is seen. However, in the venous phase both axial (**c**) and coronal MIP images (**d**) demonstrate active extravasation from varix draining to the splenic vein (arrows)

occurs concurrently with renal arteries and cortical angionephrogram as a result of rapid parenchymal contrast circulation [77].

The desired contrast attenuation in the renal arteries (approximately 300–400 HU) can be achieved by injection of contrast material with a concentration of 300 mg/mL or greater with an injection rate of 5–6 mL/s [76]. In normal weight patients, an acquisition time equal to 4 s and a delay time equal to 6 s with a total of contrast material injection duration of 10 s is optimal. In patients with larger body weights, a longer delay time with a longer injection duration is used [76]. The acquisition should cover adrenals and aortic bifurcation to evaluate pheochromocytoma arising from the adrenal medulla and extra-adrenal paraganglioma most commonly arising from the organ of Zuckerkandl located near the origin of the inferior mesenteric artery [78].

Renal artery stenosis that can be caused mostly by atherosclerosis in the elderly and fibromuscular dysplasia (FMD) in the young adult population may result in renovascular hypertension. CTA has the capability to demonstrate all but superior to MRI in the field of demonstrating FMD. A hemodynamically significant renal artery stenosis means a luminal diameter reduction of approximately 60–70% and best demonstrated with MIP images and curved planar reformations [76]. CTA is also good to demonstrate renal artery aneurysm, traumatic renal artery injury, and acute renal artery occlusive disease such as dissection and thromboembolism (Fig. 15.9). Living donor kidney imaging is important especially with increasing ratios of laparoscopic surgery and CTA is the preferred modality as it provides a better depiction of small renal arteries than MRI [79]. A non-enhanced CT is obtained to demonstrate vascular calcifications and nephrolithiasis [80]. It is recommended to take a double pass acquisition after contrast administration to show arteries, veins, and collecting system in these patients [76].

CE-MRA can be an alternative to CTA for the demonstration of renal artery stenosis. Rountas et al. showed that CE-MRA performed with a coronal 3D fast spoiled gradient-echo breath-hold sequence with fat saturation can be used for detection of renal artery stenosis and FMD with a slightly lower sensitivity compared to CTA [81]. Non-CE-MRA is a commonly used method in the assessment of renal vasculature with recent technical advances and of concerns about the safety of gadolinium-based contrast agents especially in patients with renal insufficiency. TOF-MRA, PCA, ASL, and bSSFP angiography have been used for the assessment of RAS. However, the most commonly used sequence is respiratory gated bSSFP sequence with inversion recovery saturation and was shown to have good agreement with CE-MRA and CTA for the presence of renal artery stenosis and FMD [82, 83] (Fig. 15.10).

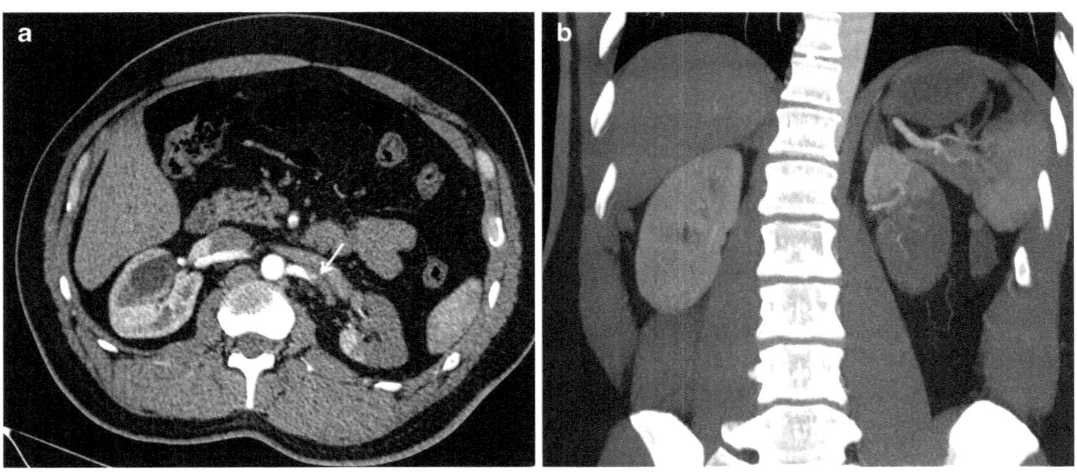

Fig. 15.9 A 42-year-old man with acute onset severe left flank pain. On the axial image (**a**) spontaneous dissection of the left renal artery is seen (arrow). On MIP images (**b**) perfusion defect is seen in the middle and lower portion of the left kidney

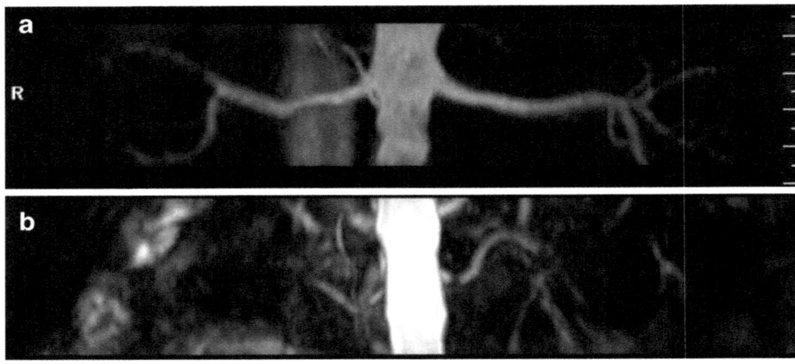

Fig. 15.10 Two patients referred for evaluation of renal artery stenosis with non-contrast MRE. bSSFP sequence was performed in both patients. Figure (**a**) shows normal renal arteries. Figure (**b**) shows severe renal artery stenosis in the left renal artery. With courtesy of Dr. Tuncay Hazirolan

References

1. Kalender WA, Seissler W, Klotz E, Vock P. Spiral volumetric CT with single-breathhold technique, continuous transport, and continuous scanner rotation. Radiology. 1990;176:181–3.
2. Rubin GD, Leipsic J, Joseph Schoepf U, Fleischmann D, Napel S. CT angiography after 20 years: a transformation in cardiovascular disease characterization continues to advance. Radiology. 2014;271(3):633–52.
3. Fleischmann D. CT angiography: injection and acquisition technique. Radiol Clin North Am. 2010;48:237–47.
4. Lusic H, Grinstaff MW. X-ray-computed tomography contrast agents. Chem Rev. 2013;113(3):1641–66.
5. Bae KT. Intravenous contrast medium administration and scan timing at CT: considerations and approaches. Radiology. 2010;256:32–61.
6. Murphy DJ, Aghayev A, Steigner ML. Vascular CT and MRI: a practical guide to imaging protocols. Insights Imaging. 2018;9(2):215–36.
7. Paparo F, Garello I, Bacigalupo L, Marziano A, Galletto Pregliasco A, Rollandi L, Puppo C, Mattioli F, Puntoni M, Rollandi GA. CT of the abdomen: degree and quality of enhancement obtained with two concentrations of the same iodinated contrast medium with fixed iodine delivery rate and total iodine load. Eur J Radiol. 2014;83:1995–2000.
8. Lell MM, Fleischmann U, Pietsch H, et al. Relationship between low tube voltage (70 kV) and the iodine delivery rate (IDR) in CT angiography: an experimental in-vivo study. PLoS One. 2017;12:e0173592–12.
9. Mihl C, Kok M, Wildberger JE, et al. Coronary CT angiography using low concentrated contrast media injected with high flow rates: feasible in clinical practice. Eur J Radiol. 2015;84:2155–60.
10. Claussen CD, Banzer D, Pfretzschner C, Kalender WA, Schörner W. Bolus geometry and dynamics after intravenous contrast medium injection. Radiology. 1984;153:365–8.
11. Oh LCW, Lau KK, Devapalaundaram A, et al. Efficacy of "fine" focal spot imaging in CT abdominal angiography. Eur Radiol. 2014;24:3010–6.
12. Fleischmann D, Chin AS, Molvin L, Wang J, Hallett R. Computed tomography angiography: a review and technical update. Radiol Clin North Am. 2016;54:1–12.
13. De Santis D, Eid M, De Cecco CN, Jacobs BE, Albrecht MH, Varga-Szemes A, Tesche C, Caruso D, Laghi A, Schoepf UJ. Dual-energy computed tomography in cardiothoracic vascular imaging. Radiol Clin North Am. 2018;56(4):521–34.
14. Morita S, Ueno E, Masukawa A, Suzuki K, Machida H, Fujimura M. Hyperattenuating signs at unenhanced CT indicating acute vascular disease. Radiographics. 2010;30(1):111–25.
15. Zhang H, Maki JH, Prince MR. 3D contrast-enhanced MR angiography. J Magn Reson Imaging. 2007;25:13–25.
16. Prince MR, Yucel EK, Kaufman JA, Harrison DC, Geller SC. Dynamic gadolinium-enhanced three-dimensional abdominal MR arteriography. J Magn Reson Imaging. 1993;3:877–81.
17. Biglands JD, Radjenovic A, Ridgway JP. Cardiovascular magnetic resonance physics for clinicians: part II. J Cardiovasc Magn Reson. 2012;14:66.
18. Frayne R, Omary RA, Unal O, Strother CM. Determination of optimal injection parameters for intraarterial gadolinium-enhanced MR angiography. J Vasc Interv Radiol. 2000;11:1277–84.
19. Frayne R, Grist TM, Swan JS, Peters DC, Korosec FR, Mistretta CA. 3D MR DSA: effects of injection protocol and image masking. J Magn Reson Imaging. 2000;12:476–87.
20. Thakor AS, Chung J, Patel P, Chan A, Ahmed A, McNeil G, Liu DM, Forster B, Klass D. Use of blood pool agents with steady-state MRI to assess the vascular system. J Magn Reson Imaging. 2017;45:1559–72.
21. Ruangwattanapaisarn N, Hsiao A, Vasanawala SS. Ferumoxytol as an off-label contrast agent in body 3T MR angiography: a pilot study in children. Pediatr Radiol. 2015;45:831–9.
22. Hope MD, Hope TA, Zhu C, et al. Vascular imaging with ferumoxytol as a contrast agent. AJR Am J Roentgenol. 2015;205:W366–73.

23. Edelman RR, Koktzoglou I. Noncontrast MR angiography: an update. J Magn Reson Imaging. 2019;49(2):355–73.
24. Dalrymple NC, Prasad SR, Freckleton MW, Chintapalli KN. Informatics in radiology (infoRAD): introduction to the language of three-dimensional imaging with multidetector CT. Radiographics. 2005;25(5):1409–28.
25. Fishman EK, Ney DR, Heath DG, Corl FM, Horton KM, Johnson PT. Volume rendering versus maximum intensity projection in CT angiography: what works best, when, and why. Radiographics. 2006;26(3):905–22.
26. Albrecht MH, Bickford MW, Nance JW Jr, Zhang L, De Cecco CN, Wichmann JL, Vogl TJ, Schoepf UJ. State-of-the-art pulmonary CT angiography for acute pulmonary embolism. AJR Am J Roentgenol. 2017;208:495–504.
27. Saade C, Bourne R, El-Merhi F, Somanathan A, Chakraborty D, Brennan P. An optimised patient specific approach to administration of contrast agent for CT pulmonary angiography. Eur Radiol. 2013;23:3205–12.
28. Hartmann IJ, Wittenberg R, Schaefer-Prokop C. Imaging of acute pulmonary embolism using multi-detector CT angiography: an update on imaging technique and interpretation. Eur J Radiol. 2010;74(1):40–9.
29. Schoellnast H, Deutschmann HA, Fritz GA, Stessel U, Schaffler GJ, Tillich M. MDCT angiography of the pulmonary arteries: influence of iodine flow concentration on vessel attenuation and visualization. AJR Am J Roentgenol. 2005;184(6):1935–9.
30. Schueller-Weidekamm C, Schaefer-Prokop CM, Weber M, Herold CJ, Prokop M. CT angiography of pulmonary arteries to detect pulmonary embolism: improvement of vascular enhancement with low kilovoltage settings. Radiology. 2006;241: 899–907.
31. Cummings KW, Bhalla S. Multidetector computed tomographic pulmonary angiography: beyond acute pulmonary embolism. Radiol Clin North Am. 2010;48(1):51–65.
32. Yıldız AE, Arıyürek OM, Akpınar E, Peynircioğlu B, Çil BE. Multidetector CT of bronchial and non-bronchial systemic arteries. Diagn Interv Radiol. 2011;17(1):10–7.
33. Johns CS, Swift AJ, Hughes PJC, Ohno Y, Schiebler M, Wild JM. Pulmonary MR angiography and perfusion imaging-a review of methods and applications. Eur J Radiol. 2017;86:361–70.
34. Aziz M, Krishnam M, Madhuranthakam AJ, Rajiah P. Update on MR imaging of the pulmonary vasculature. Int J Cardiovasc Imaging. 2019;35(8):1483–97. https://doi.org/10.1007/s10554-019-01603-y.
35. Wild JM, Marshall H, Bock M, Schad LR, Jakob PM, Puderbach M, et al. MRI of the lung (1/3): methods. Insights Imaging. 2012;3:345–53.
36. Hopkins SR, Wielpütz MO, Kauczor HU. Imaging lung perfusion. J Appl Physiol (1985). 2012;113:328–39.
37. Miyazaki M, Lee VS. Nonenhanced MR angiography. Radiology. 2008;248:20–43.
38. Abdel Razek AAK, Al-Marsafawy H, Elmansy M, El-Latif MA, Sobh D. Computed tomography angiography and magnetic resonance angiography of congenital anomalies of pulmonary veins. J Comput Assist Tomogr. 2019;43(3):399–405. https://doi.org/10.1097/RCT.0000000000000857.
39. Mueller GC, Lu JC, Mahani MG, Dorfman AL, Agarwal PP. MR imaging of thoracic veins. Magn Reson Imaging Clin N Am. 2015;23:293–307.
40. Chin AS, Fleischmann D. State-of-the-art computed tomography angiography of acute aortic syndrome. Semin Ultrasound CT MR. 2012;33(3):222–34.
41. Morgan TA, Steenburg SD, Siegel EL, Mirvis SE. Acute traumatic aortic injuries: posttherapy multidetector CT findings. Radiographics. 2010;30(4):851–67.
42. Prescott-Focht JA, Martinez-Jimenez S, Hurwitz LM, et al. Ascending thoracic aorta: postoperative imaging evaluation. Radiographics. 2013;33:73–85.
43. Chu LC, Cameron DE, Johnson PT, Fishman EK. MDCT evaluation of postoperative aortic root pseudoaneurysms: imaging pearls and pitfalls. AJR Am J Roentgenol. 2012;199:W84–90.
44. McCollough CH, Primak AN, Braun N, et al. Strategies for reducing radiation dose in CT. Radiol Clin North Am. 2009;47:27–40.
45. Bischoff B, Hein F, Meyer T, et al. Comparison of sequential and helical scanning for radiation dose and image quality: results of the prospective multicenter study on radiation dose estimates of cardiac CT angiography (PROTECTION) I study. Am J Roentgenol. 2010;194:1495–9.
46. Görich J, Rilinger N, Sokiranski R, et al. Leakages after endovascular repair of aortic aneurysms: classification based on findings at CT, angiography, and radiography. Radiology. 1999;213:767–72.
47. Golzarian J, Dussaussois L, Abada HT, et al. Helical CT of aorta after endoluminal stent-graft therapy: value of biphasic acquisition. AJR Am J Roentgenol. 1998;171:329–31.
48. Javor D, Wressnegger A, Unterhumer S, et al. Endoleak detection using single-acquisition split-bolus dual-energy computer tomography (DECT). Eur Radiol. 2017;4:1622–30.
49. Kramer CM, Budoff MJ, Fayad ZA, Ferrari VA, Goldman C, Lesser JR, Martin ET, Rajagopalan S, Reilly JP, Rodgers GP, Wechsler L, American College of Cardiology Foundation; American Heart Association; American College of Physicians-Task Force on Clinical Competence and Training. ACCF/AHA 2007 Clinical Competence Statement on vascular imaging with computed tomography and magnetic resonance. Vasc Med. 2007;12: 359–78.
50. Macura KJ, Szarf G, Fishman EK, Bluemke DA. Role of computed tomography and magnetic resonance imaging in assessment of acute aortic syndromes. Semin Ultrasound CT MR. 2003;24:232–54.

51. Murphy DJ, Keraliya AR, Agrawal MD, Aghayev A, Steigner ML. Cross-sectional imaging of aortic infections. Insights Imaging. 2016;7(6):801–18.
52. Gutberlet M, Hosten N, Vogel M, et al. Quantification of morphologic and hemodynamic severity of coarctation of the aorta by magnetic resonance imaging. Cardiol Young. 2001;11:512–20.
53. Lichtenberger JP 3rd, Franco DF, Kim JS, Carter BW. MR imaging of thoracic aortic disease. Top Magn Reson Imaging. 2018;27(2):95–102.
54. Lee JC, Branch KR, Hamilton-Craig C, et al. Evaluation of aortic regurgitation with cardiac magnetic resonance imaging: a systematic review. Heart. 2018;104(2):103–10.
55. Ishimura RA, Otto CM, Bonow RO, et al. 2014 AHA/ACC guideline for the management of patients with valvular heart disease: a report of the American College of Cardiology/American Heart Association Task Force on Practice Guidelines. J Thorac Cardiovasc Surg. 2014;148:e1–e132.
56. Groves EM, Bireley W, Dill K, et al. Quantitative analysis of ECG-gated high-resolution contrast-enhanced MR angiography of the thoracic aorta. AJR Am J Roentgenol. 2007;188:522–8.
57. Hartlage GR, Palios J, Barron BJ, et al. Multimodality imaging of aortitis. JACC Cardiovasc Imaging. 2014;7:605–19.
58. Wehrum T, Dragonu I, Strecker C, et al. Multi-contrast and three-dimensional assessment of the aortic wall using 3T MRI. Eur J Radiol. 2017;91:148–54.
59. Baliga RR, Nienaber CA, Bossone E, et al. The role of imaging in aortic dissection and related syndromes. JACC Cardiovasc Imaging. 2014;7:406–24.
60. Nikolaou K, Kramer H, Grosse C, et al. High-spatial-resolution multistation MR angiography with parallel imaging and blood pool contrast agent: initial experience. Radiology. 2006;241:861–72.
61. Rao B, Duran C, Steigner ML, Rybicki FJ. Inferior vena cava filter-associated abnormalities: MDCT findings. AJR Am J Roentgenol. 2012;198:W605–10.
62. Pandey T, Shaikh R, Viswamitra S, Jambhekar K. Use of time resolved magnetic resonance imaging in the diagnosis of pelvic congestion syndrome. J Magn Reson Imaging. 2010;32:700–4.
63. Chennur VS, Nzekwu EV, Bhayana D, Raber EL, Wong JK. MR venography using time-resolved imaging in interventional management of pelvic venous insufficiency. Abdom Radiol (NY). 2019;44:2301–7.
64. Price M, Patino M, Sahani D. Computed tomography angiography of the hepatic, pancreatic, and splenic circulation. Radiol Clin North Am. 2016;54(1):55–70.
65. Kanasaki S, Furukawa A, Fumoto K, Hamanaka Y, Ota S, Hirose T, Inoue A, Shirakawa T, Hung Nguyen LD, Tulyeubai S. Acute mesenteric ischemia: multidetector CT findings and endovascular management. Radiographics. 2018;38(3):945–61.
66. Horton KM, Fishman EK. Multidetector CT angiography in the diagnosis of mesenteric ischemia. Radiol Clin North Am. 2007;45(2):275–88.
67. Raman SP, Fishman EK. Computed tomography angiography of the small bowel and mesentery. Radiol Clin North Am. 2016;54(1):87–100.
68. Wells ML, Hansel SL, Bruining DH, Fletcher JG, Froemming AT, Barlow JM, Fidler JL. CT for evaluation of acute gastrointestinal bleeding. Radiographics. 2018;38(4):1089–107.
69. Lum DP, Busse RF, Francois CJ, et al. Increased volume of coverage for abdominal contrast-enhanced MR angiography with two-dimensional autocalibrating parallel imaging: initial experience at 3.0 Tesla. J Magn Reson Imaging. 2009;30:1093–100.
70. Hagspiel KD, Flors L, Hanley M, Norton PT. Computed tomography angiography and magnetic resonance angiography imaging of the mesenteric vasculature. Tech Vasc Interv Radiol. 2015;18(1):2–13.
71. Heverhagen JT, Reitz I, Pavlicova M, et al. The impact of the dosage of intravenous gadolinium-chelates on the vascular signal intensity in MR angiography. Eur Radiol. 2007;17:626–37.
72. Kramer U, Fenchel M, Laub G, et al. Low-dose, time-resolved, contrast-enhanced 3D MR angiography in the assessment of the abdominal aorta and its major branches at 3 Tesla. Acad Radiol. 2010;17:564–76.
73. Edelman RR, Sheehan JJ, Dunkle E, et al. Quiescent interval single shot unenhanced magnetic resonance angiography of peripheral vascular disease: technical considerations and clinical feasibility. Magn Reson Med. 2010;63(4):951–8.
74. Ayache JB, Collins JD. MR angiography of the abdomen and pelvis. Radiol Clin North Am. 2014;52:839–59.
75. Kurosaka K, Kawai T, Shimohira M, et al. Time resolved magnetic resonance angiography for assessment of recanalization after coil embolization of visceral artery aneurysms. Pol J Radiol. 2013;78:64–8.
76. Falesch LA, Foley WD. Computed tomography angiography of the renal circulation. Radiol Clin North Am. 2016;54(1):71–86.
77. Foley WD. Renal MDCT. Eur J Radiol. 2003;45(Suppl1):S73–8.
78. Kahraman D, Goretzki PE, Szangolies M, et al. Extraadrenal pheochromocytoma in the organ of Zuckerkandl: diagnosis and treatment strategies. Exp Clin Endocrinol Diabetes. 2011;119:436–9.
79. Engelken F, Friedersdorff F, Fuller TF, et al. Pre-operative assessment of living renal transplant donors with state-of-the-art imaging modalities: computed tomography angiography versus magnetic resonance angiography in 118 patients. World J Urol. 2013;31:983–90.
80. Sebastia C, Peri L, Salvador R. Multidetector CT of living renal donors: lessons learned from surgeons. Radiographics. 2010;30:1875–90.
81. Rountas C, Vlychou M, Vassiou K, Liakopoulos V, Kapsalaki E, Koukoulis G, Fezoulidis IV, Stefanidis I. Imaging modalities for renal artery stenosis in suspected renovascular hypertension: prospective intraindividual comparison of color Doppler US, CT angiography, GD-enhanced MR angiogra-

phy, and digital subtraction angiography. Ren Fail. 2007;29:295–302.
82. Glockner JF, Takahashi N, Kawashima A, Woodrum DA, Stanley DW, Takei N, Miyoshi M, Sun W. Non-contrast renal artery MRA using an inflow inversion recovery steady state free precession technique (Inhance): comparison with 3D contrast-enhanced MRA. J Magn Reson Imaging. 2010;31(6):1411–8.
83. Albert TS, Akahane M, Parienty I, Yellin N, Catalá V, Alomar X, Prot A, Tomizawa N, Xue H, Katabathina VS, Lopera JE, Jin Z. An international multicenter comparison of time-SLIP unenhanced MR angiography and contrast-enhanced CT angiography for assessing renal artery stenosis: the renal artery contrast-free trial. AJR Am J Roentgenol. 2015;204(1): 182–8.

Contrast-Enhanced CT and MR Scanning of the Brain

16

Yilmaz Onal

Abbreviations

BBB	Blood–brain barrier
CA	Contrast agent
CE	Contrast enhancement
CNS	Central nervous system
CSF	Cerebrospinal fluid
CT	Computed tomography
GBM	Glioblastoma multiforme
Gd	Gadolinium
MR	Magnetic resonance
MS	Multiple sclerosis
NSF	Nephrogenic systemic fibrosis
WHO	World Health Organization

16.1 CA Enhancement Mechanisms and Accumulation in Brain

According to endothelial structure, normal microvasculature is divided into four main categories: continuous, discontinuous, fenestrated, and tight junctional (blood-brain barrier). Brain has the most restrictive environment for CA diffusion due to the presence of the blood-brain barrier (BBB). Contrast material enhancement of the brain is compound of two primary mechanisms: intra and extravascular enhancement. After injection of contrast medium through a peripheral vein, the amount of contrast material is increased and gradient occurs between the extravascular interstitial fluid and the capillary endothelium. CA diffuses into the perivascular interstitium from the endothelial membrane where capillary permeability occurs, but an intact BBB prevents it.

Knowledge about the patterns and mechanisms of CAs is important in terms of radiological differential diagnosis. Brain enhancement is associated with both intravascular and extravascular contrast material. Intravascular enhancement might show neovascularity, vasodilatation, or hyperemia, and shortened transit time or shunting [1–6]. Although interstitial CE varies according to the permeability conditions in the BBB, intravascular CE is proportional to increased blood flow or volume. Intravascular opacification on CT can be seen simultaneously with CE. However, when we get the image 10–15 min after the injection, CE is interstitial.

Interstitial CE in MRI requires both free water protons and Gd. If there is no free water proton in a tissue, Gd involvement is not observed in T1-weighted studies. For example, the skull and dura mater often show shiny enhancement of the falx and tentorium on CE-CT images, but they do not routinely show similar enhancement on MRI [7]. Normal dura mater does not have

Y. Onal (✉)
Fatih Sultan Mehmet Training and Research Hospital, Istanbul, Turkey

S. M. Erturk et al. (eds.), *Medical Imaging Contrast Agents: A Clinical Manual*,
https://doi.org/10.1007/978-3-030-79256-5_16

a BBB, but it lacks enough water to display the T1 shortening essential for enhancement on MR images. Physiologic or pathological situations may show abnormal CE, whether or not related to the primary lesion. Angiogenesis, active inflammation, cerebral ischemia, and hypertension are all related to variation in permeability of the BBB. In addition, reactive hyperemia and neovascularity often have increased blood volume and flow that will cause a shortened mean transit time. These properties, abnormally increased capillary permeability, modified blood volume and flow, result in abnormal CE on Gd-enhanced MRI and iodine-enhanced CT examinations.

In current practice, Gd-based CAs have been taken into account safe when used at clinically recommended doses in subjects without severe renal insufficiency. The introduction of the relationship between nephrogenic systemic fibrosis with the use of Gd-based CAs and the use of new regulations about injections have led to the elimination of the NSF since 2009. But in 2014, we were first concerned with Gd accumulation in subjects with normal renal function. Kanda et al. in 2014 [8] revealed abnormal T1 shortening in the globus pallidus and the dentate nuclei in subjects who had undergone recurrent administration of Gd. And with coupled plasma mass spectrometry they demonstrate that Gd accumulation was not only in the global pallidus and dentate nuclei but also in frontal lobe cortex, frontal lobe white matter, and cerebellar white matter, at concentrations that far exceeded those seen in the control group. And of course this situation rises the question, whether the CA or agent class affects Gd deposition. Gd-based CAs can be classified as ionic and non-ionic. While ionic agents were thermodynamically more stable, no link between stabilization and Gd deposition was shown. Also, they are more commonly classified as linear or macrocyclic based on the chemical structure of the chelating agent which binds to the Gd. There are many studies investigating the effect of linear or macrocyclic agents on Gd deposition. In a study performed in subjects who underwent six or more gadopentetate dimeglumine (linear agent) or gadoterate meglumine (macrocyclic agent) enhanced MRI were compared. While no significant signal increase was observed in the subjects with macrocyclic agent, linear agent injected subjects showed increased signal in the dentate nucleus compared to the pons and in the globus pallidus compared to the thalamus [9]. In another study [10] comparing gadobenate dimeglumine and gadopentetate dimeglumine (two linear agents), a signal increase was observed in the dentate nucleus compared to pons and CSF in subjects who were administered gadobenate dimeglumine. But this signal increase was lower with gadopentetate dimeglumine than gadopentetate. Radbruch et al. [11] compared the dentate nucleus signal intensity with pons and middle cerebellar peduncle in 33 subjects. After 20 consecutive injections of macrocyclic agents (gadoterate meglumine and gadobutrol) there was no signal increase in the dentate nucleus after both agents. Radbruch and his colleagues [11] interpreted the difference in signaling, when exposed to linear and macrocyclic agents, with the fact that the two groups differ in chemical stabilization thus containing different amounts of non-chelating Gd. This hypothesis was based on the fact that the signal increase was associated with Gd deposition, as shown in autopsy series, and that some linear agents had lower thermodynamic stability.

16.1.1 Extraaxial Enhancement

Extraaxial enhancement of the CNS can be divided into pachymeningeal or leptomeningeal. The meninges that surround the CNS, origin of cranial and spinal nerves, consists of three connective layers. Pachymeningeal enhancement shows dural enhancement while leptomeningeal enhancement shows pial and arachnoidal enhancement. Pachymeninks are formed of two membranes, the periosteum of the inner layer of the skull and the meningeal layer. Pachymeningeal enhancement is come up with bone or dural reverberations of the falx cerebri, tentorium cerebelli, or cavernous sinus, while leptomeningeal enhancement is seen in surface of the brain or subarachnoid space. In pathological pachymeningeal enhancement, there is an increase in thickness as well as signal density or intensity [12, 13]. In leptomeningeal enhancement, unlike pachymeningeal, a gyriform or serpentine pattern is observed following the pial and subarachnoid spaces along the sulcus and cisterns [7].

16.1.2 Pachymeningeal Enhancement

The avid uptake of CA and enhancement in dura is the result of absent BBB within the vessels in dura, which allows diffusion of the CAs easily [14]. While normal dural enhancement is well seen on CT scans in the dural reflections, it is not well recognized in the inner table of the skull [7].

The dura mater is isointense to the cortical bone of the inner table of the skull on T1 and T2 weighted images. Dura shows thin, linear uninterrupted CE, which can be seen in half of the normal population after injection of contrast material [7–15]. Under focal or diffuse pachymeningeal enhancement, there can be many benign and malignant conditions. Intracranial hypotension, infectious or inflammatory processes (granulomatous diseases), neoplasms (menengiomas, metastasis, seconder CNS lymphoma), and iatrogenic (lumbar puncture) can be given as an example. Pachymeningeal enhancement can return to normal after the underlying cause has disappeared.

Intracranial hypotension is a rare benign condition due to low CSF pressure, generally due to CSF leakage (Fig. 16.1). When the CSF pressure decreases, there might be secondary fluid transfer that causes volume increase in capacitance veins in the subarachnoid space. Diffuse pachymeningeal enhancement is the main MRI finding and orthostatic headache is clinical finding. Except diffuse pachymeningeal enhancement, MRI might also show enhancement above and below the tentorium, expansion of the pituitary gland, low cerebellar tonsils, and subdural effusions in some subjects [16, 17].

Meningiomas represent the most common primary brain tumor and implicate three World Health Organization (WHO) grades. WHO grade I (90%) is the most frequent [18]. They are also the most common primary dural neoplasms with pachymeningeal enhancement [7–15]. The incidence increases with age and shows marked female dominance, especially in third and sixth decade [19]. Clinical findings such as personality changes, neurological deficits, sensorimotor

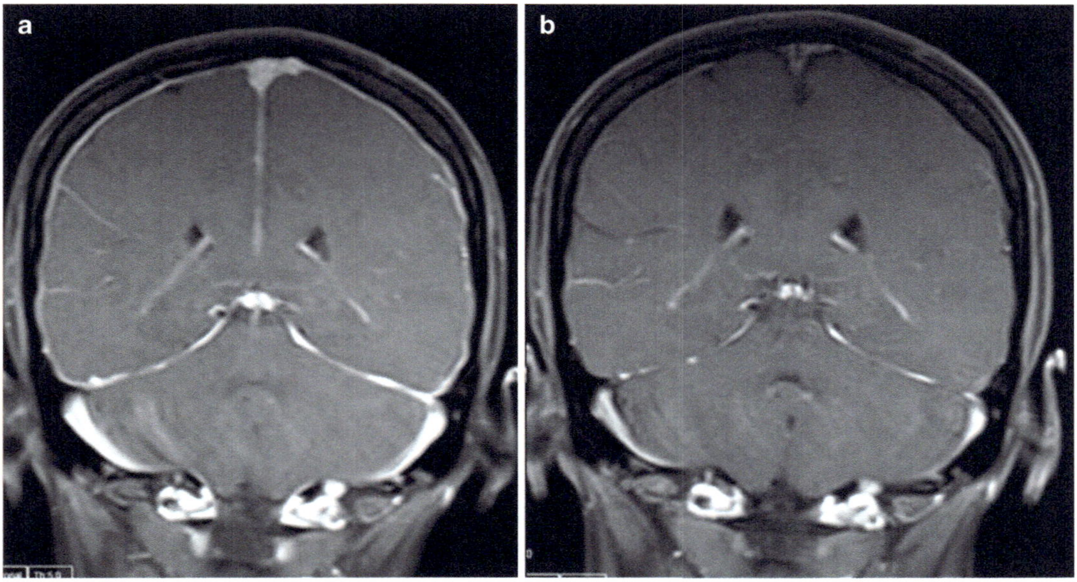

Fig. 16.1 A 34-year-old female subject with orthostatic headache, CE-MRI reveals diffuse non-nodular dural thickening at post-contrast images (**a**) and after the treatment (**b**), post-contrast images show significant decrease in dural enhancement

changes and visual symptoms, aphasia, and seizures can all be manifested by the location of the menengioma. For example, skull-based meningiomas may cause cranial nerve palsies. Despite the superiority of MRI in the evaluation of soft tissue, the combination with CT is important for the determination of bone invasion which is important in the planning of surgery and radiotherapy [20, 21]. Due to the lack of BBB, meningiomas show marked CE in CT and T1-weighted MRI examinations. Since the prognosis is directly related to the removal of the infiltrated dura, the determination of the pathological changes in the dura by assessing dural tail sign is very important for the surgical approach (Fig. 16.2).

Dural metastases of the other primary tumors may also show pachymeningeal enhancement, especially breast and prostate metastases [7, 22, 23] (Fig. 16.3). Granulomatous diseases, rheumatoid nodules, fungal diseases may cause dural

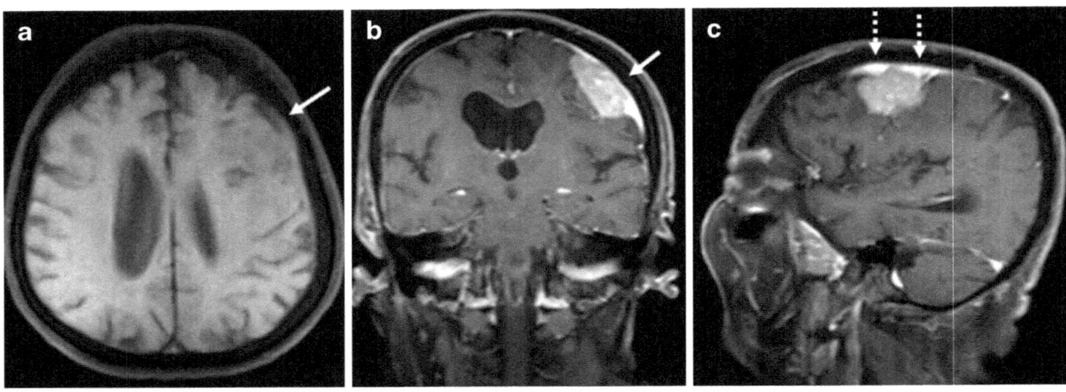

Fig. 16.2 In pre-contrast T1 images (**a**), there is a mass with heterogeneous intensity which does not allow to discriminate morphologically. In post-contrast coronal (**b**) and sagittal (**c**) images, the lesion shows diffuse homogenous CE, causes thickening of the dura in the neighborhood which indicates a menengioma

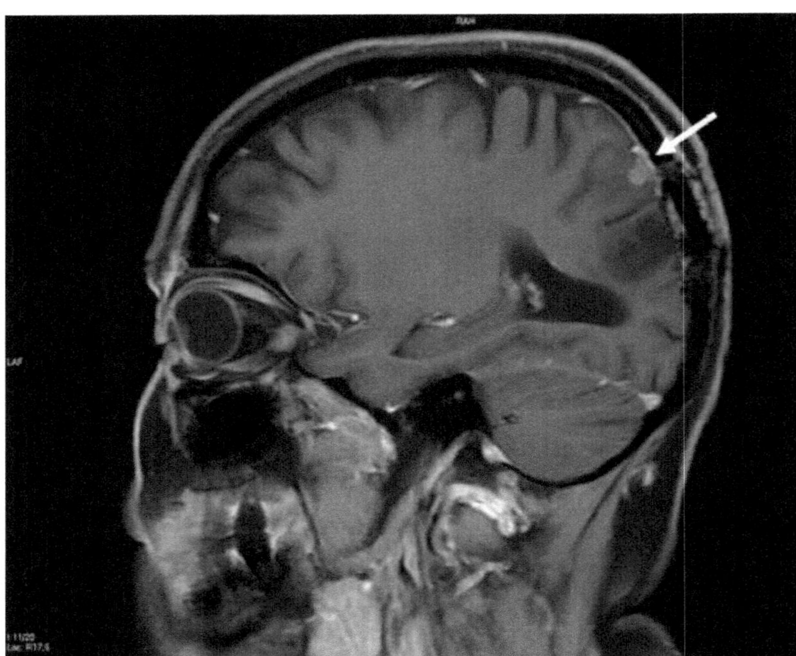

Fig. 16.3 A 67-year-old man with primary prostate cancer, post-contrast MR imaging shows nodular CE of the dura, which is a biopsy-proven metastases

involvement and pachymeningeal enhancement [7]. Chronic subdural hematoma, sinus thrombosis, carotico-cavernous fistula, and temporal arteritis have been reported to show dural enhancement [24–27].

16.1.3 Leptomeningeal Enhancement

Leptomeningeal enhancement is the enhancement of sulcus and cistern into the subarachnoid spaces or enhancement of the pia mater. Leptomeningeal CE is mostly due to meningitis which may be caused by viral, bacterial, or fungal agents. Bacterial and viral agents display thin and linear enhancement while fungal agents cause thick and nodular CE [28]. In the diagnosis of meningitis, imaging is not performed for initial diagnosis but to confirm the suspicious clinic, to eliminate meningitis mimics and increased intracranial pressure before lumbar puncture and to assess complications. CE-MR is superior to CE-CT in identification of pathological meningeal CE in basal cistern, sylvian fissure, and deep cortical sulci [29].

Tumor cells spreading along the brain surface, mostly leptomeningeal less pachymeningeal, is called meningeal carcinomatosis. Meningeal carcinomatosis may be due to both primary (medulloblastoma, ependymoma, glioblastoma) and secondary tumors (lymphoma, breast cancer) (Fig. 16.4). Neoplastic conditions, similar to fungal meningitis, may cause thick and nodular CE [7].

16.1.4 Intraaxial Enhancement

16.1.4.1 Gyral Enhancement

Superficial enhancement of the brain parenchyma is generally caused by vascular or inflammatory processes.

Reperfusion of ischemic brain, vasodilatation phase of migraine, posterior reversible encephalopathy syndrome can be given as an example of vascular causes to serpentine CE [30, 31]. Inflammatory causes include meningitis and encephalitis. The distinction between vascular and inflammatory causes can be made according to clinical history and contrast-enhancing localizations. While sudden clinical symptoms refer a vascular cause, sluggish and nonspecific headache or lethargy suggests inflammation-infection. In addition, gyral lesions in which single vessel district is affected are thought to cause by vascular pathologies, whereas multiple districts are thought to cause by inflammatory events. The most commonly affected vascular circulation district is the middle cerebral artery, but lesions in posterior reversible encephalopathy syndrome are generally in the posterior cerebral artery territory [31, 32].

The most common and the most serious form of acute encephalitis is herpes encephalitis and the agent is usually latent Herpes Simplex Virus 1. The latent virus extends along the trigeminal nerves through the leptomeninges of the anterior and posterior cranial fossa retrogradely from the trigeminal ganglion. Patients present with acute fever, headache, altered conscious level, or seizure. In the imaging, bilateral asymmetric temporal lobe

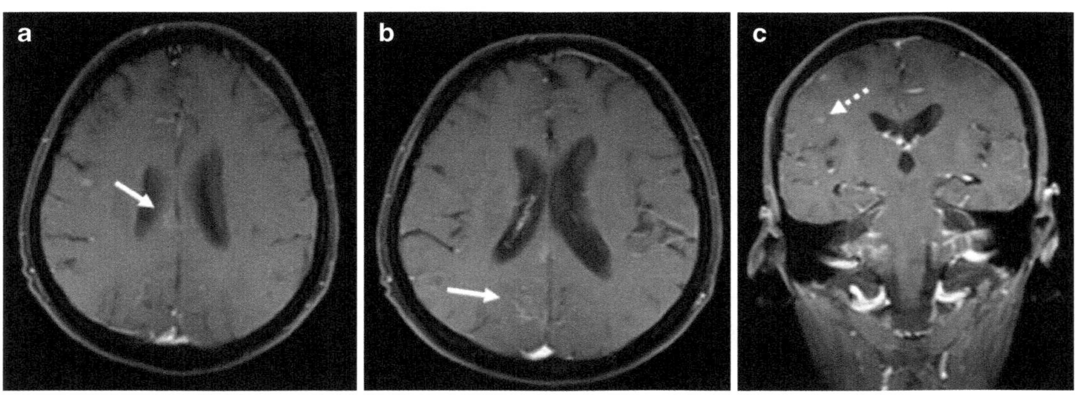

Fig. 16.4 A 65-year-old subject with a history of primary lung cancer, post-contrast axial (**a**, **b**) and coronal MR images (**c**) of the patient showed leptomeningeal enhancement (arrows) in bilateral occipital and infratentorial area consistent with diffuse linear metastasis. Also note the nodular metastatic lesions (dashed arrow)

involvement together with insula which extends to the putaminal border is observed. CT may appear normal or show edema. On MRI, gyral enhancement in cortex and white matter of the temporal lobe is typical with increased T2 signal. In T2* examination, cortical microbleedings can be seen [33]. Other sections of the brain may also be involved, such as cingulum of the frontal lobe.

The vascular causes of gyral enhancement may occur in varying periods of time with different mechanisms. Temporary disruption of BBB after ischemia with reperfusion is the earliest cause of enhancement [34, 35]. Early reperfusion also causes vasodilatation, increase in blood volume, and shortening of the mean transit time. These properties were first detected in conventional angiography [36]. Increased blood flow can be explained by the autoregulation mechanisms that develop due to increased PCO_2 pressure because of ischemia. CT or MRI images taken after ischemia with early reperfusion may show gyral enhancement within minutes. Vascular proliferation or hypertrophy is seen in the recovery phase of cerebral infarction after several days or weeks. CE returns after 1–4 months after ischemia and leaves its place to decrease in brain volume [37].

Post-ictal status imaging aspect is similar in many respects to cerebral infarct findings; increased T2 signal, gyral swelling, sulcal and gyral enhancement [38].

16.1.4.2 Nodular Cortical and Subcortical Enhancement

Subcortical or cortical parenchymal nodular enhancement refers to the hematogenous spread of metastasis or clot embolism. These lesions are usually <2 cm and located at the gray-white matter junction. Brain metastases are the most common malignant brain tumors in adults and their incidence increases [39, 40]. This may be related to prolongation of life, more effective treatment methods, and imaging techniques. Lung cancer, breast cancer, and melanoma are the most common metastatic tumors of the brain [41].

Metastatic lesions show T1 hypo-T2 hyperintensity and show CE in nodular pattern after post-contrast images (Fig. 16.5). Malign mela-

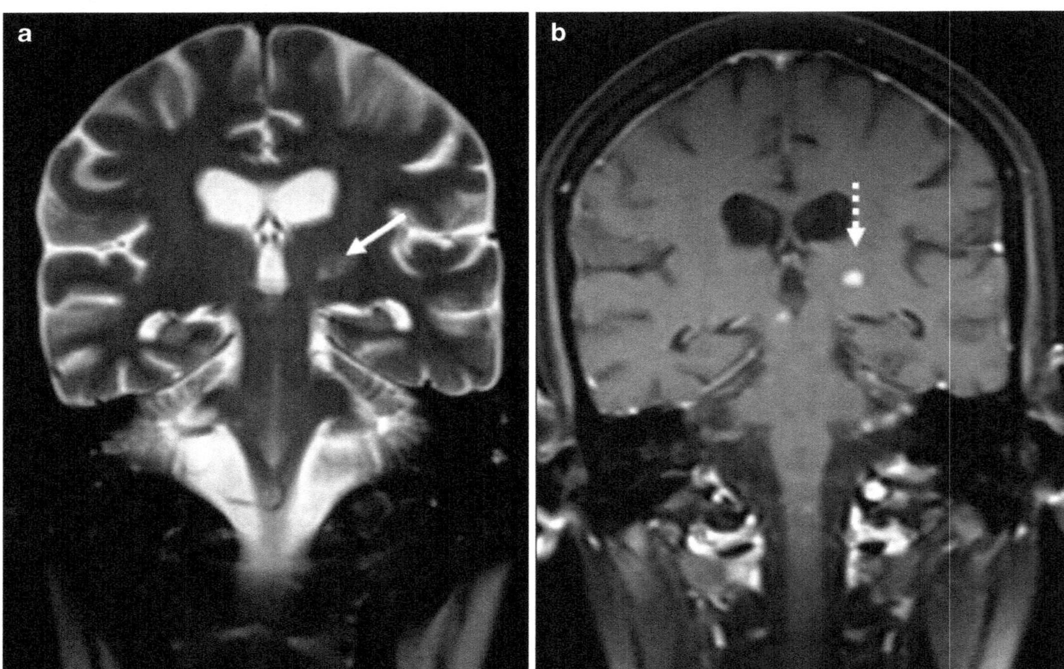

Fig. 16.5 A 54-year-old woman with primary breast cancer has a hyperintense lesion of less than 1 cm (arrow) in her left basal ganglia in T2W images (**a**). Post-contrast T1W coronal image (**b**) shows a nodular contrast-bearing lesion consistent with metastasis (dashed arrow)

noma metastases may show hyperintensity in T1 weighted images due to hemorrhage or melanin component [42]. Metastases to the brain are generally by hematogenous transmission, usually through the arterial system. They are mostly seen in gray-white matter junction where the vessel diameter decreases and embolic tumor cells are trapped [43]. While metastases are mostly to the supratentorial region, in one study 23% of colorectal cancer patients with brain metastasis were shown to have isolated cerebellar metastasis [44]. In another study, it was shown that cerebellar metastasis was detected in 31% of patients with primary gastrointestinal tumors [45]. The reason for this predisposition to posterior fossa might be related to transmission through Batson's plexus.

Routine CE CT-MRI may detect approximately 40–60% of metastases, while increasing contrast dose or taking late-phase images may demonstrate additional metastatic lesions.

16.1.4.3 Deep and Periventricular Enhancement

These deeper subcortical lesions might involve the white matter, basal ganglia, thalamus, or both white and gray matter. Metabolic diseases and toxins mostly affect deep gray matter. Many diseases which disrupt myelin construction primarily affect white matter. And most leukoencephalopathies become destructive during their natural process and cause reduction in white matter volume. These changes may cause increased water signal intensity on MRI and decreased attenuation on CT images.

16.1.5 Deep Ring Enhancing Lesions

Many etiologies of infectious, neoplastic, inflammatory, or vascular origin may cause ring-like CE in the brain. Schwartz and colleagues examined 221 lesions with a ring-style CE and found that 40% were gliomas, 30% metastasis, 8% abscesses, and 6% demyelinating disease [46]. In their study, 45% of metastases and 77% of gliomas were single lesions, whereas 77% of abscesses and 85% of MS lesions were seen as multiple lesions.

Lesions with ring CE accompanied by mass effect and edema in the deep white matter are usually primary brain tumors or abscesses [46]. Metastatic lesions may also show ring CE due to central necrosis. Infectious etiology should be considered in subjects with subacute bacterial endocarditis, permanent catheters, or cardiac valves, that have multiple cortical or subcortical ring contrast-enhancing lesions. These lesions appear to be hypo-isodense in non-contrast CT, but they exhibit homogeneous ring-like CE in the post-contrast images. These lesions, which may vary in size, are usually accompanied by perifocal edema. They are usually located at the junction of the gray-white matter, but they also can be seen in the subcortical area and deep in the brain parenchyma [7].

Abscess Brain abscess is a focal collection of purulence in the brain because of necrosis of infected tissues. It is a life-threatening condition and its diagnosis and treatment are urgent. In the etiology, infections from adjacent structures (mastoiditis, sinusitis, etc.), head trauma or surgical history can be seen. It can also develop due to hematogenous spread of infection from other parts of the body (osteomyelitis, etc.). The clinic can develop in a broad spectrum. Fever and fatigue due to the infectious state; headache, vomiting, and confusion due to increased intracranial pressure; and a variety of neurological symptoms may occur due to focal brain damage.

The abscess first begins as a focal cerebritis and usually has four stages; early cerebritis, late cerebritis, early capsule abscess, and late capsule abscess [47]. Abscess is the final stage of cerebritis resulting in a necrotic cavity which seems as an irregular-shaped rim-enhancing collection debris. At 20–40 min delayed images that gained, central CE on CT and MR suggests cerebritis rather than abscess. Because of its purulent content and liquefaction necrosis, there is no CE in abscess cavity even on the delayed images (Fig. 16.6). There are several explanations about rim T2 hypointensity on MRI. These include collagen and hemosiderin content. Nearly 90% of the abscesses have hypointense rim and 75% of them show steady hypointense rim [46].

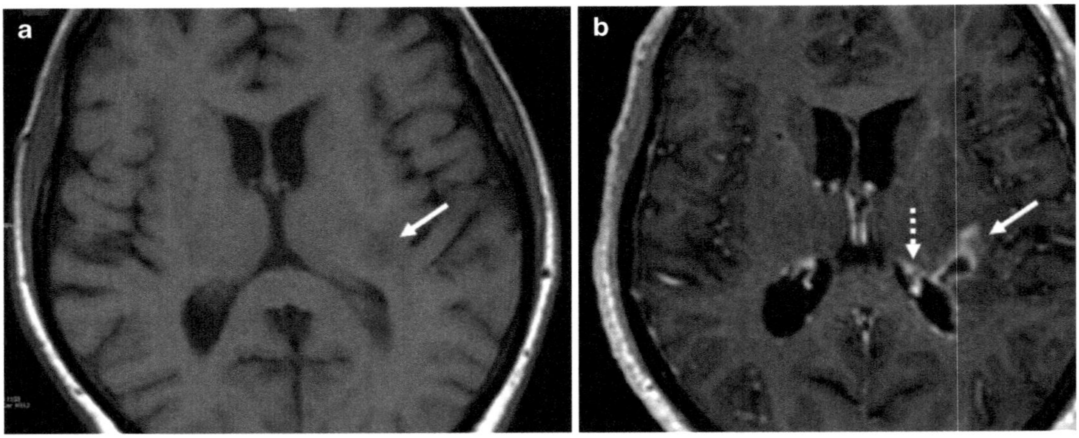

Fig. 16.6 A 39-year-old female with a history of MVR who presented with headache-fever, pre-contrast axial T1W MR image showed an obscure hypointense area with a diameter of approximately 15 mm in the white matter adjacent to the left atrial ventricular atrium (**a**). The post-contrast axial T1W MR image revealed the hypointense central necrosis, a lesion consistent with an abscess (**b**), and diffuse contrast enhancement in the adjacent ventricular wall which represents the extension of inflammation (dashed arrow)

16.1.6 Necrotic High-Grade Primary Neoplasms

Necrotic neoplasms are usually primary or metastatic malignancies. These lesions which are located deeply, especially in the corpus callosum and thalamus, suggest primary astrocytic glial neoplasms. In adults, such lesions are often diffusely infiltrating astrocytomas, with 60% high grade (glioblastoma multiforme). The most common primary malignancy in adults is glioblastoma multiforme (GBM) [48]. Although its appearance is different, the most important pathological feature that differentiates GBM from low-grade astrocytomas is the presence of central necrosis. Beside increased cellularity, atypia, and mitotic activity as other anaplastic astrocytomas, GBM also shows central necrosis, microvascular proliferation and invasion [49]. In GBM, neoplastic cells form an irregular border around the necrotic debris [50, 51]. And this characteristic pathology is fundamental of imaging findings of GBM. MRI shows thick, irregular ring of heterogeneous CE, that surrounds non-enhancing central necrosis and hyperintensity in T2-FLAIR images indicating peritumoral edema (Fig. 16.7) [52, 53].

16.1.7 Ventricular Neoplasms

Several different neoplasms can arise in the ventricular system. These neoplasms may appear from a variety of ventricular structures, including the ependymal lining (ependymoma), subependymal layer (subependymoma), choroid plexus (choroid plexus neoplasms), or they may have a cell of origin that has yet to be determined (chordoid glioma). Central neurocytoma, subependymal giant cell tumor, meningioma, rosette-forming glioneuronal tumor, and metastases are among the other neoplasms infiltrating the ventricular system. Differential diagnosis in intraventricular neoplasms are broad and most of them have similar imaging findings and CE patterns. After contrast administration, ependymomas enhance heterogeneously, subependymomas enhance non-minimal or less often moderately heterogeneous, the central neurocytomas enhance variable but generally mid-strongly, subependymal giant cell tumors and the choroid plexus neoplasms exhibit avidly CE [54]. Subjects may present clinically headache, increased intracranial pressure findings, or focal neurological deficits. In addition, ataxia or paresis may be seen in neoplasms infiltrating the fourth ventricle. The

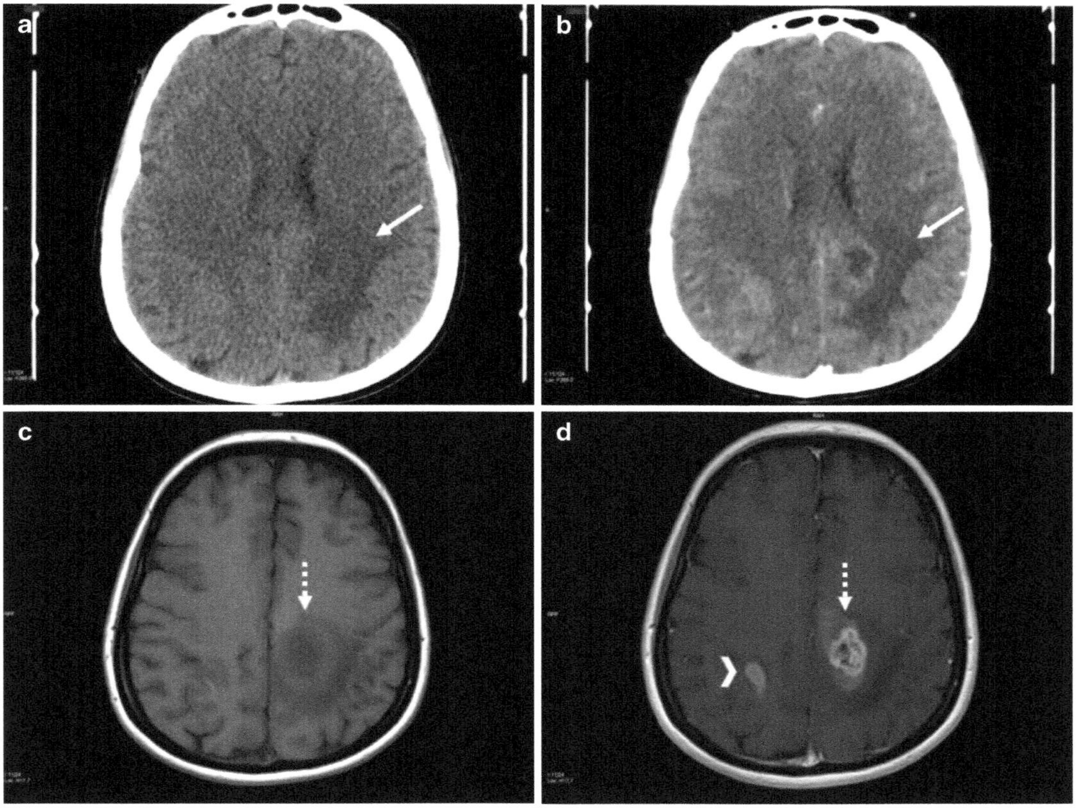

Fig. 16.7 A 57-year-old male presented with right-sided weakness. The unenhanced CT revealed amorphous hypodensity (**a**) in the left posterior fronto-parietal space. In CE-CT, vasogenic edema and environmental CE are suspicious (**b**). The pre-contrast T1W image shows hypo-isointense areas with unclear boundaries (**c**). In the post-contrast T1W image, high-grade glial tumor with heterogeneous and nonuniform enhancing with unenhanced areas compatible with necrosis at the central site and vasogenic edema can be easily selected (**d**). Note the multifocality of the tumor (arrowhead)

age, sex, and history of the subject along with the location of the lesion in the ventricular system are important in terms of differential diagnosis.

16.1.8 Cyst with a Mural Nodule Primary Neoplasms

The well-demarcated appearance is the general characteristic of "cyst within a mural nodule" primary tumors of the brain [55]. Most cysts within a mural nodule tumors display enhancement in the mural nodular part, but some may show a nodule with partial rim enhancement. Familial pilocytic astrocytoma and hemangioblastoma can be given as samples located in the cerebellum. Pilocytic astrocytoma, pleomorphic xanthoastrocytoma, ganglioglioma, and extraventricular ependymoma are the tumors that usually show settlement above the cerebellar tentorium.

16.1.9 Demyelination

Multiple sclerosis (MS) is the most common cause of demyelination which is a chronic immune moderated disorder. In MS, the diagnosis is made by the presence of neurological symptoms with the spread of the lesions over time. Subjects presenting with MS clinic should undergo MRI because almost all of them have abnormal appearance [56] and in more than 80% of subjects with clinically isolated syndrome [57]. MS plaques are hyperintense in T2 and FLAIR examinations. And they show post-contrast enhancement acutely within first 4–6 weeks as a result of perivascular inflammation and impaired BBB (Fig. 16.8) [58].

16.1.10 Deep Lesions: Periventricular Pattern

The frequent causes of periventricular enhancement contain primary CNS lymphoma, primary glial tumors, and infectious ependymitis.

Primary CNS lymphoma constitutes 4–7% of all primary brain tumors but the incidence has increased recently. Although the increase in the incidence of the acquired immunodeficiency syndrome (AIDS) has an impact on this condition, the incidence in subjects with no immune defect has also increased [59]. Primary CNS lymphoma is diffuse large B cell lymphoma in 90% of cases and is often high grade. Less common histological types are Burkitt's lymphoma and T cell lymphoma [60]. Unlike systemic lymphoma, neurological symptoms may occur in the primary CNS lymphoma. In a study performed in 248 subjects with primary CNS lymphoma, focal neurological deficits, seizures, eye, and neuropsychiatric symptoms were observed due to increased intracranial pressure [61]. In another study of 466 subjects, B symptoms such as fever, weight loss, and night sweat were observed in only 8% of the subjects [62]. Primary CNS lymphoma is usually a single and supratentorial lesion. In a study of 100 subjects with no immune deficiency, 38% were found to have the lesion in cerebral hemispheres, followed by basal ganglia and thalamus in 16% of the subjects [63]. Corpus callosum is another site of characteristic involvement [64]. Similar to GBM, the primary lymphoma disseminates throughout the corpus callosum, involve both frontal lobe and corpus callosum genus given the appearance of butterfly pattern (Fig. 16.9). These lesions are larger than the other primary CNS lymphomas [63] The cerebellum and brainstem involvement are less frequent [63–65].

Primary lymphomas are observed as hyperattenuating on non-contrast CT and after

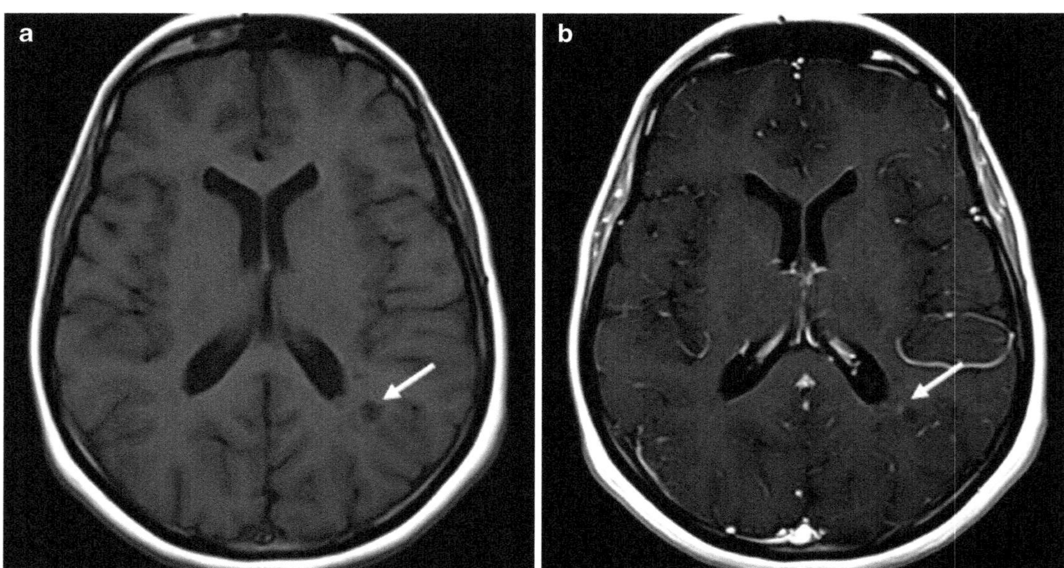

Fig. 16.8 In a subject with diagnosis of MS, T1W pre-contrast image (**a**) shows hypointense lesion, after gadolinium administration post-contrast rim enhancement of the plaque (**b**) indicating active disease

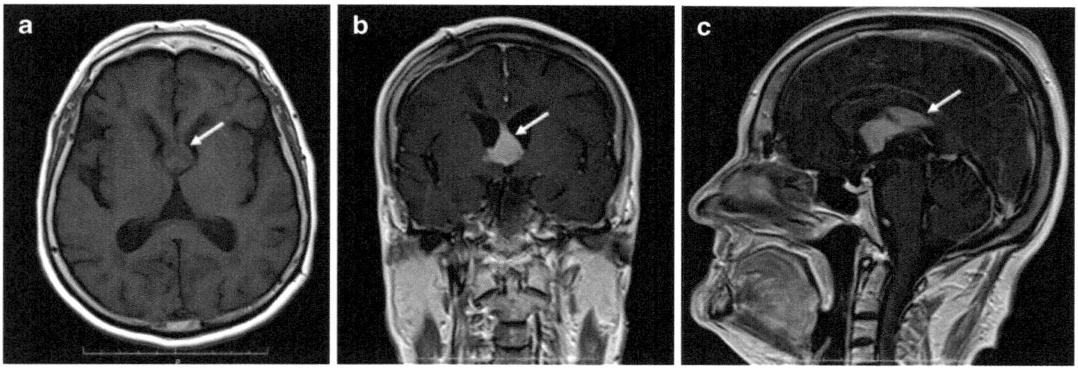

Fig. 16.9 A well-demarcated, 2 cm in diameter lesion localized at the corpus callosum genu can be seen in FLAIR image (**a**). In post-contrast coronal (**b**) and sagittal (**c**) T1W images, a diffuse homogeneous CE is observed. The expansion of the corpus callosum genu is accompanied by a space-occupying lesion consistent with the primary CNS lymphoma that crosses the midline

post-contrast images they show homogenous CE. However, a complete lack of enhancement has been reported [63]. Heterogeneous or ring CE is more common in subjects with AIDS or immune deficiency. CE-MR imaging is the optimal imaging method [66]. Primary CNS lymphomas are hypointense in T1 and also hypointense in T2 compared to gray matter. With this feature, they can be distinguished from T2 hyperintense many primary brain tumors. Because primary CNS lymphoma is rarely seen hyperintense in T2, CE tends to be homogeneous in primary CNS lymphoma.

Thin, linear enhancement along the borders of the ventricles on CT and MR images is typical of infectious ependymitis. Both ependymitis and ventriculitis can also cause thin linear enhancement along the ventricular surface of the corpus callosum. This finding may indicate CMV-induced ventriculitis in subjects with immunodeficiency. Subjects with ventricular shunt catheters may also develop ventriculitis from an ascending infection in the shunt tubing.

References

1. Beckett KR, Moriarity AK, Langer JM. Safe use of contrast media: what the radiologist needs to know. Radiographics. 2015;35(6):1738–50.
2. Lohrke J, Frenzel T, Endrikat J, et al. 25 years of contrast-enhanced MRI: developments, current challenges and future perspectives. Adv Ther. 2016;33(1):1–28.
3. Schoerner W, Kazner E, Laniado M, Sprung C, Felix R. Magnetic resonance tomography (MRT) of intracranial tumours: initial experience with the use of the contrast medium gadolinium-DTPA. Neurosurg Rev. 1984;7(4):303–12.
4. Runge VM, Clanton JA, Price AC, et al. Dyke Award. Evaluation of contrast-enhanced MR imaging in a brain-abscess model. AJNR Am J Neuroradiol. 1985;6(2):139–47.
5. Kirshner HS, Tsai SI, Runge VM, Price AC. Magnetic resonance imaging and other techniques in the diagnosis of multiple sclerosis. Arch Neurol. 1985;42(9):859–63.
6. Young IR, Hall AS, Pallis CA, Legg NJ, Bydder GM, Steiner RE. Nuclear magnetic resonance imaging of the brain in multiple sclerosis. Lancet. 1981;2(8255):1063–6.
7. Smirniotopoulos JG, Murphy FM, Rushing EJ, Rees JH, Schroeder JW. Patterns of contrast enhancement in the brain and meninges. Radiographics. 2007;27(2):525–51.
8. Kanda T, Fukusato T, Matsuda M, et al. Gadolinium-based contrast agent accumulates in the brain even in subjects without severe renal dysfunction: evaluation of autopsy brain specimens with inductively coupled plasma mass spectroscopy. Radiology. 2015;276(1):228–32.
9. Radbruch A, Weberling LD, Kieslich PJ, et al. Gadolinium retention in the dentate nucleus and globus pallidus is dependent on the class of contrast agent. Radiology. 2015;275:783–91.
10. Weberling LD, Kieslich PJ, Kickingereder P, et al. Increased signal intensity in the dentate nucleus on unenhanced T1-weighted images after gadobenate dimeglumine administration. Invest Radiol. 2015;50:743–8.

11. Radbruch A, Haase R, Kieslich PJ, et al. No signal intensity increase in 1the dentate nucleus on unenhanced T1-weighted MR images after more than 20 serial injections of macrocyclic gadolinium-based contrast agents. Radiology. 2017;282:699–707.
12. Arana E, Martí-Bonmatí L, Ricart V, Pérez-Ebrí M. Dural enhancement with primary calvarial lesions. Neuroradiology. 2004;46(11):900–5.
13. Patel N, Kirmi O. Anatomy and imaging of the normal meninges. Semin Ultrasound CT MR. 2009;30(6):559–64.
14. George U, Rathore S, Pandian JD, Singh Y. Diffuse pachymeningeal enhancement and subdural and subarachnoid space opacification on delayed post-contrast fluid-attenuated inversion recovery imaging in spontaneous intracranial hypotension: visualizing the Monro-Kellie hypothesis. Am J Neuroradiol. 2011;32(1):E16.
15. Antony J, Hacking C, Jeffree RL. Pachymeningeal enhancement—a comprehensive review of literature. Neurosurg Rev. 2015;38(4):649–59.
16. Sainani NI, Lawande MA, Pungavkar SA, Desai M, Patkar DP, Mohanty PH. Spontaneous intracranial hypotension: a study of six cases with MR findings and literature review. Australas Radiol. 2006;50(5):419–23.
17. Watanabe A, Horikoshi T, Uchida M, Koizumi H, Yagishita T, Kinouchi H. Diagnostic value of spinal MR imaging in spontaneous intracranial hypotension syndrome. Am J Neuroradiol. 2009;30(1):147–51.
18. Fathi AR, Roelcke U. Meningioma. Curr Neurol Neurosci Rep. 2013;13(4):337.
19. Wiemels J, Wrensch M, Claus EB. Epidemiology and etiology of meningioma. J Neurooncol. 2010;99(3):307–14.
20. Saloner D, Uzelac A, Hetts S, Martin A, Dillon W. Modern meningioma imaging techniques. J Neurooncol. 2010;99(3):333–40.
21. Omay SB, Barnett GH. Surgical navigation for meningioma surgery. J Neurooncol. 2010;99(3):357–64.
22. Baizabal CJF, Barragán-Campos HM, Alonso-Juárez M, et al. Dural metastases as a presentation of a Brenner tumor. J Clin Neurosci. 2010;17(4):524–6.
23. Cheng YK, Wang TC, Yang JT, Lee MH, Su CH. Dural metastasis from prostatic adenocarcinoma mimicking chronic subdural hematoma. J Clin Neurosci. 2009;16(8):1084–6.
24. Blitshteyn S, Mechtler LL, Bakshi R. Diffuse dural gadolinium MRI enhancement associated with bilateral chronic subdural hematomas. Clin Imaging. 2004;28(2):90–2.
25. Rozen TD. Pachymeningeal enhancement on MRI: a venous phenomena not always related to intracranial hypotension resolving pachymeningeal enhancement and cerebral vein thrombosis. Headache. 2013;53(4):673–5.
26. Tian CL, Pu CQ. Dural enhancement detected by magnetic resonance imaging reflecting the underlying causes of cerebral venous sinus thrombosis. Chin Med J (Engl). 2012;125(8):1513–6.
27. Joelson E, Ruthrauff B, Ali F, et al. Multifocal dural enhancement associated with temporal arteritis. Arch Neurol. 2000;57(1):119–22.
28. Sage MR, Wilson AJ, Scroop R. Contrast media and the brain. The basis of CT and MR imaging enhancement. Neuroimaging Clin N Am. 1998;8(3):695–707.
29. Wong J, Douglas JQ. Imaging of central nervous system infections. Semin Roentgenol. 1999;34(2):123–43. WB Saunders.
30. Schaefer PW. Diffusion-weighted imaging as a problem-solving tool in the evaluation of patients with acute strokelike syndromes. Top Magn Reson Imaging. 2000;11(5):300–9.
31. Silverstein AM, Alexander JA. Acute postictal cerebral imaging. Am J Neuroradiol. 1998;19(8):1485–8.
32. Muller JP, Destee A, Lozes G, Pruvo JP, Jomin M, Warot P. Transient cortical contrast enhancement on CT scan in migraine. Headache. 1987;27:578–9.
33. Noguchi T, et al. CT and MRI findings of human herpesvirus 6–associated encephalopathy: comparison with findings of herpes simplex virus encephalitis. Am J Roentgenol. 2010;194(3):754–60.
34. Elster AD, Moody DM. Early cerebral infarction: gadopentetate dimeglumine enhancement. Radiology. 1990;177:627–32.
35. Inoue Y, Takemoto K, Miyamoto T, et al. Sequential computed tomography scans in acute cerebral infarction. Radiology. 1980;135:655–62.
36. Runge VM, Kirsch JE, Wells JW, Dunworth JN, Woolfolk CE. Visualization of blood-brain barrier disruption on MR images of cats with acute cerebral infarction: value of administering a high dose of contrast material. Am J Roentgenol. 1994;162:431–5.
37. Norton GA, Kishore PR, Lin J. CT contrast enhancement in cerebral infarction. Am J Roentgenol. 1978;131:881–5.
38. Silverstein AM, Alexander JA. Acute postictal cerebral imaging. Am J Neuroradiol. 1998;19:1485–8.
39. Barnholtz-Sloan JS, Sloan AE, Davis FG, Vigneau FD, Lai P, Sawaya RE. Incidence proportions of brain metastases in patients diagnosed (1973 to 2001) in the Metropolitan Detroit Cancer Surveillance System. J Clin Oncol. 2004;22(14):2865–72.
40. Fabi A, Felici A, Metro G, et al. Brain metastases from solid tumors: disease outcome according to type of treatment and therapeutic resources of the treating center. J Exp Clin Cancer Res. 2011;30(1):10.
41. Eichler AF, Plotkin SR. Brain metastases. Curr Treat Options Neurol. 2008;10(4):308–14.
42. Young RJ, Sills AK, Brem S, Knopp EA. Neuroimaging of metastatic brain disease. Neurosurgery. 2005;57(Suppl 5):S4–10.
43. Nayak L, Lee EQ, Wen PY. Epidemiology of brain metastases. Curr Oncol Rep. 2012;14(1):48–54.
44. Mongan JP, Fadul CE, Cole BF, et al. Brain metastases from colorectal cancer: risk factors, incidence, and the possible role of chemokines. Clin Colorectal Cancer. 2009;8(2):100–5.

45. Nussbaum ES, Djalilian HR, Cho KH, Hall WA. Brain metastases: histology, multiplicity, surgery, and survival. Cancer. 1996;78(8):1781–8.
46. Schwartz KM, Erickson BJ, Lucchinetti C. Pattern of T2 hypointensity associated with ring-enhancing brain lesions can help to differentiate pathology. Neuroradiology. 2006;48(3):143–9.
47. Rozell JM, Mtui E, Pan YN, Li S. Infectious and inflammatory diseases of the central nervous system—the spectrum of imaging findings and differential diagnosis. Emerg Radiol. 2017;24(6):619–33.
48. Kikuchi K, Hiratsuka Y, Kohno S, Ohue S, Miki H, Mochizuki T. Radiological features of cerebellar glioblastoma. J Neuroradiol. 2016;43(4):260–5.
49. Agnihotri S, Burrell KE, Wolf A, et al. Glioblastoma, a brief review of history, molecular genetics, animal models and novel therapeutic strategies. Arch Immunol Ther Exp. 2013;61(1):25–41.
50. Rees JH, Smirniotopoulos JG, Jones RV, Wong K. Glioblastoma multiforme: radiologic-pathologic correlation. Radiographics. 1996;16(6):1413–38.
51. ElBanan MG, Amer AM, Zinn PO, Colen RR. Imaging genomics of glioblastoma: state of the art bridge between genomics and neuroradiology. Neuroimaging Clin N Am. 2015;25(1):141–53.
52. Zinn PO, Colen RR. Imaging genomic mapping in glioblastoma. Neurosurgery. 2013;60(Suppl 1):126–30.
53. Osborn AG, Salzman KL, Barkovich AJ. Diagnostic imaging: brain. Philadelphia: Amirsys; 2010.
54. Smith AB, Smirniotopoulos JG, Horkanyne-Szakaly I. From the radiologic pathology archives: intraventricular neoplasms: radiologic-pathologic correlation. Radiographics. 2013;33(1):21–43.
55. Raz E, Zagzag D, Saba L, et al. Cyst with a mural nodule tumor of the brain. Cancer Imaging. 2012;12(1):237.
56. Offenbacher H, Fazekas F, Schmidt R, et al. Assessment of MRI criteria for a diagnosis of MS. Neurology. 1993;43(5):905.
57. Fisniku LK, Brex PA, Altmann DR, et al. Disability and T2 MRI lesions: a 20-year follow-up of patients with relapse onset of multiple sclerosis. Brain. 2008;131(3):808–17.
58. Tillema JM, Pirko I. Neuroradiological evaluation of demyelinating disease. Ther Adv Neurol Disord. 2013;6:249–68.
59. Surawicz TS, McCarthy BJ, Kupelian V, Jukich PJ, Bruner JM, Davis FG. Descriptive epidemiology of primary brain and CNS tumors: results from the Central Brain Tumor Registry of the United States, 1990-1994. Neuro Oncol. 1999;1(1):14–25.
60. Miller DC, Hochberg FH, Harris NL, Gruber ML, Louis DN, Cohen H. Pathology with clinical correlations of primary central nervous system non-Hodgkin's lymphoma. The Massachusetts General Hospital experience 1958-1989. Cancer. 1994;74(4):1383–97.
61. Bataille B, Delwail V, Menet E, et al. Primary intracerebral malignant lymphoma: report of 248 cases. J Neurosurg. 2000;92(2):261–6.
62. Hayabuchi N, Shibamoto Y, Onizuka Y, JASTRO CNS Lymphoma Study Group Members. Primary central nervous system lymphoma in Japan: a nationwide survey. Int J Radiat Oncol Biol Phys. 1999;44(2):265–72.
63. Kuker W, Nägele T, Korfel A, et al. Primary central nervous system lymphomas (PCNSL): MRI features at presentation in 100 patients. J Neurooncol. 2005;72(2):169177.
64. Erdag N, Bhorade RM, Alberico RA, Yousuf N, Patel MR. Primary lymphoma of the central nervous system: typical and atypical CT and MR imaging appearances. Am J Roentgenol. 2001;176(5):1319–26.
65. Zhang D, Hu LB, Henning T, et al. MRI findings of primary CNS lymphoma in 26 immunocompetent patients. Korean J Radiol. 2010;11(3):269–77.
66. Batchelor T, Loeffler JS. Primary CNS lymphoma. J Clin Oncol. 2006;24(8):1281–8.

17 Perfusion CT and MR Imaging of the Brain

Emetullah Cindil, Turgut Tali, and Yusuf Oner

Abbreviations

ASL	Arterial spin labeling
BBB	Blood-brain barrier
CBF	Cerebral blood flow
CBV	Cerebral blood volume
CTP	CT perfusion
DCE-MRI	Dynamic contrast-enhanced MRI
DSC-MRI	Dynamic susceptibility contrast MRI
EGFR	Epidermal growth factor receptor
GB	Glioblastoma
HGG	High-grade glioma
IDH	Isocitrate dehydrogenase
Kep	Reverse transfer constant
Ktrans	The volume transfer constant
LGG	Low-grade glioma
MGMT	Methyl-guanine methyltransferase
MTT	Mean transit time
PS	Permeability surface-area product
PSR	Percentage of signal recovery
PW-MRI	Perfusion-weighted magnetic resonance imaging
rCBF	Relative cerebral blood flow
rCBV	Relative CBV
Ve	The volume of extracellular extravascular space
VEGF	Vascular endothelial growth factor
*V*p	Fractional plasma volume

E. Cindil (✉) · T. Tali · Y. Oner
Gazi University, Ankara, Turkey

Highlights

- Perfusion imaging allows to select patients most suitable for thrombolytic or endovascular treatment by differentiation of penumbra from ischemic core.
- In the discrimination of malign solitary intra-axial brain lesions, a perfusion curve in DSC-MRI that does not turn close to the baseline suggests metastasis rather than glioma or lymphoma.
- Differantiation of true tumor progression from treatment effects can be done by using perfusion imaging/rCBV.
- High relative cerebral blood volume may be useful to differentiate residual/recurrent tumor from treatment-related changes.

17.1 Introduction

Since the beginning of the century, brain perfusion imaging has been used with increasing interest. Perfusion imaging techniques provide valuable information about brain physiology, hemodynamics, and microvascular structure of brain lesions. Depending on modality (magnetic resonance imaging [MRI], computed tomography [CT]) and method (arterial spin labeling [ASL], dynamic contrast-enhanced [DCE], dynamic susceptibility [DSC]) used, perfusion parameters indicating different properties of perfusion algo-

S. M. Erturk et al. (eds.), *Medical Imaging Contrast Agents: A Clinical Manual*,
https://doi.org/10.1007/978-3-030-79256-5_17

rithm can be obtained and assessed qualitatively and quantitatively. The blood volume in a particular tissue region and the blood movement over time are the main parameters that are evaluated. Additionally, it is possible to evaluate vascular leakage quantitatively by measuring vascular permeability.

In clinical practice, perfusion imaging is widely used for initial diagnosis and characterization of the tumor, biopsy or surgical navigation, and monitoring and evaluation of treatment response [1]. Today, especially perfusion weighted MRI (PW-MRI) has become indispensable for initial diagnosis and monitoring of brain tumors [2]. By the emerging and development of CT perfusion (CTP) imaging, it has started to be used widely in emergencies, in particular, stroke management [3].

This chapter reviews the technical properties and the clinical applications of brain perfusion imaging.

17.2 Methods

17.2.1 Perfusion Weighted MR Imaging (PW-MRI)

The metrics of PW-MRI can be obtained from gadolinium-based contrast-enhanced and also non-contrast-enhanced (ASL) techniques. Contrast used technics are two types: dynamic contrast-enhanced (DCE)-MRI (T1-weighted) and dynamic susceptibility contrast-enhanced (DSC)-MRI (T2*-weighted) imaging [4, 5]. Although the methods used to measure cerebral perfusion by these techniques are different, both are based on the tracking of contrast material in time [6]. In DCE, the contrast bolus causes T1 shortening in the vascular structure and also in the tissues that have accumulation of contrast agent due to the leakage of vessels. The T1 shortening effect causes an increase in signal, and therefore the technique is called positive contrast permeability technique. In DSC, the contrast bolus causes a signal drop during the initial pass through the vascular structure. For this reason, this technique is called negative contrast blood volume tracking technique.

Both of these contrast-enhanced technics can be used at the same imaging session to enable as a complementary tool about microvascular changes of tissue. DSC-MRI is prone to susceptibility effects mainly caused by calcium, metals, and blood products, while DCE-MRI without these effects can be used in close bone structure neighborhoods and parenchyma-air interfaces [7]. Conversely, DSC-MRI imaging has a better signal-to-noise ratio and needs a more straightforward postprocessing procedure.

Both methods provide several perfusion parameters;

Cerebral blood volume (CBV) derived from DSC and influx transfer constant (Ktrans) derived from DCE which are mostly used [8]. Relative CBV (rCBV) a ratio of pathologic side to the contralateral side is an indicator of microvascular structure and angiogenesis [9]. Ktrans is a microvascular permeability metric, showing the transfer coefficient from plasma to the extravascular extracellular space [9]. Both CBV and Ktrans correlate with molecular markers and histopathological changes of vascular endothelial growth factor (VEGF) [10]. Besides, several studies revealed that rCBV is correlated with tumor grading and molecular markers indicating high-grade tumors [11, 12].

ASL is a relatively new technique and does not require contrast material. Perfusion imaging data is obtained using labeled inflowing arterial blood water protons at the proximal segment of the imaging area. Cerebral blood flow (CBF) maps provide quantitative measurement in a wide range of clinical conditions. ASL enables quick imaging of the whole brain parenchyma and needs little postprocessing procedure in nearly all software of manufacturers.

PW-MRI has some advantages over CTP imaging. Primarily, PW-MRI does not require ionizing radiation, which is crucial for particularly oncologic patients because these patients may require repeat imaging with short intervals for tumor surveillance. MRI is a standard imaging tool to assess treatment response or disease progression, especially in neuro-oncological imaging. The perfusion parameters obtained by PW-MRI require the inclusion of additional sequences instead of a completely separate examination as in CTP, which is another advantage.

17.2.1.1 Dynamic Contrast Enhanced-T1 MR Imaging (DCE-MRI)

DCE-MRI is technically dependent on an increase in contrast agent concentration, which shows a proportional increase in T1 relaxation rate. DCE-MRI allows to characterize the microvascular changes by the help of quantitative (model-dependent) parameters derived from various pharmacokinetic models (commonly used classic Tofts-Kermode model), including Ktrans (influx transfer constant), Kep (reverse transfer constant), Ve (volume of extracellular extravascular space), and Vp (blood plasma volume) [13]. Ktrans refers to the volume transfer coefficient from plasma to extracellular extravascular space and is the main parameter of permeability. It also indicates blood flow depending on the degree of permeability (Fig. 17.1). An increase in Ktrans shows the increase in capillary permeability and disruption of blood-brain barrier (BBB), particularly in high-grade gliomas and used to differentiate from low-grade gliomas [14, 15]. Kep refers to the volume transfer coefficient from extracellular extravascular space to plasma, a wash-out parameter, and has also been found correlated with glioma grading, tumor recurrence [16, 17]. Similar to Ktrans, elevated Ve, elevated fractional volume of the extravascular extracellular space is indicative of a wider BBB disruption and higher tumoral grade.

DCE has some advantages compared to DSC imaging, such as a smaller dose of contrast agent and better temporal resolution. But, in contrast to DSC-MRI, DCE has not been extensively studied in the diagnosis and grading of tumors and the differentiation of true progression from pseudoprogression. However, it has been reported that it can differentiate recurrent/residual tumor from treatment response using the maximum slope of initial enhancement [18]. Both absolute and normalized values of maximum slope of initial enhancement in progressive and recurrent tumors show significantly higher values than those in treatment-related necrosis [18].

The clinical use of quantitative metrics of DCE-MRI is usually limited to the complex, multi-compartmental physiological models needed to achieve quantitative measurements. To increase clinical benefit, semi-quantitative metrics (model-free) were developed to evaluate tissue perfusion. This method is easy to apply without fitting complicated pharmacokinetic models and semi-quantitative parameters derived from signal intensity-acquisition time curve. On the other hand, lower temporal resolution and limited knowledge of lesion vascular pathophysi-

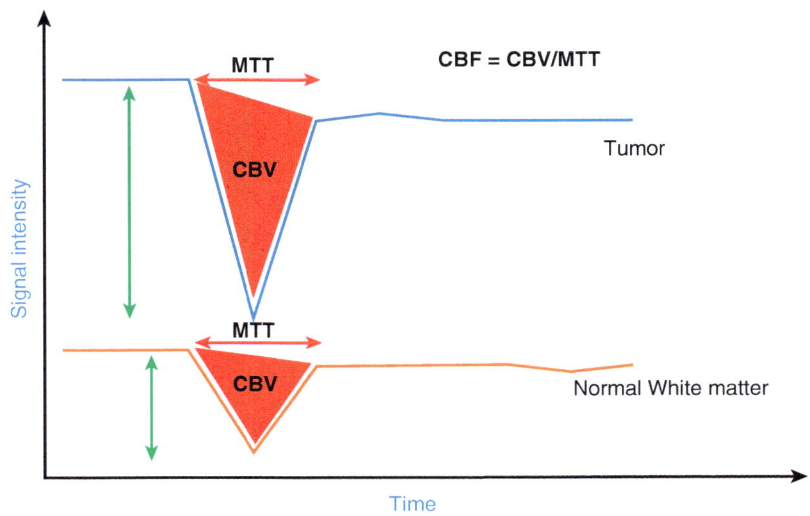

Fig. 17.1 Primary central nervous system lymphoma in the splenium of corpus callosum. Ktrans map shows remarkable increase in Ktrans value (mean value = 0.654 min^{-1})

ology are the main limitations [19]. The initial and wash-out phase of contrast distribution has been evaluating to provide objective indices by the help of signal intensity-time curve which provides a slope of wash-in, wash-out slopes and also the initial area under the time–intensity curve (IAUC).

Technical issues

- It is recommended to include whole brain with maximum field of view with no gap.
- To obtain baseline T1 signal, several non-contrast series should be obtained initially.

17.2.1.2 Dynamic Susceptibility Contrast Enhanced T2* Imaging (DSC-MRI)

DSC-MR imaging is the most used perfusion technique in clinical practice [4–6, 8, 20, 21]. The technique uses T2* susceptibility-weighted imaging with the help of the initial pass effect of contrast material through tissue to constitute a signal intensity-time curve and a postcontrast time-concentration curve. Once the contrast material reaches the tissue, there is an abrupt drop in signal intensity due to the shortening effect of T2 *, but over time signal intensity recovers as the contrast material disperses within the tissue [4–6, 8, 20, 21].

Since the first-pass effect of the contrast agent for DSC-MRI is very short, rapid imaging techniques such as echo-planar imaging (EPI) should be used to accurately characterize the decrease in signal intensity [20]. Gradient echo (GRE) techniques also are preferred over spin echo techniques due to the sensitivity to wider range of vessel size [6]. However, susceptibility artifacts, particularly due to the close neighborhood of bone and air or blood contents of tumors, are main disadvantages of these sequences. DSC-MRI is also vulnerable to errors associated with contrast leakage from disrupted BBB, especially in high-grade hypervascularized tumors or meningiomas. Low molecular weight extravascular contrast materials make this effect even more prominent by causing a rapid contrast extravasation from the vascular compartment to the interstitium. Consequently, the leakage produces a strong T1 relaxation effect (T1 shine-through effect) [22] and increasing or decreasing of T2* effect, which may result in misestimation of rCBV. Several methods, such as pre-bolus contrast material administration, baseline correction, and gamma-variate fitting, are being used to decrease T1 contamination [5, 7, 23].

Perfusion parameters derived from DSC-MR are CBF, CBV, and mean transit time (MTT). CBV is the most widely used parameter and is calculated using the area under the time-concentration curve (Fig. 17.2), CBV indicates the amount of blood in a particular tissue region over a given period of time, and usually defined in milliliter per 100 g of tissue. CBF calculation is more complex and is obtained by dividing CBV by MTT. MTT is defined as the average time to pass through the interested tissue and calculated in seconds. CBF is expressed in milliliters of blood per 100 g in 1 min. In addition, another time-dependent parameter map, time to

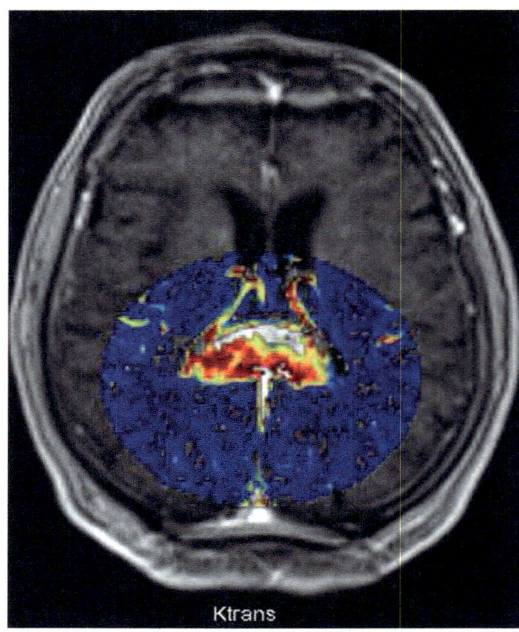

Fig. 17.2 Signal intensity-time curve illustration of normal white matter and tumor. Red colored triangular shapes indicate CBV for both regions. CBV is significantly higher in tumor area than that in normal white matter. Signal drop at initial phase (green lines) is related to vascularity. Higher vascularity shows higher signal drop

peak (TTP), can be measured for the detection of abnormal signals in the tissue. Because the use of absolute quantities is not optimal due to the nonlinear relationship between signal change and gadolinium contrast, in daily practice the relative values of these parameters (ratio of pathologic tissue value to the contralateral normal tissue value; rCBV, rCBF, rMTT) are used. On signal intensity-time curve, the amount of signal decrease is correlated tissue vascularity. Highly vascular lesions such as glioblastomas (GBs), metastasis, or meningiomas show more signal loss than low-grade gliomas and normal white matter. Accordingly, increased CBV is a marker of higher tumor aggressiveness due to increased neoangiogenesis. On the other hand, the amount of signal recovery (percentage signal recovery [PSR]) depends on whether the blood-brain barrier is intact or disrupted. In metastasis, signal recovery is lower than those in lymphoma and glioblastoma due to the disruption of BBB.

Technical Issues

- Perfusion imaging is performed during the injection of contrast material via an automatic injector at a minimum rate of 4 mL/s.

17.2.1.3 Arterial Spin Labeling (ASL)

ASL perfusion technique uses the tagging or labeling of arterial blood as an endogen tracer. After this labeling procedure, a so-called labeling delay is required to allow time for the labeled blood to reach the targeted tissue. For ASL imaging, both labeled and unlabeled images are taken and subtracted. The signal obtained from the subtraction of the labeled images from unlabeled images is used to generate the CBF maps. Labeling arterial water varied in methodology, and take these names according to these methods; continuous ASL, pseuducontinuous ASL, pulsed ASL, and velocity selective [24]. A long-term RF pulse in continuous ASL (CASL). Continually tags arterial blood water at a specific proximal segment of the imaging area [4]. CASL has higher perfusion sensitivity than the other. But, prolonged RF may cause higher energy accumulation and lead to magnetization transfer effect, which cause overestimation of perfusion [24]. Conversely, Pulsed ASL uses a single short RF pulse to tag the vessel [24]. Although PASL shows better labeling performance with single RF pulse, perfusion sensitivity is lower compared to CASL.

After arterial blood labeling, ASL is obtained using fast EPI techniques, similar to DSC-MRI imaging. Again, similar to DSC-MRI, EPI sequences are prone to susceptibility artifacts caused by close neighboring bone, and air or blood contents of lesion.

As an easily applicable technique, ASL has some advantages compared with other perfusion imaging methods. Similiarly with other MR perfusion techniques, ASL does not require radiation. The most important advantage is that, unlike other MR and CT perfusion methods, ASL does not require an exogenous tracer to generate perfusion imaging which is beneficial for patients with renal failure.

In recent years, increased number of studies have reported the diagnostic value in the diagnosis of high-grade gliomas, metastases, and meningiomas due to increased CBFs [25–29].

The authors found that ASL is a very useful and easy-to-use technique with several advantages compared to other perfusion techniques.

Technical Issues

- After the labeling procedure, a delay time is required for the labeled blood to reach the targeted tissue.

17.2.2 CT Perfusion (CTP) Imaging

CTP is based on the principle of the transit of iodinated contrast material through brain parenchyma. The main purpose is to evaluate the distribution of the contrast agent in tissue over time. This technique requires the acquisition of multiple series in short intervals after intravenous injection of contrast agent. CTP enables both CBV, CBF, MTT, and also permeability (permeability surface [PS]) to be evaluated in a single scan. Direct measurement of quantitative parameters helps in interpretation of CTP. CTP protocols vary depending on the cause of the examination, such as brain tumor or ischemia.

Technical Issues

- Hemorrhage should be ruled out with low-dose radiation non-contrast CT prior to perfusion screening.
- Perfusion maps are obtained by the use of a number of commercially available software applications. An input artery is used to obtain the time-attenuation curve to determine the arterial input function, and venous sinus, usually superior sagittal sinus, is used to determine the venous output [30].

17.3 Clinical Applications

17.3.1 Neuro-oncologic Imaging

In recent years, increasing interest and published articles focused on cranial neoplasms revealed that the perfusion imaging of brain has an important role in differentiation of tumor subgroups (lymphoma, metastasis, glial tumors, e.g.), glial tumor grading, discrimination of benign and malign tumors. The relationship between neoangiogenesis and tumor aggressiveness has been demonstrated by both CT and MR perfusion methods. Increased permeability and CBV are related to higher grade tumors [12, 31]. DSC-MRI can also be helpful in brain tumor monitoring and evaluation of response to therapy.

17.3.1.1 Tumor Grading

The main method in grading tumors is the histopathological evaluation of the tissue which is based on the World Health Organization grading system. However, grading systems based on histopathology and molecular imaging are confronted with several limitations, in particular sampling error and interobserver variation. Furthermore, the biopsy material may not fully represent the tumor characteristics due to inappropriate resection and tumoral heterogeneity, which can lead to incorrect grading and classifications especially for high-grade gliomas (HGG) [30]. If surgical removal of the lesion is not necessary or if it is located in a critical area that cannot be surgically removed, it is very important to make a definitive diagnosis without a biopsy. Conventional MRI is limited for glioma grading. Approximately 45% of non-enhanced gliomas are malignant and approximately 20% of the enhanced oligodendrogliomas (ODG) are benign [32, 33]. MR PWI and CT PWI have been successfully used in grading of gliomas and targeted biopsy.

Tumor vessels in low-grade gliomas (LGGs) are constituted of normal endothelial cells with a relatively intact BBB [34]. Malignant gliomas have aberrant neovascularization consist of disorganized, irregular, large caliber vascular structure with immature endothelial cells, and disrupted BBB [35]. This abnormal vascular structure results in increasing permeability and perfusion in malignant gliomas. Many researchers have shown that increased rCBV is related to increased angiogenesis and higher tumor grades and is a potential noninvasive biomarker in assessing tumor grade [12]. Using a threshold value of 1.75 for rCBV, Law et al. achieved to distinguish low- and high-grade gliomas with 95% sensitivity and 57.5% specificity [12].

rCBV correlates is the most reliable hemodynamic parameter in overall MR PWI parameters. Studies based on CT PWI also revealed a good diagnostic performance in the differentiation of low-grade tumors from high-grade tumors (Fig. 17.3). Ellika et al. reported that a threshold of 1.92 for rCBV derived from CT PWI showed 85.7% sensitivity and 100% specificity in distinguishing between low- and high-grade gliomas [36]. For ODG, this approach could be challenging due to the ODGs can also have high rCBV values [5, 37, 38].

Tumor grade is also reported to correlate with Ktrans which represents the larger extension of BBB disruption, but the correlation value is lower compared to the value of rCBV [15, 31, 39]. PSR derived from signal intensity-time curve is negatively correlated with vascular permeability and tumor grade. In other words, lower PSR represents higher vascular permeability and higher tumor grade [40, 41].

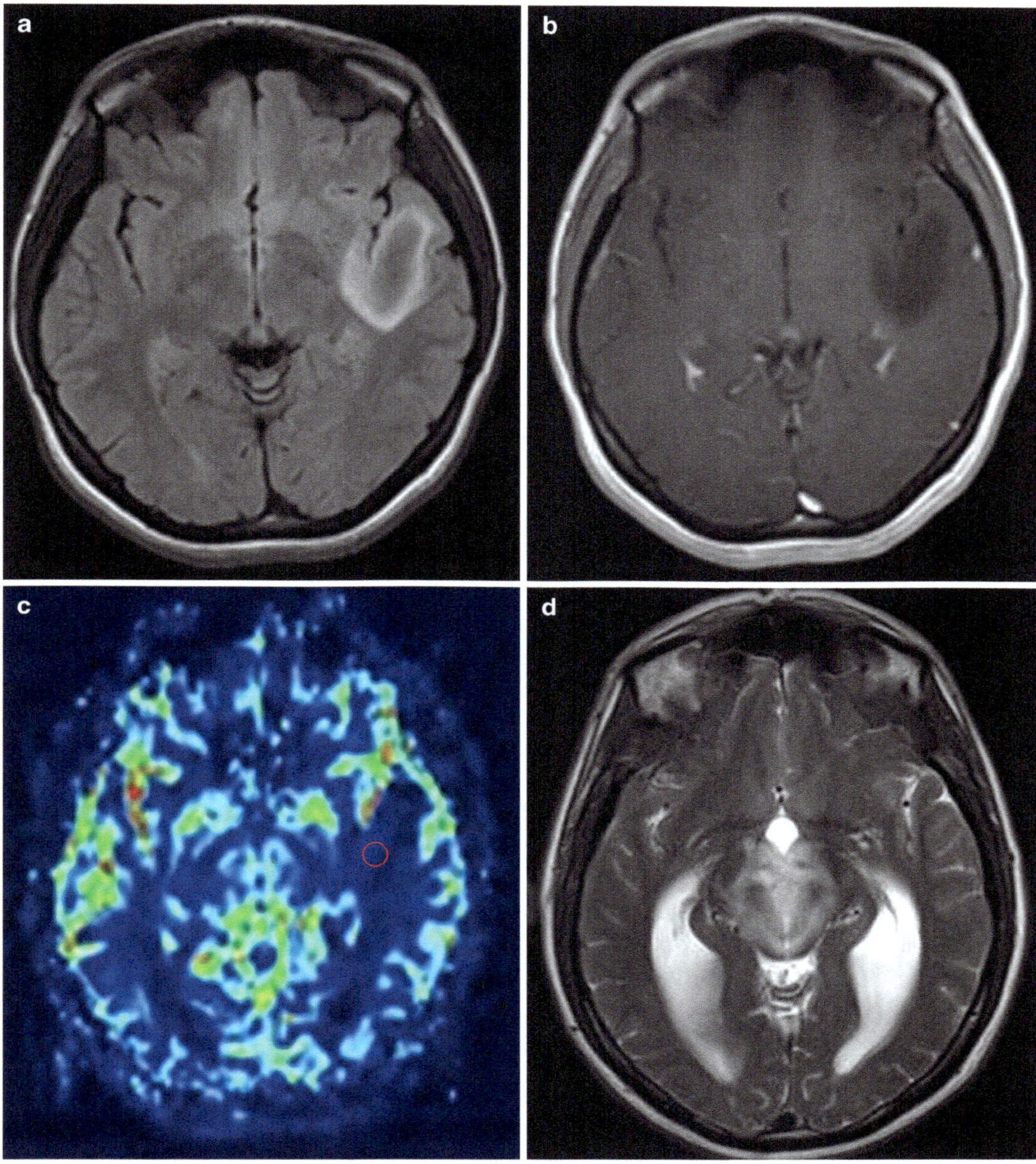

Fig. 17.3 Axial FLAIR (**a**), axial T1 postcontrast (**b**), DSC perfusion cerebral blood volume map (**c**) of diffuse astrocytoma in left temporal lobe. Axial FLAIR (**d**), axial T1 postcontrast (**e**), DSC perfusion cerebral blood volume map (**f**) of anaplastic astrocytoma in talamomesancephalic region. Axial FLAIR (**g**), axial T1 postcontrast (**h**), DSC perfusion cerebral blood volume map (**i**) of glioblastoma in left frontal lobe. Anaplastic astrocytoma (**f**) and glioblastoma (**i**) demonstrate high perfusion on cerebral blood volume map, while no increase was observed for diffuse astrocytoma (**c**)

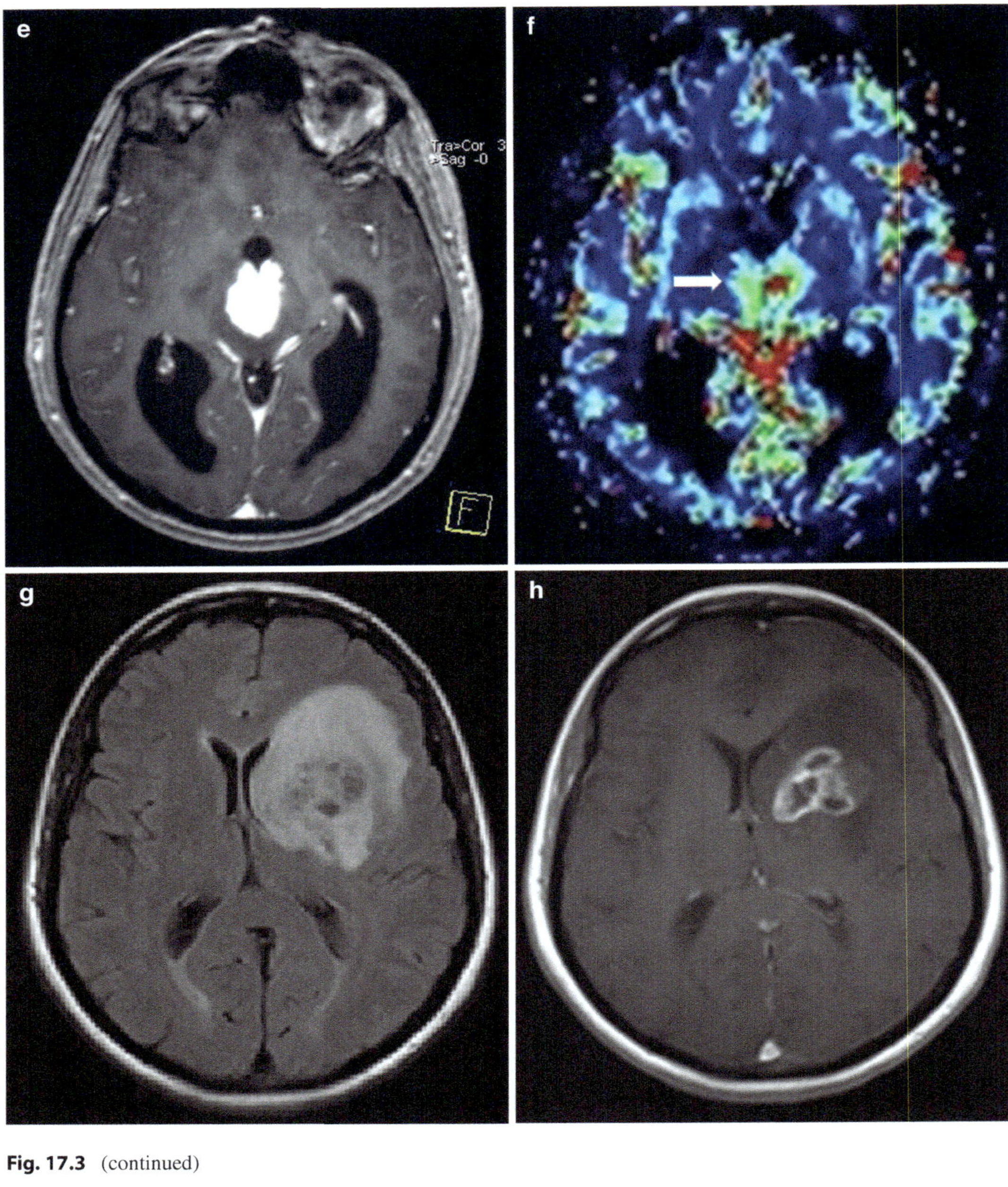

Fig. 17.3 (continued)

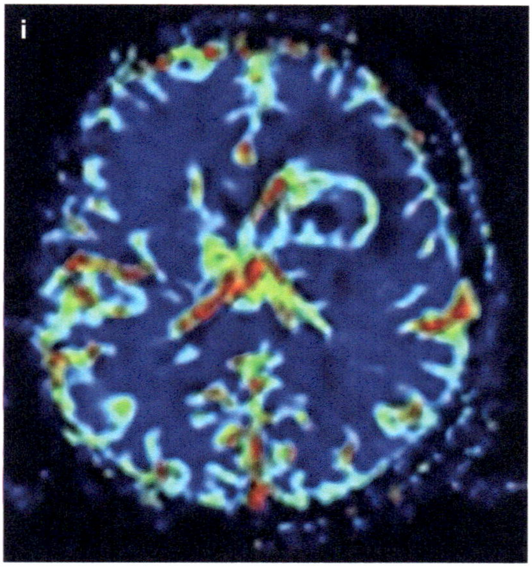

Fig. 17.3 (continued)

Low-grade gliomas can continue to differentiate through malignant transformation. This differentiation time can be shown in rCBV maps before they occur in conventional MR imaging. "Angiogenic switch" refers to the time when a low-grade tumor becomes angiogenic and shows malignant transformation [35, 42]. The angiogenic switch may be determined in perfusion imaging by an increase in rCBV 12 months prior to the appearance of contrast enhancement in T1-weighted images [43].

17.3.1.2 Molecular/Genetic Characteristics

2016 update of WHO classification of brain tumors integrates molecular/genetic criteria with histological diagnosis [44]. Molecular classification for gliomas encompasses various molecular and genetic markers, such as isocitrate dehydrogenase (IDH) gene mutation, methyl-guanine methyltransferase (MGMT) promoter methylation status, chromosome 1p/19q codeletion, and epidermal growth factor receptor (EGFR) status. Identification of these molecular/genetic properties before surgery can be very useful in differential diagnosis, treatment planning, and monitoring. Recent studies have focused on the discrimination ability of perfusion MRI in the setting of genotypic characteristics of gliomas [45].

IDH mutation is present approximately in 50–80% of grade II–III gliomas and nearly in all secondary GBs. In general, IDH-1 mutations are much more seen than IDH-2 mutation [46, 47]. Patients with IDH-1 gene mutation have a better prognosis than those with wild type gliomas, which indicates IDH-1 mutations can be accepted as an independent prognostic factor [46, 48]. The detection of IDH gene mutations by noninvasive methods is very useful in the management of treatment in gliomas. Several studies revealed that the rCBV has the potential to predict IDH mutation status in all grades of astrocytoma [49–52]. Wild type gliomas have much more neoangiogenesis with a less heterogeneous microenvironment. rCBV may be a reliable imaging marker to predict the IDH mutation status [53]. On the other hand, DCE-MRI-derived Ktrans also showed significant differences between IDH-mutated and IDH-wild type high-grade gliomas. IDH-wild type tumors have higher Ktrans values than IDH-mutant types [39].

GBs with EGFRvIII mutation have poor prognosis [54]. EGFR has been considered to be a potential target for immune therapy [55]. The establishment of reliable imaging biomarkers is important in determining EGFR status of gliomas to assist in treatment plan [54]. The publications suggest that tumor angiogenesis characterized by increased perfusion and permeability may reflect EGFR status [56]. Gupta et al. [57] reported that GB with EGFR amplification positive showed higher rCBV and lower PSR values in preoperative DSC-MRI measurements. Another study with DCE-MRI reported that Ktrans and Vp values in EGFRvIII-positive GBs were significantly higher than negative group. The predictive power of Vp has been reported as better than that of Ktrans [58].

MGMT is a DNA repair enzyme in glioma cells. MGMT methylation may inhibit the functioning of this gene and cause DNA damage [59]. Patients with MGMT methylation have better prognosis and long-term survival [60], better responding to temozolomide chemotherapy

[61], and increased pseudoprogression formation [62]. Biopsy procedures today often show inadequate biopsy due to tumor heterogeneity [63]. Noninvasive prediction of MGMT methylation by imaging methods is very important. Several studies have been studied on perfusion parameters as a noninvasive tool to predict MGMT methylation in GB. Lower rCBV values were found with 73.3% sensitivity and 85.7% specificity for MGMT methylation in GB [64]. In another study, Ahn et al. [65] indicated that only Ktrans was associated with the MGMT methylation status in GB. Interestingly, GB with MGMT methylation showed higher Ktrans indicating that MGMT methylation may have an impact on the angiogenesis of glioma characterized by vascular structures with high endothelial permeability. Larger studies are needed to clarify the relationship between imaging characteristics and MGMT status.

17.3.1.3 Differentiation of Solitary Brain Tumors

Perfusion MRI has been shown as an effective tool in the characterization and differentiation of solitary brain lesions. It is very important to determine the histologic features of a lesion, to guide treatment plans and to determine the prognosis. High-grade glioma, primary central nervous system lymphoma (PCNSL), and solitary brain metastasis have similar imaging characteristics on conventional MRI, and the differential diagnosis is difficult with this method alone. Advanced MRI techniques may add physiological information that was not previously found in the evaluation of brain lesions. Perfusion parameters indicating microvascular changes can be used to facilitate diagnosis and differentiation of brain tumors (Table 17.1) [11, 31, 67].

Perfusion imaging can be used in discrimination between HGG and PCNSL. PCNSL is known to show markedly impaired vascular integrity and less neovascularization, and therefore low blood perfusion and increased vascular permeability in comparison with other tumors [68, 69].

GBs have high rCBV values while lymphoma does not show a significant increase in perfusion (Fig. 17.4). And also lower PSR is suggestive of GB (Fig. 17.4) [66, 70]. Despite similar findings, cut-off values of rCBV and PSR vary between the studies [66, 69, 71]. The difference between imaging protocols can cause this variability.

Perfusion imaging may also help in the differentiation of GB from solitary metastasis where other sequences are limited. Perfusion imaging has been used on the basis of the fact that microstructure of tumor capillaries varies greatly between glioma and brain metastasis [72]. Metastasis generally has no disruption of BBB in contrast to GBs, which causes relatively lower rCBV but increased more capillary permeability throughout the tumor [73]. Besides, vasogenic edema around metastasis has no infiltrative tumor cells or angiogenesis [74, 75]. Metastasis's signal intensity curve does not return close to baseline due to the leakage of contrast material within leaky capillaries in contrast to gliomas whose signal intensity curve comes to close after

Table 17.1 CBV and Ktrans parameters changes in common cranial tumors

	CBV	Ktrans
PCNSL	Not increased or minimal	↑↑ (severe vascular leakage)
Metastasis	↑↑	↑↑ (absence of BBB component)
High-grade glioma	↑↑	↑ (disruption of BBB)
Low-grade glioma	Not increased	Not increased
Radiation necrosis	↓	↓
Meningioma	↑↑	↑↑
Ependymoma	↑↑	↑↑
Medulloblastoma	↑↑	↑↑
Hemangioblastoma	↑	↑

CBV cerebral blood volume, *Ktrans* volüme transfer constant, *BBB* blood-brain barrier, *PCNSL* primary cranial nervous system lymphoma

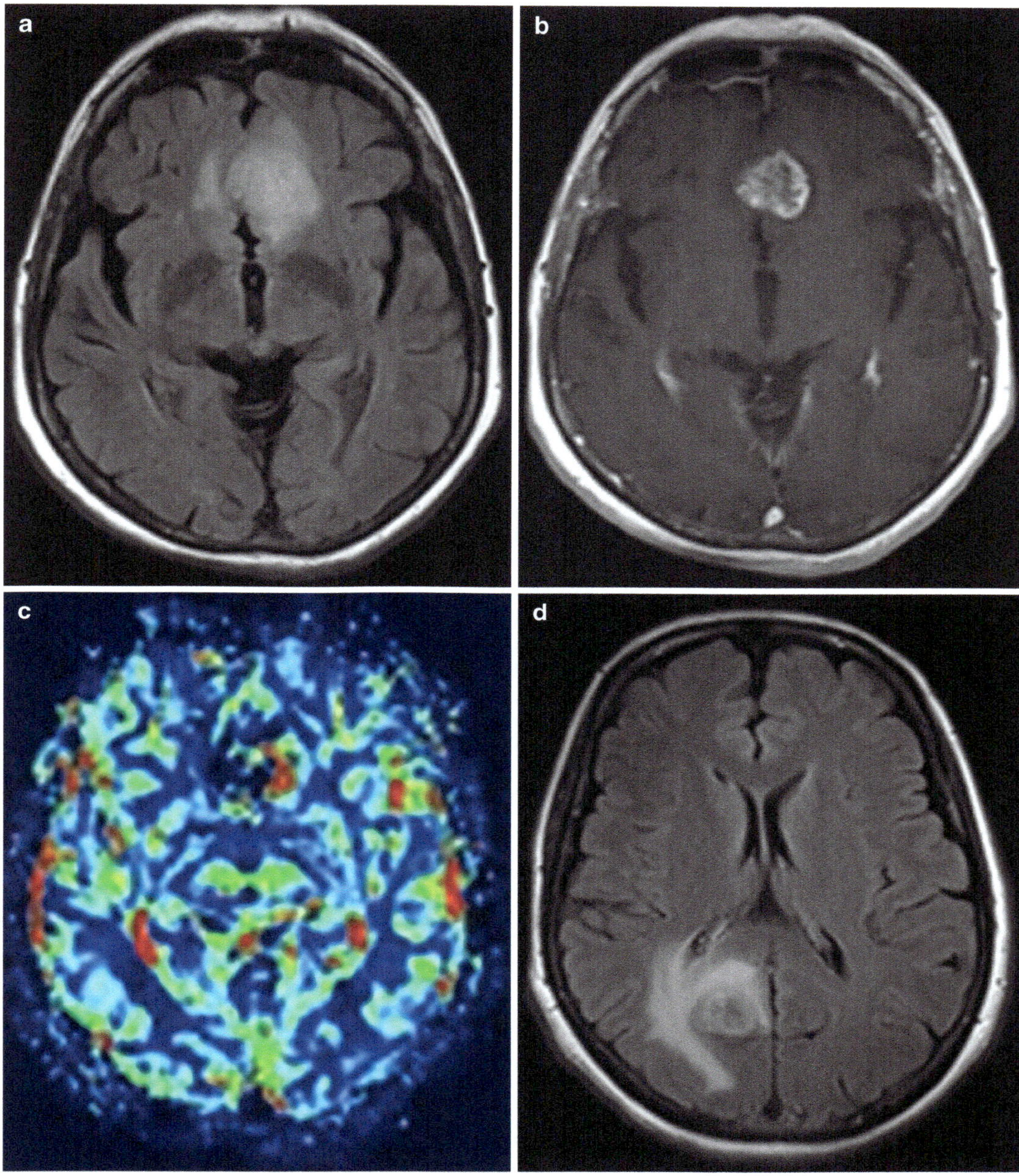

Fig. 17.4 Axial FLAIR (**a**), axial T1 postcontrast (**b**), DSC perfusion cerebral blood volume map (**c**) of glioblastoma in left temporal lobe. Axial FLAIR (**d**), axial T1 postcontrast (**e**), DSC perfusion cerebral blood volume map (**f**) of breast carcinoma metastasis in parietooccipital region. Axial T2 (**g**), axial T1 postcontrast (**h**), DSC perfusion cerebral blood volume map (**i**) of lymphoma in corpus callosum and neighboring bifrontal area. Glioblastoma (**c**) and metastasis (**f**) showed an increase in relative cerebral volume, while no increase was observed in lymphoma (**i**). Illustrations of signal intensity-time curves of dynamic susceptibility contrast MR represent significant differences in percentage signal recovery (**j**). In metastasis (gray curve), the curve does not return close to baseline due to leaky capillaries in contrast to the one in glioblastoma (blue curve). On the other hand, the signal recovery showed higher values for lymphoma (orange curve) in contrary to the others

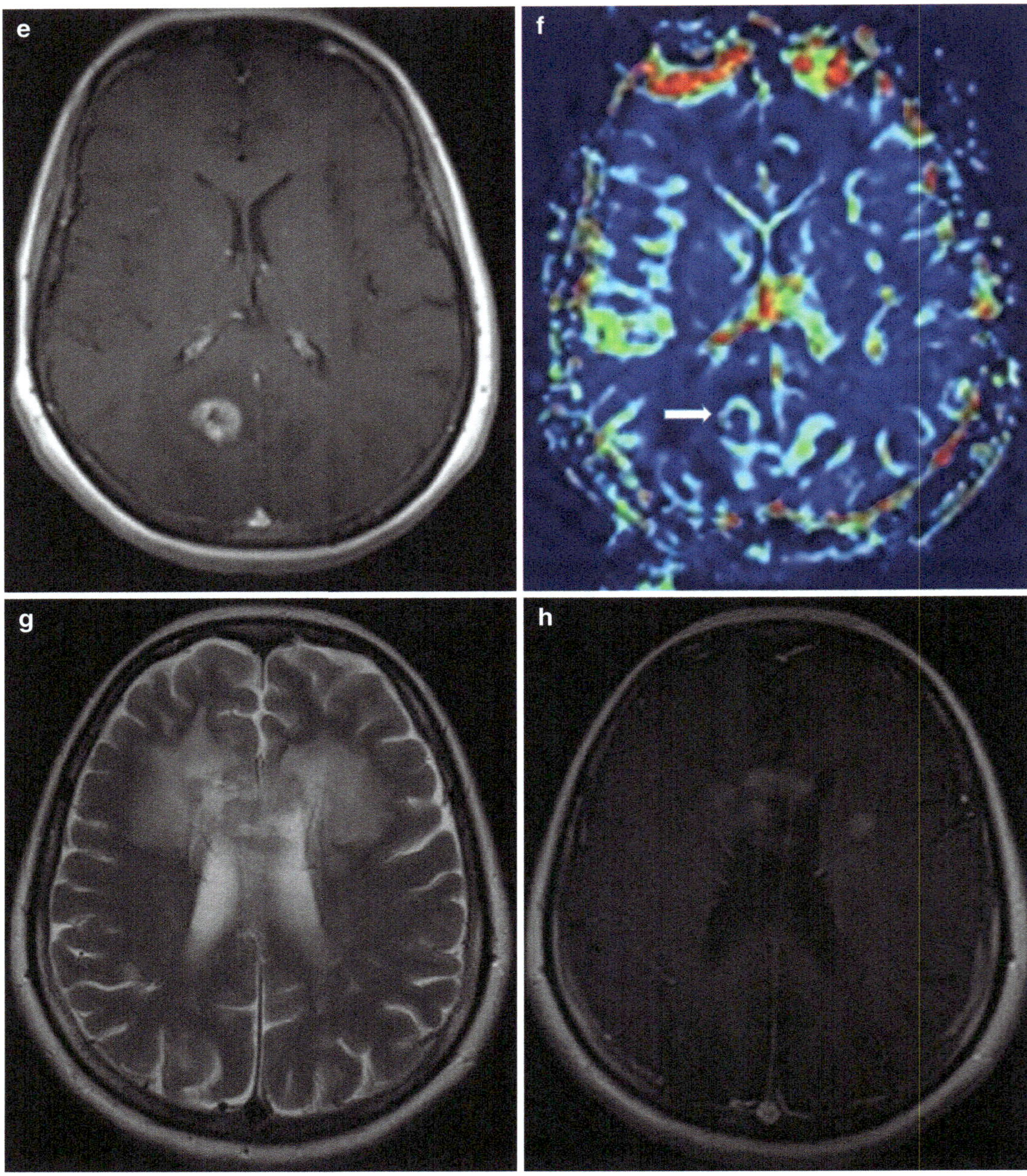

Fig. 17.4 (continued)

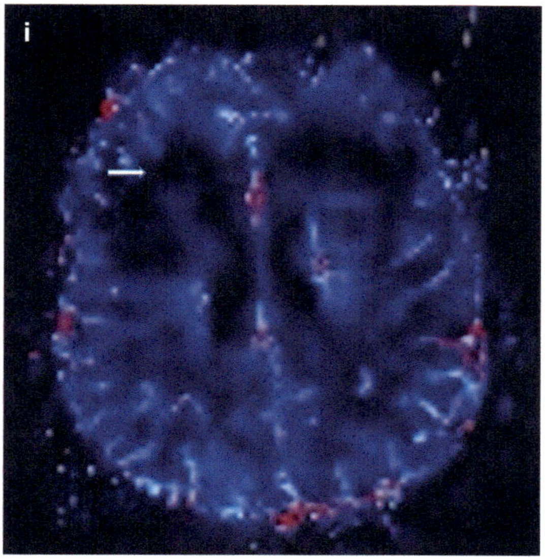

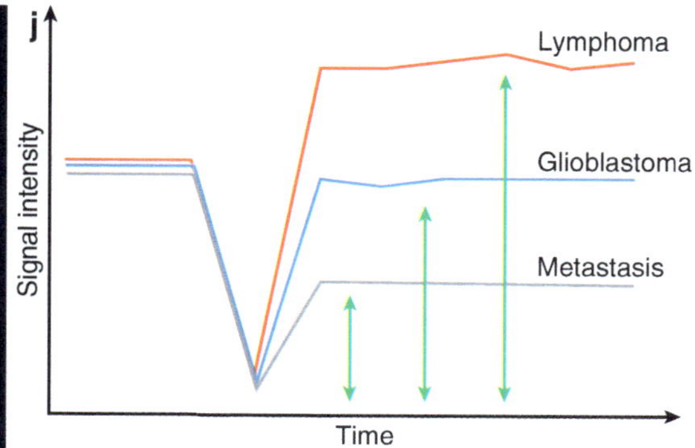

Fig. 17.4 (continued)

a while of contrast administration (Fig. 17.4). Statistically significant differences were reported between values of PSR between metastasis and glioma. It has been reported that rCBV is further increased in the infiltrating peritumoral edema of high-grade gliomas compared to the vasogenic edema surrounding the metastasis. Compared with metastasis, higher rCBV and higher PSR were present in the peritumoral region of HGG [71, 73, 76–80]. On the other hand, DSC-MRI is not sufficient in differentiating high vascular brain metastasis, such as melanoma metastasis from HGG, due to similar vascular features. Studies based on Ktrans value derived from DCE-MRI showed significant overlaps between lymphoma, metastasis, and high-grade gliomas (Fig. 17.4) [81].

Ependymomas and medulloblastomas can have increased rCBV and Ktrans values (Fig. 17.5). Evaluation of the PSRs may be useful in differentiation. Ependymoma shows a poor return to the baseline in PSR curve due to fenestrated blood vessels and focal deficits in the BBB [82].

Although hemangioblastoma (HB) and pilocytic astrocytoma (PA) have similar imaging findings in conventional MRI, perfusion imaging can be used in differentiation. PA showed high rCBV and permeability values, but HB has higher rCBV values when compared. Meningioma and choroid plexus tumors show increased rCBV values due to highly leaky capillaries (Fig. 17.6) [5, 83, 84].

17.3.1.4 Differentiating Primary Gliomas from Tumefactive Demyelinating Lesions

Perfusion imaging is useful in differentiating brain tumors from tumefactive active demyelinating plaques. Tumefactive demyelinating lesions (TDL) with a larger size, accompanying perilesional edema, and mass effect with atypical enhancement, particularly ring-shaped enhancement, can be challenging in differentiation from tumoral lesions [85]. These imaging findings are frequently seen in glial tumors, often in glioblastoma, and in some cases, a biopsy is required for diagnosis. On the other hand, some studies revealed that tumefactive demyelinating lesions could mimic gliomas on pathologic examinations [86]. Differences in vascularity on perfusion imaging can lead to differentiate these entities. High-grade gliomas show increased perfusion dynamics due to neoangiogenesis. TDLs contain inflammatory vessels that show mild to moderate angiogenesis, and thus resulting in lower permeability surface and CBV values compared to high-grade gliomas on CTP imaging [4,

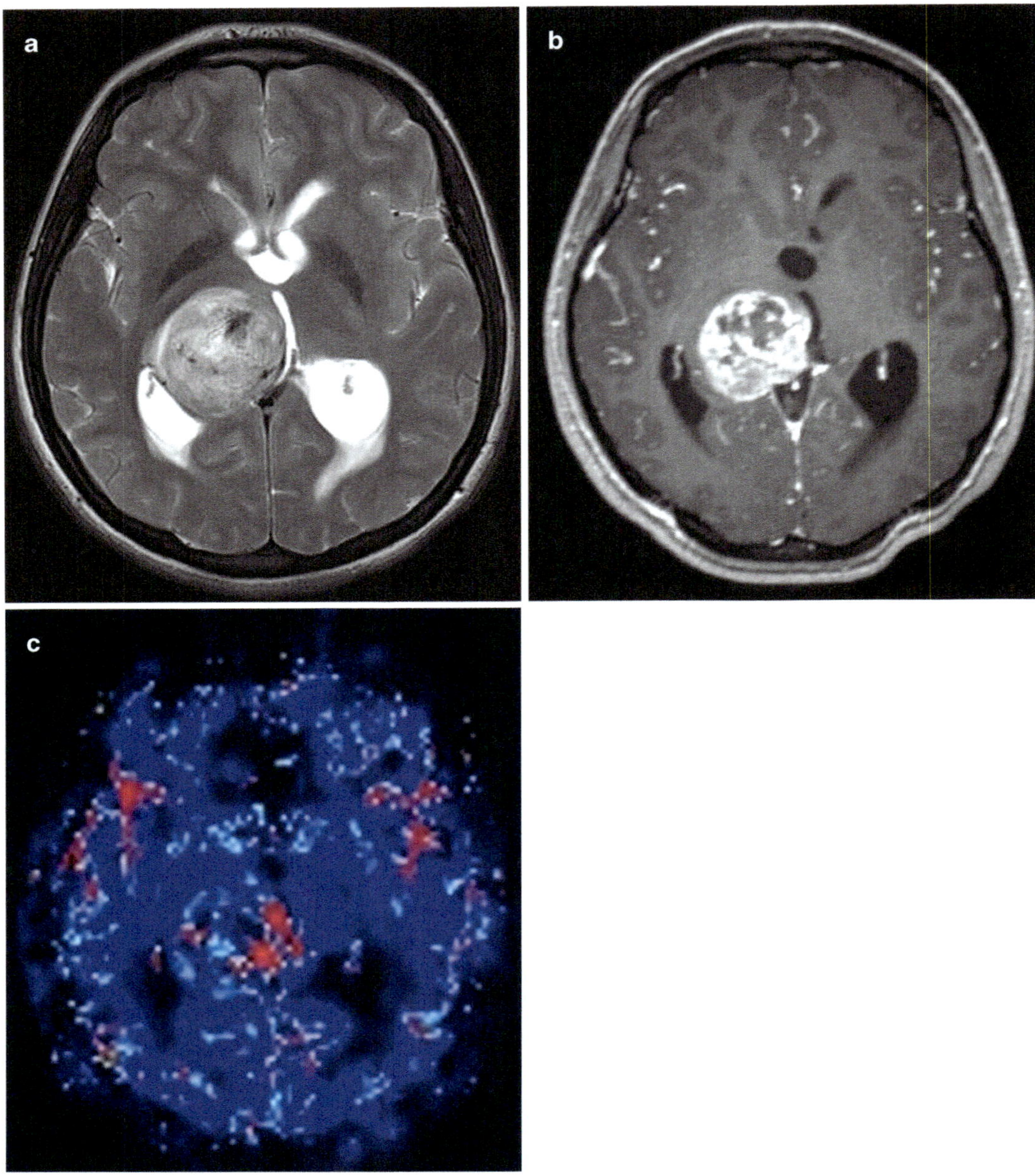

Fig. 17.5 Intraventricular ependymoma. Axial T2 (**a**), axial T1 postcontrast (**b**), DSC perfusion cerebral blood volume map (**c**). Relative cerebral blood volume increased at a significant level

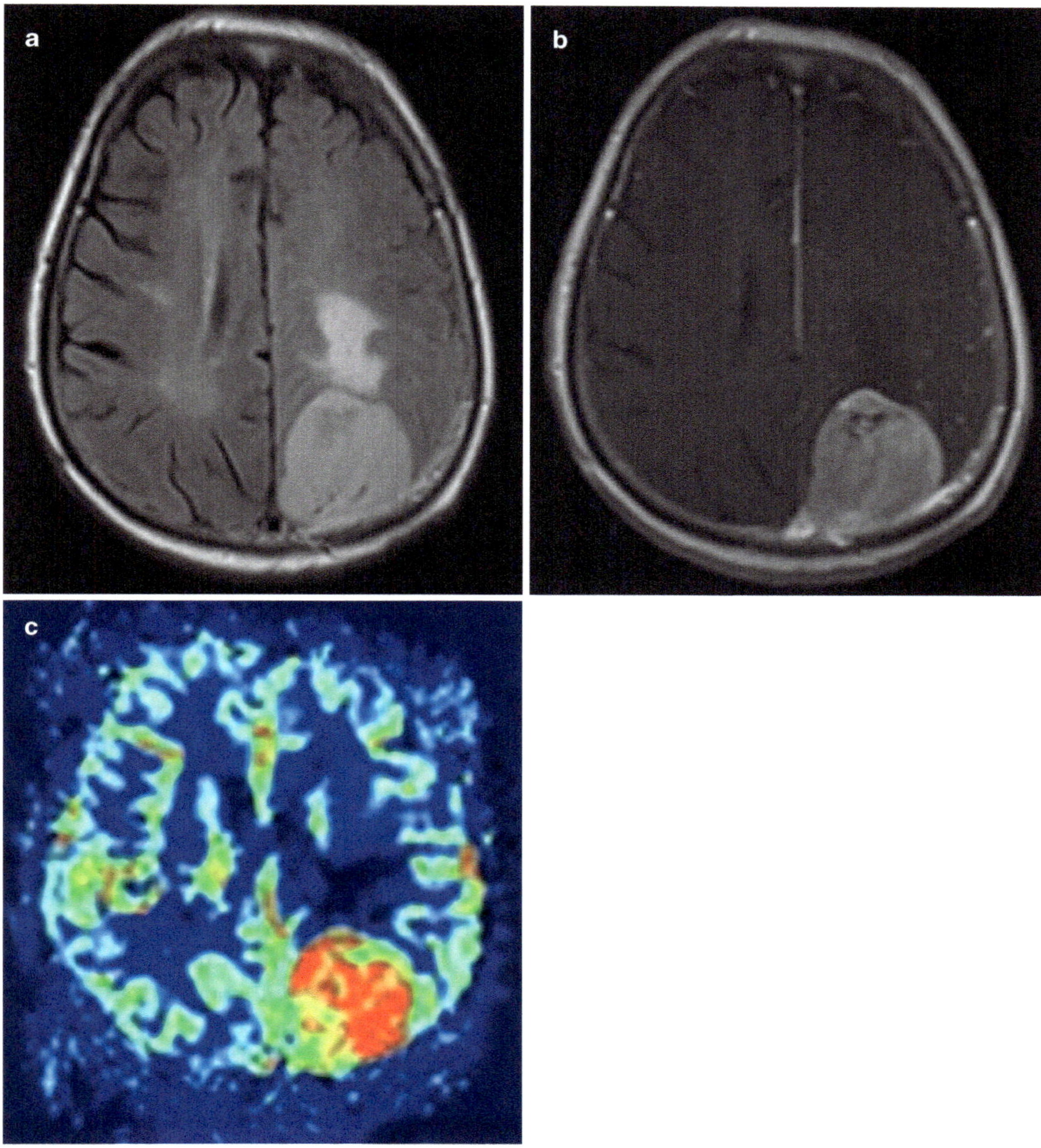

Fig. 17.6 Meningioma. Axial FLAIR (**a**), axial T1 post-contrast (**b**), DSC perfusion cerebral blood volume map (**c**). This large enhancing extra-axial meningioma developing on parietal region shows increased cerebral blood flow at a significant level

87]. rCBV values obtained from MR perfusion also demonstrate significant difference between high-grade gliomas and TDLs [88]. However, perfusion imaging is limited in the differentiation of grade 2–3 glial tumors and TDL, due to both of these entities have a similar increase in the level of rCBV [89].

17.3.1.5 Guiding Biopsy and Radiosurgery

Misclassification of gliomas is a common problem affecting treatment management and outcomes. Tumor heterogeneity is an important cause of sampling errors. Contrast enhancement has a limited specificity in tumor grading, although it has a widely used MR imaging feature to evaluate GBs.

Because of the heterogeneity of the lesion, it is known that GB contains areas of different grades. Recent data suggest that angiogenesis and high cellularity-related rCBV values are increased in high-grade areas of GBs [90]. Therefore, areas with a high rCBV value in perfusion imaging should be preferred for biopsy sampling. It can also be used to identify the most malignant regions of irradiated tumors.

17.3.1.6 Differentiation of Recurrent Tumor and Response to Treatment

Recent studies have demonstrated that perfusion imaging, particularly MR perfusion imaging, has a vital role in discrimination between treatment effects and disease progression because accurate differentiation results in changes to the treatment approach. Determining the progress or response of the disease by conventional imaging depended on the evaluation of the contrast enhancing lesion using MacDonald criteria [91]. By recognizing the importance of the non-enhancing region in monitoring the treatment response, the non-enhancing region of the tumor is considered in the updated guidelines for Response Evaluation in Neuro-Oncology (RANO) [92]. Postoperative infarcts, treatment-related inflammatory processes, and postictal changes, related to tumor physiopathology can disrupt the BBB, and lead to contrast enhancement, and mimics recurrent or residual tumor, today has been named pseudoprogression. On the other hand, steroid and antiangiogenic drug therapies stabilize the BBB, and cause a decrease in contrast enhancement even there is no true treatment response. This condition is called pseudoresponse [93, 94].

Pseudoprogression

Pseudoprogression is the name given to an increase in enhancing lesion size and/or edema due to treatment without a real increase in tumor component. These findings do not show improvement on follow-up imaging. Pseudoprogression caused by increased fluid of interstitial space due to increased vessel permeability and inflammation in tissue and perilesional edema area, and usually is seen in the 2- to 6-months after chemoradiation therapy. Discrimination between pseudoprogression and true tumor progression is not possible with conventional MRI because they both can show similar imaging findings, including increased enhancement and edema. By the way, perfusion imaging, which provides information on changes in the level of the microvascular system, is very helpful in distinguishing these two conditions. In pseudoprogression, contrast-enhanced lesions lack neoangiogenesis and do not show increased perfusion in contrast to true tumor progression (Fig. 17.7) [95–99].

Pseudoresponse

Antiangiogenic drugs (anti-VEGF antibody bevacizumab and VEGF receptor tyrosine kinase inhibitor cediranib) have been used as a second choice in high-grade glioma treatment protocols. These drugs restore the integrity of the BBB, causing a marked and rapid decrease in contrast enhancement and lesion circumference edema. Although antiangiogenic drugs provide a 6-month progression-free survival with this effect, they do not have a significant effect on overall survival [100–102]. High-grade gliomas are usually multicentric at the time of diagnosis and malignant infiltrating cells are found in the area of peripheral edema. Therefore, total excision of tumor is difficult. Non-enhanced infiltrating brain parenchyma adjacent to the surgical bed is observed as hyperintense on fluid-attenuated inversion recovery (FLAIR) and T2-weighted images. These areas continue to expand with disease progression. When tumor cells in these regions progress and transform a more malignant form, an angiogenic switch occurs, which leads to contrast enhancement. However, if antiangiogenic agents are used in this process, by reducing the vascular permeability and correcting the BBB decreases the contrast enhancement even if there is real tumor progress (Fig. 17.8). These effects can be

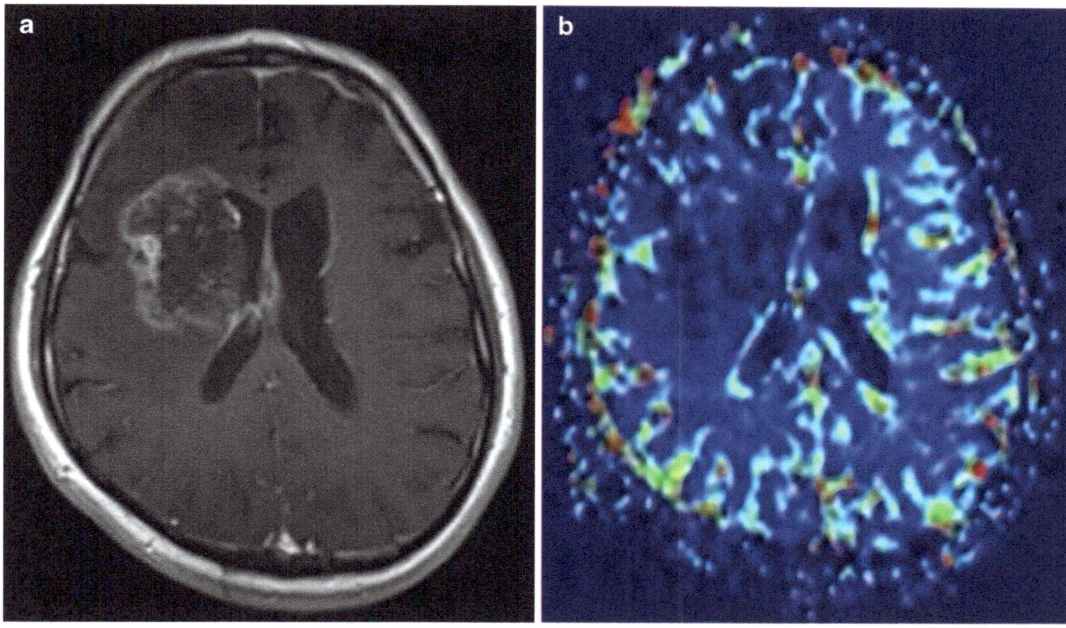

Fig. 17.7 Pseudoprogression in a treated glioblastoma. Axial T1 postcontrast (**a**), DSC perfusion cerebral blood volume map (**b**) obtained after chemo-radiotherapy. Contrast enhancement is prominent due to the changes caused by treatment regime. Cerebral blood volume did not show any increase consistent with pseudoprogression

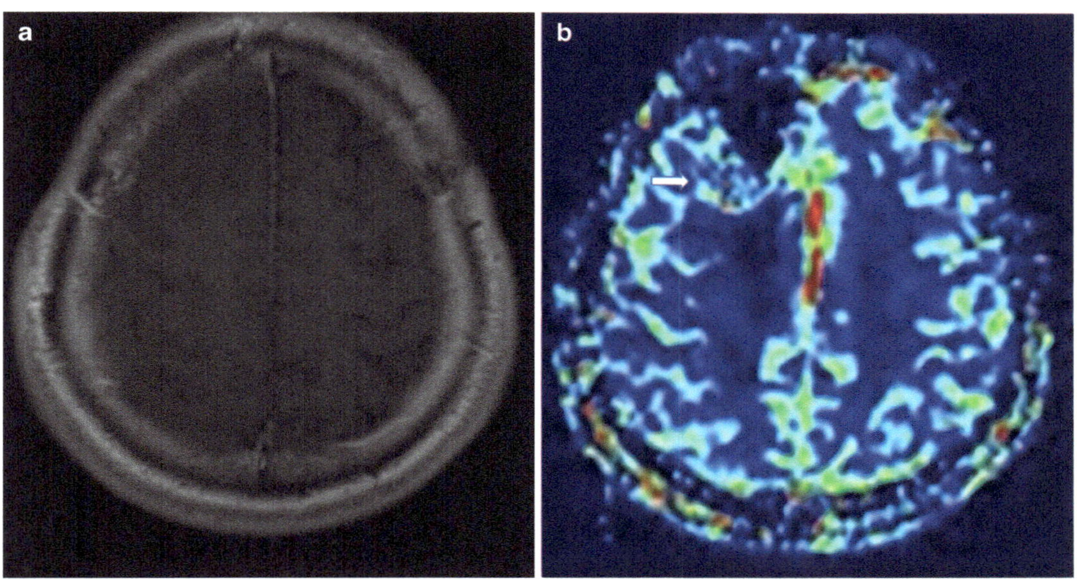

Fig. 17.8 Pseudoresponse. Axial T1 postcontrast (**a**), color DSC perfusion cerebral blood volume map (**b**) of glioblastoma after the treatment with bevacizumab. No contrast enhancement is seen due to the treatment effect of antiangiogenic agent. But increased cerebral blood volume reveals recurrent tumor

detected within hours after the start of treatment. When the use of medication is discontinued due to toxicity concerns, this reverses vascular normalization, resulting in rebound enhancement and edema [103].

Radiation Necrosis

Radiation necrosis is a late effect of radiation injury and occurs in about 3–24% of patients who had received standard radiation therapy. Radiation necrosis usually occurs around the original tumor and in the region of the maximum radiation dose surrounding the surgical cavity usually between 3 and 12 months after radiation treatment [104].

Radiation necrosis is caused by obstructive vasculopathy leading to stroke-like attacks. Radiation necrosis is associated with endothelial proliferation, hyalinization, and consequently vascular thrombosis and fibrinoid necrosis of small vessels. By the way, recurrent/residual tumors are related to vascular proliferation and neoangiogenesis without vascular luminal obstruction [105].

The clinical findings of radiation necrosis and true tumor progression are similar and complicate patient management. It is also difficult to distinguish true tumor progression and radiation necrosis in conventional imaging because they both occur around the original tumor, enhance after contrast administration, and grows in time with peripheral edema. Necrosis caused by chemoradiotherapy and tumor recurrence/progress may also coexist.

Perfusion imaging techniques are quite helpful in distinguishing radiation necrosis from true tumor progression. rCBV increases in the area of the tumor and decreases in the area of radiation necrosis (Table 17.1) [21, 84, 104]. Ktrans with PW-MRI or permeability surface (PS) in CTP imaging as an indicator of vascular leakage has also been used in differentiation tumor progression from radiation necrosis. Blood vessels of irradiated tissue are prone to sustain patency of BBB which results in lower Ktrans compared to recurrent tumor with neoangiogenesis which tends to have leaky BBB (Table 17.1).

17.3.1.7 Tumor Surveillance

In the light of current information, standard conventional imaging methods do not provide sufficient information about the pathophysiological characteristics of the tumor and therefore are not sufficient to accurately assess the success of treatment. Perfusion imaging has a significant effect when used in conjunction with conventional imaging in the detection of treatment response. CBV is a hot topic in distinguishing treatment effects from true tumor progression [106], and a definitive cut-off point is still needed for discrimination in larger studies. Roughly, it can be said that a progressively increasing rCBV may suggest tumor progression, and a decreasing rCBV may suggest treatment effects [106].

17.3.2 Stroke Management

Non-contrast CT, cranial CT angiography, and then diffusion-weighted imaging of brain are the first imaging modalities in the suspicious of ischemic stroke. After determining the arterial occlusion, it is critical to evaluate the presence and size of the hypoperfused tissue with a risk of necrosis, called penumbra, around the infarct core. The aim of thrombolytic therapy in acute stroke is to rescue the hypoperfused penumbra under the risk of ischemia which surrounds the infarct core. The time of clinical onset of symptoms is so crucial to apply anti-thrombolytic therapy to survive penumbra. The main point is to identify and define the patients that may benefit from anti-thrombolytic therapy.

17.3.2.1 CT Perfusion

Maps computed for perfusion imaging include CBV, CBF, MTT, and time to maximum (Tmax) [107]. The definition of the penumbra and the infarct core depend on the measurement of CBF on CT PWI. The CBF varied according to the age of the patient and is approximately three times higher in gray matter than white matter. In general, the CBF of the normal perfused area is greater than 50 mL/100 g/min. The CBF value is between 20 and 40 mL/100 g/min in the oligemia, 10 and 20 mL/100 g/min in the penumbrae, and 10 mL/100 g/min in the ischemic area. The vascular autoregulation is lost in the ischemic area, and CBV value also reduces while MTT value prolongs. In the penumbra, there is a decrease in CBF when trying to protect CBV by vasodilatation and collateral pathways. In critically hypoperfused tissue, the Tmax duration is longer than 6 s [16]. The mismatch between the critically hypoperfused tissue and the ischemic core is used to predict the penumbra.

17.3.2.2 MR Perfusion

DWI is useful in the determination of the ischemic core by defining cytotoxic edema. The decrease in the ADC indicates that there is an irreversible necrosis. It is critical to determine the tissue at risk. In the last decade, there has been an effort to determine thresholds to define the penumbra with MRI diffusion/perfusion mismatch and also CT perfusion values. In a study using diffusion and perfusion mismatch, better neurological recovery was reported with early reperfusion (patients who received tPa for 3–6 h after the onset of symptoms) [108]. The criteria for mismatch include: a lesion with Tmax over 2 s and the lesion size at least 20% greater than that measured in DWI. Another study showed [109] that tPA had no significant effect on the growth of the ischemic area but significantly improved reperfusion in patients with mismatch and improved clinical outcome. Consequently, patients who have a lesion with Tmax of more than 2 s and at least 20% greater than that measured in DWI may benefit from tPA therapy within 6 h of the onset of symptoms. The mismatch approach also helps eliminate poor candidates who will not benefit from treatment.

Lansberg et al. [110] proposed three groups of patients with newly defined thresholds. The first group consists of patients with mismatch benefit from reperfusion, resulting in a better clinical outcome and a reduction in the size of the infarction. The second group without mismatch does not show a significant clinical response and the size of the infarct does not decrease. The third group of patients with the worst profile (volume of infarct core is over100 mL in DWI or Tmax is superior 8 s on perfusion imaging) show no improvement in clinical and image findings after reperfusion.

17.3.3 Delayed Cerebral Ischemia (DCI) due to a Vasospasm

DCI may occur due to a complication of subarachnoid hemorrhage. In half of the patients with severe vasospasm, ischemia occurs in the progressive process. The use of perfusion CT in delayed ischemia has increased. If the MTT is above 6.4 s on perfusion imaging, it can be said that the risk of DCI increases [111].

17.4 Conclusion

Perfusion imaging tools today are invaluable in the setting of differential diagnosis of a wide range of brain pathologies. Understanding of these techniques and wide application in routine clinical practice will make an impact especially in the interpretation of challenging conditions.

References

1. Mabray MC, Barajas RF Jr, Cha S. Modern brain tumor imaging. Brain Tumor Res Treat. 2015;3:8–23.
2. Petrella JR, Provenzale JM. MR perfusion imaging of the brain: techniques and applications. AJR Am J Roentgenol. 2000;175(1):207–19.
3. Wintermark M, Flanders AE, Velthuis B, et al. Perfusion-CT assessment of infarct core and penumbra: receiver operating characteristic curve analysis in 130 patients suspected of acute hemispheric stroke. Stroke. 2006;37(4):979–85.
4. Essig M, Shiroishi MS, Nguyen TB, et al. Perfusion MRI: the five most frequently asked technical questions. AJR Am J Roentgenol. 2013;200(1):24–34.
5. Welker K, Boxerman J, Kalnin A, et al. ASFNR recommendations for clinical performance of MR dynamic susceptibility contrast perfusion imaging of the brain. AJNR Am J Neuroradiol. 2015;36:E41–51.
6. Shiroishi MS, Castellazzi G, Boxerman JL, et al. Principles of T2*-weighted dynamic susceptibility contrast MRI technique in brain tumor imaging. J Magn Reson Imaging. 2015;41:296–313.
7. Hu LS, Baxter LC, Pinnaduwage DS, et al. Optimized preload leakage correction methods to improve

the diagnostic accuracy of dynamic susceptibility-weighted contrast-enhanced perfusion MR imaging in posttreatment gliomas. AJNR Am J Neuroradiol. 2010;31(1):40–8.
8. Zaharchuk G. Theoretical basis of hemodynamic MR imaging techniques to measure cerebral blood volume, cerebral blood flow, and permeability. AJNR Am J Neuroradiol. 2007;28:1850–8.
9. Cha S, Yang L, Johnson G, et al. Comparison of microvascular permeability measurements, Ktrans, determined with conventional steady-state T1-weighted and first-pass T2*-weighted MR imaging methods in gliomas and meningiomas. AJNR Am J Neuroradiol. 2006;27(2):409–17.
10. Maia ACM Jr, Malheiros SMF, da Rocha AJ, et al. MR cerebral blood volume maps correlated with vascular endothelial growth factor expression and tumor grade in nonenhancing gliomas. AJNR Am J Neuroradiol. 2005;26(4):777–83.
11. Sugahara T, Korogi Y, Kochi M, et al. Correlation of MR imaging-determined cerebral blood volume maps with histologic and angiographic determination of vascularity of gliomas. AJR Am J Roentgenol. 1998;171(6):1479–86.
12. Law M, Yang S, Wang H, et al. Glioma grading: sensitivity, specificity, and predictive values of perfusionMRimagingand proton MR spectroscopic imaging compared with conventional MR imaging. AJNR Am J Neuroradiol. 2003;24(10):1989–98.
13. Hylton N. Dynamic contrast-enhanced magnetic resonance imaging as an imaging biomarker. J Clin Oncol. 2006;24:3293–8.
14. Roberts HC, Roberts TP, Ley S, et al. Quantitative estimation of microvascular permeability in human brain tumors: correlation of dynamic Gd-DTPAenhanced MR imaging with histopathologic grading. Acad Radiol. 2002;9(Suppl 1):S151–5.
15. Patankar TF, Haroon HA, Mills SJ, et al. Is volume transfer coefficient (K(trans)) related to histologic grade in human gliomas? AJNR Am J Neuroradiol. 2005;26:2455–65.
16. Nelson SJ. Assessment of therapeutic response and treatment planning for brain tumors using metabolic and physiological MRI. NMR Biomed. 2011;24(6):734–49.
17. Weber M, Giesel F, Stieltjes B. MRI for identification of progression in brain tumors: from morphology to function. Expert Rev Neurother. 2008;8(10):1507–25.
18. Narang J, Jain R, Arbab AS, et al. Differentiating treatment-induced necrosis from recurrent/progressive brain tumor using nonmodel-based semiquantitative indices derived from dynamic contrast-enhanced T1-weighted MR perfusion. Neuro Oncol. 2011;13:1037–46.
19. O'Connor JP, Tofts PS, Miles KA, et al. Dynamic contrast-enhanced imaging techniques: CT and MRI. Br J Radiol. 2011;84(2):112–20.
20. Shiroishi MS, Lacerda S, Tang X, et al. Physical principles of MR perfusion and permeability imaging: gadolinium bolus technique. Functional neuroradiology. Springer, Boston, MA. 2011 https://doi.org/10.1007/978-1-4419-0345-7_3.
21. Jain R, Narang J, Arbab AS, et al. Role of nonmodel-based semi-quantitative indices obtained from DCE T1 MR Perfusion in differentiating pseudoprogression from true-progression [meeting abstract]. Neuro Oncol. 2011;13:140.
22. Thompson G, Mills SJ, Coope DJ, et al. Imaging biomarkers of angiogenesis and the microvascular environment in cerebral tumours. Br J Radiol. 2011;84:127–44.
23. Boxerman JL, Paulson ES, Prah MA, et al. The effect of pulse sequence parameters and contrast agent dose on percentage signal recovery in DSC-MRI: implications for clinical applications. Am J Neuroradiol. 2013;34:1364–9.
24. Watts JM, Whitlow CT, Maldjian JA. Clinical applications of arterial spin labeling. NMR Biomed. 2013;26(8):892–900.
25. Detre JA, Rao H, Wang DJ, et al. Applications of arterial spin labeled MRI in the brain. J Magn Reson Imaging. 2012;35:1026–37.
26. Hirai T, Kitajima M, Nakamura H, et al. Quantitative blood flow measurements in gliomas using arterial spin-labeling at 3T: intermodality agreement and inter- and intraobserver reproducibility study. AJNR Am J Neuroradiol. 2011;32:2073–9.
27. Jiang J, Zhao L, Zhang Y, et al. Comparative analysis of arterial spin labeling and dynamic susceptibility contrast perfusion imaging for quantitative perfusion measurements of brain tumors. Int J Clin Exp Pathol. 2014;7:2790–9.
28. Ata ES, Turgut M, Eraslan C, et al. Comparison between dynamic susceptibility contrast magnetic resonance imaging and arterial spin labeling techniques in distinguishing malignant from benign brain tumors. Eur J Radiol. 2016;85:1545–53.
29. Soni N, Dhanota DPS, Kumar S, et al. Perfusion MR imaging of enhancing brain tumors: comparison of arterial spin labeling technique with dynamic susceptibility contrast technique. Neurol India. 2017;65:1046–52.
30. Jain R. Perfusion CT imaging of brain tumors: an overview. AJNR Am J Neuroradiol. 2011;32(9):1570–7.
31. Law M, Yang S, Babb JS, et al. Comparison of cerebral blood volume and vascular permeability from dynamic susceptibility contrast-enhanced perfusion MR imaging with glioma grade. AJNR Am J Neuroradiol. 2004;25:746–55.
32. Scott JN, Brasher PMA, Sevick RJ, et al. How often are nonenhancing supratentorial gliomas malignant? A population study. Neurology. 2002;59(6):947–9.
33. Whittle IR. The dilemma of low grade glioma. J Neurol Neurosurg Psychiatry. 2004;75:ii31–6.

34. Wolburg H, Noell S, Fallier-Becker P, et al. The disturbed blood-brain barrier in human glioblastoma. Mol Asp Med. 2012;33(5–6):579–89.
35. Jain RK, Di Tomaso E, Duda DG, et al. Angiogenesis in brain tumours. Nat Rev Neurosci. 2007;8(8):610–22.
36. Ellika SK, Jain R, Patel SC, et al. Role of perfusion CT in glioma grading and comparison with conventional MR imaging features. AJNR Am J Neuroradiol. 2007;28(10):1981–7.
37. Lev MH, Ozsunar Y, Henson JW, et al. Glial tumor grading and outcome prediction using dynamic spin-echo MR susceptibility mapping compared with conventional contrast-enhanced MR: confounding effect of elevated rCBV of oligodendrogliomas [corrected]. AJNR Am J Neuroradiol. 2004;25:214–21.
38. Cha S, Tihan T, Crawford F, et al. Differentiation of low-grade oligodendrogliomas from low-grade astrocytomas by using quantitative blood-volume measurements derived from dynamic susceptibility contrast-enhanced MR imaging. AJNR Am J Neuroradiol. 2005;26:266–73.
39. Hilario A, Hernandez-Lain A, Sepulveda JM, et al. Perfusion MRI grading diffuse gliomas: impact of permeability parameters on molecular biomarkers and survival. Neurocirugia. 2019;30(1):11–8.
40. Aprile I, Giovannelli G, Fiaschini P, et al. High- and low-grade glioma differentiation: the role of percentage signal recovery evaluation in MR dynamic susceptibility contrast imaging. Radiol Med. 2015;120(10):967–74.
41. Smitha KA, Gupta AK, Jayasree RS. Relative percentage signal intensity recovery of perfusion metrics—an efficient tool for differentiating grades of glioma. Br J Radiol. 2015;88:1052.
42. Kerbel RS. Tumor angiogenesis. N Engl J Med. 2008;358(19):2039–49.
43. Danchaivijitr N, Waldman AD, Tozer DJ, et al. Low grade gliomas: do changes in rCBV measurements at longitudinal perfusion-weighted MR imaging predict malignant transformation? Radiology. 2008;247(1):170–8.
44. Louis DN, Perry A, Reifenberger G, et al. The 2016 World Health Organization Classification of Tumors of the Central Nervous System: a summary. Acta Neuropathol. 2016;131(6):803–20.
45. Itakura H, Achrol AS, Mitchell LA, et al. Magnetic resonance image features identify glioblastoma phenotypic subtypes with distinct molecular pathway activities. Sci Transl Med. 2015;7(303):303.
46. Yan H, Parsons DW, Jin G, et al. IDH1 and IDH2 mutations in gliomas. N Engl J Med. 2009;360(8):765–73.
47. Lai A, Kharbanda S, Pope WB, et al. Evidence for sequenced molecular evolution of IDH1 mutant glioblastoma from a distinct cell of origin. J Clin Oncol. 2011;29(34):4482–90.
48. SongTao Q, Lei Y, Si G, et al. IDH mutations predict longer survival and response to temozolomide in secondary glioblastoma. Cancer Sci. 2012;103(2):269–73.
49. Kickingereder P, Sahm F, Radbruch A, et al. IDH mutation status is associated with a distinct hypoxia/angiogenesis transcriptome signature which is non-invasively predictable with rCBV imaging in human glioma. Sci Rep. 2015;5:16238.
50. Lee S, Choi SH, Ryoo I, et al. Evaluation of the microenvironmental heterogeneity in high-grade gliomas with IDH1/2 gene mutation using histogram analysis of diffusion-weighted imaging and dynamic-susceptibility contrast perfusion imaging. J Neurooncol. 2015;121(1):141–50.
51. Yamashita K, Hiwatashi A, Togao O, et al. MR imaging based analysis of glioblastoma multiforme: estimation of IDH1 mutation status. Am J Neuroradiol. 2016;37(1):58–65.
52. Tan W, Xiong J, Huang W, et al. Noninvasively detecting Isocitrate dehydrogenase 1 gene status in astrocytoma by dynamic susceptibility contrast MRI. J Magn Reson Imaging. 2017;45(2):492–9.
53. Zhang J, Liu H, Tong H, et al. Clinical applications of contrast-enhanced perfusion MRI techniques in gliomas: recent advances and current challenges. Contrast Media Mol Imaging. 2017;2017:7064120.
54. Siegal T. Clinical impact of molecular biomarkers in gliomas. J Clin Neurosci. 2015;22(3):437–44.
55. Swartz AM, Batich KA, Fecci PE, et al. Peptide vaccines for the treatment of glioblastoma. J Neurooncol. 2015;123(3):433–40.
56. Aghi M, Gaviani P, Henson JW, et al. Magnetic resonance imaging characteristics predict epidermal growth factor receptor amplification status in glioblastoma. Clin Cancer Res. 2005;11(24):8600–5.
57. Gupta A, Young RJ, Shah AD, et al. Pretreatment dynamic susceptibility contrast MRI perfusion in glioblastoma: prediction of EGFR gene amplification. Clin Neuroradiol. 2015;25(2):143–50.
58. Arevalo-Perez J, Thomas AA, Kaley T, et al. T1-weighted dynamic contrast-enhanced MRI as a noninvasive biomarker of epidermal growth factor receptor VIII status. Am J Neuroradiol. 2015;36(12):2256–61.
59. Riemenschneider MJ, Hegi ME, Reifenberger G. MGMTpromoter methylation in malignant gliomas. Target Oncol. 2010;5(3):161–5.
60. Weller M, Tabatabai G, Kästner B, et al. MGMT promoter methylation is a strong prognostic biomarker for benefit from dose-intensified temozolomide rechallenge in progressive glioblastoma: the DIRECTOR trial. Clin Cancer Res. 2015;21(9):2057–64.
61. Rapkins RW, Wang F, Nguyen HTN, et al. The MGMT promoter SNP rs16906252 is a risk factor for MGMT methylation in glioblastoma and is predictive of response to temozolomide. Neuro Oncol. 2015;17(12):1589–98.
62. Li H, Li J, Cheng G, et al. IDH mutation and MGMT promoter methylation are associated with

the pseudoprogression and improved prognosis of glioblastoma multiforme patients who have undergone concurrent and adjuvant temozolomide-based chemoradiotherapy. Clin Neurol Neurosurg. 2016;151:31–6.
63. Della Puppa A, Persano L, Masi G, et al. MGMT expression and promoter methylation status may depend on the site of surgical sample collection within glioblastoma: a possible pitfall in stratification of patients? J Neurooncol. 2012;106(1):33–41.
64. Jung SC, Choi SH, Yeom JA, et al. Cerebral blood volume analysis in glioblastomas using dynamic susceptibility contrast enhanced perfusion MRI: a comparison of manual and semiautomatic segmentation methods. PLoS One. 2013;8(8):69323.
65. Ahn SS, Shin NY, Chang JH, et al. Prediction of methylguanine methyltransferase promoter methylation in glioblastoma using dynamic contrast-enhanced magnetic resonance and diffusion tensor imaging. J Neurosurg. 2014;121(2):367–73.
66. Xing Z, You RX, Li J, et al. Differentiation of primary central nervous system lymphomas from high-grade gliomas by rCBV and percentage of signal intensity recovery derived from dynamic susceptibility-weighted contrast-enhanced perfusion MR imaging. Clin Neuroradiol. 2014;24:329–36.
67. Kickingereder P, Wiestler B, Sahm F, et al. Primary central nervous system lymphoma and atypical glioblastoma: multiparametric differentiation by using diffusion-, perfusion-, and susceptibility weighted MR imaging. Radiology. 2014;272:843–50.
68. Takeuchi H, Matsuda K, Kitai R, et al. Angiogenesis in primary central nervous system lymphoma (PCNSL). J Neurooncol. 2007;84(2):141–5.
69. Toh CH, Wei KC, Chang CN, et al. Differentiation of primary central nervous system lymphomas and glioblastomas: comparisons of diagnostic performance of dynamic susceptibility contrast-enhanced perfusion mr imaging without and with contrast-leakage correction. Am J Neuroradiol. 2013;34(6):1145–9.
70. Nakajima S, Okada T, Yamamoto T, et al. Differentiation between primary central nervous system lymphoma and glioblastoma: a comparative study of parameters derived from dynamic susceptibility contrast-enhanced perfusion-weighted MRI. Clin Radiol. 2015;70(12):1393–9.
71. Mangla R, Kolar B, Zhu T, et al. Percentage signal recovery derived from MR dynamic susceptibility contrast imaging is useful to differentiate common enhancing malignant lesions of the brain. Am J Neuroradiol. 2011;32(6):1004–10.
72. Wesseling P, Ruiter DJ, Burger PC. Angiogenesis in brain tumors; pathobiological and clinical aspects. J Neurooncol. 1997;32:253–65.
73. Cha S, Lupo JM, Chen MH, et al. Differentiation of glioblastoma multiforme and single brain metastasis by peak height and percentage of signal intensity recovery derived from dynamic susceptibility-weighted contrast-enhanced perfusion MR imaging. AJNR Am J Neuroradiol. 2007;28:1078–84.
74. Blasel S, Jurcoane A, Franz K, et al. Elevated peritumoural rCBV values as a mean to differentiate metastases from high-grade gliomas. Acta Neurochir. 2010;152:1893–9.
75. Lin L, Xue Y, Duan Q, et al. The role of cerebral blood flow gradient in peritumoral edema for differentiation of glioblastomas from solitary metastatic lesions. Oncotarget. 2016;7:69051–9.
76. Nduom EK, Yang C, Merrill MJ, et al. Characterization of the blood-brain barrier of metastatic and primary malignant neoplasms. J Neurosurg. 2013;119(2):427–33.
77. Fidler IJ. The biology of brain metastasis: challenges for therapy. Cancer J. 2015;21(4):284–93.
78. Bauer AH, Erly W, Moser FG, et al. Differentiation of solitary brain metastasis from glioblastoma multiforme: a predictive multiparametric approach using combined MR diffusion and perfusion. Neuroradiology. 2015;57:697–703.
79. Bulakbasi N, Kocaoglu M, Farzaliyev A, et al. Assessment of diagnostic accuracy of perfusion MR imaging in primary and metastatic solitary malignant brain tumors. AJNR Am J Neuroradiol. 2005;26:2187–99.
80. Ganbold M, Harada M, Khashbat D, et al. Differences in high-intensity signal volume between arterial spin labeling and contrast-enhanced T1-weighted imaging may be useful for differentiating glioblastoma from brain metastasis. J Med Invest. 2017;64:58–63.
81. Abe T, Mizobuchi Y, Nakajima K, et al. Diagnosis of brain tumors using dynamic contrast-enhanced perfusion imaging with a short acquisition time. Springerplus. 2015;4:88.
82. Yuh EL, Barkovich AJ, Gupta N. Imaging of ependymomas: MRI and CT. Childs Nerv Syst. 2009;25:1203–13.
83. Saloner D, Uzelac A, Hetts S, et al. Modern meningioma imaging techniques. J Neurooncol. 2010;99:333–40.
84. Cha S. Update on brain tumor imaging: from anatomy to physiology. AJNR Am J Neuroradiol. 2006;27:475–87.
85. Lucchinetti CF, Gavrilova RH, Metz I, et al. Clinical and radiographic spectrum of pathologically confirmed tumefactive multiple sclerosis. Brain. 2008;131(Pt 7):1759–75.
86. Sugita Y, Terasaki M, Shigemori M, et al. Acute focal demyelinating disease simulating brain tumors: histopathologic guidelines for an accurate diagnosis. Neuropathology. 2001;21(1):25–31.
87. Jain R, Ellika S, Lehman NL, et al. Can permeability measurements add to blood volume measurements in differentiating tumefactive demyelinating lesions from high grade gliomas using perfusion CT? J Neurooncol. 2010;97(3):383–8.
88. Hourani R, Brant LJ, Rizk T, et al. Can proton MR spectroscopic and perfusion imaging dif-

ferentiate between neoplastic and nonneoplastic brain lesions in adults? AJNR Am J Neuroradiol. 2008;29(2):366–72.
89. Blasel S, Pfeilschifter W, Jansen V, et al. Metabolism and regional cerebral blood volume in autoimmune inflammatory demyelinating lesions mimicking malignant gliomas. J Neurol. 2011;258(1):113–22.
90. Barajas RF, Hodgson JG, Chang JS, et al. Glioblastoma multiform regional genetic and cellular expression patterns: influence on anatomic and physiologic MR imaging. Radiology. 2010;254(2):564–76.
91. Macdonald DR, Cascino TL, Schold SC, et al. Response criteria for phase II studies of supratentorial malignant glioma. J Clin Oncol. 1990;8(7):1277–80.
92. Wen PY, Macdonald DR, Reardon DA, et al. Updated response assessment criteria for high-grade gliomas: response assessment in neuro-oncology working group. J Clin Oncol. 2010;28(11):1963–72.
93. Clarke JL, Chang S. Pseudoprogression and pseudoresponse: challenges in brain tumor imaging. Curr Neurol Neurosci Rep. 2009;9(3):241–6.
94. Vogelbaum MA, Jost S, Aghi MK, et al. Application of novel response/progression measures for surgically delivered therapies for gliomas: Response Assessment in Neuro-Oncology (RANO) Working Group. Neurosurgery. 2012;70(1):234–43; discussion: 243–4.
95. Young RJ, Gupta A, Shah AD, et al. MRI perfusion in determining pseudoprogression in patients with glioblastoma. Clin Imaging. 2013;37(1):41–9.
96. Mangla R, Singh G, Ziegelitz D, et al. Changes in relative cerebral blood volume 1 month after radiation-temozolomide therapy can help predict overall survival in patients with glioblastoma. Radiology. 2010;256(2):575–84.
97. Kong DS, Kim ST, Kim EH, et al. Diagnostic dilemma of pseudoprogression in the treatment of newly diagnosed glioblastomas: the role of assessing relative cerebral blood flow volume and oxygen-6-methylguanine-DNA methyltransferase promoter methylation status. AJNR Am J Neuroradiol. 2011;32:382–7.
98. Brandsma D, Stalpers L, Taal W, et al. Clinical features, mechanisms, and management of pseudoprogression in malignant gliomas. Lancet Oncol. 2008;9(5):453–61.
99. Shiroishi MS, Boxerman JL, Pope WB. Physiologic MRI for assessment of response to therapy and prognosis in glioblastoma. Neuro-Oncology. 2016;18(4):467–78.
100. Batchelor TT, Sorensen AG, di Tomaso E, et al. AZD2171, a pan-VEGF receptor tyrosine kinase inhibitor, normalizes tumor vasculature and alleviates edema in glioblastoma patients. Cancer Cell. 2007;11:83–95.
101. Gerstner ER, Duda DG, di Tomaso E, et al. VEGF inhibitors in the treatment of cerebral edema in patients with brain cancer. Nat Rev Clin Oncol. 2009;6:229–36.
102. Carmeliet P, Jain RK. Principles and mechanisms of vessel normalization for cancer and other angiogenic diseases. Nat Rev Drug Discov. 2011;10(6):417–27.
103. Hygino da Cruz LC Jr, Rodriguez I, Domingues RC, et al. Pseudoprogression and pseudoresponse: imaging challenges in the assessment of post treatment glioma. AJNR Am J Neuroradiol. 2011;32(11):1978–85.
104. Barajas RF Jr, Chang JS, Segal MR, et al. Differentiation of recurrent glioblastoma multiforme from radiation necrosis after external beam radiation therapy with dynamic susceptibility-weighted contrast-enhanced perfusion MR imaging. Radiology. 2009;253:486–96.
105. Lacerda S, Law M. Magnetic resonance perfusion and permeability imaging in brain tumors. Neuroimaging Clin N Am. 2009;19:527–57.
106. White ML, Zhang Y, Yu F, et al. Post-operative perfusion and diffusion MR imaging and tumor progression in high-grade gliomas. PLoS One. 2019;14(3):e0213905.
107. Srinivasan A, Goyal M, Azri FA, et al. State-of-the-art imaging of acute stroke. Radiographics. 2006;26:75–95.
108. Albers GW, Thijs VN, Wechsler L, et al. Magnetic resonance imaging profiles predict clinical response to early reperfusion: the diffusion and perfusion imaging evaluation for understanding stroke evolution (DEFUSE) study. Ann Neurol. 2006;60(5):508–17.
109. Davis SM, Donnan GA, Parsons MW, et al. Effects of alteplase beyond 3 h after stroke in the echoplanar imaging thrombolytic evaluation trial (EPI-THET): a placebo-controlled randomised trial. Lancet Neurol. 2008;7(4):299–309.
110. Lansberg MG, Lee J, Christensen S, et al. RAPID automated patient selection for reperfusion therapy: a pooled analysis of the echoplanar imaging thrombolytic evaluation trial (EPITHET) and the diffusion and perfusion imaging evaluation for understanding stroke evolution (DEFUSE) study. Stroke. 2011;42(6):1608–14.
111. Wintermark M, Ko NU, Smith WS, Liu S, Higashida RT, Dillon WP. Vasospasm after subarachnoid hemorrhage: utility of perfusion CT and CT angiography on diagnosis and management. AJNR Am J Neuroradiol. 2006;27(1):26–34.

CT and MR Angiography of the Brain and Carotid Arteries

18

Cesur Samanci

18.1 CT Angiography of the Brain and Carotid Arteries

The brain CTA is from C1 to vertex and the neck CTA is from the aortic arch to C1. In stroke imaging, head and neck CTA is performed from aortic arch to vertex, including Willis. For reducing the volume of contrast material (CM) and to prevent venous opacification, CT scannings are caudocranial [1–5]. CTA is a must in acute cerebrovascular disease. It is important to demonstrate the patency of intracranial vascular structures and the stenosis in the carotid artery in transient ischemic attack or stroke patients. The stenosis-forming plaque in the carotid artery may be the source of emboli. Besides, CTA shows exactly which segment of the vessel is occluded in patients undergoing mechanical thrombectomy [6–8]. CTA is more preferred than MRA in acute cases because of its speed. Evaluation of CTA in the evaluation of carotid artery stenosis (more than 70%) has a high specificity and sensitivity [9–17]. Single section CTA is not widely used in patients with CAS (Fig. 18.1). This may be due to the use of more than 100 mL of CM and a slice thickness of more than 2 mm. MDCT has eliminated most of these limitations. In addition to the use of less dose of CA, it allows obtaining less than 1 mm slice thickness and high resolution (HR) images [18–20]. In addition, MDCTA can show carotid arteries from the aortic arch to Willis in <15 seconds (s), with 1 mm slice thickness, HR, and most importantly low-dose CA [19, 20]. As the technology progresses in radiology, it has become important to reduce the dose of the CA, along with the radiation dose, in such a way as not to affect the image quality. Another way to reduce the amount of contrast agent (CA) is to give saline bolus immediately after administration [21–25]. de Monyé et al. [18] compared different volumes of CM at 16 detector row computed tomographic CTA of the carotid arteries. Patients included in the study were divided into three groups: Group 1 80 mL CA, Group 2 80 mL CA followed by 40 mL saline, and Group 3 60 mL CA followed by 40 mL saline. The Hounsfield unit was measured from the ascending aorta and arteries from the aorta at 1-s intervals. The attenuation was measured more than the other groups in patients who received 40 mL of the saline bolus in 80 mL of contrast. In the group with 60 mL CA, attenuation was lower than the other groups. Kim and colleagues [26] developed a contrast dose protocol for CTA at 64 detector CT for the diagnosis of acute cerebrovascular disease. A 70 mL CA (iohexol, Omnipaque 350 mgI/mL) and 25 mL saline bolus were given at a rate of 5 mL/s for CTA. About 1 min after CTA, CE brain CT was performed. The purpose of this brain CT after CTA is to demonstrate incidental lesions, sub-

C. Samanci (✉)
Istanbul University Cerrahpaşa Medical Faculty
Radiology Department, Istanbul, Turkey

S. M. Erturk et al. (eds.), *Medical Imaging Contrast Agents: A Clinical Manual*,
https://doi.org/10.1007/978-3-030-79256-5_18

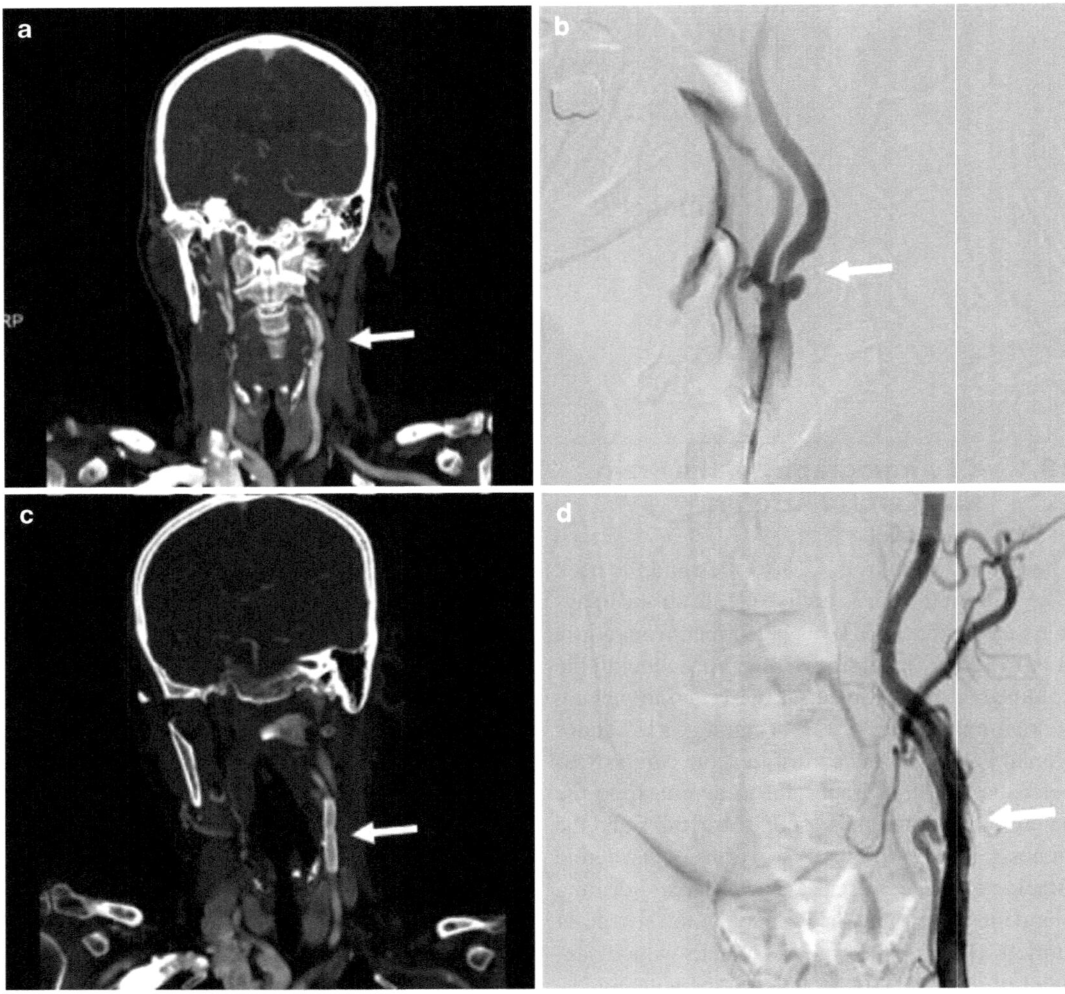

Fig. 18.1 CTA and digital subtraction angiography (DSA) of the carotid arteries before and after stenting. CTA MIP image (**a**) and DSA (**b**) of the left carotid artery stenosis before stenting. CTA MIP image (**c**) and DSA (**d**) of the left carotid artery after stenting

acute infarctions, hematoma, or contrast extravasation in aneurysm rupture. 150 mL of contrast medium (CM) is used (2 × 40 mL for CT perfusion and 70 mL for CTA). The total time of the procedure is approximately 8 min and the timing of contrast injection is very important for the best filling of the arteries. CA can be given with a delay of approximately 25 s. Since blood flow dynamics will change from patient to patient, it is useful to use the bolus tracking method especially in 64 section CT [26–29]. In a study by Kayan et al. [30], image resolution of carotid and cerebral CTA with a low voltage and low dose of CA was evaluated. Subjects were divided into two groups. CTA was performed with high-dose CA (1 mL/kg) and high-voltage (100 kv) in the first group and with low-dose CA (0.5 mL/kg) and low voltage (80 kv) in the second group. CA (iopromide, Ultravist 370, Bayer Schering Pharma, Berlin, Germany) with 370 mg iodine was used in both groups. The attenuation values were measured as HU from the lumen of the arteries and 300 HU and above were accepted as good image quality. The attenuation values were over 300 in both groups. In other words, it is possible to perform carotid and cerebral CTA with low voltage and low CA with 128-detector CT. Thus, possible nephropathy and possible damaging effects of radiation are reduced. In another study about the reduction of the dose of CA, in one group cerebral CTA was performed with a moderate concentration of CA and 80 kV protocol, while the other group received a high concentration of CA with 120 kV [31]. Moderate concentration of CA with 80 kV protocol has better arterial opacification, has better signal to noise and contrast to noise ratios than a high concentration of CA with 120 kV protocol. Also, the iodine used in the low contrast group is about 18.9% less than the other group. Besides, subjective image quality is better, although less iodine is used. So giving less CA can reduce the risk of CIN, because it has less osmolality and less viscosity [31]. Similar to these studies, Nagayama et al. [32] demonstrate that under the 80 kVp (296 mgI/kg) with sinogram affirmed iterative reconstruction protocol, both the radiation and the CM dose were substantially reduced at cerebral bone subtraction CTA and that the image quality was better than on scans obtained with the standard 120 kVp (CA was 370 mgI/kg) with FBP protocol. In another study [33], the authors investigated results of low concentration CAs in craniocervical dual-energy CTA using a monoenergetic reconstruction method. In the first group, high concentration CA was used (iopromide 370) and in the second group low concentration CA was used (iopromide 270). Image qualities were comparable. So contrast dose could be reduced by the monoenergetic reconstruction method in craniocervical dual-energy CTA. Hinkmann et al. [34] evaluated the efficacy of low-dose contrast in carotid CTA using 128 slice ultra-fast (with a gantry rotation time of 300 ms) spiral CT. One group was studied with 80 mL contrast at a rate of 5 mL/s, while another group was studied with a 30 mL contrast, at a rate of 4 mL/s, followed by saline flushes in two groups. They used the test-bolus technique to calculate transit time in both groups. They showed that 30 mL of CM was sufficient to show arterial stenosis, vascular contrast density, and image quality.

In MDCTA volume of CA is related to the time of the procedure which is dependent on detector numbers [35].

50–100 mL CA containing about 350–370 mg iodine are used in carotid and cerebral CTAs depending on the patient size and speed of the scanner [36]. To achieve CTA attenuation of 250–350 HU for a 70 kg patient, 35 g iodine was administered at 1.4 g of iodine/s (100 mL of 350 mg of iodine/mL concentration at 4 mL/s) over 25 s is suggested for 16 detector CT, while 25 g of iodine injected at 1.6 g of iodine/s (75 mL of 350 mg of iodine/mL concentration at 4.5–5.0 mL/s) over 15 s is suggested for 64 detector CT, followed by a saline flush. When administration rates are decreased for a given CM volume to prolong the injection time for slower CT scanners, the magnitude of contrast enhancement will decline, if a higher iodine concentration CA is not given. Injection time appropriate to scan time may be estimated by using an approach, 15 s + (1/2) scan time. Speed of 4 mL/s is suggested for a 70 kg adult (slower injection for a smaller subject but faster for a larger subject), with a saline flush. In MDCT, a fixed delay time of 18–20 s is used for the cerebral CTA, 15 s for the carotid CTA [5]. Although the values are not certain, the duration of the injection is 15–20 s and the screening time can be 5–15 s. However, these values may not be appropriate even in an individual with normal circulation parameters. Therefore, it is important to use variable scan delays that allow variations to the patient while shooting. If it was assumed that the time to the peak contrast enhancement at the carotid artery is similar to the ascending aorta, the variable scan delay for carotid CTA may be determined as injection time + 5 − (1/2) scan time for an injection time more than 15 s or as 15 + (1/2) injection time − (1/2) scan time for an injection time 15 s or less (for a short injection, the CM transit time is governed more by intrinsic physiological circulation time of CM bolus than the injection time). Scan delay for cerebral CTA only is obtained by adding 3–5 s to carotid CTA. According to the patient's circulation, we use region of interest (ROI) to determine the scan delay. If we are going to perform carotid and cerebral CTA, we put the ROI in ascending aorta, if we want to perform a cerebral only CTA, we place ROI over the aortic arch or mid carotid artery. When 12 s is used as the normal default value for CM arrival time in aortic arch, the time to peak aortic enhancement corresponds to injection time + (CM arrival time − 12) + (5 s) or injection time + CM arrival time − (7 s). So, at CM arrival time equals 12, the circulation adjusted and variable delay approaches become equivalent. CM arrival time would increase in subjects with slow circulation. From the equation, scan delay can be computed as injection time + CM arrival time − (7 s) − (1/2) scan time. For example, for a 10-s scan with a 20-s injection, scan delay would be 20 + CM arrival time − 7 − (10/2) or CM arrival time + 8. So, scan delay is determined by adding 8 s to CM arrival time measured from a test-bolus technique. On the other hand, when a bolus tracking technique is used, CM arrival time is not estimated prior to the injection of a full bolus of CM. CT scan will start at CM arrival time + 8, that is, 8 s of additional diagnostic delay after a time of reaching 50 HU enhancement threshold [36, 37]. A longer diagnostic delay will be required for a faster scan, a longer injection, and the brain-only CTA triggered at aorta but the scan started more distally at C1 level. MDCTA is a widely used method for brain imaging, especially in stroke (Fig. 18.2). However, in the 64-detector CT, the *z*-axis coverage is 3.2 cm and only allows for perfusion in small brain tissue around Willis and does not permit the evaluation of whole-brain circulation by dynamic angiography. Ruiz et al. [38] performed a whole head dynamic CTA using a 16 cm *z*-axis coverage with 320 detector MDCT in a patient with stenosis in the carotid. In addition to perfusion of the whole brain, all the vascular structures in the brain were demonstrated with dynamic subtracted angiography. CT with 320 detectors has uniquely increased *z*-axis coverage and is a very important innovation for all brain perfusion and subtracted dynamic angiography. It has a very important place in the first intention imaging of neurovascular diseases, especially in stroke [38].

When talking about CAs, it is even important that the CA is delivered from the right arm or the left arm. The purpose of the authors in a paper was to demonstrate the results of right and left-sided CA injection and mutual effects on the subject's age, gender, body weight, and arterial opacification in carotid and cerebral angiography. Their findings support preferential right-sided injection in subjects older than 40 years who have higher body mass index and weight in CTA procedures [39].

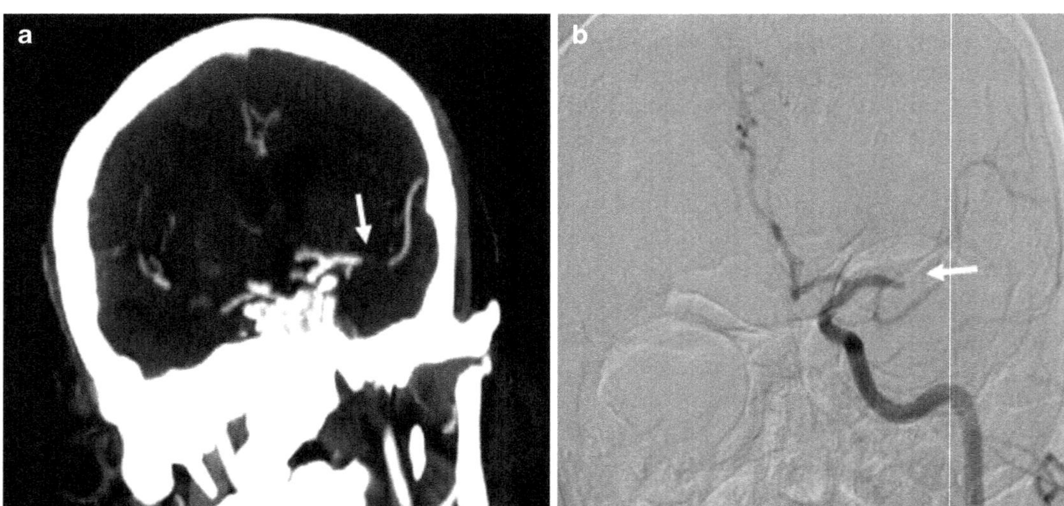

Fig. 18.2 CTA MIP image (**a**) and DSA (**b**) showing occlusion of left MCA M1segment

CE cone-beam CT plays an important role in stent imaging especially in patients with stent implantation due to intracranial aneurysm. Currently applied CE cone-beam CT images require a quantitative dilution of the CA to improve image quality. In a study, it was shown that this technique could be performed without quantitative contrast dilution. CM dilution for high image quality can be achieved from quantitative contrast infusion (0.2 cm^3/s) with saline flushes through a guiding catheter and using normal blood flow. Saline flush with a 300 mmHg pressure bag is suggested to show the relationship between stent strut and the parent artery and stent architecture [40].

Doerfler et al. [41] wanted to clarify whether iopromide, a nonionic CA, is safe in stroke. In their study rats underwent endovascular occlusion of the middle cerebral artery. Four hours later, they received iothalamate sodium and iopromide. Iopromide (Ultravist 370; Schering, Berlin, Germany) is available as a stable, clean, and colorless aqueous solution for parenteral injection; it has an iodine content of 370 mg/mL. The osmolality of the nonionic, monomeric solution was 770 mOsm per kilogram of water. Iothalamate sodium (Conray 70; Mallinckrodt, Hennef, Germany) is an ionic, iodinated CA that is available as an aqueous solution for parenteral injection; it has 420 mg/mL iodine. Lothalamate sodium contains sodium salt of iothalamic acid. The adequate dose is 588 mg of iodine per kilogram body weight. The osmolality of the solution was 2520 mOsm per kilogram of water. Bolus injection of the nonionic iopromide does not statistically significantly affect infarction volume or cerebral ischemia symptoms. The ionic CA iothalamate sodium caused higher mortality and morbidity and increased infarction volume in rats. Nonionic rather than ionic CAs should be preferred during acute cerebral ischemia.

While the carotid CTA is performed, the CA from the arm is not yet diluent, so it causes perivenous artifacts especially at the level of the subclavian vein, brachiocephalic vein, and superior vena cava [42, 43]. These artifacts cause a possible pathology to be missed in the main arteries originating from the aortic arch. In one study, the authors tested how these perivenous artifacts were affected by the craniocaudal scan direction and the caudocranial scan direction. In CTAs with 16-detector MDCT, low attenuation in the carotid artery and low attenuation in superior vena cava were obtained in the craniocaudal direction. Streak artifacts were significantly decreased and a better evaluation was obtained in the arteries originating from the arch [44].

Since the autopsy is highly traumatic for the family of the deceased person, it is particularly undesirable for the relatives of the deceased. Postmortem imaging may be a good alternative to autopsy and is now becoming increasingly popular. There is a lot of research on this subject, for example, Ross et al. [45] have tried to establish a contrast protocol for whole body CTA. They evaluated the results by comparing lipophilic and hydrophilic CAs. In the first group, paraffin oil and iodized oil (Lipiodol Ultra Fluide, Guerbet) were used in a ratio of 15/1. In the other group, the PEG solution (PEG 200, Schaerer-Schlaepfer AG) and iopentol (Imagopaque 300, GE-Healthcare) were perfused to be 10/1 (average density 600 HU). In these images, end portions of vascular structures and small extravasations were shown better than those in alive patients.

An inguinal incision was made before imaging and retrograde cannulation in femoral artery and antegrade cannulation in femoral vein was performed. 2000 mL was perfusion volume, 80 mmHg was perfusion pressure, 800 mL/min was flow rate for head and neck CTA. Postmortem angiography using PEG is successful in visualizing tissues showing good vascularization and prevents unintended gastrointestinal extravasation [45].

18.2 MR Angiography of the Brain and Carotid Arteries

CE MRI can show many pathologies that are not seen in non-CE imaging [46–52]. In 1988, Gd-DTPA (Magnevist), the first specific CA that is compatible with MRI, was released [53]. These MR-compatible CAs showed considerable variation over time. These extracellular, gadolinium-based CAs show kidney excretion and are increasingly used in routine clinical practice over the years. Gadoterate was introduced in 1989, gadoteridol in 1992, gadodiamide (Omniscan) in 1993, gadobutrol in 1998, and gadoversetamide (Optimark) in 1999. In addition to these CAs, gadobenate which was received by hepatocytes in the liver was released in 1998 and gadoxetic acid was introduced in 2005. CAs that contain gadofosveset and very small super-paramagnetic iron oxide (USPIO) particles can be used in MRA because they can remain in the vessel for a long time [54]. Gadolinium-based CAs are divided according to their ability to shorten relaxation time and their level of accumulation in tissue. Gadobutrol is the only gadolinium-based CA formulated as 1.0 m, which accumulates more in tissue and is twice the concentration of other agents. Due to its high relaxation, it is the maximum T1 shortening CA per volume [55–57].

When using the CA in MRA, the SNR increases, the flow and motion artifacts are reduced, because the paramagnetic Gd reduces the T1 relaxation time [58]. Evaluating the vessel lumen using the T1 sequence which is not affected by flow artifacts removes many problems in TOF or flow-based MR sequences. Turbulence decreases, resolution increases, high-speed MRA images with high SNR are obtained. If Gd is given at a high injection rate, the concentration increases, SNR increases, but if the concentration increases too much, it can reduce the signal with T2* effect. The T2* effects start if the injection is faster than 5 mL/s. It is necessary not to change the Gd concentration during the process because this may cause a ringing artifact. Also, if we make an injection with high speed for a long time, this causes too much Gd usage and high cost. It should also not exceed the FDA limit. For this reason, it would be correct to make an injection at a rate of 2–3 mL/s in less than the scan time to maximize the injection rate while keeping the dose minimum.

Although DSA is the gold standard in CS evaluation [59], it is an invasive method and non-invasive methods such as Doppler US, MRA, and CTA have come to the fore. Although there is no clear consensus about exactly what is the best option, MRA, CTA, and Doppler US is widely used in the diagnosis of CS. Since the 1990s, TOF MR has been used to detect CS with a specificity and sensitivity of more than 70% [60–62]. CE MRA can cover more of the carotid artery distribution in a fraction of time that TOF MRA is needed. Although there are plenty of papers, the optimal protocol for carotid CE MRA is still controversial.

Willinek et al. [63] compared CE MRA and DSA in the evaluation of lesions in supra-aortic arteries. They found the specificity, sensitivity, positive predictive value, and negative predictive value of CE MRA in detecting 70–90% stenosis was 99.3%, 100%, 93.6%, 100%, respectively. The same parameters were calculated as 100%, 100%, 100%, and 100% in the same order when evaluating the CE MRA occlusion. In this study, 0.2 mmol/kg Gd was used with an infusion rate of 3 mL/s, followed by 30 mL saline bolus. CE MRA, which is a noninvasive method in supra-aortic strictures, seems to be a good alternative to replace DSA.

Because of the complications such as nephrogenic systemic fibrosis which may develop after the use of CA, CAs should be used at the lowest dose or as low as possible. For this reason, methods such as TOF, which is an MRA protocol without CA become popular.

Fellner et al. [64] compared 3D TOF MRI with HR CE MRI and time-resolved CE MRA in the evaluation of carotid stenosis. When evaluating these three methods, they used DSA and endarterectomy specimens as the gold standard. The sensitivity of all MR methods in severe stenosis was 100%, while the specificity of 3D TOF MRI, HR CE MRI, and time-resolved CE MRA were 96.7%, 80.6%, and 83.9%, respectively. While 3D TOF MRI is better than others in grading stenosis at carotid bifurcation level, the best option should be to combine these methods. However, according to this study, TOF MRI seems to be adequate when evaluating the carotid arteries if the contrast administration is risky. If we evaluate how CA is used in contrast-enhanced MRA sequences in this study: In HR CE MRA, 25 mL of Gd-DTPA was given with a speed of 2 mL/s. Timing for the HR CE sequence was performed with fluoroscopic triggering at one image/s. 3D MRA sequence was started manually when CA was seen in the common carotid arteries on the fluoroscopy. In time-resolved CE MRA four data sets were acquired consecutively, resulting in a timing interval of 10 s between successive data sets; no data sharing or temporal interpolation was employed. Instead of a dedicated timing procedure, measurement of the sequence and the injection of 15 mL of Gd-DTPA (2 mL/s) were started simultaneously. The data set showing the optimal arterial phase was selected afterward.

For the more widespread use of MRI in patients with stroke, the speed of MRI acquisition should be increased. In a study [65] conducted on the feasibility of low-dose CE MRA and dynamic contrast perfusion without extra CM, a total of 0.1 mmol/kg of Gd was given to patients (0.05 mmol/kg for CE MRA, 0.05 mmol/kg for dynamic contrast perfusion). This 0.1 mmol/kg CM was diluted with saline to a total of 50 mL. Transit time to the carotid artery was calculated with 3 mL of this 50 mL CM by flashing 20 mL of saline, and then 22 mL of contrast was flushed with 20 mL saline and CE MRA was performed. In this process, the contrast rate is set to 1.5 mL/s. The remaining 25 mL contrast was flushed with 20 mL saline and MR perfusion was performed. Here, the speed of contrast is set to 5 mL/s. In the full-dose group, the same procedure was performed without dilution. The half-dose CM group and full-dose CM group were compared with the DSA results and there was no significant difference between the two groups in terms of SNR, maximum T2 * effect, and detecting the degree of arterial stenosis.

In a study comparing 2D TOF MRA and CE MRA in patients with hemodynamically significant carotid stenosis [66], no significant difference was found between these two methods. In CE MRA, they gave 0.01 mmol/kg (or 0.2 mg/kg) CM as a single dose of 20 mL at a rate of 3 mL/s. Although CE MRA showed neurovascular structures better than 2D TOF MRA in this study, Gd administration did not provide any advantage in carotid stenosis requiring surgical treatment. Therefore, 2D TOF MRI may be sufficient to evaluate carotid stenosis patients with renal problems.

In a study [67], 3D HR MRA of supra-aortic arteries was performed with 3 T MRI scanner with three different contrast regimens, and patients were divided into three groups: high dose (group A), moderate dose (group B), and low dose (group C). Group A received 0.154 mmol/kg, group B received 0.097 mmol/kg, and group C received 0.047 mmol/kg Gd-DTPA. Incrementally, CA dose decreased from an initial dose of 12.5 mmol Gd-DTPA (0.5 mmol/mL in 25 mL) to 7.5 mmol and then to 3.875 mmol, based on clinical observation of the stability of image quality. In all dose levels, infusion time was fixed at 15 s, corresponding to 0.8 mmol/s for group A, 0.5 mmol/s for group B, and 0.25 mmol/s for group C. For the group B and C, CM was diluted with normal saline by factors of two and three, respectively, to maintain equivalent injected volumes and rates. According to the results of the study, it is possible to demonstrate the supra-aortic arteries at 3 T MRI with 3D CE MRA at a low CM dose of 0.047 mmol/kg without reducing the image quality.

Jung et al. [68] performed a study to determine the optimal dose of Gd-DTPA for CE MRA of intracranial vascular diseases. In this study, subjects suspected of having intracranial vascular diseases had cerebral MR angiograms on a 1.5 T unit. Patients were randomly assigned to receive one of four doses of Gd-DTPA (Magnevist; Schering, Berlin, Germany): 36 subjects received no injection, 37 received 5 mL (0.04 0.06 mmoVkg), 38 received 10 mL (0.08 0.12 mmoVkg), and 11 received 20 mL (0.15 0.25 mmol/kg). The other 30 subjects had unenhanced and CE MR angiography (10 subjects each for the 5 ml, 10 ml, and 20 ml groups). CE MR angiograms were obtained immediately after IV injection of a bolus of gadopentetate dimeglumine. 5–10 mL of Gd-DTPA appears to be sufficient for CE cerebral MR angiography. Injection of 20 mL of the CM frequently limited visualization of the major arteries because of venous overlap. 5–10 mL of Gd-DTPA appears to be an optimal dose range for CE cerebral MRA. Use of this dose can help in differentiating true stenosis of large arteries from artifactual narrowing and in depicting small arteriovenous malformation with a slow flow.

TOF MRI is a very popular method since it does not require contrast and is used in the diagnosis of cerebral aneurysms. In a study [69], authors compared TOF MRA and CE MRA using the elliptical centric method with the 3 T MR scanner for the diagnosis of cerebral aneurysms. Using 2 mL of gadoteridol and 20 mL of saline flush, the time between injection and reaching of CM to the skull base level was calculated. 25 mL of gadoteridol followed by 25 mL of saline flush was given at 2 mL/s. In terms of image quality, TOF MRA was shown to be superior (Fig. 18.3).

In another similar study, 3D TOF MRA and CE MRA were used to evaluate cerebral aneurysms treated with flow diverter stents [70]. In the CE MRA process, 20 mL bolus CM followed by 30 mL saline flush was used. This time, CE MRA was found to be superior to TOF MRI in subjects such as the presence of residual filling in the aneurysm and parent artery patency (Fig. 18.4). If we look at how the contrast should be used in the MRA when grading cerebral AVMs [71], in 3 T MRI, with a two-cylinder injector, the Gd-DTPA in one cylinder and saline in the other cylinder is prepared then 20 mL Gd is given at 5 mL/s, followed by 40 mL of saline flush. With this protocol, in the CE MRA, the feeders, draining veins, and nidus of the AVM can be shown clearly.

There is a manganese-based alternative to Gd. Gale et al. [72] compared iv contrast enhancement produced by the manganese-based MRI CA manganese N picolyl N,N′,N′ trans 1,2 cyclohexenediaminetriacetate (Mn PyC3A) to Gd-DTPA and evaluated the excretion, pharmacokinetics, and metabolism of Mn PyC3A in baboons. Mn PyC3A was eliminated via renal and hepatobiliary excretion with similar pharmacokinetics to Gd-DTPA. High-performance liquid chromatography revealed no evidence of Mn PyC3A biotransformation. Mn PyC3A enables CE MRA with comparable contrast enhancement to Gd-based agents and may overcome concerns regarding Gd-associated toxicity and retention. Mn PyC3A may enable CE MRA in subjects with renal insufficiency who are currently contraindicated for Gd-based CAs.

New MR protocols and new CAs that are constantly evolving provide the opportunity to

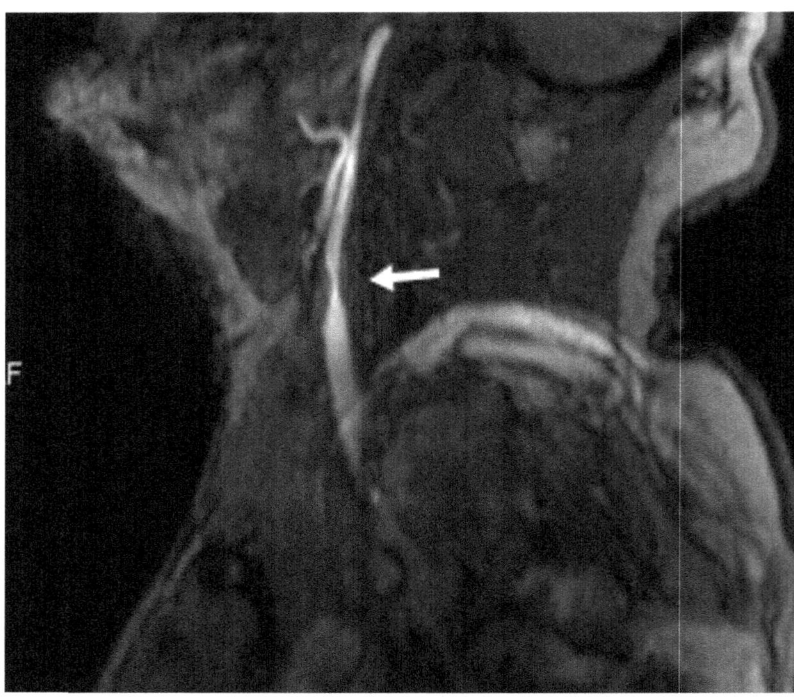

Fig. 18.3 2D TOF MRA showing stenosis in left ICA (arrow)

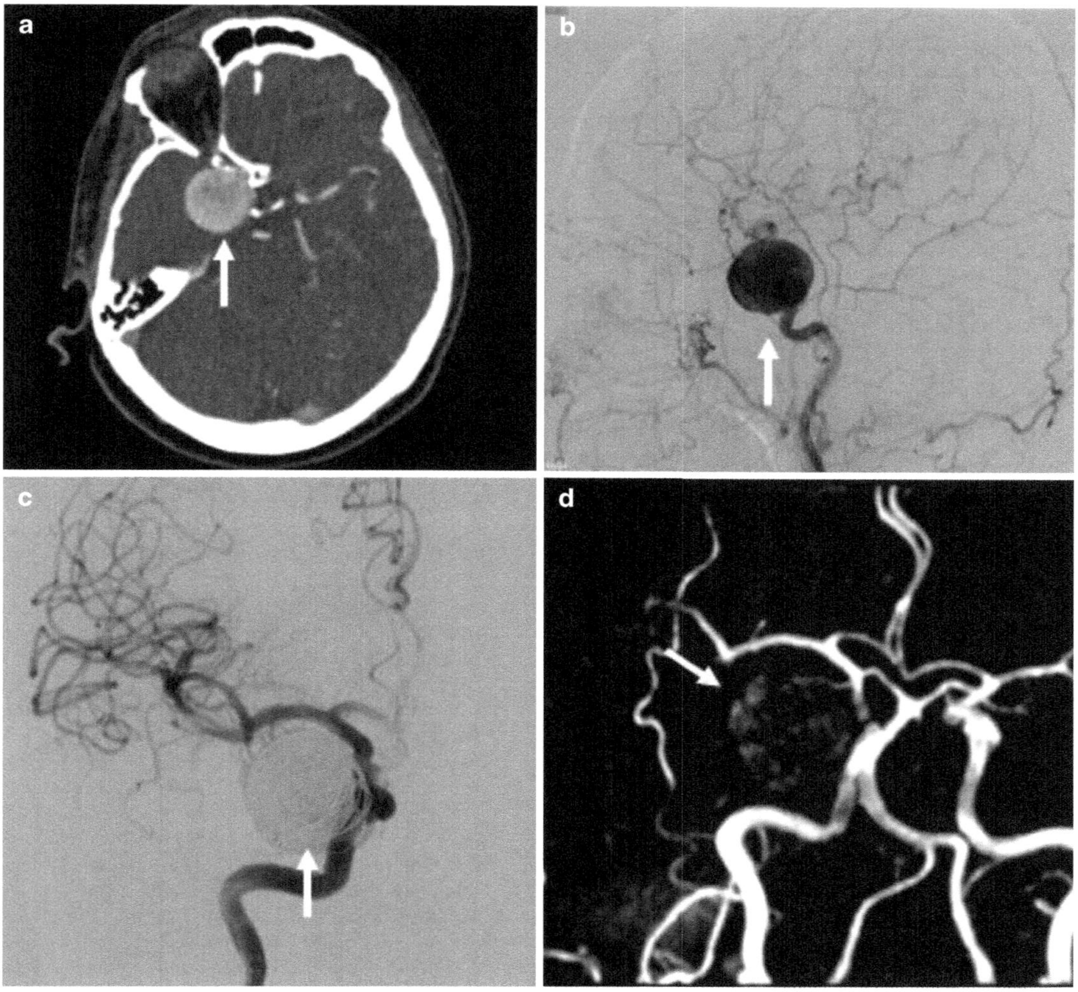

Fig. 18.4 CTA (**a**) and selective DSA of the right internal carotid artery (**b**) before treatment reveals a giant carotid ophthalmic aneurysm. DSA (**c**) and 2D TOF MRA (**d**) of the same aneurysm after coil embolization

receive radio anatomic or physiopathological additional information. It is extremely wrong to think that the positive acceleration progress in radiology especially in recent years has come to an end. We believe that new developments will cause a revision of some information in this section in the near future.

References

1. Orrison WW Jr, Snyder KV, Hopkins LN, et al. Whole-brain dynamic CT angiography and perfusion imaging. Clin Radiol. 2011;66(6):566–74.
2. Creasy JL, Price RR, Presbrey T, Goins D, Partain CL, Kessler RM. Gadolinium-enhanced MR angiography. Radiology. 1990;175(1):280–3.
3. Marchal G, Bosmans H, Van PH, Jiang YB, Aerts P, Bauer H. Experimental Gd-DTPA polylysine enhanced MR angiography: sequence optimization. J Comput Assist Tomogr. 1991;15(4):711–5.
4. Brenner DJ, Hricak H. Radiation exposure from medical imaging: time to regulate? JAMA. 2010;304(2):208–9.
5. Enterline DS, Kapoor G. A practical approach to CT angiography of the neck and brain. Tech Vasc Interv Radiol. 2006;9(4):192–204.
6. Koelemay MJ, Nederkoorn PJ, Reitsma JB, Majoie CB. Systematic review of computed tomographic angiography for assessment of carotid artery disease. Stroke. 2004;35(10):2306–12.

7. Schellinger PD, Fiebach JB, Hacke W. Imaging-based decision making in thrombolytic therapy for ischemic stroke: present status. Stroke. 2003;34(2):575–83.
8. Truwit CL. CT angiography versus MR angiography in the evaluation of acute neurovascular disease. Radiology. 2007;245(2):362–6.
9. Nederkoorn PJ, Mali WPTM, Eikelboom BC, et al. Preoperative diagnosis of carotid artery stenosis: accuracy of noninvasive testing. Stroke. 2002;33(8):2003–8.
10. Napel S, Marks MP, Rubin GD, et al. CT angiography with spiral CT and maximum intensity projection. Radiology. 1992;185(2):607–10.
11. Katz DA, Marks MP, Napel SA, Bracci PM, Roberts SL. Circle of Willis: evaluation with spiral CT angiography, MR angiography, and conventional angiography. Radiology. 1995;195(2):445–9.
12. Hollingworth W, Nathens AB, Kanne JP, et al. The diagnostic accuracy of computed tomography angiography for traumatic or atherosclerotic lesions of the carotid and vertebral arteries: a systematic review. Eur J Radiol. 2003;48(1):88–102.
13. Dillon EH, Van Leeuwen MS, Fernandez MA, Eikelboom BC, Mali WP. CT angiography: application to the evaluation of carotid artery stenosis. Radiology. 1993;189(1):211–9.
14. Cumming MJ, Morrow IM. Carotid artery stenosis: a prospective comparison of CT angiography and conventional angiography. AJR Am J Roentgenol. 1994;163(3):517–23.
15. Link J, Brossmann J, Grabener M, et al. Spiral CT angiography and selective digital subtraction angiography of internal carotid artery stenosis. Am J Neuroradiol. 1996;17(1):89–94.
16. Marcus CD, Ladam-Marcus VJ, Bigot JL, Clement C, Baehrel B, Menanteau BP. Carotid arterial stenosis: evaluation at CT angiography with the volume-rendering technique. Radiology. 1999;211(3):775–80.
17. Leclerc X, Godefroy O, Lucas C, et al. Internal carotid arterial stenosis: CT angiography with volume rendering. Radiology. 1999;210(3):673–82.
18. de Monyé C, Cademartiri F, de Weert TT, Siepman DA, Dippel DW, van Der Lugt A. Sixteen–detector row CT angiography of carotid arteries: comparison of different volumes of contrast material with and without a bolus chaser. Radiology. 2005;237(2):555–62.
19. Lell M, Wildberger JE, Heuschmid M, et al. CT-angiographie der A. carotis: erste erfahrungen mit einem 16-schicht-spiral-CT. In: RöFo-Fortschritte auf dem Gebiet der Röntgenstrahlen und der bildgebenden Verfahren 2002. Vol. 174, No. 09, p. 1165–69.
20. Ertl-Wagner B, Hoffmann RT, Brüning R, Dichgans M, Reiser MF. Supraaortale Gefäßdiagnostik mit dem 16-Zeilen-Multidetektor-Spiral-CT. Untersuchungsprotokoll und erste Erfahrungen. Radiologe. 2002;42(9):728–32.
21. Irie T, Kajitani M, Yamaguchi M, Itai Y. Contrast-enhanced CT with saline flush technique using two automated injectors: how much contrast medium does it save? J Comput Assist Tomogr. 2002;26(2):287–91.
22. Cademartiri F, van der Lugt A, Luccichenti G, Pavone P, Krestin GP. Parameters affecting bolus geometry in CTA: a review. J Comput Assist Tomogr. 2002;26(4):598–607.
23. Haage P, Schmitz-Rode T, Hübner D, Piroth W, Gunther RW. Reduction of contrast material dose and artifacts by a saline flush using a double power injector in helical CT of the thorax. Am J Roentgenol. 2000;174(4):1049–53.
24. Hopper KD, Mosher TJ, Kasales CJ, TenHave TR, Tully DA, Weaver JS. Thoracic spiral CT: delivery of contrast material pushed with injectable saline solution in a power injector. Radiology. 1997;205(1):269–71.
25. Cademartiri F, Mollet N, van der Lugt A, et al. Non-invasive 16-row multislice CT coronary angiography: usefulness of saline chaser. Eur Radiol. 2004;14(2):178–83.
26. Kim JJ, Dillon WP, Glastonbury CM, Provenzale JM, Wintermark M. Sixty-four-section multidetector CT angiography of carotid arteries: a systematic analysis of image quality and artifacts. Am J Neuroradiol. 2010;31(1):91–9.
27. Bae KT. Test-bolus versus bolus-tracking techniques for CT angiographic timing. Radiology. 2005;236(1):369.
28. Cademartiri F, Nieman K, van der Lugt A, et al. Intravenous contrast material administration at 16–detector row helical CT coronary angiography: test bolus versus bolus-tracking technique. Radiology. 2004;233(3):817–23.
29. Hallett RL, Fleischmann D. Tools of the trade for CTA: MDCT scanners and contrast medium injection protocols. Tech Vasc Interv Radiol. 2006;9(4):134–42.
30. Kayan M, Demirtas H, Türker Y, et al. Carotid and cerebral CT angiography using low volume of iodinated contrast material and low tube voltage. Diagn Interv Imaging. 2016;97(11):1173–9.
31. Cho ES, Chung TS, Oh DK, et al. Computed tomography angiography using a low tube voltage (80 kVp) and a moderate concentration of iodine contrast material: a quantitative and qualitative comparison with conventional computed tomography angiography. Invest Radiol. 2012;47(2):142–7.
32. Nagayama Y, Nakaura T, Tsuji A, et al. Cerebral bone subtraction CT angiography using 80 kVp and sinogram-affirmed iterative reconstruction: contrast medium and radiation dose reduction with improvement of image quality. Neuroradiology. 2017;59(2):127–34.
33. Zhao L, Li F, Zhang Z. Assessment of an advanced virtual monoenergetic reconstruction technique in cerebral and cervical angiography with third-generation dual-source CT: feasibility of using low-concentration contrast medium. Eur Radiol. 2018;28(10):4379–88.
34. Hinkmann FM, Voit HL, Anders K. Ultra-fast carotid CT-angiography: low versus standard volume contrast material protocol for a 128-slice CT-system. Invest Radiol. 2009;44(5):257–64.

35. Saba L, Sanfilippo R, Pirisi R, Pascalis L, Montisci R, Mallarini G. Multidetector-row CT angiography in the study of atherosclerotic carotid arteries. Neuroradiology. 2007;49(8):623–37.
36. Bae KT. Intravenous contrast medium administration and scan timing at CT: considerations and approaches. Radiology. 2010;256(1):32–61.
37. Bae KT, Heiken JP. Computer modeling approach to contrast medium administration and scan timing for multislice computed tomography. In: Multislice CT: a practical guide. Berlin, Heidelberg: Springer; 2001. p. 28–36.
38. Ruíz DSM, Murphy K, Gailloud P. 320-Multidetector row whole-head dynamic subtracted CT angiography and whole-brain CT perfusion before and after carotid artery stenting. Eur J Radiol. 2010;74(3):413–9.
39. Chang YM, Tsai AC, Gutierrez A. Effect of right-sided versus left-sided contrast injection on intra-arterial opacification characteristics of head and neck computed tomography angiograms and interactions with patient sex, weight, and cardiac output. J Comput Assist Tomogr. 2015;39(5):752–9.
40. Jo KI, Kim SR, Choi JH, Kim KH, Jeon P. Contrast-enhanced angiographic cone-beam computed tomography without pre-diluted contrast medium. Neuroradiology. 2015;57(11):1121–6.
41. Doerfler A, Engelhorn T, Von Kummer R. Are iodinated contrast agents detrimental in acute cerebral ischemia? An experimental study in rats. Radiology. 1998;206(1):211–7.
42. Rubin GD, Lane MJ, Bloch DA, Leung AN, Stark P. Optimization of thoracic spiral CT: effects of iodinated contrast medium concentration. Radiology. 1996;201(3):785–91.
43. Loubeyre P, Debard I, Nemoz C, Minh VAT. High opacification of hilar pulmonary vessels with a small amount of nonionic contrast medium for general thoracic CT: a prospective study. Am J Roentgenol. 2002;178(6):1377–81.
44. de Monyé C, de Weert TT, Zaalberg W, et al. Optimization of CT angiography of the carotid artery with a 16-MDCT scanner: craniocaudal scan direction reduces contrast material-related perivenous artifacts. Am J Roentgenol. 2006;186(6):1737–45.
45. Ross S, Spendlove D, Bolliger S, et al. Postmortem whole-body CT angiography: evaluation of two contrast media solutions. Am J Roentgenol. 2008;190(5):1380–9.
46. Moon M, Cornfeld D, Weinreb J. Dynamic contrast-enhanced breast MR imaging. Magn Reson Imaging Clin N Am. 2009;17(2):351–62.
47. Essig M, Dinkel J, Gutierrez JE. Use of contrast media in neuroimaging. Magn Reson Imaging Clin. 2012;20(4):633–48.
48. Yang S, Law M, Zagzag D, et al. Dynamic contrast-enhanced perfusion MR imaging measurements of endothelial permeability: differentiation between atypical and typical meningiomas. Am J Neuroradiol. 2003;24(8):1554–9.
49. Leiner T, Michaely H. Advances in contrast-enhanced MR angiography of the renal arteries. Magn Reson Imaging Clin N Am. 2008;16(4):561–72.
50. Keston P, Murray AD, Jackson A. Cerebral perfusion imaging using contrast-enhanced MRI. Clin Radiol. 2003;58(7):505–13.
51. Lima JA. Myocardial viability assessment by contrast-enhanced magnetic resonance imaging. J Am Coll Cardiol. 2003;42(5):902–4.
52. Catalano OA, Manfredi R, Vanzulli A, et al. MR arthrography of the glenohumeral joint: modified posterior approach without imaging guidance. Radiology. 2007;242(2):550–4.
53. Lohrke J, Frenzel T, Endrikat J, et al. 25 years of contrast-enhanced MRI: developments, current challenges and future perspectives. Adv Ther. 2016;33(1):1–28.
54. Bremerich J, Bilecen D, Reimer P. MR angiography with blood pool contrast agents. Eur Radiol. 2007;17(12):3017.
55. Sieber MA. Pharmaceutical and safety aspects of gadolinium-based contrast agents. 2009;15(6):24–6.
56. Rohrer M, Bauer H, Mintorovitch J, Requardt M, Weinmann HJ. Comparison of magnetic properties of MRI contrast media solutions at different magnetic field strengths. Invest Radiol. 2005;40(11):715–24.
57. Cheng KT, Cheng HY, Leung K. Clinical use of gadobutrol for contrast-enhanced magnetic resonance imaging of neurological diseases. Rep Med Imaging. 2012;5:15–22.
58. Zhang H, Maki JH, Prince MR. 3D contrast-enhanced MR angiography. J Magn Reson Imaging. 2007;25(1):13–25.
59. DeMarco JK, Huston J, Nash AK. Extracranial carotid MR imaging at 3T. Magn Reson Imaging Clin. 2006;14(1):109–21.
60. Anderson CM, Lee RE, Levin DL, De la Torre Alonso S, Saloner D. Measurement of internal carotid artery stenosis from source MR angiograms. Radiology. 1994;193(1):219–26.
61. Kent KC, Kuntz KM, Patel MR, et al. Perioperative imaging strategies for carotid endarterectomy: an analysis of morbidity and cost-effectiveness in symptomatic patients. JAMA. 1995;274(11):888–93.
62. Patel MR, Kuntz KM, Klufas RA, et al. Preoperative assessment of the carotid bifurcation: can magnetic resonance angiography and duplex ultrasonography replace contrast arteriography? Stroke. 1995;26(10):1753–8.
63. Willinek WA, von Falkenhausen M, Born M, et al. Noninvasive detection of steno-occlusive disease of the supra-aortic arteries with three-dimensional contrast-enhanced magnetic resonance angiography: a prospective, intra-individual comparative analysis with digital subtraction angiography. Stroke. 2005;36(1):38–43.
64. Fellner C, Lang W, Janka R, et al. Magnetic resonance angiography of the carotid arteries using three different techniques: accuracy compared with intraarterial

x-ray angiography and endarterectomy specimens. J Magn Reson Imaging. 2005;21(4):424–31.
65. Nael K, Meshksar A, Ellingson B, et al. Combined low-dose contrast-enhanced MR angiography and perfusion for acute ischemic stroke at 3T: a more efficient stroke protocol. Am J Neuroradiol. 2014;35(6):1078–84.
66. Babiarz LS, Romero JM, Murphy EK, et al. Contrast-enhanced MR angiography is not more accurate than unenhanced 2D time-of-flight MR angiography for determining ≥ 70% internal carotid artery stenosis. Am J Neuroradiol. 2009;30(4):761–8.
67. Tomasian A, Salamon N, Lohan DG, Jalili M, Villablanca JP, Finn JP. Supraaortic arteries: contrast material dose reduction at 3.0-T high-spatial-resolution MR angiography—feasibility study. Radiology. 2008;249(3):980–90.
68. Jung HW, Chang KH, Choi DS, Han MH, Han MC. Contrast-enhanced MR angiography for the diagnosis of intracranial vascular disease: optimal dose of gadopentetate dimeglumine. AJR Am J Roentgenol. 1995;165(5):1251–5.
69. Gibbs GF, Huston J III, Bernstein MA, Riederer SJ, Brown RD Jr. 3.0-Tesla MR angiography of intracranial aneurysms: comparison of time-of-flight and contrast-enhanced techniques. J Magn Reson Imaging. 2005;21(2):97–102.
70. Attali J, Benaissa A, Soize S, Kadziolka K, Portefaix C, Pierot L. Follow-up of intracranial aneurysms treated by flow diverter: comparison of three-dimensional time-of-flight MR angiography (3D-TOF-MRA) and contrast-enhanced MR angiography (CE-MRA) sequences with digital subtraction angiography as the gold standard. J Neurointerv Surg. 2016;8(1):81–6.
71. Oleaga L, Dalal SS, Weigele JB, et al. The role of time-resolved 3D contrast-enhanced MR angiography in the assessment and grading of cerebral arteriovenous malformations. Eur J Radiol. 2010;74(3):e117–21.
72. Gale EM, Wey HY, Ramsay I, Yen YF, Sosnovik DE, Caravan P. A manganese-based alternative to gadolinium: contrast-enhanced MR angiography, excretion, pharmacokinetics, and metabolism. Radiology. 2017;286(3):865–72.

Peripheral Contrast-Enhanced CT and MR Angiography

19

Shintaro Ichikawa

19.1 Introduction

Peripheral arterial occlusive disease (PAOD) is a common condition associated with arteriosclerosis that most commonly affects the lower extremities [1]. Luminal narrowing of the peripheral arteries is caused by progressive accumulation of plaque on the arterial wall. PAOD is a chronic, progressive disease in which the first and typical symptom is intermittent claudication that ultimately leads to organ ischemia or severe infection. The most severe forms of PAOD will require lower limb amputation, which markedly reduces the patient's quality of life. Diabetes mellitus is a major risk factor for PAOD, and its prevalence is increasing worldwide [2]. Therefore, the number of patients with PAOD will continue to increase in the future. Traditionally, surgical bypass has been the mainstream therapeutic choice for PAOD. Recently, endovascular treatment has become widely accepted as a routine treatment [3]. Along with the development of interventional techniques, detailed assessment of lesion localization or severity has been required before treatment. Digital subtraction angiography (DSA) has long been considered the reference standard for the assessment of PAOD; however, noninvasive imaging diagnostic tests such as computed tomography (CT) and magnetic resonance (MR) angiography have recently begun to play a crucial role in the planning and follow-up of treatment. Both of them provide complementary information; therefore, it is necessary to use both methods depending on the intended purpose. General features of contrast-enhanced CT and MR angiography are summarized in Table 19.1. This chapter focuses on imaging techniques,

Table 19.1 General features of contrast-enhanced CT and MR angiography

	CT angiography	MR angiography
Contrast agents	Iodine-based	Gadolinium-based
Availability	High	Low
Scan time	Shorter	Longer
Radiation exposure	With	Without
Toxicity of contrast agents	Contrast-induced nephropathy	Nephrogenic systemic fibrosis
Cost	Cost-effective	Costly
Diagnostic accuracy	High	High
Evaluation of calcification	Possible	Impossible
Evaluation of severely calcified lesions	Difficult	Possible
Evaluation of critical limb ischemia	Difficult	Possible

S. Ichikawa (✉)
Department of Radiology, Hamamatsu University School of Medicine, Hamamatsu, Japan
e-mail: shintaro@hama-med.ac.jp

S. M. Erturk et al. (eds.), *Medical Imaging Contrast Agents: A Clinical Manual*,
https://doi.org/10.1007/978-3-030-79256-5_19

advantages, and drawbacks of peripheral contrast-enhanced CT and MR angiography.

19.2 CT Angiography (Fig. 19.1)

19.2.1 General Features

CT angiography is a quick, noninvasive imaging modality with excellent spatial and temporal resolution. Recent CT scanners can provide submillimeter isotropic three-dimensional (3D) datasets during the first pass of intravenous iodine-based contrast medium, and 3D visualization of the vascular abnormalities using the datasets helps to plan and guide interventions. The diagnostic performance of CT angiography in PAOD has been reported to be very high (sensitivity and specificity were 92–99% and 93–99%, respectively) [4–7]. However, the image quality of the peripheral artery tends to be lower than that of abdominal level arteries (Fig. 19.2). CT angiography is excellent in the detection of calcification and useful for evaluating the properties of arterial walls. In patients with indications for surgery or endovascular treatment, the presence or absence of calcification and its degree are indispensable information. For example, vascular anastomosis at severe calcification sites is difficult. In the case of percutaneous transluminal angioplasty, when a balloon with a larger diameter is selected at severe calcification sites, vascular injuries may result. On the other hand, CT angiography has some drawbacks such as radiation exposure, use of nephrotoxic iodine-based contrast medium, and blooming artifacts.

19.2.2 Protocol

More than 16-row CT scanners are adequate for CT angiography. Obtaining satisfactory arterial enhancement is crucial for CT angiography. Optimizing intravenous contrast medium administration is important in obtaining strong arterial enhancement during CT angiography. There are three adjustable factors that determine arterial

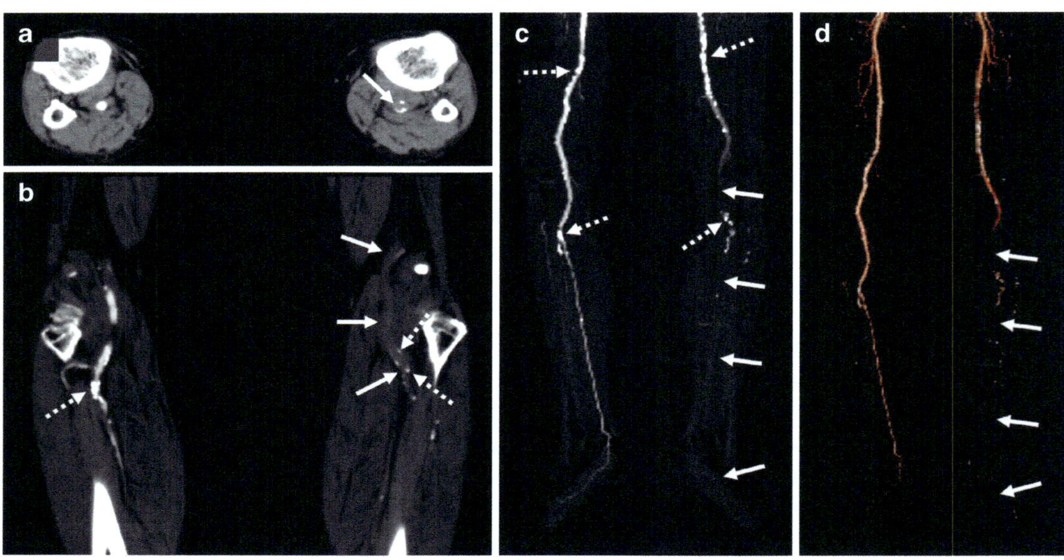

Fig. 19.1 CT angiography of an 80-year-old man with PAOD. (**a**) Axial image, (**b**) coronal image, (**c**) MIP image, (**d**) VR image. CT angiography shows a lengthy left popliteal artery to below-the-knee artery occlusion (arrows) with severe arterial wall calcification (dotted arrows). CT angiography demonstrates diffuse severe arterial wall calcification in the bilateral superficial femoral arteries thus rendering the evaluation of the arterial lumen very difficult (**c**). It is difficult to evaluate the foot arteries in detail because of their low contrast (**c**, **d**). *CT* computed tomography, *PAOD* peripheral arterial occlusive disease, *MIP* maximum intensity projection, *VR* volume rendering

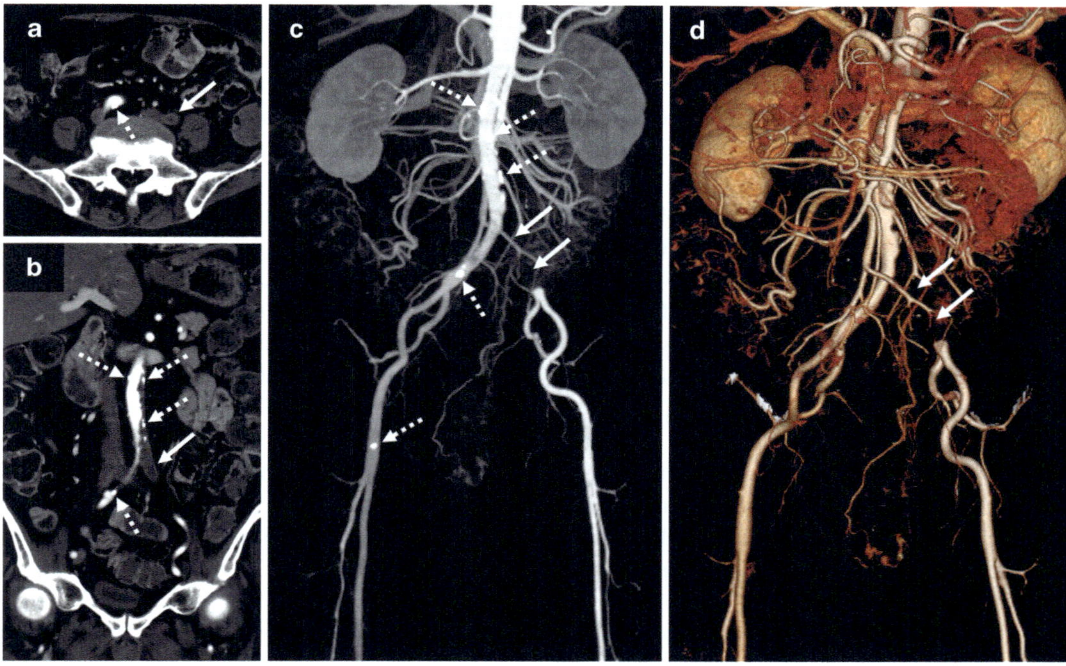

Fig. 19.2 CT angiography of a 75-year-old man with a common iliac artery occlusion. (**a**) Axial image, (**b**) coronal image, (**c**) MIP image, (**d**) VR image. CT angiography shows a lengthy left common iliac artery occlusion (arrows). CT is excellent in detection of arterial wall calcification (dotted arrows). The image quality is better than Fig. 19.1. *CT* computed tomography, *MIP* maximum intensity projection, *VR* volume rendering

enhancement: iodine concentration, iodine dose, and injection rate when the injection duration is fixed. High iodine delivery rates determined by the iodine concentration of the contrast medium and the injection rate are important in obtaining adequate enhancement of arteries in CT angiography [8]. If contrast medium preparations with lower iodine concentrations are used, a greater amount of contrast medium and a higher injection rate are required to maintain the same degree of enhancement achieved as when contrast medium preparations with higher iodine concentrations are used. Therefore, contrast medium preparations with higher iodine concentrations such as 370 mg/mL are recommended for CT angiography. The strength of arterial enhancement is proportional to the injection rate. Increasing the injection rate leads to a faster accumulation of contrast medium in the aorta, increasing peak aortic enhancement. With recent CT scanners, an injection rate of 4–5 mL/s is usually sufficient to provide excellent arterial enhancement for most vascular studies [9]. It needs to be tailored to the individual because patient-related factors can influence arterial enhancement. For example, lower cardiac output causes delayed peak arterial enhancement. The bolus tracking technique is commonly used to obtain accurate scan timing. It involves acquiring a pre-contrast image at a reference level with the placement of a region of interest (ROI) over a target vessel. After the contrast medium injection is started, a low-dose monitoring scan is performed at a predetermined level after a fixed time delay (usually 5 s) and thereafter every 1–3 s, until the enhancement in the ROI reaches a specified level (typically 150 Hounsfield Units). The CT angiography then begins after a prespecified adjustable delay to allow peak arterial enhancement (approximately 8 s) [9].

19.2.3 Image Processing

In CT angiography, processing is performed by volume rendering (VR), maximum intensity projection (MIP), and multi-planar reconstruction (MPR)/curved MPR. VR involves a color display that gives images with a stereoscopic effect and is suitable for overviewing (Figs. 19.1d and 19.2d). In VR, small arteries or arteries with low enhancement cannot be visualized due to the display settings; therefore, there is a possibility of overestimating lesions. By removing bone, MIP obtains a projection image similar to DSA and is usually displayed in gray scale (Figs. 19.1c and 19.2c). Recently, automated CT angiography analysis software has been developed to measure the vascular lumen. It can automatically measure diameters on the short axial section in the post-processing workstation [10]. Measurement of vascular diameter is useful in planning endovascular treatment of PAOD.

19.2.4 Drawbacks of CT Angiography

19.2.4.1 Evaluation of Severe Calcified Lesion

CT angiography is excellent in the detection of calcification and useful for evaluating the properties of the arterial walls however blooming artifacts can arise from heavily calcified arterial walls. These artifacts have been reported to result in the overdiagnosis of the severity of stenotic lesions and significantly decrease diagnostic accuracy, especially in the peripheral arteries to the knee arteries [4]. The following two methods may be effective as solutions against the problem: dual energy CT and ultra-high-resolution CT. Several dual energy CT systems are available for each vendor, but all the techniques provide different spectral data acquired from two different voltages. The settings of 80 and 140 kV are commonly used because they provide the maximum difference and least amount of overlap between the spectra with standard tubes [11]. The spectral data enable the separation of contrast medium and calcification. The luminal image is obtained by subtraction between these two datasets. There are several reports about the utility of diagnosing PAOD using dual energy CT [12–14]; however, there are still some problems. The processing of subtraction using the different spectral data might introduce some artifacts. Moreover, dual energy CT remains limited in the evaluation of poorly opacified lumen or small arteries [12, 15]. Recently, an ultra-high-resolution CT system has been released by Canon Medical Systems, and it allows more than twofold increase in spatial resolution. The high spatial resolution may be particularly beneficial in the visualization of small arteries [16].

19.2.4.2 Evaluation of Critical Limb Ischemia

For severely ischemic limbs, it is necessary to evaluate the lower leg arteries with poor blood flow or the arteries below the ankle, but these are often difficult to evaluate with CT angiography due to its low contrast (Fig. 19.2c, d). Ultra-high-resolution CT systems may help in such cases. Small vasculature such as the pedal arch, digital arteries, and collateral arteries can be observed by using a reconstruction field of view [16]. Another solution for such cases is MR angiography. As will be described later, MR angiography has good contrast, and there is the possibility that contrast enhancement can be evaluated even in peripheral arteries in which the blood flow has decreased (Fig. 19.3).

19.2.4.3 Radiation Exposure

Wide range and thinner section images are required for CT angiography; therefore, it has gained widespread concern because of the radiation dose. Various methods of reducing the radiation dose for CT angiography have been developed such as low tube voltage [17–20] and dual energy CT. Using low tube voltage is an effective method to reduce radiation doses because of the exponential relationship between tube voltage and radiation dose. It has been reported that a 30–91% radiation dose reduction was achieved using 80 kVp instead of 120 kVp for CT angiography [17, 18, 20]. The main disadvantage of using low tube voltage is that it diminishes image quality by increasing image noise

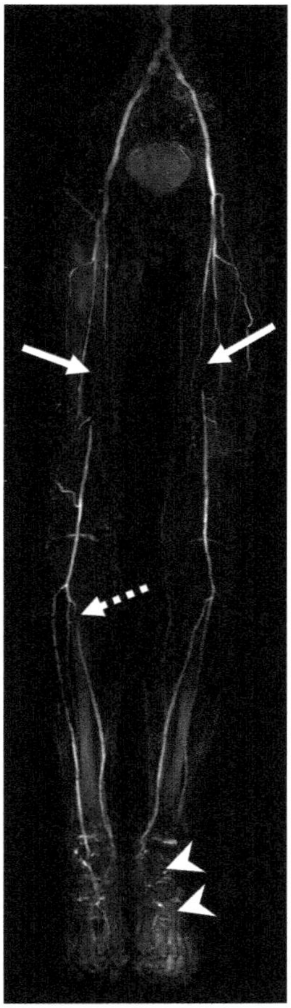

Fig. 19.3 CE-MR angiography of a 57-year-old man with PAOD. CE-MR angiography shows lengthy bilateral superficial femoral artery occlusion (arrows), as well as severe stenosis of the right posterior tibial artery (dotted arrow). CE-MR angiography has good contrast, and therefore stenosis/occlusion of the arteries of the foot can be evaluated in detail (arrowheads). *CE-MR* contrast-enhanced magnetic resonance, *PAOD* peripheral arterial occlusive disease

however iterative model reconstruction (IMR) can solve the problem. IMR is a knowledge-based reconstruction method that has the potential to improve image quality by decreasing image noise through iterative minimization of the difference between measured raw data and the estimated image [21]. In general, with the currently available high-end scanners, radiation doses from dual energy CT are lower or no more than 10–15% higher than single energy CT [22]. However, dual energy CT can significantly decrease radiation doses much lower than in single energy CT without significantly affecting image quality, using an optimized protocol and IMR [22].

19.2.4.4 Toxicity of Contrast Agents: Contrast-Induced Nephropathy

Iodine-based contrast medium has been considered as the common cause of hospital-acquired acute kidney injury [23]. Post-contrast acute kidney injury (PC-AKI) is defined as an increase in serum creatinine level >0.3 mg/dL (or >26.5 μmol/L), or >1.5 times the baseline value, within 48–72 h of intravascular administration of a contrast agent [24]. The most important risk factor for PC-AKI is renal dysfunction without dialysis, namely an estimated glomerular filtration rate (eGFR) < 30 mL/min/1.73 m^2 before intravenous contrast medium. Patients on dialysis can receive iodine-based contrast medium, and early post-procedural dialysis is not routinely required. Patients with PAOD often have renal dysfunction because diabetes mellitus is a major risk factor for PAOD. The association between intravenous contrast dose and nephrotoxicity is controversial, but in general, it is desirable to reduce the amount of contrast medium in patients with renal dysfunction. Using low tube voltage or dual energy CT is also an effective method to reduce contrast dose. Enhancement of iodine-based contrast medium substantially increases at lower tube voltage, as the effective energy of the x-ray beam approaches the absorption k-edge of iodine (33.2 keV) [25]. The concept of using low tube voltage examinations to achieve high contrast-to-noise ratios in the evaluation of peripheral arteries while reducing iodine dose (and radiation dose) has been widely investigated [17, 19, 26, 27]. However, lowering the tube voltage causes an increase in image noise, for which dual energy CT may be a solution. Low-energy virtual monochromatic datasets generated from dual energy CT can yield more than double the iodine attenuation of single energy CT [28], enabling reduction of iodine load for CT angiography without decreasing the contrast-to-noise ratio. Recent studies have reported that a 50% reduction of iodine dose for peripheral CT angiography was achieved by using dual energy CT [29].

19.3 MR Angiography (Fig. 19.3)

19.3.1 General Features

MR angiography is a multiparametric imaging modality with excellent contrast resolution. Contrast-enhanced (CE-) MR angiography relies on the T1 shortening effect of gadolinium-based contrast agents (GBCAs), accurately diagnosing the anatomic location and extent of stenosis in PAOD. CE-MR angiography has equal performance to CT angiography in the detection of arterial stenosis and occlusion [30]. CE-MR angiography is often preferable to CT angiography, especially in patients with distal disease, and in those with heavily calcified vessels which can hinder stenosis assessment on CT angiography [31]. Time-resolved CE-MR angiography (see below for details) is an excellent method of assessing the patency of small arteries and is particularly useful when imaging below-the-knee arteries [32, 33]. On the other hand, MR angiography has some drawbacks, such as not being able to evaluate calcification and toxicity from GBCAs (resulting in nephrogenic systemic fibrosis [NSF]).

19.3.2 Protocol

A rapid 3D T1-weighted spoiled gradient echo (GRE) pulse sequence with a short repetition time and echo time is ideal for CE-MR angiography. This sequence provides images with high signal-to-noise ratio, good spatial resolution, and with no flow-related artifacts [9, 34]. In general, an injection rate of 1.5 mL/s provides arterial imaging with high vessel-to-background contrast. Two different acquisition modes are common in CE-MR angiography: single phase and time-resolved MR angiography [9]. Single phase MR angiography captures vascular images at a single point in time. On the other hand, time-resolved MR angiography consists of multiple acquisitions of an imaged volume over successive time points post GBCAs administration. This technique is particularly useful in displaying the passage of the contrast bolus through smaller vessels including severely ischemic limbs. The core of time-resolved MR angiography is a 3D-spoiled GRE sequence employing k-space filling tricks to quicken image acquisition, such as view sharing, in which central k-space (responsible for image contrast) can be sampled more frequently than peripheral k-space (responsible for spatial resolution), providing improvement in apparent temporal resolution [9, 35, 36]. These techniques, aligned with the use of parallel imaging, improve acquisition speed [36]. For routine MR angiography, the standard protocol is to begin with localizers of the anatomical area in question, followed by coronal and axial T2-weighted imaging, which allows for a global anatomic assessment. This is then followed by 3D CE-MR angiography providing anisotropic images that allow for reconstruction of the dataset on a 3D workstation. Finally, an axial T1-weighted 3D spoiled GRE sequence of the anatomical area can be acquired, allowing for the assessment of significant incidental findings [9].

19.3.3 Image Processing

Subtraction technique improves contrast resolution in CE-MR angiography. This reduces signal from background tissues by acquiring a mask image prior to GBCAs administration and subtracting it from the post-contrast imaging [9]. Similar to CT angiography, MPR/curved MPR and MIP images are required for MR angiography because arteries tend to not follow anatomical axial, coronal, or sagittal planes.

19.3.4 Drawbacks of MR Angiography

19.3.4.1 Evaluation of Calcification

MR angiography is advantageous since it is not affected by calcification, but it also has a problem that it cannot visualize calcification. The reason this is problematic is that in patients with indications for surgery or endovascular treatment, the presence or absence of calcification and the degree of calcification are indispensable information. It is important to use CT and MR angiography complementarily for each case.

19.3.4.2 Toxicity of Contrast Agents: Nephrogenic Systemic Fibrosis

NSF is a very late adverse reaction to GBCAs (see Chap. 2 for details). Patients with renal dysfunction, particularly with an eGFR <15 mL/min/1.73 m^2 or on dialysis are at risk for NSF [24]. Although patients on dialysis can undergo CT angiography, neither examination can be performed in patients with severe renal dysfunction without dialysis. The following two methods may be effective as solutions for such patients: non-contrast MR angiography and ferumoxytol-enhanced MR angiography.

There are several different contrast mechanisms available for non-contrast MR angiography [37]. The optimal contrast mechanism and associated imaging technique are highly dependent on the individual clinical indication since no single mechanism or imaging technique is yet ideal in all situations. There are several sequences that are currently available in non-contrast MR angiography, such as balanced steady-state free precession, time-of-flight, inflow-dependent inversion recovery, quiescent-interval slice-selective (QISS), cardiac-gated 3D fast spin-echo, flow sensitive dephasing (FSD), arterial spin labeling, 2D/3D phase contrast, 4D phase contrast, and velocity selective [38]. Among them, QISS, cardiac-gated 3D fast spin-echo, and FSD are useful for lower extremity MR angiography, and they have a comparable diagnostic ability to CE-MR angiography [39–44].

Ferumoxytol, an iron-based material that is United States Food and Drug Administration (FDA) approved for the treatment of iron deficiency anemia in adult patients with chronic kidney disease, has been proposed as an alternative to GBCAs for CE-MR angiography [38]. Ferumoxytol poses no risk for NSF. Due to its large size, once it is injected intravenously, ferumoxytol is trapped within the intravascular space producing dramatic enhancement of blood vessels, but virtually no enhancement of extravascular spaces [45]. These properties make it a vascular contrast agent that is highly suited for MR angiography (first-pass image). Moreover, the plasma half-life of ferumoxytol is about 14–21 h [46]. This means that once the steady-state is achieved in approximately 2 min, a steady-state image can be obtained anytime within several hours afterwards, and adequate images can be generated up to a day later [45]. There are several reports that have examined the usefulness of ferumoxytol-enhanced MR angiography for PAOD [47–49]. While ferumoxytol has great potential for use in CE-MR angiography, there are serious drawbacks including (1) high cost, (2) non-FDA approval for use as an MR contrast agent, and (3) a boxed warning (the strongest type of FDA warning) because of reports of serious and potentially fatal allergic reactions [50]. This warning includes a recommendation to only administer diluted ferumoxytol as an intravenous infusion over a minimum of 15 min, which is problematic for first-pass imaging [38].

19.4 Conclusion

CE-CT and MR angiography are very useful noninvasive diagnostic methods for PAOD. MR angiography has the advantage of superior observation of the vessel lumen, but evaluation of calcification is only possible with CT angiography. Both of them provide complementary information thus which technique to use depends on the desired outcome. It is thought that these techniques will continue to be developed in the future as the technology progresses, and therefore we have to continue to update ourselves with the latest knowledge.

References

1. Hirsch AT, Criqui MH, Treat-Jacobson D, et al. Peripheral arterial disease detection, awareness, and treatment in primary care. JAMA. 2001;286(11):1317–24.
2. Collaboration NCDRF. Worldwide trends in diabetes since 1980: a pooled analysis of 751 population-based studies with 4.4 million participants. Lancet. 2016;387(10027):1513–30.
3. Behrendt CA, Heidemann F, Haustein K, et al. Percutaneous endovascular treatment of infrainguinal PAOD: results of the PSI register study in 74 German vascular centers. Gefasschirurgie. 2017;22(Suppl 1):17–27.
4. Heijenbrok-Kal MH, Kock MC, Hunink MG. Lower extremity arterial disease: multidetector CT angiography meta-analysis. Radiology. 2007;245(2):433–9.
5. Met R, Bipat S, Legemate DA, et al. Diagnostic performance of computed tomography angiography in peripheral arterial disease: a systematic review and meta-analysis. JAMA. 2009;301(4):415–24.
6. Jakobs TF, Wintersperger BJ, Becker CR. MDCT-imaging of peripheral arterial disease. Semin Ultrasound CT MR. 2004;25(2):145–55.
7. Ota H, Takase K, Igarashi K, et al. MDCT compared with digital subtraction angiography for assessment of lower extremity arterial occlusive disease: importance of reviewing cross-sectional images. AJR Am J Roentgenol. 2004;182(1):201–9.
8. Hansmann J, Fink C, Jost G, et al. Impact of iodine delivery rate with varying flow rates on image quality in dual-energy CT of patients with suspected pulmonary embolism. Acad Radiol. 2013;20(8):962–71.
9. Murphy DJ, Aghayev A, Steigner ML. Vascular CT and MRI: a practical guide to imaging protocols. Insights Imaging. 2018;9(2):215–36.
10. Keller D, Wildermuth S, Boehm T, et al. CT angiography of peripheral arterial bypass grafts: accuracy and time-effectiveness of quantitative image analysis with an automated software tool. Acad Radiol. 2006;13(5):610–20.
11. Johnson TR. Dual-energy CT: general principles. AJR Am J Roentgenol. 2012;199(5 Suppl):S3–8.
12. Klink T, Wilhelm T, Roth C, et al. Dual-energy CTA in patients with symptomatic peripheral arterial occlusive disease: study of diagnostic accuracy and impeding factors. Rofo. 2017;189(5):441–52.
13. Kau T, Eicher W, Reiterer C, et al. Dual-energy CT angiography in peripheral arterial occlusive disease-accuracy of maximum intensity projections in clinical routine and subgroup analysis. Eur Radiol. 2011;21(8):1677–86.
14. Sommer WH, Johnson TR, Becker CR, et al. The value of dual-energy bone removal in maximum intensity projections of lower extremity computed tomography angiography. Invest Radiol. 2009;44(5):285–92.
15. Werncke T, Albrecht T, Wolf KJ, et al. Dual energy CT of the peripheral arteries: a phantom study to assess the effect of automatic plaque removal on stenosis grading. Rofo. 2010;182(8):682–9.
16. Tanaka R, Yoshioka K, Takagi H, et al. Novel developments in non-invasive imaging of peripheral arterial disease with CT: experience with state-of-the-art, ultra-high-resolution CT and subtraction imaging. Clin Radiol. 2019;74(1):51–8.
17. Liu B, Gao S, Chang Z, et al. Lower extremity CT angiography at 80 kVp using iterative model reconstruction. Diagn Interv Imaging. 2018;99(9):561–8.
18. Qian WL, Zhou DJ, Jiang Y, et al. Ultra-low radiation dose CT angiography of the lower extremity using the iterative model reconstruction (IMR) algorithm. Clin Radiol. 2018;73(11):985.e13–9.
19. Qi L, Zhao Y, Zhou CS, et al. Image quality and radiation dose of lower extremity CT angiography at 70 kVp on an integrated circuit detector dual-source computed tomography. Acta Radiol. 2015;56(6):659–65.
20. Utsunomiya D, Oda S, Funama Y, et al. Comparison of standard- and low-tube voltage MDCT angiography in patients with peripheral arterial disease. Eur Radiol. 2010;20(11):2758–65.
21. Eck BL, Fahmi R, Brown KM, et al. Computational and human observer image quality evaluation of low dose, knowledge-based CT iterative reconstruction. Med Phys. 2015;42(10):6098–111.
22. Parakh A, Macri F, Sahani D. Dual-energy computed tomography: dose reduction, series reduction, and contrast load reduction in dual-energy computed tomography. Radiol Clin North Am. 2018;56(4):601–24.
23. Mohammed NM, Mahfouz A, Achkar K, et al. Contrast-induced nephropathy. Heart Views. 2013;14(3):106–16.
24. ESUR guidelines on contrast agents v10.0. 2018. http://www.esur-cm.org/index.php/en/.
25. Szucs-Farkas Z, Verdun FR, von Allmen G, et al. Effect of X-ray tube parameters, iodine concentration, and patient size on image quality in pulmonary computed tomography angiography: a chest-phantom-study. Invest Radiol. 2008;43(6):374–81.
26. Duan Y, Wang X, Yang X, et al. Diagnostic efficiency of low-dose CT angiography compared with conventional angiography in peripheral arterial occlusions. AJR Am J Roentgenol. 2013;201(6):W906–14.
27. Kim JW, Choo KS, Jeon UB, et al. Diagnostic performance and radiation dose of lower extremity CT angiography using a 128-slice dual source CT at 80 kVp and high pitch. Acta Radiol. 2016;57(7):822–8.
28. Pinho DF, Kulkarni NM, Krishnaraj A, et al. Initial experience with single-source dual-energy CT abdominal angiography and comparison with single-energy CT angiography: image quality, enhancement, diagnosis and radiation dose. Eur Radiol. 2013;23(2):351–9.
29. Almutairi A, Sun Z, Poovathumkadavi A, et al. Dual energy CT angiography of peripheral arterial disease: feasibility of using lower contrast medium volume. PLoS One. 2015;10(9):e0139275.
30. Jens S, Koelemay MJ, Reekers JA, et al. Diagnostic performance of computed tomography angiography

and contrast-enhanced magnetic resonance angiography in patients with critical limb ischaemia and intermittent claudication: systematic review and meta-analysis. Eur Radiol. 2013;23(11):3104–14.
31. Iglesias J, Pena C. Computed tomography angiography and magnetic resonance angiography imaging in critical limb ischemia: an overview. Tech Vasc Interv Radiol. 2014;17(3):147–54.
32. Andreisek G, Pfammatter T, Goepfert K, et al. Peripheral arteries in diabetic patients: standard bolus-chase and time-resolved MR angiography. Radiology. 2007;242(2):610–20.
33. Eshed I, Rimon U, Novikov I, et al. Time-resolved MR angiography of the calf arteries using a phased array cardiac coil: comparison of visibility with standard three-step bolus chase MR angiography. Acta Radiol. 2011;52(9):973–7.
34. Nielsen YW, Thomsen HS. Contrast-enhanced peripheral MRA: technique and contrast agents. Acta Radiol. 2012;53(7):769–77.
35. Riederer SJ, Haider CR, Borisch EA, et al. Recent advances in 3D time-resolved contrast-enhanced MR angiography. J Magn Reson Imaging. 2015;42(1):3–22.
36. Riederer SJ, Stinson EG, Weavers PT. Technical aspects of contrast-enhanced MR angiography: current status and new applications. Magn Reson Med Sci. 2018;17(1):3–12.
37. Wheaton AJ, Miyazaki M. Non-contrast enhanced MR angiography: physical principles. J Magn Reson Imaging. 2012;36(2):286–304.
38. Edelman RR, Koktzoglou I. Noncontrast MR angiography: an update. J Magn Reson Imaging. 2019;49(2):355–73.
39. Amin P, Collins JD, Koktzoglou I, et al. Evaluating peripheral arterial disease with unenhanced quiescent-interval single-shot MR angiography at 3 T. AJR Am J Roentgenol. 2014;202(4):886–93.
40. Hodnett PA, Koktzoglou I, Davarpanah AH, et al. Evaluation of peripheral arterial disease with nonenhanced quiescent-interval single-shot MR angiography. Radiology. 2011;260(1):282–93.
41. Schubert T, Takes M, Aschwanden M, et al. Non-enhanced, ECG-gated MR angiography of the pedal vasculature: comparison with contrast-enhanced MR angiography and digital subtraction angiography in peripheral arterial occlusive disease. Eur Radiol. 2016;26(8):2705–13.
42. Rasper M, Wildgruber M, Settles M, et al. 3D non-contrast-enhanced ECG-gated MR angiography of the lower extremities with dual-source radiofrequency transmission at 3.0 T: intraindividual comparison with contrast-enhanced MR angiography in PAOD patients. Eur Radiol. 2016;26(9):2871–80.
43. Liu X, Fan Z, Zhang N, et al. Unenhanced MR angiography of the foot: initial experience of using flow-sensitive dephasing-prepared steady-state free precession in patients with diabetes. Radiology. 2014;272(3):885–94.
44. Zhang N, Fan Z, Luo N, et al. Noncontrast MR angiography (MRA) of infragenual arteries using flow-sensitive dephasing (FSD)-prepared steady-state free precession (SSFP) at 3.0 Tesla: comparison with contrast-enhanced MRA. J Magn Reson Imaging. 2016;43(2):364–72.
45. Lehrman ED, Plotnik AN, Hope T, et al. Ferumoxytol-enhanced MRI in the peripheral vasculature. Clin Radiol. 2019;74(1):37–50.
46. Toth GB, Varallyay CG, Horvath A, et al. Current and potential imaging applications of ferumoxytol for magnetic resonance imaging. Kidney Int. 2017;92(1):47–66.
47. Hope MD, Hope TA, Zhu C, et al. Vascular imaging with ferumoxytol as a contrast agent. AJR Am J Roentgenol. 2015;205(3):W366–73.
48. Li W, Tutton S, Vu AT, et al. First-pass contrast-enhanced magnetic resonance angiography in humans using ferumoxytol, a novel ultrasmall superparamagnetic iron oxide (USPIO)-based blood pool agent. J Magn Reson Imaging. 2005;21(1):46–52.
49. Walker JP, Nosova E, Sigovan M, et al. Ferumoxytol-enhanced magnetic resonance angiography is a feasible method for the clinical evaluation of lower extremity arterial disease. Ann Vasc Surg. 2015;29(1):63–8.
50. FDA Drug Safety Communication: FDA strengthens warnings and changes prescribing instructions to decrease the risk of serious allergic reactions with anemia drug Feraheme (ferumoxytol). 2015. https://www.fda.gov/Drugs/DrugSafety/ucm440138.htm.

Contrast Agent Use and Safety in Pediatric Patients

20

Evrim Özmen and Sukru Mehmet Erturk

20.1 Introduction

Contrast agents are widely used in routine clinical practice for enhancing the diagnostic value of radiologic modalities, including fluoroscopy, computed tomography (CT), magnetic resonance (MR) imaging, and ultrasonography (US) both for pediatric and adult patients. Barium sulfate and iodinated contrast agents can be used for fluoroscopic studies and for computed tomography via oral or rectal administration. Low osmolality contrast agents can be used via intravenous administration in computed tomography examination. Gadolinium-containing contrast agents can be used for magnetic resonance imaging. Each one of the contrast agents has advantages and disadvantages for pediatric patients.

20.2 Barium Sulfate

Barium suspension is the most widely used contrast agent in fluoroscopic studies in pediatric patients for demonstrating and evaluating the gastrointestinal tract (Fig. 20.1). These agents can be administered orally, rectally, or via ostomies and catheters.

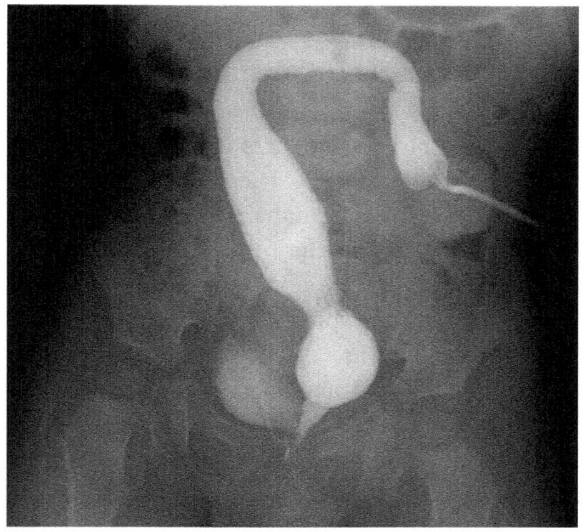

Fig. 20.1 In fluoroscopic image of the 2-year-old boy with anorectal malformation who received iodinated contrast agent from his ostomy a rectovesical fistula could be seen (arrow)

Barium sulfate is derived from barium that has an atomic number of 56 [1]. Barium suspension could not be absorbed or metabolized and is excreted with feces [1]. Barium sulfate is generally well tolerated orally by pediatric patients. Barium-based contrast agents are considerably less expensive than most iodine-based nonionic contrast agents for a given volume of contrast [1]. However, barium-based contrast agents have

E. Özmen (✉)
Department of Radiology, Koç University Hospital, Istanbul, Turkey

S. M. Erturk
Department of Radiology, Istanbul University School of Medicine, Istanbul, Turkey

S. M. Erturk et al. (eds.), *Medical Imaging Contrast Agents: A Clinical Manual*,
https://doi.org/10.1007/978-3-030-79256-5_20

some disadvantages. They may convert partial intestinal obstructions to a total of one [2]. If barium sulfate suspension leaks into surrounding soft tissues from the gastrointestinal tract, it may produce an inflammatory response and will remain there permanently [1]. These agents should not be given in the suspicion of gastrointestinal perforation, toxic megacolon, and within 10 days after a biopsy. In these circumstances, iodine-based contrast agents should be considered for the fluoroscopic evaluation of the gastrointestinal tract, especially if gastrointestinal perforation is suspected.

20.3 Iodinated Contrast Agents

Iodinated contrast agents are the most frequently used contrast materials. These agents are either water-soluble or oil-soluble. Lipiodol, which is an oil-soluble agent, can be used for lymphangiography, sialography, and chemoembolization. Most of the water-soluble forms are used intravascularly. They are often preferred for procedures, including CT and angiography, while these agents could be used for gastrointestinal imaging and voiding cystourethrography. Contrast administration for CT examinations is beneficial in most of the diseases, including the differential diagnosis of pulmonary nodules, malignancies, infections, and inflammatory diseases (Figs. 20.2 and 20.3). The ionic iodinated contrast agents have a high osmolality and limited use, including the treatment of meconium ileus and voiding cystourethrography in pediatric patients. The osmolality of the contrast agents should be considered when deciding which iodinated contrast material to administer orally since the high-osmolality contrast agents may lead to a fluid shift into the gastrointestinal cavity and thus may cause hypotension, dehydration, and electrolyte imbalance [2–7]. Likewise, any injected hyperosmolar material creates an osmotic gradient in blood and leads to a fluid shift into the vessels [8]. The osmotic load and fluid shift into the vessels may cause complications such as congestive heart failure and pulmonary edema, especially in infants who have underlying diseases such as congenital heart disease and renal failure [8]. Thus, low osmolality contrast material should be preferred in those patients [9]. High-osmolality iodinated contrast agents should be avoided in children who are at risk for aspiration, as well. The aspirated hyperosmolality contrast agent may cause fluid shifts into the pulmonary alveolus and chemical pneumonitis with resultant pulmonary edema [10–12].

In 1968, the carboxyl group, which is responsible for the adverse events, was removed from the structure of the contrast agents and replaced with the amide component. Since it does not dissolve in blood, the era of nonionic contrast agents began [2]. Adverse reactions, including nausea and vomiting, allergic reactions, and fatal reactions are less with nonionic contrast agents when compared with the ionic ones [2].

Viscosity is another essential feature, especially for the administration of the contrast agents

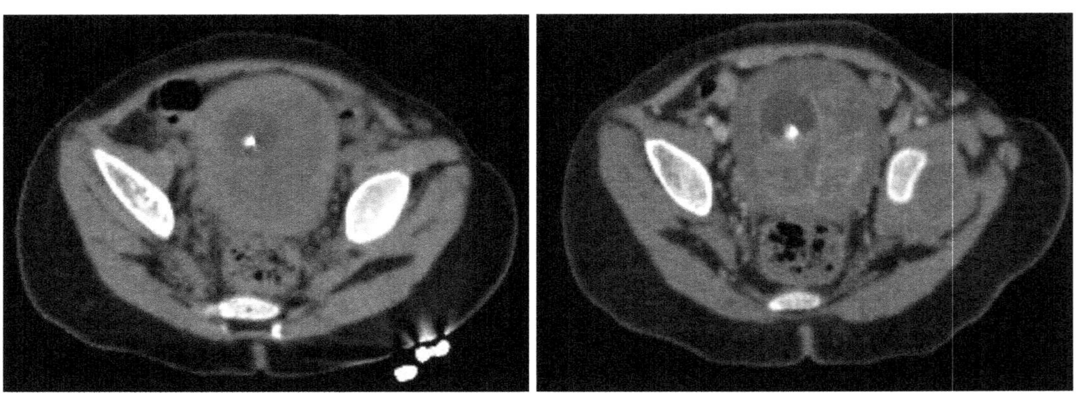

Fig. 20.2 Axial CT images with and without contrast administration of a 3-year-old boy with rhabdomyosarcoma in bladder reveal a mass enhancing with contrast agent

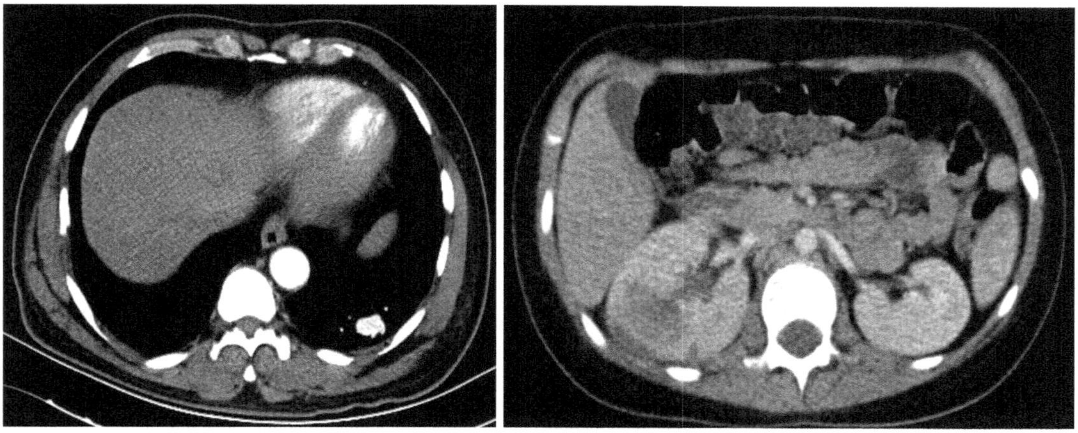

Fig. 20.3 In the left figure; contrast-enhanced axial CT image of an adolescent patient demonstrated a contrast-enhanced nodular lesion which is indicating a vascular lesion. The contrast-enhanced CT findings save the patient from biopsy procedure which could lead to over-bleeding. In the right axial contrast-enhanced CT image of the 9-year-old girl who had fever and abdominal pain, there is a hypodense area compatible with the absence of contrast enhancement and enlargement of the kidney indicating pyelonephritis

intravenously. An increase in viscosity makes the contrast agent injection more challenging. The viscosity of the contrast agents is variable similar to their osmolality. While using high viscosity agents, especially in pediatric patients, since the catheters' and needles' sizes are small, the desired flow rates might not be reached, and catheter rupture or vascular injuries might occur [8]. Viscosity generally varies with temperature and decreases with increasing temperatures. Thus, it is recommended to warm up the contrast agents to the body temperature before the administration in pediatric patients [8]. Another method is diluting the contrast agents with saline to decrease the viscosity. This method is useful, particularly in CT angiography. It also reduces the beam hardening effect on CT images [13].

20.4 Allergic-Like Reactions and Chemotoxicity with Iodine-Based Contrast Agents

The majority of allergic-like reactions are related to the release of histamine or the other mediators from basophils, eosinophils, and mast cells, not connected with Ig E [9]. Low osmolality non-ionic contrast agents cause less histamine release than the high osmolality ones [14]. Although some complications are milder for adults, the same complications might be severe for children. For example, warmth at the injection site may cause the child to cry and move. This may lead to bad quality images, recurrent examinations, and increased radiation exposure [8]. Besides, nausea and vomiting can lead to aspiration of gastric contents. They can also cause delay in the examination time and skip the optimal phase for the contrast-enhanced images [8]. Low osmolality nonionic monomers lead to nonallergic-like reactions such as nausea and vomiting less than the high-osmolality ionic iodine-based contrast agents [9]. In 2007, Dillman et al. [15] reported the acute allergic reactions in pediatric patients in whom nonionic contrast agents were used; they detected 20 allergic reactions among >11,000 intravenous injections. Sixteen of those 20 allergic reactions were mild, one of them was moderate, and three of them were severe reactions. There were no deaths reported. The patient with moderate reaction experienced wheezing. Severe reactions included wheezing and facial edema. Dillman et al. reported that allergic reactions are less common in pediatric patients when compared with adults. Other authors did not detect any difference between the children and adults about adverse reactions [16, 17].

The predicted incidence of allergic-like reactions related to iodine-based contrast agents is between 0.18 and 0.46% in the pediatric population [15, 18]. Contrast media reactions are highest in pediatric patients between 16 and 18 years of age. These reactions are infrequent under the age of three [18].

The premedication approach in pediatric patients is similar to adults. There is only dose change [9]. There are two choices for premedication: steroid use alone or combined steroid and antihistamine use. Usually, the oral application is preferred well than the intravenous route [9]. Steroids should be given at least 6–12 h before the examination [8]. However, one should know that premedication could not prevent life-threatening reactions. Antihistamine (e.g., diphenhydramine) orally 1 h before contrast agent administration may reduce the frequency of urticaria, angioedema, and respiratory symptoms [9].

20.5 Contrast-Induced Renal Toxicity

Although the incidence of contrast-induced nephropathy (CIN) has not been well established in the pediatric population, it is considered extremely rare in children with normal renal functions. In children, CIN occurs only in the use of iodine-based contrast agents. It is not seen in the use of gadolinium-based contrast materials in their recommended amounts [13].

Serum creatinine levels should be observed before the contrast material administration in children with abnormal renal function [19]. A normal serum creatinine level is different in children compared to adults and changes with age. Serum creatinine levels should be 0.6 under the age of 1, 0.7 between 1 and 5 years, and 1.0 between 6 and 10 years, 1.2 between 10 and 18 years, and 1.4 above 18 years. However, serum creatinine level does not directly reflect renal function. It only shows the creatinine balance between that produced by muscles and excreted from the kidney [8]. A normal serum creatinine level cannot exclude acute renal failure because it starts to increase when the glomerular filtration rate (GFR) decreased by 50%. An increase in serum creatinine level can be seen only after a few days in patients with acute renal failure. GFR is considered a gold standard in predicting and demonstrating renal function. However, GFR detection with routine laboratory examination is both time-consuming and expensive. Thus, several formulas are produced for estimating GFR from the serum creatinine value. Among them, the Schwartz equation is recommended for calculating GFR in the pediatric population. According to this formula; GFR (mL/min/1.73 m^2) = (k × height in cm)/serum creatinine (mg/dL) [20]. In this formula, k is a constant and equal to 0.33 in preterm infants, 0.45 in up to 1 year, 0.55 in 1–13 years, and 0.7 in older children. According to this formula, GFR below 30 mL/min/1.73 m^2 indicates renal failure and GFR between 30 and 60 mL/min/1.73 m^2 indicates renal insufficiency [8]. Contrast-dependent nephropathy may be defined as a 50% increase or >0.5 mg/dL increase in the creatinine value over 72 h following the contrast agent administration.

The most important recommendation for preventing contrast-induced nephropathy in children who have mild or moderate renal function impairment is hydrating the patient sufficiently. The other suggestions are including using low osmolality contrast agents, decreasing the amount of administered contrast material, and avoiding the nephrotoxic and diuretic drugs. A premedication with acetylcysteine could also be considered. Patients with more severe renal dysfunction should have aggressive therapy, including oral and intravenous liquid replacement that started 12 h before the examination [8].

Dialysis can be preferred in two cases the first is in patients with chronic renal insufficiency who receive regular dialysis. These patients do not need urgent dialysis and intravenous administration of contrast material and contrast-enhanced examinations could be planned before the dialysis session. The second is in patients with mild to moderate renal dysfunction. These patients should receive urgent dialysis just after the contrast agent administration since the removal of contrast materials reduces renal toxicity. However, one should consider that the benefit of dialysis is not proven [8].

In pediatric patients with implanted ports or peripherally inserted central catheters that are not designed for use with a power injector, complications including catheter fragmentation and embolization may develop. Injection by hand or using pressure-limiting power injectors are recommended in those patients. Placement of peripheral intravenous catheters may be required for contrast-enhanced CT examinations in children with implanted ports or peripherally inserted central catheters [21]. Especially pressure-limiting power injectors significantly reduce complications due to administration of contrast agents through central lines and provide consistent injection rates [22]. A maximum injection rate varies with different catheter sizes. Maximum injection rate is 0.5 mL/s for 16–18 gauge catheters, 4.0 mL/s for 20 gauge, 2.5 mL/s for 22 gauge, and 1.0 mL/s for 24 gauge catheters [21]. Contrast media injection rates also change according to the examination type, and this should be below or equal to 2.0 mL/s in routine CT examinations while it should be between 2.0 mL/s and 4.0 mL/s in CT angiography examinations.

20.6 Contrast Agent Extravasation

Contrast media administration has a risk of extravasation of the contrast agent to the soft tissue in addition to allergy and renal toxicity. This is a rare condition with an incidence of 0.1–0.9% [21]. Contrast material extravasation can lead to complications such as tissue ulceration, necrosis, and neurovascular injury, as well as serious complications such as compartment syndrome. It is important to decide when the patient should be referred to the surgery. Radiologists should establish the approximate amount of extravasated contrast medium. If this amount is small, elevation of the extremity and applying an ice pack would be sufficient for the treatment. However, if symptoms are suggesting a clinic of compartment syndrome, including blistering, abnormal tissue perfusion, severe pain, or neurologic symptoms, surgical consultation is required [21].

20.7 Gadolinium-Containing Contrast Agents

Contrast-enhanced magnetic resonance (MR) examinations play an important role in detection and evaluation of tumors, infections and inflammations, metastases, differentiation of benign lesions from malignancies, evaluation of congenital vascular malformations and detection of arterial supply and venous drainage in vascular malformations, evaluation of neurocutaneous diseases and metabolic diseases (Figs. 20.4, 20.5, and 20.6). Contrast media administration is also required for congenital cardiac malformation imaging and advanced MR practice, including MR urography, perfusion MR.

The recommended dose is 0.1 mmol/kg for the use of this contrast agent in pediatric patients. The majority of gadolinium-based contrast agents are available as 0.5 molar formulations while gadobutrol is a new generation 1 molar contrast medium [23]. Higher gadolinium concentration is advantageous because a smaller injection volume may be used for contrast-enhanced MR imaging procedures. Besides, gadobutrol has higher relaxivity compared to the other contrast agents. The most critical disadvantage of gadolinium-based contrast substances is the risk of nephrogenic systemic fibrosis (NSF) development. NSF is a disease characterized by progressive tissue fibrosis with deposition of collagen and fibroblast [24, 25]. As far we know, there is not any reported NSF case related to gadolinium-based contrast media in patients under 8 years of age [26, 27]. However, one should consider the risk of NSF in the pediatric population [19].

The use of gadolinium-based contrast agents has the risk of free gadolinium deposition in addition to NSF development. Free gadolinium

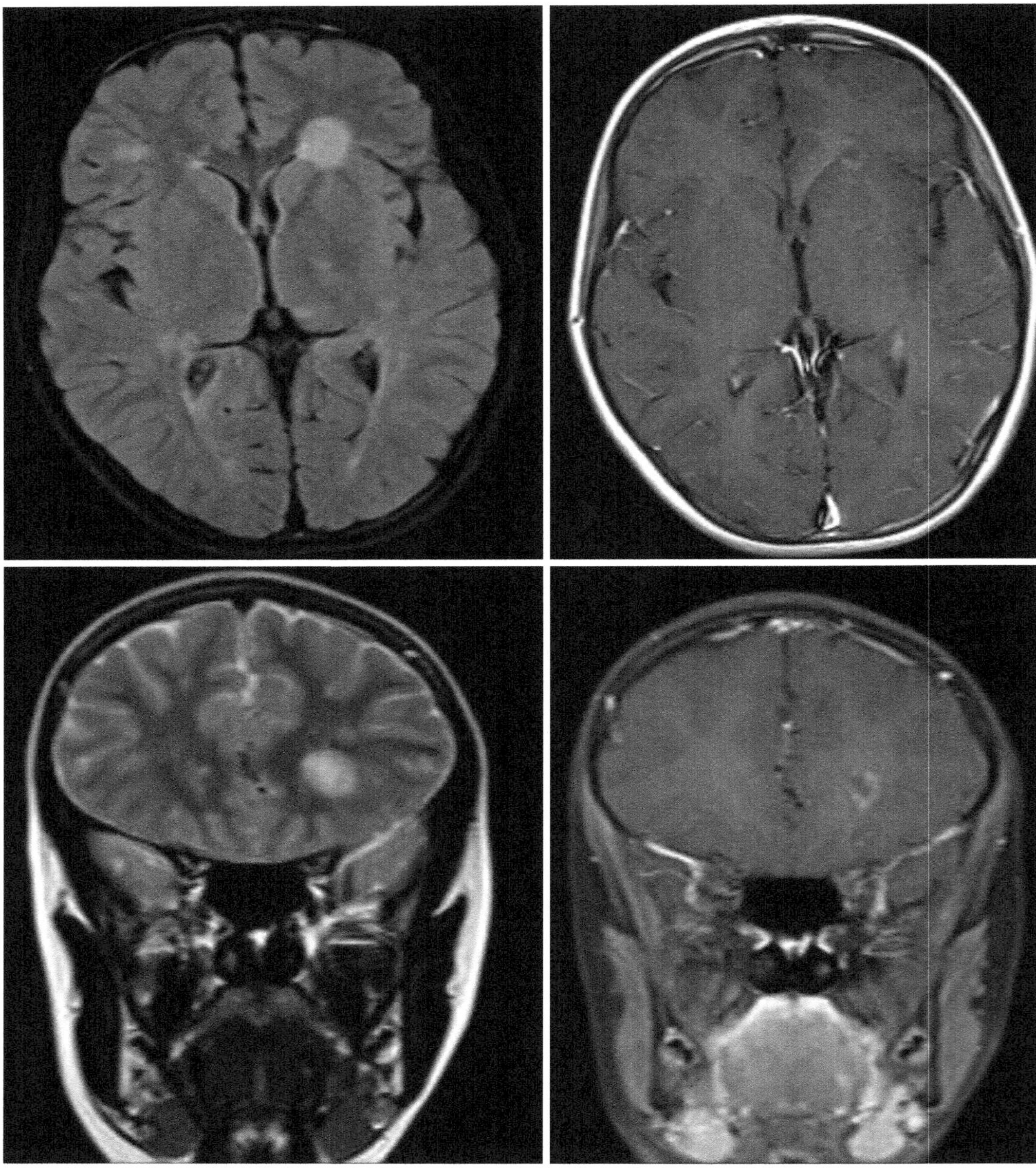

Fig. 20.4 In 16-year-old girl with the diagnosis of multiple sclerosis MR examination was performed to detect the activity of the disease. Axial FLAIR and coronal T2-weighted images demonstrate a demyelinating area in the periventricular white matter in the left frontal lobe. Contrast-enhanced axial and coronal images show contrast enhancement in this area indicating disease activity.

may deposit in human tissues even in patients with a normal renal function who had gadolinium-based contrast media administration [28, 29]. Free gadolinium may accumulate in the metaphysis of bones in addition to globus pallidus ve dentate nucleus, especially in patients who have multiple gadolinium-based media administration [30, 31]. The long-term effects of gadolinium deposition are not yet known. Pediatric patients may be more vulnerable to gadolinium deposition

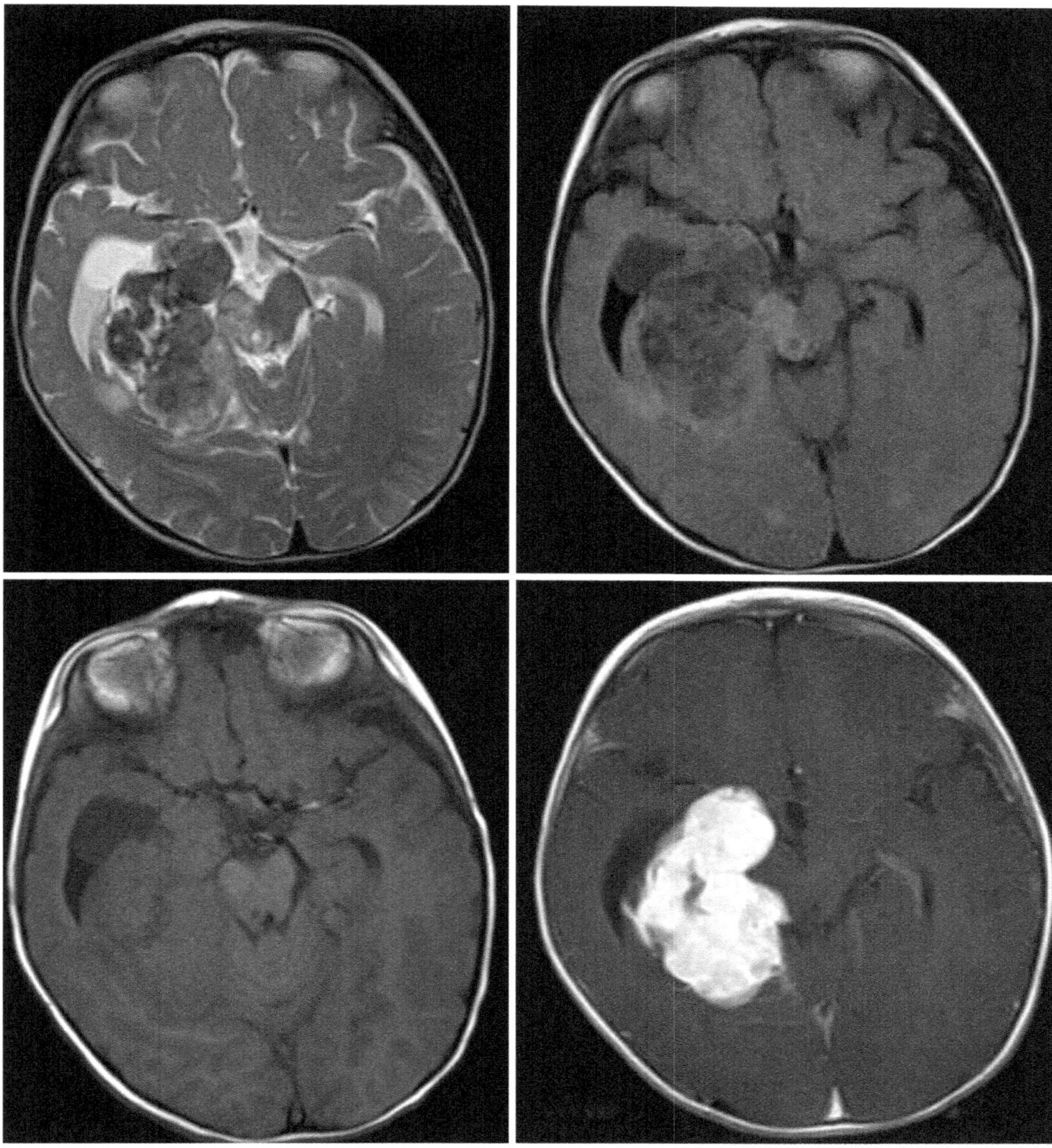

Fig. 20.5 MR images of a 9-year-old girl with anaplastic astrocytoma are shown. Axial T2-weighted, FLAIR, and T1-weighted images show a mass in temporal lobe adjacent to temporal horn of right lateral ventricle invading the right hipocampus and mesencephalus. T1-weighted axial image with contrast administration demonstrate the demarcation of lesion better than the conventional sequences and show the avid enhancement of the lesion with the contrast media

since free gadolinium may have much more toxic effects on the developing brain or bones [19]. Active myelination and bone ossification could be affected by gadolinium in children. Besides, the risk of complications related to gadolinium accumulation is higher in children due to their longer life span. While osmolality and viscosity are critical characteristics of the iodine-based contrast agents, they are not that important regarding the gadolinium-based ones because

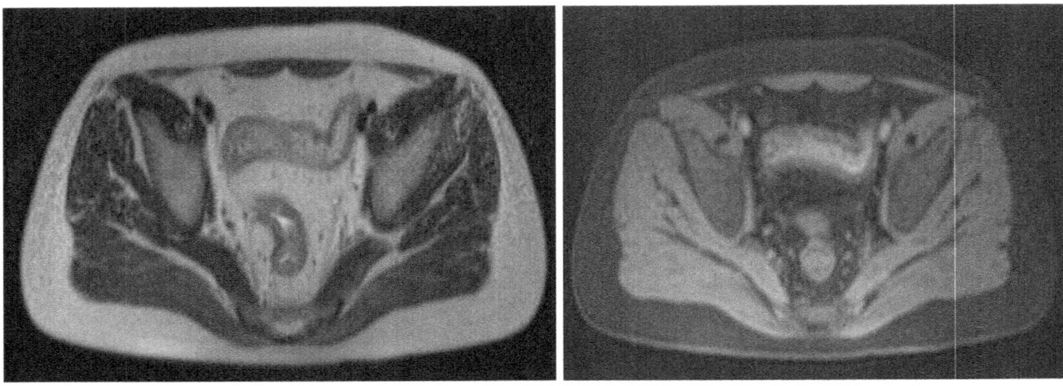

Fig. 20.6 Axial T2-weighted image of the 15-year-old girl with inflammatory bowel disease reveals a mild increase in the thickness of sigmoid segment of colon. Contrast-enhanced axial T1-weighted image with fat suppression shows significant mucosal enhancement with contrast media and increase in vasculature in the mesentery

they are administered in smaller volumes. Besides, high injection rates are not needed in pediatric patients [8, 13]. Thus, the risk of vascular injury and contrast extravasation is lower as well [13].

Regarding the allergic-like reactions, it was reported that only 6 of the 13.344 children injected with gadolinium-based contrast agents had mild reactions including coldness at the injection site, nausea, headache, warmth, and dizziness [32]. To the best of our knowledge, renal toxicity related to the gadolinium-based contrast agents is not reported in the literature [8].

In conclusion, in fluoroscopic studies, barium suspension is the most widely used oral contrast material in the examination of the gastrointestinal tract since it is well tolerated and creates a good image quality in pediatric patients. Regarding the use of intravenous contrast agents in CT imaging, low osmolality iodinated contrast materials are preferable since they are safer compared to high osmolality ones. High-osmolality contrast agents can lead to a fluid shift and heart and renal failure. Regarding the MR imaging, macrocyclic chelates have a lower risk of gadolinium accumulation, and therefore are safer to use compared to the linear ones. Finally, it should be remembered that children are not just small adults.

References

1. Callahan MJ, Talmadge JM, MacDougall RD, Kleinman PL, Taylor GA, Buonomo C. Selecting appropriate gastroenteric contrast media for diagnostic fluoroscopic imaging in infants and children: a practical approach. Pediatr Radiol. 2017;47(4):372–81. https://doi.org/10.1007/s00247-016-3709-5. Epub 2016 Oct 10.
2. Erdogan N. Radyolojik kontrast maddeler ve aşırı duyarlık tepkimeleri. In: Balci P, Pabuscu Y, editors. Temel radyoloji fiziği. 2008.
3. Harris PD, Neuhauser EB, Gerth R. The osmotic effect of water soluble contrast media on circulating plasma volume. AJR Am J Roentgenol. 1964;91:694–8.
4. Johansen JG, Kolmannskog S. Osmotic effect and solubility of amipaque (metrizamide) in the gastrointestinal tract. Invest Radiol. 1978;13(632053):93–7.
5. Cohen MD. Choosing contrast media for the evaluation of the gastrointestinal tract of neonates and infants. Radiology. 1987;162:447–56.
6. Poole CA, Rowe MI. Clinical evidence of intestinal absorption of Gastrografin. Radiology. 1976;118(1244649):151–3.
7. Rowe MI, Seagram G, Weinberger M. Gastrografin-induced hypertonicity. The pathogenesis of a neonatal hazard. Am J Surg. 1973;125(4687998):185–8.
8. Cohen MD. Safe use of imaging contrast agents in children. J Am Coll Radiol. 2009;6:576–81.
9. Contrast media in children ACR manual on contrast media—version 10.3/May 31, 2017.
10. Frech RS, Davie JM, Adatepe M, Feldhaus R, McAlister WH. Comparison of barium sulfate and oral 40 percent diatrizoate injected into the trachea of dogs. Radiology. 1970;95(5439432):299–303.

11. Friedman BI, Hartenberg MA, Mulroy JJ, Tong TK, Mickell JJ. Gastrografin aspiration in a 3 3/4-year-old girl. Pediatr Radiol. 1986;16(3774397):506–7.
12. McAlister WH, Siegel MJ. Fatal aspirations in infancy during gastrointestinal series. Pediatr Radiol. 1984;14(6728539):81–3.
13. Soares BP, Lequin MH, Huisman TAGM. Safety of contrast material use in children. Magn Reson Imaging Clin N Am. 2017;25:779–85.
14. Peachell PT, Morcos SK. Effect of radiographic contrast media on histamine release from human mast cells and basophils. Br J Radiol. 1998;71(841):24–30.
15. Dillman JR, Strouse PJ, Ellis JH, Cohan RH, Jan SC. Incidence and severity of acute allergic-like reactions to i.v. non-ionic iodinated contrast material in children. AJR Am J Roentgenol. 2007;188:1643–7.
16. Shehadi WH. Adverse reactions to intravascularly administered contrast media. A comprehensive study based on a prospective survey. Am J Roentgenol Radium Ther Nucl Med. 1975;124:145–52.
17. Katayama H, Yamaguchi K, Kozuka T, Takashima T, Seez P, Matsura K. Adverse reactions to ionic and non-ionic contrast media. A report from the Japanese Committee on the Safety of contrast media. Radiology. 1990;175:621–8.
18. Callahan MJ, Poznauskis L, Zurakowski D, Taylor GA. Non-ionic iodinated intravenous contrast-material related reactions: incidence in large urban children's hospital-retrospective analysis of data in 12,494 patients. Radiology. 2009;250:674–81.
19. Rozenfeld MN, Podberesky DJ. Gadolinium-based contrast agents in children. Pediatr Radiol. 2018;48(9):1188–96.
20. Schwartz GJ, Munoz A, Schneider MF, et al. New equations to estimate GFR in children with CKD. J Am Soc Nephrol. 2009;20(3):629–37.
21. Callahan MJ, Servaes S, Lee EY, Towbin AJ, Westra SJ, Frush DP. Practice patterns for the use of iodinated IV contrast media for pediatric CT studies: a survey of the society for pediatric radiology. AJR. 2014;202:872–9.
22. Rigsby CK, Gasber E, Seshadri R, Sullivan C, Wyers M, Ben-Ami T. Safety and efficacy of pressure-limited power injection of iodinated contrast medium through central lines in children. AJR Am J Roentgenol. 2007;188:726–32.
23. Bhargava R, Hahn G, Hirsch W, Kim MJ, Mentzel HJ, Olsen QE. Contrast-enhanced magnetic resonance imaging in pediatric patients: review and recommendations for current practice. Magn Reson Insights. 2013;6:95–111.
24. Grobner T. Gadolinium: a specific trigger for the development of nephrogenic fibrosing dermatopathy and nephrogenic systemic fibrosis? Nephrol Dial Transplant. 2006;21(4):1104–8.
25. Marckmann P, Skov L, Rossen K, et al. Nephrogenic systemic fibrosis: suspected causative role of gadodiamide used for contrast-enhanced magnetic resonance imaging. J Am Soc Nephrol. 2006;17(9):2359–62.
26. Nardone B, Saddleton E, Laumann AE, et al. Pediatric nephrogenic systemic fibrosis is rarely reported: a RADAR report. Pediatr Radiol. 2014;44(2):173–80.
27. Roberts DR, Chatterjee R, Yazdani M, Marebwa B, Brown T, Collins HT. Pediatric patients demonstrate progressive T1-weighted hyperintensity in the dentate nucleus following multiple doses of gadolinium-based contrast agent. AJNR Am J Neuroradiol. 2016;37(12):2340–7.
28. Kanda T, Fukusato T, Matsuda M, et al. Gadolinium-based contrast agent accumulates in the brain even in subjects without severe renal dysfunction: evaluation of autopsy brain specimens with inductively coupled plasma mass spectroscopy. Radiology. 2015;276(1):228–32.
29. Mc Donald RJ, McDonald JS, Kallmes DF, et al. Intracranial gadolinium deposition after contrast-enhanced MR imaging. Radiology. 2015;275(3):772–82.
30. Kanda T, Ishii K, Kawaguchi H, et al. High signal intensity in the dentate nucleus and globus pallidus on unenhanced T1 weighted MR images: relationship with increasing cumulative dose of a gadolinium based contrast material. Radiology. 2014;270:834–41.
31. Darrah TH, Prutsman-Pfeiffer JJ, Poreda RJ, et al. Incorporation of excess gadolinium into human bone from medical contrast agents. Metallomics. 2009;1:479–88.
32. Dillman JR, Ellis JH, Cohan RH, Strause PJ, Jan SC. Frequency and severity acute allergic-like reactions to gadolinium containing i.v. contrast media in children and adults. AJR Am J Roentgenol. 2007;189:1533–8.

21 Contrast-Enhanced Breast MR Imaging

Suzan Saylisoy

Breast cancer (BC) is still the most common cancer among women. Breast cancer mortality has decreased substantially in recent decades, due both to early detection of BC through improved imaging techniques and improved therapeutics [1]. The common clinical indications for contrast-enhanced (CE) breast magnetic resonance imaging (MRI) include preoperative BC staging, screening for high-risk patients, assessment of BC response to neoadjuvant chemotherapy, differentiation between scar and recurrence, evaluation of breast implants, assessment of patients with cancer of unknown primary [2–4]. Breast MRI appears to be more useful than mammography and ultrasound, especially for the assessment of invasive lobular cancer, ductal carcinoma in situ, multifocal/multicentric disease, and lesions with suspected associated extensive intraductal component [5].

Abnormal breast tissue demonstrates differences in longitudinal (T1) and transverse (T2) relaxation times in vitro compared with normal tissue [6]. Contrast-enhanced MRI evaluates the permeability of blood vessels by using intravenous gadolinium that shortens the local T1 time, leading to a higher signal on T1-weighted images (WI). The underlying principle is that neoangiogenesis leads to the formation of leaky vessels that allow for faster extravasation of contrast agents thus leading to rapid local enhancement [7].

The sensitivity of MRI for BC is relatively high (reported to approach 100%) [2]; however, specificity is moderately low (ranging from 47 to 97%) due to overlap in the imaging features of benign and malignant lesions [8]. Its modest specificity can lead to unnecessary biopsies, follow-ups, and patient anxiety [9]. To overcome limitations in specificity, several functional MRI parameters such as diffusion-weighted imaging (DWI) and magnetic resonance spectroscopy can be combined with dynamic contrast-enhanced (DCE) MRI to visualize specific biological properties, such as cellularity and chemical composition; this approach is defined as multiparametric MRI [6].

21.1 Breast MR Imaging

MR imaging should include an acquisition using a high-field magnet that is bilateral with complete breast and axilla coverage. Only dedicated breast surface coils are appropriate for breast MR imaging to provide enough signal-to-noise (SNR) for high-quality breast imaging [6]. The use of high-resolution protocol allows the more accurate assessment of tumor morphology and neoangiogenesis. Its diagnostic value can be further improved by parallel imaging techniques and higher field strengths leading to higher spatial

S. Saylisoy (✉)
Department of Radiology, Eskişehir Osmangazi University, Eskisehir, Turkey

S. M. Erturk et al. (eds.), *Medical Imaging Contrast Agents: A Clinical Manual*,
https://doi.org/10.1007/978-3-030-79256-5_21

and temporal resolution; therefore, breast MRI is increasingly moving towards 3 T. Breast MRI should be ideally performed in the second week of the menstrual cycle to reduce background enhancement of normal parenchyma [10].

Although there is a wide variation among centers with respect to the number of post-contrast phases acquired, the ACR Breast MRI Accreditation Program requires acquisition of at least two post-contrast T1-WI, with the first post-contrast sequence acquired within 4 min of after contrast injection [11].

DCE-MR imaging provides two primary imaging features that can be used to evaluate breast lesions: morphology and kinetic enhancement features [10]. Both assessment of tumor morphology and enhancement kinetics are necessary for the optimal diagnosis of breast lesions.

21.1.1 Assessment of Morphology

The ACR BI-RADS atlas describes three general lesion types: foci, masses, and non-mass enhancements (NMEs) [12]. Masses and NMEs should be reported with additional descriptors that can further refine an interpreting radiologist's suspicion for malignancy. Typically benign morphological features include round or oval shape, circumscribed margins, dark septa, and homogeneous slow-to-medium/persistent enhancement. Irregular shape, irregular or spiculated margins, heterogeneous or rim enhancement, and a wash-out curve are descriptors that most strongly indicate malignancy [13, 14]. According to a modified interpretation scheme, a lesion should be assigned as BI-RADS category 4 if both shape and margin are suspicious but enhancement kinetics suggest a benign lesion, or if lesion shape and margin are both non-suspicious but a wash-out is observed [10].

21.1.2 Semiquantitative Kinetic Enhancement Features

Cancers typically develop an abnormal vasculature and increased vessel permeability to support its high metabolic demand for oxygen and nutrients. The DCE-MRI is able to visualize and characterize this abnormal vasculature and permeability as a tumor-specific feature through the measurement of semiquantitative kinetic features [10]. Breast kinetic enhancement features are measured semi-quantitatively using a modest temporal resolution with at least two post-contrast T1-WI, with k-space centered at approximately 90–120 s after contrast injection for the first post-contrast images [6]. Using the data obtained at each of these time points, a time–signal intensity curves can be determined for a given lesion or region of interest (ROI), allowing assessment of two phases of enhancement: initial phase, within approximately 2 min of contrast injection, and delayed phase, after 2 min or after peak enhancement (Fig. 21.1) [15].

In the initial phase, enhancement classifications of slow, medium, and fast are determined by signal intensity increase ($SI_{\%increase}$) defined by the following enhancement formula: $SI_{\%increase}$ $[(SI_{post\ contrast} - SI_{precontrast})/SI_{precontrast}] \times 100\%$ [16].

In the delayed phase, enhancement curves can be described using three curve types: persistent, plateau, and wash-out [17]. Persistent enhancement is generally considered a benign curve type, whereas plateau enhancement is of intermediate suspicion for malignancy, and wash-out enhancement is the most suggestive of malignancy. The most classic combined curve type for malignant breast lesions is fast initial enhancement followed by early wash-out [6].

21.1.3 Quantitative Kinetic Enhancement Features

MR imaging techniques that acquire post-contrast images with high temporal resolution can allow a quantitative kinetic enhancement analysis through pharmacokinetic modeling [6]. Pharmacokinetic model, also known as two-compartment model first proposed by Tofts and Kermode, allows the quantification of the contrast agent exchange between the intravascular and the interstitial space, providing MRI pharmacokinetic parameters of K_{trans}, K_{ep}, and V_e (%).

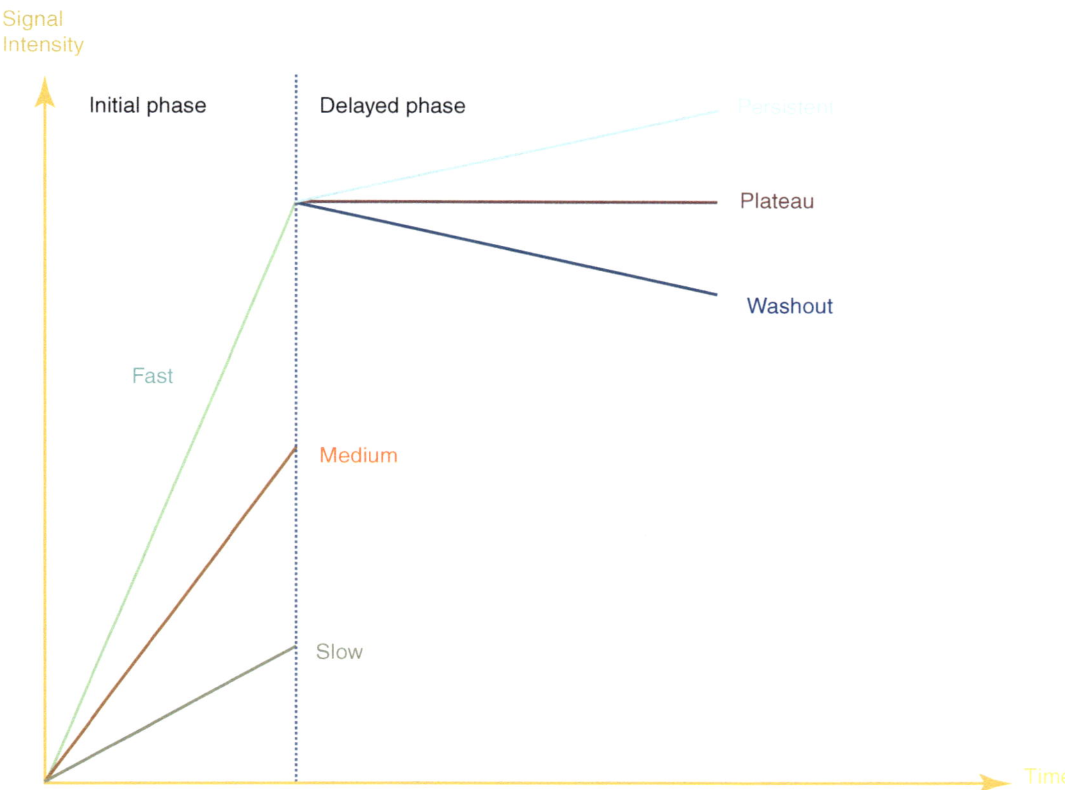

Fig. 21.1 Kinetic curve analysis of breast lesions. The enhancement kinetics is evaluated by assessing the time–signal intensity curve with its initial and delayed phases

Contrast agent concentrations for each compartment vary with time after bolus injection [18].

$\boldsymbol{K_{trans}}$ is the volume transfer constant, which describes the rate of contrast agent uptake into tumor from plasma.

$\boldsymbol{K_{ep}}$ is the transfer rate constant, which describes the reflux of the contrast agent from tumor to the plasma.

$\boldsymbol{V_e}$ **(%)** is the leakage of fractional volume from the extravascular extracellular space into the plasma [8].

Pharmacokinetic MRI parameters can potentially improve the differentiation of benign and malignant breast tumors. $K_{trans} > 0.25$/min and $K_{ep} > 1$/min are associated with malignancy, and, therefore, have been suggested as parameters to aid in the differentiation between benign and malignant breast tumors [10].

Pharmacokinetic MRI parameters have also been investigated to distinguish different BC subtypes. Yim et al. found that V_e values were significantly lower in BC with high tumor/stroma ratio, whereas K_{ep} values were significantly lower in BC with dominant collagen type and higher in BC with high nuclear grade [19].

21.1.4 Intravoxel Incoherent Motion DWI

Intravoxel incoherent motion (IVIM) DWI is sensitive to perfusion because the flow of blood in randomly oriented capillaries mimics a diffusion process through the IVIM effect. Several studies have investigated IVIM in breast tumors and preliminary data suggest that it may provide valuable information about both tissue microstructure and the microvasculature for improved BC diagnosis and for differentiation of different BC subtypes and molecular prognostic factors [6].

21.1.5 Abbreviated MRI

Recently, abbreviated as well as ultrafast dynamic imaging protocols have been evaluated for both BC diagnosis and screening. Several studies have investigated whether a shortened protocol, consisting of either a pre-contrast T1-WI and a single early post-contrast T1-WI or high-resolution ultrafast dynamic imaging is suitable for BC detection. All authors concluded that the abbreviated MRI protocol for breast MRI screening allows detection of breast lesions and classification with high accuracy. These results suggest that a significant shortening of scan protocols is possible and support the possibility of refining breast MRI screening protocols [20, 21].

References

1. Le-Petross HT, Lim B. Role of MR imaging in neoadjuvant therapy monitoring. Magn Reson Imaging Clin N Am. 2018;26(2):207–20.
2. Kilic F, Ogul H, Bayraktutan U, Gumus H, Unal O, Kantarci M, et al. Diagnostic magnetic resonance imaging of the breast. Eurasian J Med. 2012;44(2):106–14.
3. Schoub PK. Understanding indications and defining guidelines for breast magnetic resonance imaging. SA J Radiol. 2018;22(2):1353.
4. Tan S, David J, Lalonde L, El Khoury M, Labelle M, Younan R, et al. Breast magnetic resonance imaging: are those who need it getting it? Curr Oncol. 2017;24(3):e205–13.
5. Gilbert FJ, Pinker-Domenig K. Chapter 13: Diagnosis and staging of breast cancer: when and how to use mammography, tomosynthesis, ultrasound, contrast-enhanced mammography, and magnetic resonance imaging. In: Hodler J, Kubik-Huch RA, von Schulthess GK, editors. Diseases of the chest, breast, heart and vessels 2019-2022: diagnostic and interventional imaging [Internet]. Cham: Springer; 2019. http://www.ncbi.nlm.nih.gov/books/NBK553859/.
6. Rahbar H, Partridge SC. Multiparametric MR imaging of breast cancer. Magn Reson Imaging Clin N Am. 2016;24(1):223–38.
7. Lohrke J, Frenzel T, Endrikat J, Alves FC, Grist TM, Law M, et al. 25 years of contrast-enhanced MRI: developments, current challenges and future perspectives. Adv Ther. 2016;33(1):1–28.
8. Pinker K, Helbich TH, Morris EA. The potential of multiparametric MRI of the breast. Br J Radiol. 2017;90(1069):20160715.
9. Taşkın F, Polat Y, Erdoğdu İH, Türkdoğan FT, Öztürk VS, Özbaş S. Problem-solving breast MRI: useful or a source of new problems? Diagn Interv Radiol. 2018;24(5):255–61.
10. Leithner D, Wengert GJ, Helbich TH, Thakur S, Ochoa-Albiztegui RE, Morris EA, et al. Clinical role of breast MRI now and going forward. Clin Radiol. 2018;73(8):700–14.
11. Radiology ACo. Breast magnetic resonance imaging (MRI) accreditation program requirements. Reston: ACR; 2011. p. 13.
12. D'Orsi CJ, Sickles EA, Mendelson EB, Morris EA. ACR BI-RADS atlas, breast imaging reporting and data system. Reston: American College of Radiology; 2013.
13. Palestrant S, Comstock CE, Moy L. Approach to breast magnetic resonance imaging interpretation. Radiol Clin North Am. 2014;52(3):563–83.
14. Agrawal G, Su MY, Nalcioglu O, Feig SA, Chen JH. Significance of breast lesion descriptors in the ACR BI-RADS MRI lexicon. Cancer. 2009;115(7):1363–80.
15. Macura KJ, Ouwerkerk R, Jacobs MA, Bluemke DA. Patterns of enhancement on breast MR images: interpretation and imaging pitfalls. Radiographics. 2006;26(6):1719–34.
16. Cheng L, Li X. Breast magnetic resonance imaging: kinetic curve assessment. Gland Surg. 2013;2(1):50–3.
17. El Khouli RH, Macura KJ, Jacobs MA, Khalil TH, Kamel IR, Dwyer A, et al. Dynamic contrast-enhanced MRI of the breast: quantitative method for kinetic curve type assessment. AJR Am J Roentgenol. 2009;193(4):W295–300.
18. Seuss C, Heller SL. Breast Oncology: techniques, indications and interpretation. Springer. 2017;49–63.
19. Yim H, Kang DK, Jung YS, Jeon GS, Kim TH. Analysis of kinetic curve and model-based perfusion parameters on dynamic contrast enhanced MRI in breast cancer patients: correlations with dominant stroma type. Magn Reson Imaging. 2016;34(1):60–5.
20. Leithner D, Moy L, Morris EA, Marino MA, Helbich TH, Pinker K. Abbreviated MRI of the breast: does it provide value? J Magn Reson Imaging. 2019;49(7):e85–e100.
21. Ko ES, Morris EA. Abbreviated magnetic resonance imaging for breast cancer screening: concept, early results, and considerations. Korean J Radiol. 2019;20(4):533–41.

Musculoskeletal Imaging and Contrast Agents

22

Fethi Emre Ustabasioglu

Abbreviations

CA	Contrast agent
CBCT	Cone-beam computed tomography
CE-US	Contrast-enhanced ultrasound
CT	Computed tomography
CTA	Computed tomography arthrography
dCTA	Delayed CT arthrography
dGEMRIC	Delayed gadolinium-enhanced MRI of cartilage
Gd	Gadolinium
IV	Intravenous
MCP	Metacarpophalangeal
MDCT	Multi-detector computed tomography
MPR	Multiplanar reformat
MRA	Magnetic resonance arthrography
MRI	Magnetic resonance imaging
MSK	Musculoskeletal
OA	Osteoarthritis
PD	Power Doppler
RA	Rheumatoid arthritis
T1W	T1-weighted
T2W	T2-weighted
TFCC	Triangular fibrocartilage complex
US	Ultrasound

F. E. Ustabasioglu (✉)
Trakya University, Edirne, Turkey

22.1 Sonography of Musculoskeletal Imaging

US is an important tool for the imaging of MSK pathologies. For example, in a patient with inflammatory arthritis, US may show inflammation in the synovium, or in non-inflammatory arthritis, US can show the soft tissue pathologies. Contrary to MRI and CT, CAs are frequently used in US imaging. CAs have a role in US and Doppler US evaluation of synovial inflammation, especially in superficial soft tissue lesions and inflammatory arthritis.

Contrast-enhanced ultrasound (CE-US) is a modality which can assess the flow in tumors and to support Doppler US examinations [1]. US CAs are gas-filled micro-bubbles composed of a shell of biocompatible materials which contain gases of low solubility and diffusivity [2]. Szkudlarek et al. [3] showed that the IV CAs increase the sensitivity of power Doppler (PD) examination, especially in the evaluation of synovitis in hand and finger in RA patients.

The first published studies regarding CE-US used 7–15 mL bolus, first-generation CA (Levovist) ~400 mg/mL [4], within 1 min [5], or in slow 15–20 min perfusion [6]. In new studies, second-generation CA (SonoVue), 2.4 mL [7–9] or 4.8 mL [10, 11] was used. The appearance of micro-bubbles in the joint from the injection of the CA shows a high variability time interval. Microbubble appearances in articular and periar-

S. M. Erturk et al. (eds.), *Medical Imaging Contrast Agents: A Clinical Manual*,
https://doi.org/10.1007/978-3-030-79256-5_22

ticular tissues were identified by bolus administration in 20 s which is typical for small joint inflammation [12]. On the other hand, this time is usually up to 30 s for the hand and foot joints, because of the small calibration of the vessels. The presence of micro-bubbles for the inflamed synovium in large joints such as the knee is approximately 15 s after the use of the CA [12].

In bolus CA use, the examination window is 3–5 min. The slow 15–20 min IV perfusion allows the examination of the joints in this time period. This technique provides an increase in uniform CA over a longer time period and allows for the imaging of a greater number of joints [6]. Slow perfusion allows the penetration of micro-bubbles to small vessels [13]. No more than one or two joints can be examined by the bolus administration technique however this technique provides quantifying of inflammation analyzing time–intensity curve. It is a significant purpose of arthritis CE-US monitoring of the disease evolution and treatment response. The mean duration of an examination should be approximately 20 min. With the help of technological developments, the time allocated to a patient was decreased by computer programs that analyze time–intensity curves faster [12].

Both CE-US and gadolinium (Gd)-enhanced MRI are key techniques for the evaluation of joint diseases. Although MRI examination was the mainstay of joint imaging, it was found that CE-US results were significantly correlated with MRI in some studies [14].

In a paper by Szkudlarek et al. [3] it was revealed that the synovial color coding of the metacarpophalangeal (MCP) joint in RA patients after IV injection of the US contrast medium (Levovist) (Schering, Berlin, Germany) was significantly increased compared to non-contrast PD examinations. Besides, Klauser et al. [15] detected active synovitis and inactive intra-articular thickening in RA patients using CE-US.

Although CE-US is not used often for the knee in comparison with contrast-enhanced MRI, Song et al. [16] demonstrated synovium hypervascularization in osteoarthritis (OA) patients treated with intrauterine bradykinin receptor 2 antagonist and found the results were consistent with contrast-enhanced MRI.

Loizides et al. [17] stated that tumor characterization can be achieved with CE-US according to the enhancement pattern of soft tissue masses. Although the definitive diagnosis of soft tissue masses is made by biopsy, CE-US can provide great convenience to determine where the biopsy should be made. In a study, the authors determined the viable tumor region of the mass by CE-US for biopsy targeting with a 100% diagnostic yield [18].

22.2 Computed Tomography in Musculoskeletal Imaging

CT is a useful tool in MSK pathologies because it has the ability to detect most of the bone lesions correctly. MRI with the competence of producing MPR imaging and its high ST characterization has an important role. Also, multidetector computed tomography (MDCT) has a significant role in MSK pathologies, it has apparent superiorities when compared to MRI in acute trauma and evaluation of the postoperative patients [19].

Contrast administration for CT examinations is very helpful in most of the MSK diseases including malignancies, infections, and inflammatory diseases. Computed tomographic arthrography (CTA) has a high spatial resolution so it is a remarkable imaging technique in the diagnosis of a wide spectrum of joint disorders. CTA is a good alternative to magnetic resonance arthrography (MRA) in a failed MRI examination, in obese or claustrophobic patients, or when the medical device is not compatible with MRI [20].

Iodinated CA with single- or double-contrast administration into the joint shows articular surface perfectly in CTA. A single contrast technique can be applied with CA or air; whereas a double-contrast technique can be used by injecting minimal CA followed by air. Evaluation of a loose body and cartilage is superior using double-contrast method; but with the advancement of technology, CT has gone quite far, and there is nearly no difference between these two techniques [20].

CTA is highly good at showing cartilage and bone pathologies, many of which can not be displayed with other modalities. CTA provides the classification of traumatic tears of the interosseous ligaments as complete or incomplete and as partial or full thickness tears in the wrist and also differentiates that from asymptomatic degenerative lesions. In a paper by Moser et al. [21], it is recommended that 5 mL of iodinated CA should be used for wrist CTA [21].

The foremost defect in CTA is that the detection of soft tissue abnormalities, which may be shown by other imaging methods like US and MRI [21].

Contrast-enhanced tomography is very good for rheumatologic diseases. The sensitivity of CT is higher when compared to MRI in the diagnosis of RA erosions [22–25]. Polster et al. [26] indicate that IV contrast-enhanced CT can be used to demonstrate synovitis, tenosynovitis, and bone erosion in RA patients.

Delayed CT arthrography (dCTA) [27] can be used for the detection of tissue changes of bone and cartilage. Myller et al. [28] have shown that delayed CBCT arthrography is very successful in evaluating cartilage and bones in the knee joint in patients with osteoarthritis. They were also able to evaluate the fissures in the cartilage with the CA given to the joint. In dCBCTA, CA is injected intra-articularly, similarly as in clinical MRI of the rotator cuff of the shoulder, whereas in dGEMRIC, the CA is injected intravenously.

22.3 Magnetic Resonance Imaging in Musculoskeletal Imaging

MRI as a noninvasive method without ionizing radiation is the first choice in musculoskeletal imaging with capabilities such as providing high-resolution images in cartilage and soft tissues with an ability to acquire images in every desired angle or plane [29–31]. Major indications of contrast-enhanced MRI broadly include assessment of bone and soft tissue tumors, infections and inflammatory processes, and MRA.

MRA has increased the diagnostic confidence for the assessment of tendon tears and complex labral abnormalities. MRA of many joints is routinely performed in current clinical practice, common joints being the shoulder, hips, wrist, and elbow [32] (Figs. 22.1 and 22.2).

Elbow is a complex joint formed by three separate joints and these joints are connected by several ligaments and a large capsule. Because of its complex structure, the elbow represents a challenge in terms of diagnosis, therapy, and rehabilitation [33]. Currently, MRI is the most preferred method to evaluate cartilage lesions noninvasively [34, 35]. On the other hand, most

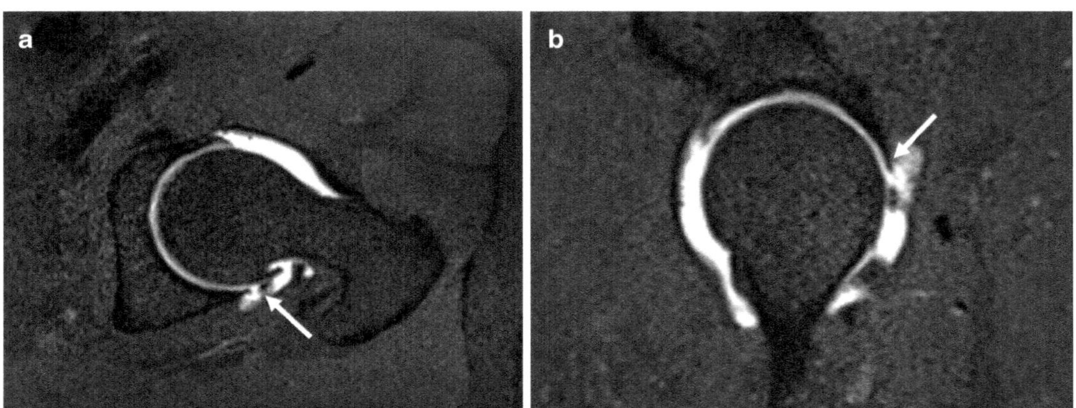

Fig. 22.1 MR arthrography (axial (**a**) and sagittal (**b**) T1W-fat sat) imaging of left hip reveals posterior acetabular labral tear with and paralabral lobulated cyst (*arrow*)

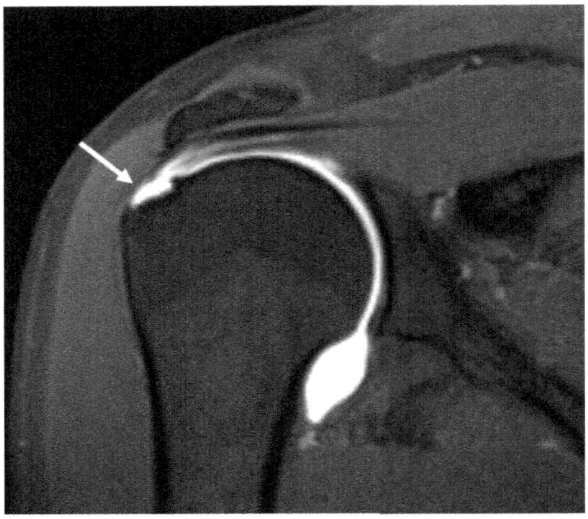

Fig. 22.2 Fat suppressed T1W coronal oblique MR arthrography image reveals articular surface tear of the supraspinatus tendon (*arrow*)

studies on conventional MRI techniques point out limitations in the diagnosis of early chondromalacia [36–38]. MRA is more sensitive than conventional MRI in surface lesions of articular cartilage [39–41]. Also, several authors who investigated the value of MRI of articular cartilage recommended the use of intra-articular contrast media to improve the detectability of small surface lesions [39, 40].

In the wrist, MRA improves the detection rate for diagnosis of both interosseous ligament and TFCC tears [42–45]. Intra-articular injection of Gd-based CAs is a reliable method [46]. The image quality for diagnostic purposes becomes critical 45 min after contrast injection for the wrist joint and after 90 min for the shoulder and hip joints [47].

Gd-chelates which are administered intra-articularly are eliminated with trans synovial diffusion [48–51]. The mechanism of trans synovial diffusion of Gd is complex and it can be affected by various factors, including the permeability, vascularity, and surface area of the synovial membrane; the volume of articular fluid; the concentration gradient of plasma and contrast-enhanced joint fluid; and intra-articular pressure [52, 53]. In patients with inflammatory rheumatologic disorders, synovial perfusion is significantly increased secondary to inflammation. Therefore, diffusion of the intra-articular Gd-chelates in MRA may be faster in these patients, that results from shorter time window during MRA [47].

In the evaluation of the hip joint, MRA provides more data than conventional MRI [54]. In routine clinical practice, the diluted Gd is usually injected into the hip joint space with US guidance. Gd can be injected under palpation or under a scopy but palpation is not very reliable. US is the most preferred method since the scopy also contains radiation. The fact that US is the most preferred method because it is fast, radiation-free, and practical.

MRA and CTA of the shoulder are considered the best-performing imaging techniques in diagnosing shoulder diseases if prospectively compared with arthroscopic and open surgical findings. Both of the modalities are certainly superior to plain CT or MRI of the shoulder because of the contrast resolution due to the presence of intra-articular diluted paramagnetic contrast or iodinated agent, respectively, and to the distension of the joint capsule [55, 56]. The evaluation of the site, type, grade, and extent of the disease is more reliable, in particular for rotator cuff tears [57, 58] and congenital or traumatic glenohumeral instability [59, 60]. The two methods represent different information due to a higher CT sensitivity for calcifications and bone injuries [61, 62] and an optimal MR contrast resolution for soft tissue abnormalities [57]. The stability of the mixture of Gd-chelates and iodinated CAs are well-known [63] while its clinical safety has been reported for performing CTA and MRA of the ankle as a one-shot exam (CTA-MRA) [64]. Aliprandi et al. [65] performed CTA and MRA of the shoulder as a one-shot exam using a mixture of iodinated and paramagnetic CAs and to test the value of this CTA-MRA exam compared with each of the two modalities used separately, using arthroscopy as a standard of reference. Their experience confirms the reliability of intra-articular administration of a mixture of iodinated and paramagnetic CA and provides the feasibility of CTA and MRA as a one-shot exam. Furthermore, CTA-MRA provides more data than CTA or MRA separately.

22.3.1 MSK Infections

MSK infections which are considered a therapeutic emergency affect bones, soft tissues, and joints. MRI is currently the best technique to determine the presence or absence of disease and its extent. It is recommended to administer IV Gd in MRI of all possible MSK infections. IV Gd contrast allows a better description of fluid collections, joint effusions, and soft tissue inflammation on soft tissue infections also it is useful for detecting soft tissue abscesses and sinus tracts, distinguishing synovial thickening from fluid and evaluating spine infections [66].

MRI of cellulitis reveals thickening of the subcutaneous tissues, diffuse linear or ill-defined increased signal intensity of superficial soft tissue on fluid-sensitive sequences, and corresponding low signal intensity on T1-weighted (T1W) sequences consistent with edema. Imaging after IV administration of CA is useful to demonstrate diffuse enhancement of the same areas, consistent with inflammation, although the extent and degree of enhancement are variable [67–69].

Even though STIR sequences in MRI enable for detecting inflammation and edema, contrast-enhanced T1W images have a remarkable higher signal-to-noise-ratio, which may have better identifiability of pathologic findings [70].

22.3.2 MSK Tumor Imaging

MRI is a valuable method for noninvasively imaging and evaluating MSK tumors [71]. Although unenhanced MRI can be a diagnostic solving method in evaluating MSK masses [72–74] gd-CM is often needed and plays an important role in the characterization of a lesion, in staging the extent of MSK masses, in biopsy planning, in monitoring chemotherapy, and in the detection of local recurrence [71].

MRI is also particularly helpful in the assessment of bone tumors when the lesion is indeterminate (e.g., solitary versus aneurysmal bone cyst) or likely to be biopsied (e.g., eosinophilic granuloma versus Ewing's sarcoma, acute osteomyelitis versus Ewing's sarcoma, enchondroma versus low-grade chondrosarcoma) [75]. All suspected bone sarcoma should be staged with MRI before biopsy [71].

The use of CA in MRI may be helpful in demonstrating tumor characteristics and also shows different characteristics of tumor in two different localizations. For instance, predominantly spindle cell variants encountered in the MSK system reveals higher CA enhancement both at CT and MRI, lower T2-signal at MRI. On the other hand, its gastrointestinal counterpart, consisting predominantly of the myxoid vascular type, shows a higher T2 signal at MRI and a lesser CA enhancement with CT and MRI [76].

Administration of Gd can help to distinguish between cystic and aneurysmal tumor components. Generally, cystic components of tumor have a homogeneous high signal intensity, whereas aneurysmal tumor components reveal a fluid-fluid level on T2-weighted (T2W) images. Therefore, T2W images are often sufficient to differentiate an aneurysmal from a simple bone cyst. The presence of non-enhancing, cystic-appearing zones, filled with lymphatic fluid, differentiate lymphangioma from hemangioma, which enhances entirely because it is perfused with Gd containing blood [71].

Contrast administration provides identification of solid, cystic, necrotic, myxoid, and cartilaginous components in MSK masses. All these components have a decreased signal intensity on T1W images and an increased signal intensity on T2W images but have different enhancement patterns [71]. Seromas, cysts, and cystic tumor components have homogeneous increased signal intensity on T2W images and show no enhancement or negligible enhancement of a thin wall. Tumor necrosis or abscess has a homogeneous or heterogeneous increased signal intensity on T2W images and reveals no enhancement [71].

Administration of Gd is also significant in managing biopsy to solid, vascularized areas that provide diagnostic tissue rather than nondiagnostic areas of hemorrhage, necrosis, or highly myxoid regions. If only static contrast-enhanced MRI is performed to find an appropriate biopsy area, the most intense enhancement regions should be selected (Fig. 22.3).

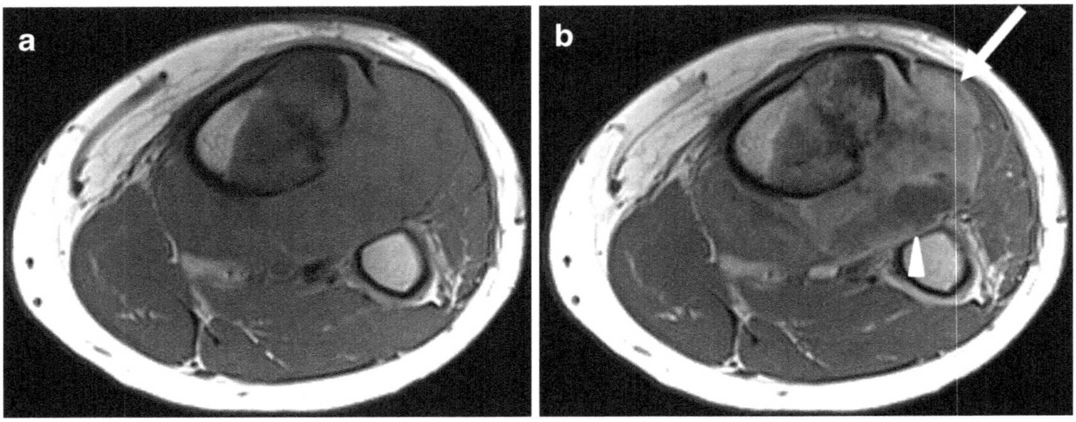

Fig. 22.3 Osteosarcoma of the left tibia in a 12-year-old girl. (**a**) Axial T1-weighted precontrast MR image shows a large mass in the proximal tibial metaphysis. The tumor is almost isointense to muscle. (**b**) Axial T1-weighted postcontrast MR image shows non-enhancing necrosis (arrowhead) and enhancing viable tumor (arrow). The biopsy was taken along the course of the arrow, distant from the necrotic area

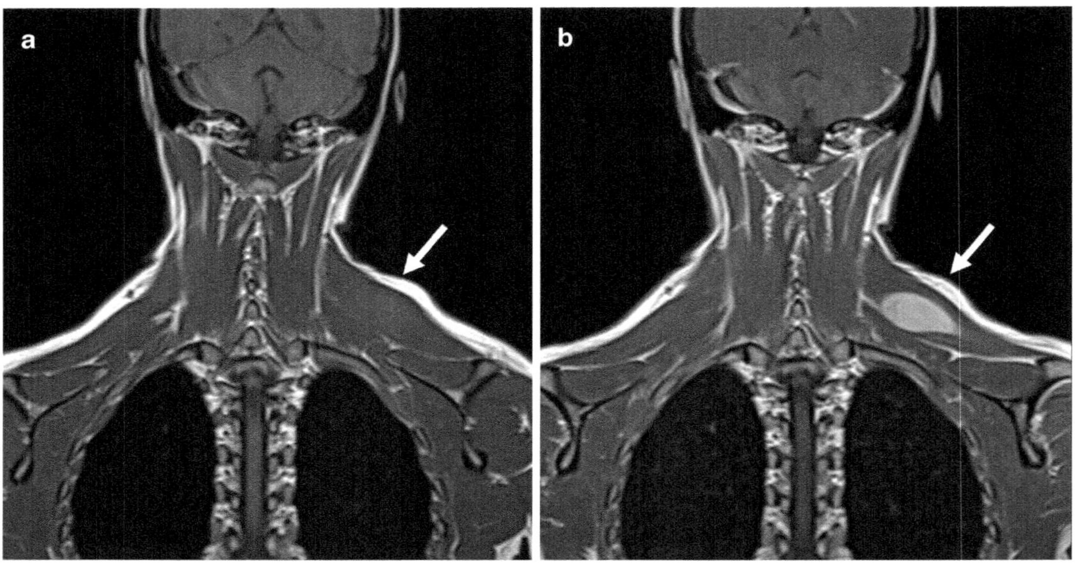

Fig. 22.4 MR images of a 35-year-old woman with low-grade myofibroblastic sarcoma are shown. Coronal T1WI (**a**) shows an isointense mass (*arrow*) in the left trapezius muscle. T1W coronal image with contrast administration (**b**) demonstrates the demarcation of lesion better than the T1W coronal image without contrast sequence and shows the avid enhancement of the lesion with the contrast media

Administration of Gd is a powerful choice to detect viable tumor components and suggest the diagnosis of sarcoma in extensive hemorrhages, where solid, cellular tumor components might be overlooked (Fig. 22.4).

The pharmacokinetic behavior of Gd-chelates CA is equal to that of the well-known, iodinated angiographic and urographic CAs in radiographic examinations. After rapid intravascular distribution, Gd diffuses into the extracellular space and is completely excreted through the kidneys. The standard dose for MSK applications is 0.1 mmol per kilogram of body weight at a concentration of 0.5 M [77].

Dynamic MRI is very useful to detect and to differentiate viable tumor from reactive changes after treatment. This method is recommended to distinguish recurrent neoplastic nodules from small seromas or reactive changes. Also, it is very useful to differentiate acute marrow infarction from tumor, because infarction is avascular, and will show no or only late enhancement [78]. In dynamic contrast-enhanced MRI, the early intravascular and interstitial distribution of Gd in MSK masses can be followed. Ultra-fast, T1W snap-shot sequences are applied after IV bolus injection, to trace the early contrast-enhancement during and immediately after the first pass of the Gd through the lesion [79]. This technique provides physiologic information, such as tissue perfusion, tissue vascularization, capillary permeability, and volume of the interstitial space, that is not available on the anatomic images obtained with routine static imaging sequences [80].

References

1. Harvey CJ, Blomley MJ, Eckersley RJ, Cosgrove DO. Developments in ultrasound contrast media. Eur Radiol. 2001;11(4):675–89.
2. Dalla LP, Bertolotto M. Introduction to ultrasound contrast agents: physics overview. Eur Radiol. 1999;9:S338–42.
3. Szkudlarek M, Strandberg C, Klarlund M, Klausen T, Østergaard M. Contrast-enhanced power Doppler ultrasonography of the metacarpophalangeal joints in rheumatoid arthritis. Eur Radiol. 2003;13(1):163–8.
4. Albrecht K, Muller-Ladner U, Strunk J. Quantification of the synovial perfusion in rheumatoid arthritis using Doppler ultrasonography. Clin Exp Rheumatol. 2007;25(4):630.
5. Salaffi F, Carotti M, Manganelli P, Filippucci E, Giuseppetti GM, Grassi W. Contrast-enhanced power Doppler sonography of knee synovitis in rheumatoid arthritis: assessment of therapeutic response. Clin Rheumatol. 2004;23(4):285–90.
6. Klauser A, Frauscher F, Schirmer M, Halpern E, Pallwein L, Herold M, et al. The value of contrast-enhanced color Doppler ultrasound in the detection of vascularization of finger joints in patients with rheumatoid arthritis. Arthritis Rheum. 2002;46(3):647–53.
7. Rees JD, Pilcher J, Heron C, Kiely PDW. A comparison of clinical vs ultrasound determined synovitis in rheumatoid arthritis utilizing gray-scale, power Doppler and the intravenous microbubble contrast agent 'Sono-Vue'®. Rheumatology. 2006;46(3):454–9.
8. Schueller-Weidekamm C, Krestan C, Schueller G, Kapral T, Aletaha D, Kainberger F. Power Doppler sonography and pulse-inversion harmonic imaging in evaluation of rheumatoid arthritis synovitis. Am J Roentgenol. 2007;188(2):504–8.
9. Klauser AS, De Zordo T, Bellmann-Weiler R, Feuchtner GM, Sailer-Höck M, Sögner P, et al. Feasibility of second-generation ultrasound contrast media in the detection of active sacroiliitis. Arthritis Care Res. 2009;61(7):909–16.
10. Platzgummer H, Schueller G, Grisar J, Weber M, Schueller-Weidekamm C. Quantification of synovitis in rheumatoid arthritis: do we really need quantitative measurement of contrast-enhanced ultrasound? Eur J Radiol. 2009;71(2):237–41.
11. Solivetti FM, Elia F, Teoli M, De Mutiis C, Chimenti S, Berardesca E, et al. Role of contrast-enhanced ultrasound in early diagnosis of psoriatic arthritis. Dermatology. 2010;220(1):25–31.
12. Rednic N, Tamas MM, Rednic S. Contrast-enhanced ultrasonography in inflammatory arthritis. Med Ultrasonogr. 2011;13(3):220–7.
13. Klauser A, Frauscher F, Schirmer M. Value of contrast-enhanced power Doppler ultrasonography (US) of the metacarpophalangeal joints on rheumatoid arthritis. Eur Radiol. 2004;14(3):545–6.
14. Ohrndorf S, Hensch A, Naumann L, Hermann KG, Scheurig-Münkler C, Meier S, et al. Contrast-enhanced ultrasonography is more sensitive than grayscale and power Doppler ultrasonography compared to MRI in therapy monitoring of rheumatoid arthritis patients. Ultraschall Med. 2011;32(Suppl 2):E38–44.
15. Klauser A, Demharter J, De Marchi A, Sureda D, Barile A, Masciocchi C, et al. Contrast enhanced gray-scale sonography in assessment of joint vascularity in rheumatoid arthritis: results from the IACUS study group. Eur Radiol. 2005;15(12):2404–10.
16. Song IH, Althoff CE, Hermann KG, Scheel AK, Knetsch T, Burmester GR, et al. Contrast-enhanced ultrasound in monitoring the efficacy of a bradykinin receptor 2 antagonist in painful knee osteoarthritis compared with MRI. Ann Rheum Dis. 2009;68(1):75–83.
17. Loizides A, Peer S, Plaikner M, Djurdjevic T, Gruber H. Perfusion pattern of musculoskeletal masses using contrast-enhanced ultrasound: a helpful tool for characterisation? Eur Radiol. 2012;22(8):1803–11.
18. Loizides A, Widmann G, Freuis T, Peer S, Gruber H. Optimizing ultrasound-guided biopsy of musculoskeletal masses by application of an ultrasound contrast agent. Ultraschall Med. 2011;32(03):307–10.
19. West ATH, Marshall TJ, Bearcroft PW. CT of the musculoskeletal system: what is left is the days of MRI? Eur Radiol. 2009;19(1):152.
20. Rydberg J, Buckwalter KA, Caldemeyer KS, Phillips MD, Conces DJ Jr, Aisen AM, et al. Multisection CT: scanning techniques and clinical applications. Radiographics. 2000;20(6):1787–806.

21. Moser T, Dosch JC, Moussaoui A, Buy X, Gangi A, Dietemann JL. Multidetector CT arthrography of the wrist joint: how to do it. Radiographics. 2008;28(3):787–800.
22. Farrant JM, Grainger AJ, O'Connor PJ. Advanced imaging in rheumatoid arthritis: part 2: erosions. Skelet Radiol. 2007;36(5):381–9.
23. Døhn UM, Ejbjerg BJ, Hasselquist M, Narvestad E, Szkudlarek M, Møller J, et al. Rheumatoid arthritis bone erosion volumes on CT and MRI: reliability and correlations with erosion scores on CT, MRI and radiography. Ann Rheum Dis. 2007;66(10):1388–92.
24. Døhn UM, Ejbjerg BJ, Hasselquist M, Narvestad E, Szkudlarek M, Møller JM, et al. Are bone erosions detected by magnetic resonance imaging and ultrasonography true erosions? A comparison with computed tomography in rheumatoid arthritis metacarpophalangeal joints. Arthritis Res Ther. 2006;8(4):R110.
25. Perry D, Stewart N, Benton N, Robinson E, Yeoman S, Crabbe J, et al. Detection of erosions in the rheumatoid hand; a comparative study of multidetector computerized tomography versus magnetic resonance scanning. J Rheumatol. 2005;32(2):256–67.
26. Polster JM, Winalski CS, Sundaram M, Lieber ML, Schils J, Ilaslan H, et al. Rheumatoid arthritis: evaluation with contrast-enhanced CT with digital bone masking. Radiology. 2009;252(1):225–31.
27. Hirvasniemi J, Kulmala KAM, Lammentausta E, Ojala R, Lehenkari P, Kamel A, et al. In vivo comparison of delayed gadolinium-enhanced MRI of cartilage and delayed quantitative CT arthrography in imaging of articular cartilage. Osteoarthr Cartil. 2013;21(3):434–42.
28. Myller KA, Turunen MJ, Honkanen JT, Väänänen SP, Iivarinen JT, Salo J, et al. In vivo contrast-enhanced cone beam CT provides quantitative information on articular cartilage and subchondral bone. Ann Biomed Eng. 2017;45(3):811–8.
29. Crues J, Bydder G. Frontiers in musculoskeletal imaging. J Magn Reson Imaging. 2007;25(2):232–3.
30. O'Neill W. The physician-owned imaging center. Orthop Clin N Am. 2008;39(1):37–48.
31. Koltzenburg M, Yousry T. Magnetic resonance imaging of skeletal muscle. Curr Opin Neurol. 2007;20(5):595–9.
32. Steinbach LS, Palmer WE, Schweitzer ME. Special focus session: MR arthrography. Radiographics. 2002;22(5):1223–46.
33. Aliprandi A, Poloni A. Approach to the radiological imaging of the elbow. In: The elbow. Cham: Springer; 2018. p. 59–66.
34. Hodler J, Resnick D. Current status of imaging of articular cartilage. Skelet Radiol. 1996;25(8):703–9.
35. McCauley TR. MR imaging of chondral and osteochondral injuries of the knee. Radiol Clin. 2002;40(5):1095–107.
36. Disler DG, Recht MP, McCauley TR. MR imaging of articular cartilage. Skelet Radiol. 2000;29(7):367–77.
37. Waldschmidt JG, Rilling RJ, Kajdacsy-Balla AA, Boynton MD, Erickson SJ. In vitro and in vivo MR imaging of hyaline cartilage: zonal anatomy, imaging pitfalls, and pathologic conditions. Radiographics. 1997;17(6):1387–402.
38. Trattnig S, Mlynarik V, Huber M, Ba-Ssalamah A, Stefan PUIG, Imhof H. Magnetic resonance imaging of articular cartilage and evaluation of cartilage disease. Invest Radiol. 2000;35(10):595–601.
39. Gagliardi JA, Chung EM, Chandnani VP, Kesling KL, Christensen KP, Null RN, et al. Detection and staging of chondromalacia patellae: relative efficacies of conventional MR imaging, MR arthrography, and CT arthrography. AJR Am J Roentgenol. 1994;163(3):629–36.
40. Gylys-Morin VM, Hajek PC, Sartoris DJ, Resnick D. Articular cartilage defects: detectability in cadaver knees with MR. Am J Roentgenol. 1987;148(6):1153–7.
41. Kramer J, Recht MP, Imhof H, Stiglbaüer R, Engel A. Postcontrast MR arthrography in assessment of cartilage lesions. J Comput Assist Tomogr. 1994;18(2):218–24.
42. Hodler J, Kursunoglu-Brahme S, Snyder SJ, Cervilla V, Karzel RP, Schweitzer ME, et al. Rotator cuff disease: assessment with MR arthrography versus standard MR imaging in 36 patients with arthroscopic confirmation. Radiology. 1992;182(2):431–6.
43. Hodler J, Yu JS, Goodwin D, Haghighi P, Trudell D, Resnick D. MR arthrography of the hip: improved imaging of the acetabular labrum with histologic correlation in cadavers. AJR Am J Roentgenol. 1995;165(4):887–91.
44. Petersilge CA. MR arthrography for evaluation of the acetabular labrum. Skelet Radiol. 2001;30(8):423–30.
45. White LM, Schweitzer ME, Weishaupt D, Kramer J, Davis A, Marks PH. Diagnosis of recurrent meniscal tears: prospective evaluation of conventional MR imaging, indirect MR arthrography, and direct MR arthrography. Radiology. 2002;222(2):421–9.
46. Schulte-Altedorneburg G, Gebhard M, Wohlgemuth W, Fischer W, Zentner J, Wegener R, et al. MR arthrography: pharmacology, efficacy and safety in clinical trials. Skelet Radiol. 2003;32(1):1–12.
47. Andreisek G, Duc SR, Froehlich JM, Hodler J, Weishaupt D. MR arthrography of the shoulder, hip, and wrist: evaluation of contrast dynamics and image quality with increasing injection-to-imaging time. Am J Roentgenol. 2007;188(4):1081–8.
48. Wagner SC, Schweitzer ME, Weishaupt D. Temporal behavior of intraarticular gadolinium. J Comput Assist Tomogr. 2001;25(5):661–70.
49. Hadler NM. Synovial fluids facilitate small solute diffusivity. Ann Rheum Dis. 1980;39(6):580–5.
50. Hall FM. Epinephrine-enhanced knee arthrography. Radiology. 1974;111(1):215–7.
51. Weishaupt D, Schweitzer ME, Rawool NM, Nazarian LN, Morrison WB, Natale PM, et al. Indirect MR arthrography of the knee: effects of low-intensity ultrasound on the diffusion rate of intravenously administered Gd-DTPA in healthy volunteers. Invest Radiol. 2001;36(8):493–9.

52. Drape JL, Thelen P, Gay-Depassier P, Silbermann O, Benacerraf R. Intraarticular diffusion of Gd-DOTA after intravenous injection in the knee: MR imaging evaluation. Radiology. 1993;188(1):227–34.
53. Schweitzer ME, Falk A, Berthoty D, Mitchell M, ReSnick D. Knee effusion: normal distribution of fluid. AJR Am J Roentgenol. 1992;159(2):361–3.
54. Messina C, Banfi G, Aliprandi A, Mauri G, Secchi F, Sardanelli F, et al. Ultrasound guidance to perform intra-articular injection of gadolinium-based contrast material for magnetic resonance arthrography as an alternative to fluoroscopy: the time is now. Eur Radiol. 2016;26(5):1221–5.
55. Flannigan B, Kursunoglu-Brahme S, Snyder S, Karzel R, Del Pizzo W, Resnick D. MR arthrography of the shoulder: comparison with conventional MR imaging. AJR Am J Roentgenol. 1990;155(4):829–32.
56. Bachmann G, Bauer T, Jürgensen I, Schwab J, Weimar B, Rau WS. The diagnostic accuracy and therapeutic relevance of CT arthrography and MR arthrography of the shoulder. RoFo. 1998;168(2):149–56.
57. Palmer WE, Brown JH, Rosenthal DI. Rotator cuff: evaluation with fat-suppressed MR arthrography. Radiology. 1993;188(3):683–7.
58. Funke M, Kopka L, Vosshenrich R, Oestmann JW, Grabbe E. MR arthrography in the diagnosis of rotator cuff tears: standard spin-echo alone or with fat suppression? Acta Radiol. 1996;37(3P2):627–32.
59. Tirman PF, Bost FW, Garvin GJ, Peterfy CG, Mall JC, Steinbach LS. Posterosuperior glenoid impingement of the shoulder: findings at MR imaging and MR arthrography with arthroscopic correlation. Radiology. 1994;193(2):431–6.
60. Bencardino JT, Beltran J, Rosenberg ZS, Rokito A, Schmahmann S, Mota J, et al. Superior labrum anterior-posterior lesions: diagnosis with MR arthrography of the shoulder. Radiology. 2000;214(1):267–71.
61. Godefroy D, Sarazin L, Rousselin B, Dupont AM, Drape JL, Chevrot A. Shoulder imaging: what is the best modality? J Radiol. 2001;82(3 Suppl):317–34.
62. Roger B, Skaf A, Hooper AW, Lektrakul N, Yeh L, Resnick D. Imaging findings in the dominant shoulder of throwing athletes: comparison of radiography, arthrography, CT arthrography, and MR arthrography with arthroscopic correlation. AJR Am J Roentgenol. 1999;172(5):1371–80.
63. Kopka L, Funke M, Fischer U, Vosshenrich R, Schröder M, Grabbe E. Signal characteristics of x-ray contrast media and their interaction with gadolinium-DTPA in MRT. RoFo. 1994;160(4):349–52.
64. Schmid MR, Pfirrmann CWA, Hodler J, Vienne P, Zanetti M. Cartilage lesions in the ankle joint: comparison of MR arthrography and CT arthrography. Skelet Radiol. 2003;32(5):259–65.
65. Aliprandi A, Fausto A, Quarenghi M, Modestino S, Randelli P, Sardanelli F. One-shot CT and MR arthrography of the shoulder with a mixture of iodinated and paramagnetic contrast agents using arthroscopy as a gold standard. Radiol Med. 2006;111(1):53–60.
66. Simpfendorfer CS. Radiologic approach to musculoskeletal infections. Infect Dis Clin. 2017;31(2):299–324.
67. Struk DW, Munk PL, Lee MJ, Ho SG, Worsley DF. Imaging of soft tissue infections. Radiol Clin N Am. 2001;39(2):277–303.
68. Towers JD. The use of intravenous contrast in MRI of extremity infection. In: Seminars in ultrasound, CT and MRI. Vol. 18, No. 4. WB Saunders; 1997. p. 269–75.
69. Gylys-Morin VM. MR imaging of pediatric musculoskeletal inflammatory and infectious disorders. Magn Reson Imaging Clin N Am. 1998;6(3):537–59.
70. Schmid MR, Hodler J, Vienne P, Binkert CA, Zanetti M. Bone marrow abnormalities of foot and ankle: STIR versus T1-weighted contrast-enhanced fat-suppressed spin-echo MR imaging. Radiology. 2002;224(2):463–9.
71. Verstraete KL, Lang P. Bone and soft tissue tumors: the role of contrast agents for MR imaging. Eur J Radiol. 2000;34(3):229–46.
72. Sundaram M, McLeod RA. MR imaging of tumor and tumorlike lesions of bone and soft tissue. AJR Am J Roentgenol. 1990;155(4):817–24.
73. Härle A, Reiser M, Erlemann R, Wuisman P. The value of nuclear magnetic resonance tomography in staging of bone and soft tissue sarcomas. Orthopade. 1989;18(1):34–40.
74. Vanel D, Verstraete KL, Shapeero LG. Primary tumors of the musculoskeletal system. Radiol Clin N Am. 1997;35(1):213–37.
75. Sundaram M. The use of gadolinium in the MR imaging of bone tumors. In: Seminars in ultrasound, CT and MRI. Vol. 18, No. 4. WB Saunders; 1997. p. 307–11.
76. Horger M, Pfannenberg C, Bitzer M, Wehrmann M, Claussen CD. Synchronous gastrointestinal and musculoskeletal manifestations of different subtypes of inflammatory myofibroblastic tumor: CT, MRI and pathological features. Eur Radiol. 2005;15(8):1713–6.
77. Beltran J, Chandnani V, McGhee RA Jr, Kursunoglu-Brahme S. Gadopentetate dimeglumine-enhanced MR imaging of the musculoskeletal system. AJR Am J Roentgenol. 1991;156(3):457–66.
78. Park SY, Chung HW, Chae SY, Lee JS. Comparison of MRI and PET-CT in detecting the loco-regional recurrence of soft tissue sarcomas during surveillance. Skelet Radiol. 2016;45(10):1375–84.
79. Sujlana P, Skrok J, Fayad LM. Review of dynamic contrast-enhanced MRI: technical aspects and applications in the musculoskeletal system. J Magn Reson Imaging. 2018;47(4):875–90.
80. Choi YJ, Lee IS, Song YS, Kim JI, Choi KU, Song JW. Diagnostic performance of diffusion-weighted (DWI) and dynamic contrast-enhanced (DCE) MRI for the differentiation of benign from malignant soft-tissue tumors. J Magn Reson Imaging. 2019;50(3):798–809.

23 Optimal Contrast-Enhanced Computed Tomography and Magnetic Resonance Cardiac Imaging

Cemile Ayşe Görmeli and Tuncay Hazırolan

Abbreviations

ARVC	Arrhythmogenic right ventricular cardiomyopathy
CAD	Coronary artery disease
CT	Computed tomography
DCM	Dilated cardiomyopathy
ECV	Extracellular volume
EMA	European Medicines Agency
FBP	Filtered back projection
HCM	Hypertrophic cardiomyopathy
HU	Hounsfield Units
IR	Inversion recovery
IR	Iterative reconstruction
IV	Intravenous
LGE	Late gadolinium enhancement
MOLLI	Modified Look-Locker inversion recovery
MRA	Magnetic resonance angiography
MRI	Magnetic resonance imaging
PSIR	Phase-sensitive inversion recovery
ROI	Region of interest
TAVR	Transcatheter aortic valve replacement
TI	Inversion time

C. A. Görmeli
Department of Radiology, School of Medicine, Halic University, Istanbul, Turkey

T. Hazırolan (✉)
Department of Radiology, School of Medicine, Hacettepe University, Ankara, Turkey

The field of cardiac imaging using computed tomography (CT) and magnetic resonance imaging (MRI) is expected to detect the complicated nature of heart and coronary vessels anatomy and diagnose the pathologic cases. Mostly, contrast enhancement is needed for the evaluation of coronary vessels and soft tissues of the heart. Therefore, as cardiac CT and cardiac MRI become widespread, the usage of contrast medium is increasing. According to a key component of cardiac imaging is effective contrast protocol that concerted to existent cardiac imaging technique [1, 2]. The aim of this section is to provide main information for the optimal contrast-enhanced CT and MRI in cardiac imaging.

23.1 Contrast Optimization in Cardiac CT

Optimal contrast enhancement for cardiac CT has been the subject of various studies; the goal is to achieve uniform contrast enhancement in the target structures, use the least amount of contrast material as possible to reduce the risk of nephropathy, and avoid streak artifacts caused by the contrast bolus. A slender technical balance is required to achieve each of these goals.

Innumerable coacting factors have influence on contrast enhancement at CT which can be labeled as patient-dependent parameters, CT

S. M. Erturk et al. (eds.), *Medical Imaging Contrast Agents: A Clinical Manual*,
https://doi.org/10.1007/978-3-030-79256-5_23

scanner-dependent parameters, and contrast medium-dependent parameters [3–5] (Fig. 23.1).

The patient and contrast medium-related parameters are well correlated with the distribution of contrast medium. Contrast enhancement is unrelated to CT scanning process and is influenced purely by the patient and contrast medium-dependent parameters. Howbeit, CT scanner-dependent parameters have a discriminative position in the acquisition of images at a special time of enhancement [3, 6, 7].

The body size (weight, height, body surface area) and cardiac output are the major patient-dependent parameter on contrast enhancement [3, 7].

The body size effect may be explained on the principle of the relation of blood volume and body weight. Since patients with large size have larger blood volumes than the patients with smaller size, the contrast medium applied to the bloodstream is more diluted in a larger size patient than in a smaller size patient [8]. Accordingly, low iodine concentration and low contrast increase occur. It would be ideal to adapt the quantity of iodine to the patient's weight or body surface area. Whereas, because of the easier management in clinical use, in most cardiac CT studies a constant amount of contrast medium has notified [2, 3].

Cardiac output and characteristics of the circulatory system effect the timing of contrast enhancement [9].

The circulation of contrast medium decelerates with a decrease in cardiac output. The bolus of contrast medium reaches leisurely and clears leisurely. The timing of contrast enhancement and peak contrast time in all organs is directly proportional to the decrease in cardiac output [10]. Therefore, the scan delay should be individualized using a test bolus or bolus monitoring

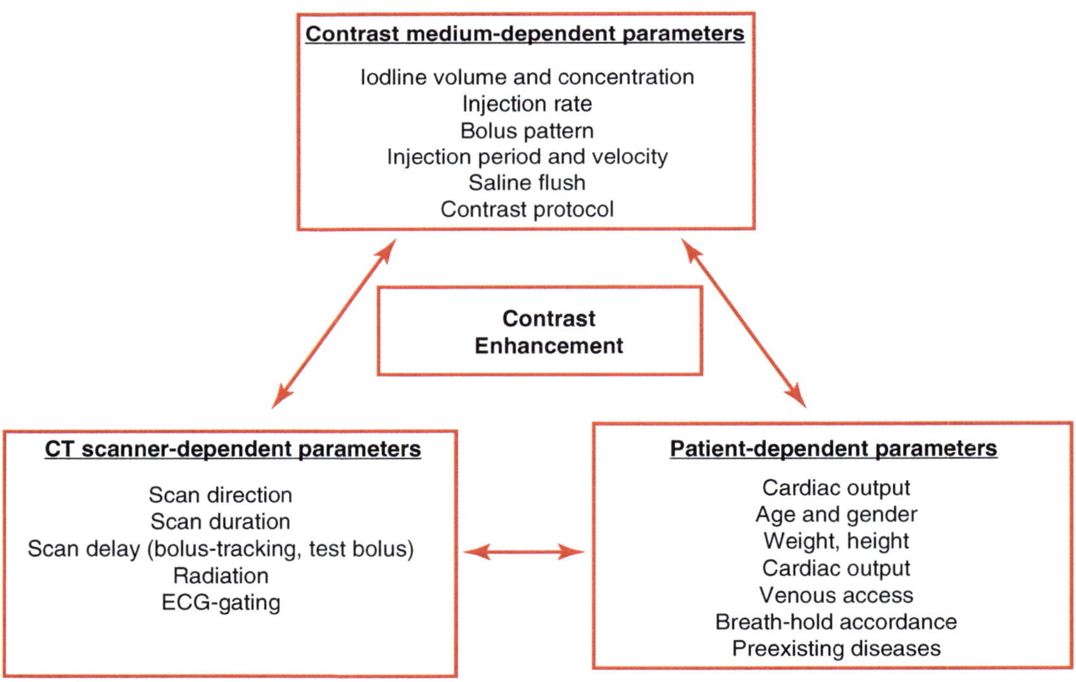

Fig. 23.1 Contrast-enhancement-dependent parameters

technique, as the scan delay is crucial for cardiac CT imaging [3].

Though with entirely defined patient and injection-depended parameters for contrast enhancement, unsatisfactory performed CT acquisition factors will end as an inefficient enhanced study. A long contrast medium injection is needed for a long CT scan period. For this reason, the duration of scan time affects the duration of injection and the injection rate or contrast agent volume immediately. The duration of scan time is connected to the quickness of the CT scanner, scanning mode, and the clinical application [2, 6].

23.1.1 Contrast Injection Protocols

The quality of cardiac CT images is subject to contrast to noise ratio. In coronary CT angiography, it is preferable that optimal contrast enhancement is between 250 and 300 Hounsfield Units (HU) to distinguish low-density atherosclerotic plaques, middle-density fibrous plaques, and high-density calcified plaques with over 130 HU. It should be avoided to exceed 350 HU to beware the difficulty in distinguishing coronary calcifications. As optimum images need high intra-arterial contrast enhancement, contrast agents with high iodine concentrations are chosen (270–400 mg Iodine/cc). Also, albeit low injection rates may be proper for lower kVp scans that depending on body habitus or intravenous (IV) catheter size (18–20 G), in most patients an injection rate of 5–7 cc/s is preferred for coronary CT angiography [11–13].

In order to prevent streak artifacts that may occur in the left subclavian vein, contrast injection is preferred from the 18 G IV catheter placed in the right antecubital vein instead of the left. In case of necessity central catheter can be used. Depending on the body habitus, 20 G catheters may be sufficient in some patients [3, 13].

Total contrast material volume is defined as a function of injection flow rate and injection time and is the primary determinant of contrast enhancement. In coronary CT angiography, high iodine concentration is used in a combination with high injection rate [14]. As a consequence of the increase in the injection rate, an earlier and higher arterial contrast enhancement is obtained. Therefore, an increased rate of contrast injection is used at higher cardiac outputs. The injection time should be as long as the estimated scan time or slightly longer. In very short scan times, the injection time should be at least 10 s. This is because the minimum bolus required for coronary contrast enhancement can be provided, although very short scan times are possible with current CT scanners [2, 3, 15, 16].

23.1.1.1 Contrast Infusion Method

In the coronary CT angiography examinations, different contrast injection protocols are used, varying from center to center, except for standard protocols.

Coronary artery enhancement can be achieved by monophasic injection protocol. A single head power injector is sufficient in this method. However, this protocol causes many artifacts related to flow, especially streak artifacts. It is also disadvantageous because it requires a high contrast medium volume and can not provide contrast differentiation between the right heart chamber and the right coronary artery. To overcome some of these deficiencies, a biphasic injection protocol has been developed [17, 18].

In the biphasic injection protocol, a saline chaser is used after contrast agent injection that permits decreased contrast agent use and provides better images than the monophasic injection protocol. This can be achieved by dual head power injectors which have separate receptacles for saline and contrast medium. The risk of nephropathy is reduced with the use of lower amount of contrast agent. This injection protocol also provides excellent contrast enhancement in coronary arteries with reduced streak artifacts in superior vena cava. Nevertheless, in many patients, an effective flushing is achieved in the right heart chambers where it is impossible to distinguish the lumen from walls, valve, and papillary muscles [19]. This prevents the appearance of the right ventricular contour required for right ventricular evaluation. The biphasic contrast injection protocol is the most plausible method if the aim is only to perform coronary artery assessment and if ventricular and functional cardiac evaluation is not needed [19–21].

For the triphasic injection protocol, the dual head power injector is also required like the biphasic protocol. The triphasic injection protocol is applied by first administering the contrast medium followed by the contrast-saline mixture and then followed by the saline flush. This technique allows right ventricular imaging in addition to uniform contrast enhancement in the coronary arteries. Recent literature studies have shown that by using the triphasic injection protocol, coronary artery evaluation can be performed with an adequate attenuation, besides right ventricular imaging with a significant reduction in streak artifacts [21–23].

23.1.1.2 Timing Method: Test Bolus Versus Bolus Tracking

The definite timing for data acquisition is the moment when the IV contrast medium reaches the target structure, in CT angiography technique. Under normal conditions, the scan delay time required to fill the whole coronary arteries is calculated by adding 2–4 s to the transit time of the contrast medium from the access vein to the ascending aorta [13]. In recent days, as CT scanners became faster and scan times decreased, the time interval required for optimal coronary artery development has significantly been shortened. For this reason, the fixed delay method is not recommended for cardiac CT angiography. In determining the scan start time, commonly two techniques are used which are called test bolus and automatic bolus tracking [2, 9].

The test bolus technique is based on minimal (10–20 mL) contrast medium injection prior to the actual CT scan with full bolus injection. Instantaneously following the test bolus injection, dynamic imaging is performed at a low radiation dose. The contrast-time curve is plotted by the region of interest (ROI) placed in the aorta. The optimal delay time is calculated after the peak contrast time is determined. Eventually, the diagnostic CT scan is performed according to the calculated time [3, 24]. The favorable feature of the test bolus method is that it gives a trial opportunity for IV catheter function and injection rate.

The bolus tracking method is based on the principle of low dose real-time serial imaging from a ROI while IV contrast medium is injected. When the contrast threshold is reached to a predefined value between 100 and 150 HU then the scan is automatically triggered [13] (Fig. 23.2). The advantage of the bolus tracking technique is that it is efficient and practical. Because less contrast medium usage is sufficient and can be scanned at a single injection phase. Also, it has been shown that the bolus tracking technique provides more homogenous contrast enhancement than the test bolus method, in the literature [25]. Notwithstanding, this method has a significant disadvantage. The breath-hold command, which should be given when threshold attenuation value is reached, can delay the initiation of the CT scan. Therefore, optimal enhancement moment may be missed [2, 3]. Except that, if the selected threshold value is too low, the contrast medium in the background can not be distinguished from the artifact and the attenuation value can not be measured. Similarly, a very high threshold is also impractical. The threshold value may never be reached, or the time to reach may be prolonged, resulting in a long scan delay or an improper enhancement [26].

Recently, a new method called dual-ROI tracker technique has been developed, which improves contrast enhancement. The threshold for the first ROI is 100 HU, at which breath-hold command is given. The threshold value for the second ROI is selected near 300 HU and triggers the CT scan [27, 28].

23.1.2 CT Scanning Factors

CT scan factors play a crucial role in the acquisition of contrast-enhanced images in a specified time frame. Though the factors of the patient and contrast injection protocols are excellently planned, images obtained with inadequate CT scanner parameters will not reach optimal quality. Technical advances that make the CT scanner

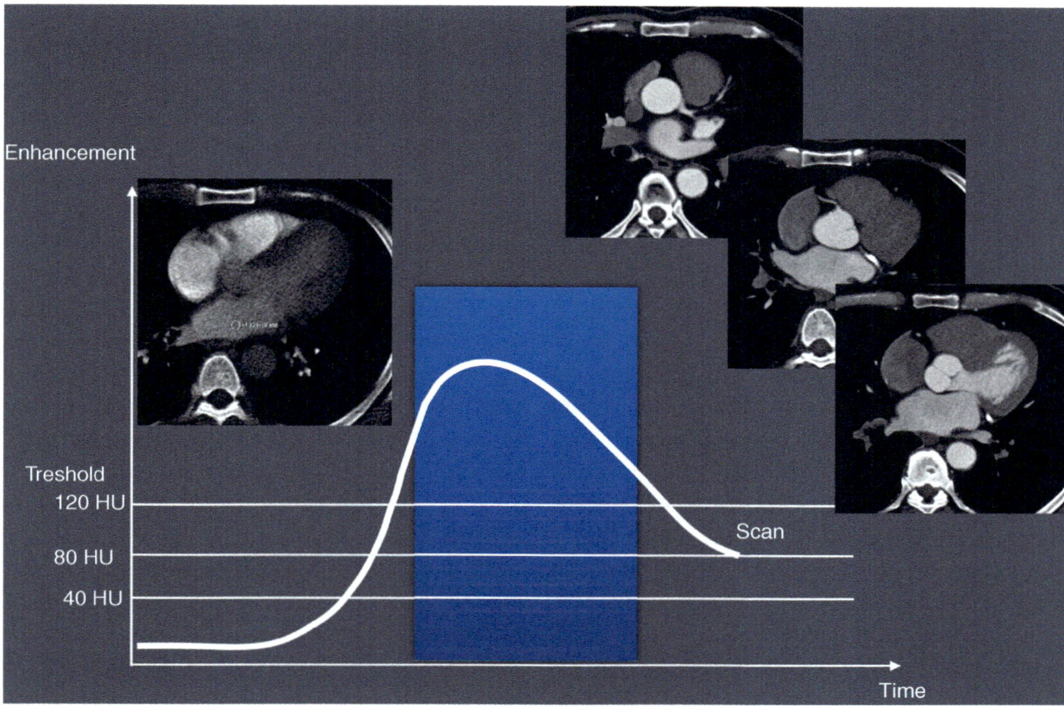

Fig. 23.2 Bolus tracking method

convenient for optimal cardiac CT imaging have occurred, especially in recent years. It is important to learn and track the novel technical advances to improve the cardiac CT image quality and diagnostic value, and also to determine the radiation dose [3, 13]. Depending on the 320 detector rows structure or depending on the high pitch characteristics of the dual-source technique, new generation CT scanners offer high spatial and temporal resolution in short scan times that can be reduced to a single heartbeat. On the other hand, the precision of the time of contrast agent bolus has a critical importance for cardiac CT scanning. Both the adaptation of old techniques and the application of new techniques have also played a critical role in the contrast injection protocols [2].

Iodine contrast medium attenuation is higher in the low tube voltages because the k-edge is closer to tube voltage of 70–80 kVp than 120 kVp tube voltage. Further, it has been shown in the literature that CT angiography can be performed at low tube voltages [29]. However, the noise of the images that are scanned with the low tube voltage is increased when compared with the high tube voltage scans, at the same display preset [2, 29]. Also, the image noise can be reduced advantageously by the iterative reconstruction (IR) technique, which is an alternative to the filtered back projection (FBP) technique, that are the algorithms developed by CT vendors [29, 30]. The coexistence of the IR technique and the low radiation dose protocol may result in a 60% reduction in dose while the FBP reconstruction technique maintains image quality compared to conventional radiation dose at the tube voltage of 120 kVp [31, 32]. The combination of low kVp and IR algorithm paves the way for reduction in the amount or concentration of iodine contrast medium. There is no significant difference between the CT images at low iodine contrast medium concentration (270 mgI/mL) with 100 kVp tube voltage and the CT images at standard iodine contrast medium concentration (370 mgI/mL) with 120 kVp tube voltage, in terms of vessel attenuation [33–35]. Also, Oda

Table 23.1 Comparison of tube voltage and contrast medium dose for similar image qualities

	CT protocol I	CT protocol II	CT protocol III
Tube voltage (kVp)	120	100	80
Contrast medium dose (mgI/kg)	370	270	210

et al. demonstrated that using 80 kVp makes it possible to reduce the dose of radiation and contrast agent. Coronary vascular enhancement and quality of images are satisfactory in not only proximal but also distal segments of coronary arteries [28] (Table 23.1). However, if the standard tube voltage of 120 kVp is selected depending on the body habitus during the scan with the automatic tube voltage system, the low contrast medium dose will weaken the vessel attenuation. Thus, optimal enhancement cannot be achieved. Conversely, if the contrast medium concentration is not reduced while scanning with low kVp, calcified plaques may be missed as the vessel attenuation increases significantly [2].

23.1.3 Optimal Contrast Enhancement for Specific Imaging Protocols

23.1.3.1 Pulmonary Vein Demonstration

Progression in imaging technology has led CT to gain an important place in pre-procedural planning and guidance in atrial fibrillation patients. Cardiac CT plays an important role in the anatomical and dimensional evaluation of pulmonary veins, and also provides the imaging and dimensional measuring of left atrium. Retrospective gating is preferred for atrial fibrillation and ROI is usually placed in the left atrium to provide optimal contrast [36].

23.1.3.2 Congenital Heart Diseases

Imaging in congenital heart diseases is now more confronted by better surgical and interventional techniques. Cardiac CT also plays an important role in this disease group, in preoperative evaluation and postoperative follow-up, as an alternative to MRI [37]. Compared to MRI, CT has several advantages, especially great spatial resolution, high temporal resolution, multi-plane reconstruction aptitudes at isotropic resolution, wide field of view, and fast and short scanning time. Due to remarkable rapid acquisition time, CT allows avoidance of anesthesia in young children or patients with disabilities or when there is a contraindication to sedation. One of the most important reasons for staying away from CT is the presence of ionizing radiation [38–40]. But with today's technology, a clear reduction in radiation dose can be achieved as significant dose reduction methods have been developed by CT vendors and also CT scanners are now able to scan in a single heartbeat [39, 40]. In congenital heart diseases, the complex anatomy and postoperative changes cause difficulties in the stages of scanning and interpretation. Contrast injection protocols also vary individually in these patients [41–43].

Congenital coronary anomalies seen in 0.2–2% of the population can be investigated by CT angiography in the best appropriate way since CT allows monitoring of coronary vascularies obviously from the origin to the distally. In patients with atrial or ventricular septal defects may require cardiac CT rarely if there is an additional major vascular pathology. MRI is usually used for postoperative evaluation and follow-up in the patient with tetralogy of Fallot. But in preoperative planning, unique anatomical information can be obtained with CT, such as aortic root, pulmonary trunk and branches, coronary arteries [42, 43].

The largest IV catheter that is available for the patient should be used for contrast media injection. The maximum amount of contrast medium that can be used in children is 1–2 cc per kg of the body weight. Also, according to the size of the selected IV catheter, the injection rate of contrast medium varies between 0.5 and 6 mL/s. Patient's age, hemodynamic parameters, type of cardiac pathology, postoperative changes are important factors in determining the acquisition time following the contrast medium injection. Because of the rapid contrast medium flow in the neonatal patient group, the bolus time can be extended by starting the acquisition following the half or one-third of contrast medium injection that mixed with saline. The test bolus technique can be preferred especially if the patient has pulmonary venous anomaly, cardiac shunt, or ventricular functional insufficiency. But this method requires additional contrast and time [37, 42, 43].

23.1.3.3 Triple Rule-Out

The triple rule-out protocol is intended to assess three main vascular that causing acute pathologies that appeared with chest pain as coronary arteries, aorta, and pulmonary arteries, in a single session. To scan these three vascular together, a greater amount of contrast material is required. It has been shown that very good images can be achieved with only 60 mL volume of 370 mg/mL contrast medium and triphasic injection protocol, in a study which was performed using the bolus tracking method with ROI placed at pulmonary trunk level by 320-row detector scanner [44]. A better enhancement can be achieved by the dual-ROI tracker technique, if the first ROI is placed for pulmonary artery evaluation and the second ROI for coronary arteries [2].

23.1.3.4 Pre-procedural Transcatheter Aortic Valve Replacement Planning

Transcatheter aortic valve replacement (TAVR) is an alternative treatment method in patients with a high risk of open surgery. Pre-TAVR CT angiography consists of two acquisitions, that is, for the selection of device size and evaluation of coronary arteries and also for the assessment of the vascular access that extend from the thoracic, abdominal, and pelvic arteries to the level of the femoral artery (Fig. 23.3). For this patient group, more attention should be paid in using contrast medium, as the risk of nephropathy is higher than the normal population. Although a few studies have shown that pre-TAVR imaging can be performed with a contrast medium volume of 20 mL, in many studies optimal enhancement has been reported with 370 mg/mL contrast medium in a volume of approximately 60 mL [45, 46].

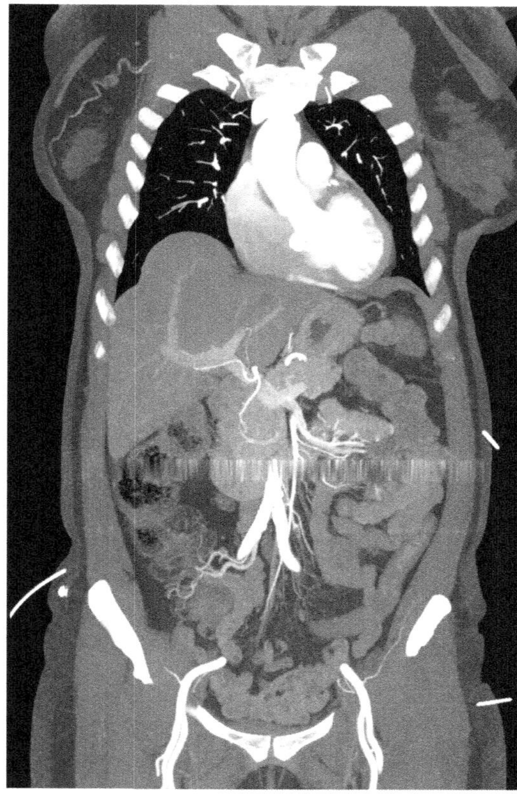

Fig. 23.3 Pre-TAVR CT angiography

23.2 Contrast Optimization in Cardiac MRI

The use of cardiac MRI in diseases such as cardiac tumors, ischemic heart diseases, cardiomyopathies, myocardial viability, and congenital heart diseases is becoming increasingly widespread. Present imaging modalities used in non-invasive cardiac imaging are listed as echocardiography, CT, and MRI. MRI has superior sides to echocardiography because of the less operator dependence and the absence of constraints like acoustic window and bowel gas. It also has the advantage over CT because it does not contain ionizing radiation and has a high soft tissue resolution [47]. Also, contrast enhancement plays a crucial role in diagnostic and follow-up evaluation by cardiac MRI. In cardiac MRI, the innate contrast of the blood and myocardium is dependent on the relaxation time of T1 and T2 and the proton density. Using contrast medium with varied MRI sequences may cause differentiation in this innate contrast [47, 48].

Extracellular contrast medium, which is mostly gadolinium chelates, is injected into the intravascular cavity. These contrast mediums, with a half-life of about 20 min, are rapidly dispersed in the extracellular space. The extracellular contrast mediums have similar effects because the relaxation times of T1 and T2 are close to each other. In addition to cardiac mass and viability evaluation in MRI, it is also used in magnetic resonance angiography (MRA) for the assessment of main vascular structures [47]. However, in 2017, the European Medicines Agency (EMA) reviewed gadolinium contrast agents which found that gadolinium deposition in brain tissue. And EMA confirmed the recommendation to restrict (gadoxetic acid, gadobenic acid, and gadopentetic acid) or suspend the permission (gadodiamide and gadoversetamide) of some linear gadolinium agents used in MRI scans. On the other hand, according to EMA, gadolinium-based macrocyclic agents (gadobutrol, gadoteric acid, and gadoteridol) are more stable than linear agents. So these agents may be used at the lowest doses that permitting adequate enhancement of the images which must be scanned with contrast medium.

A dose of approximately 0.1 mmol/kg body weight contrast medium is recommended for most imaging protocols except cardiac MRI. However, the preferred dose for cardiac MRI is about twice that (circa 0.2 mmol/kg), especially for late gadolinium enhancement and perfusion [48, 49]. Though it has been demonstrated that the myocardial enhancement also improves as the contrast medium dose increases, there is no significant change in diagnostic accuracy due to false-negative results depending on the susceptibility artifact [50, 51].

23.2.1 Late Gadolinium Enhancement

Late gadolinium enhancement (LGE) is an important entity while the area of myocardial infarction is indicated by MRI. Depending on the expansion in the extracellular space and due to the occluded capillaries that cause decrease in the surface area needed for transport, the time to arrive and clean the contrast medium in the myocardial tissue become longer. Tissue T1 relaxation time increases by the washout of the contrast medium At this stage, the infarcted myocardium area appears relatively hyperintense while normal tissue is hypointense [52, 53].

The contrast to noise ratio in LGE imaging has been improved and the clinical usage has become widespread with the introduction of the inversion recovery (IR) technique. IR sequence requires selection of inversion time (TI) to null healthy myocardium (seen as low signal and dark image). Optimal TI selection is critical to achieve diagnostic accuracy. Therefore, TI scout scans must be added prior to IR sequence to define the optimal TI in each patient. The LGE technique based on an injection protocol of a 0.1–0.2 mmol/kg bolus of Gd-containing contrast, and after 10–20 min the initiation of acquisition with an adequate TI to null the signal from healthy myocardium. The infarcted region of the myocardium may be visualized less than the actual size, if the acquisition is started earlier than the required waiting period. Whereas, if the acquisition is started too late, whole myocardial contrast medium enhancement will disappear and cause poor signal-to-noise ratio. Phase-sensitive inversion recovery (PSIR) techniques have been developed to overcome the disadvantages of the TI selection. PSIR reconstruction maintains the positive and negative polarities of tissue and negative longitudinal magnetizations seem darker than positive magnetizations. For this reason, contrast-enhanced tissue always has a higher signal than the normal myocardium without setting TI to null myocardium. Nevertheless, although the PSIR sequence allows to acquire good quality images without using TI value, PSIR images will be better by setting selected TI [54–56].

Since the T1 mapping with modified Look-Locker inversion recovery (MOLLI) technique has been introduced, synthetic IR images can also be produced besides mapping. The images of synthetic IR can be determined retrospectively by using tissue T1 values from any TI images that are scanned with a MOLLI technique retrospectively. If T1 mapping is included in the acquisition protocol, the LGE step can be omitted [57].

23.2.2 Myocardial Perfusion Imaging

Myocardial perfusion imaging is the first pass perfusion scanning method, which is performed by using gadolinium-chelated contrast agent. Due to the paramagnetic effect of gadolinium, well-perfused myocardial tissues show contrast enhancement on T1-weighted images. Since low doses of gadolinium are administered, T2 and T2* effects are not visible and myocardial tissue signal is not affected in this technique. The first pass perfusion is performed in the stress and the rest phases to determine the reversible and irreversible myocardial ischemic tissue in chronic ischemic heart diseases [52, 58].

During rest, coronary arteries can regulate the blood flow with vasodilatation compensation up to about 85% stenosis. However, with the application of pharmacological stress, relative perfusion defects in the stenosis of 50% and over can be detected owing to increased myocardial flow demand cannot be satisfied [59, 60].

Even a low dose contrast medium such as 0.025–0.05 mmol/kg is sufficient for myocardial perfusion, much better contrast enhancement can be obtained at the total dose of 0.1–0.2 mmol/kg. A high rate contrast medium infusion of 3–7 mL/s is performed and followed by at least 30 mL saline chasing bolus [49, 61].

23.2.3 Extracellular Volume Mapping

Extracellular volume (ECV) mapping is a new and important technique for examining myocardium to detect the physiologic and pathophysiologic biologic modifications. Native and post-contrast T1 maps make calculation of ECV maps possible. Even though native T1 mapping is able to detect the sum of intracellular and extracellular area, ECV mapping can focus on the extracellular space advantageously, which gives a clear idea about edema, fibrosis, or amyloid involvement. ECV mapping values can be calculated by the measurement of native and post-contrast T1 images, blood T1, and hematocrit values [62, 63] (Fig. 23.4).

It has been demonstrated that the "bolus only" contrast injection protocol is sufficient for ECV measurement. In addition, ECV values should be measured after a delay of at least 15 min after a

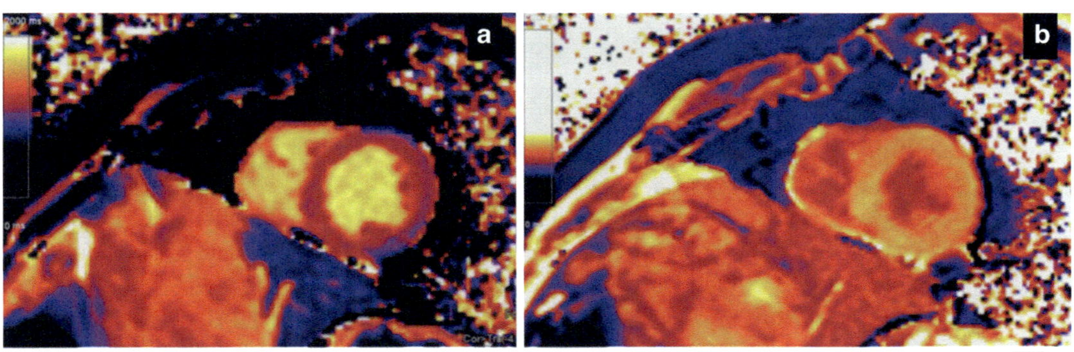

c

$$\boxed{\text{ECV}} = (1 - \text{hematocrit}) \frac{\dfrac{1}{\text{post-contrast } T1_{\text{myocardium}}} - \dfrac{1}{\text{native } T1_{\text{myocardium}}}}{\dfrac{1}{\text{post-contrast } T1_{\text{blood}}} - \dfrac{1}{\text{native } T1_{\text{blood}}}}$$

Fig. 23.4 (**a**) Native and (**b**) post-contrast T1 mapping images, (**c**) ECV formula bolus of 0.2 mmol/kg gadolinium-based contrast medium injection. Also to create accurate maps, hematocrit value required for ECV mapping calculation should be measured at the same time period of the cardiac MRI [64, 65].

23.2.4 Coronary MRI Angiography with Contrast Medium

MRA acquisition by gradient echo sequence using gadolinium-based contrast medium provides high signal-to-noise ratio and significant enhancement in the vessel lumen. In coronary MRA with contrast medium administration, gadolinium-based contrast mediums extravasate to the extracellular area from the intravascular space in 10–15 min. Due to this restrictive effect of gadolinium-based contrast medium, a slow infusion technique is recommended in coronary MRA. In this technique, contrast medium infusion is administered at 0.3 mL/s rate to prolong the blood signal coming from the coronary artery with the accompanying of respiratory navigators and ECG-gating [66].

Except the evaluation of the coronary artery lumen, vessel wall remodeling and inflammation may also be visualized by coronary MRA with contrast medium [67].

23.2.5 Appropriate Use of Contrast-Enhanced Sequences in Specific Imaging Protocols

23.2.5.1 Myocardial Infarction and Ischemia

Myocardial infarction emerges when coronary arteries do not adequately supply the blood to the myocardium. When the extracellular space gets enlarged due to cellular death, extracellular distribution of the contrast medium also increases. One of the most satisfying method to evaluate the infarct area is the LGE imaging [47, 56] (Fig. 23.5). By LGE protocol, the location and size of the acute or chronic infarct area can be determined with high accuracy and reproducibility rates. The presence of a strong correlation between the delineations of the MR-visualized contrast area and histological findings of myocardial infarction has been verified in many studies [68–70]. Furthermore, ECV mapping also shows accuracy on diagnostic evaluation in the discrimination of myocardial infarction from healthy myocardium. Besides infarcted tissue, subclinical pathologies in areas that are defined as healthy in LGE images can be detected by ECV mapping. Although ECV mapping is superior to the LGE method in this respect, it needs to be improved due to artifacts and unclear cut-off values [71].

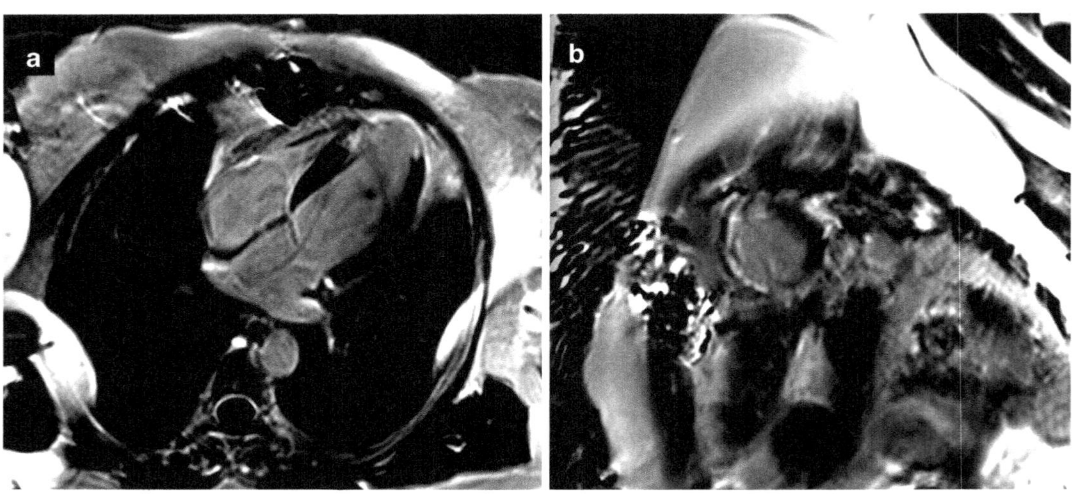

Fig. 23.5 (**a**) Four chambers and (**b**) short axis views showing contrast enhancement in apex and apical septal segments in LGE sequences

Cardiac MRI provides crucial information about the evaluation of myocardial ischemia by perfusion imaging. CMR stress perfusion allows defining the ischemic heart disease in patients who are unable to exercise or the patients with resting ECG abnormalities. Also this technique lets to determine the candidates for interventional procedures [72, 73]. This asserts that myocardial perfusion imaging allows an effective prognostic evaluation in the patient population with coronary artery disease (CAD), besides it is an alternative diagnostic method for the diagnosis of CAD [73–76].

Stress perfusion imaging is usually performed along with LGE imaging. Following the amount of 0.05 mmol/kg contrast medium that is used for perfusion imaging, the additional contrast medium should be administrated to complete the total dose of 0.1–0.2 mmol/kg during LGE acquisition [49].

Also, coronary MRA with contrast medium is an alternative method for CT angiography. In comparison to the diagnostic accuracy of coronary MRA with and without contrast medium, the contrast noise ratio and visualization of the coronal segments show superiority in the group that used contrast medium.

23.2.5.2 Nonischemic Cardiomyopathy

Nonischemic cardiomyopathies can be grouped as genetic, acquired, and mixed type. While hypertrophic cardiomyopathy (HCM) and arrhythmogenic right ventricular cardiomyopathy (ARVC) are genetic subgroups, dilated cardiomyopathy (DCM) is a component of mixed subgroup and myocarditis is in the acquired group [72].

HCM is a disorder characterized by hypertrophy and fibrotic changes in the myocardium. A strong correlation has been demonstrated between the regional contrast patterns determined by LGE imaging and perfusion defects. Also, assessment of contrast enhancement with LGE imaging is enounced as a prognostic indicator in several studies in HCM patients [77–79].

ARVC occurs as a global or regional dysfunction associated with fatty or fibrous replacement and usually involves the right ventricle. LGE on the right ventricular wall is a more specific indicator than myocardial fat, for this disease. If the right ventricular tissue characterization and wall motion assessment are performed together, high diagnostic accuracy can be obtained [80, 81].

In DCM disorder, left ventricular systolic function and septal midwall fibrosis can be evaluated by cardiac MRI. Midwall fibrosis can be detected with LGE and it was found to be associated with unwanted clinical situations [82, 83].

Fifty percent of sarcoidosis patients have cardiac involvement, with only 5% symptomatic. However, heart involvement is the most important cause of mortality. Cardiac MRI can be used to show inflammation with early contrast enhancement and ECV mapping, and also define scar tissue by LGE technique [84, 85].

23.2.5.3 Cardiac Masses

Cardiac MRI performed in the presence of a cardiac mass suspicion is useful in distinguishing mass from thrombus or benign tumor from malignant tumor [85]. The LGE method for mass and thrombus differentiation provides critical information. Cardiac masses are usually contrast-enhanced lesions as opposed to the thrombus (Fig. 23.6). However, conventional post-contrast T1-weighted sequences may be affected by paramagnetic artifacts due to blood pool [49, 86]. An avascular tissue nulling sequence that is specially improved for thrombus estimation uses a 600 ms long inversion time. By using this method, the vascularized tissue appears gray while the nulling effect is seen in the avascular thrombus [87, 88].

Most of the primary tumors of the heart are benign (myxoma, papillary fibroelastoma, and fibroma) and also the most common cardiac malign tumors are sarcomas and primary cardiac lymphomas. It is noteworthy that the malignant tumors show heterogeneous contrast enhancement. Furthermore, by first pass imaging, vascularized metastases such as renal cell carcinoma can be distinguished from nonvascularized lesions [72].

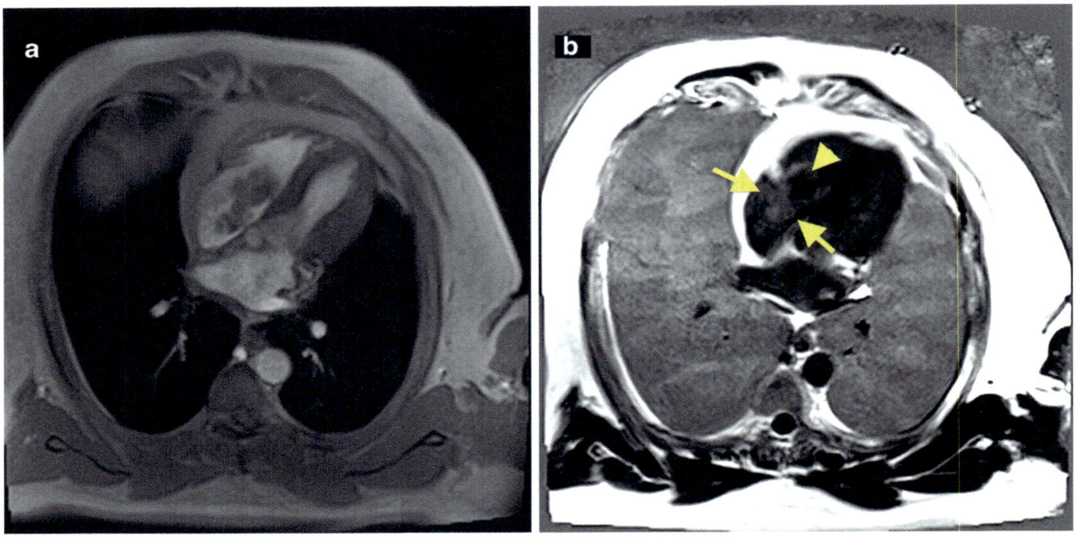

Fig. 23.6 (**a**) SSFP CINE and (**b**) LGE images in four chambers view; right atrial myxoma (arrows) showing contrast enhancement but thrombus (arrowhead) is hypointense in LGE sequence

References

1. Jinzaki M, Kitagawa K, et al. ASCI 2010 contrast media guideline for cardiac imaging: a report of the Asian Society of Cardiovascular Imaging cardiac computed tomography and cardiac magnetic resonance imaging guideline working group. Int J Cardiovasc Imaging. 2010;26(Suppl 2):203.
2. Scholtz J-E, Ghoshhajra B. Advances in cardiac CT contrast injection and acquisition protocols. Cardiovasc Diagn Ther. 2017;7(5):439–51.
3. Bae KT. Intravenous contrast medium administration and scan timing at CT: considerations and approaches. Radiology. 2010;256(1):32–61.
4. Cademartiri F, van der Lugt A, Luccichenti G, Pavone P, Krestin GP. Parameters affecting bolus geometry in CTA: a review. J Comput Assist Tomogr. 2002;26(4):598–607.
5. Hsu RM. Computed tomographic angiography: conceptual review of injection and acquisition parameters with a brief overview of rendering technique. Appl Radiol. 2002;31(6):33–9.
6. Bae KT. Technical aspects of contrast delivery in advanced CT. Appl Radiol. 2003;32:12–9.
7. Han JK, Choi BI, Kim AY, Kim SJ. Contrast media in abdominal computed tomography: optimization of delivery methods. Korean J Radiol. 2001;2(1):28–36.
8. Takeshita K. Prediction of maximum hepatic enhancement on computed tomography from dose of contrast material and patient weight: proposal of a new formula and evaluation of its accuracy. Radiat Med. 2001;19(2):75–9.
9. Bae KT, Heiken JP, Brink JA. Aortic and hepatic contrast medium enhancement at CT. II. Effect of reduced cardiac output in a porcine model. Radiology. 1998;207(3):657–62.
10. Chu LL, Joe BN, Westphalen ACA, Webb EM, Coakley FV, Yeh BM. Patient-specific time to peak abdominal organ enhancement varies with time to peak aortic enhancement at MR imaging. Radiology. 2007;245(3):779–87.
11. Hutchison SJ, Merchant N. Principles of cardiac and vascular computed tomography: expert consult. Elsevier Health Sciences; 2014.
12. Nikolaou K, Sagmeister S, Knez A, et al. Multidetector-row computed tomography of the coronary arteries: predictive value and quantitative assessment of non-calcified vessel-wall changes. Eur Radiol. 2003;13:2505–12.
13. Abbara S, Blanke P, Maroules CD, et al. SCCT guidelines for the performance and acquisition of coronary computed tomographic angiography: a report of the society of Cardiovascular Computed Tomography Guidelines Committee: endorsed by the North American Society for Cardiovascular Imaging (NASCI). J Cardiovasc Comput Tomogr. 2016;10:435–49.
14. ASCI CCT & CMR Guideline Working Group, Jinzaki M, Kitagawa K, Tsai IC, et al. ASCI 2010 contrast media guideline for cardiac imaging: a report of the Asian Society of Cardiovascular Imaging cardiac computed tomography and cardiac magnetic resonance imaging guideline working group. Int J Cardiovasc Imaging. 2010;26:203–12.
15. Abbara S, Arbab-Zadeh A, Callister TQ, et al. SCCT guidelines for performance of coronary computed

tomographic angiography: a report of the Society of Cardiovascular Computed Tomography Guidelines Committee. J Cardiovasc Comput Tomogr. 2009;3:190–204.
16. Fleischmann D, Kamaya A. Optimal vascular and parenchymal contrast enhancement: the current state of the art. Radiol Clin North Am. 2009;47(1):13–26.
17. Haage P, Schmitz-Rode T, Hubner D, Piroth W, Gunther RW. Reduction of contrast material dose and artifacts by saline flush using a double power injector in helical CT of the thorax. Am J Radiol. 2000;174:1049–53.
18. Schoellnast H, Tillich M, Deutschmann HA, Stessel U, Deutschmann MJ, Schaffler GJ, et al. Improvement of parenchymal and vascular enhancement using saline flush and power injection for multiple-detector-row abdominal CT. Eur Radiol. 2004;14:659–64.
19. Kerl JM, Ravenel JG, Nguyen SA, Suranyi P, Thilo C, Costello P. Right heart: split-bolus injection of diluted contrast medium for visualization at coronary CT angiography. Radiology. 2008;247(2):356–64.
20. Juergens KU, Grude M, Fallenberg EM, et al. Using ECG-gated multidetector CT to evaluate global left ventricular myocardial function in patients with coronary artery disease. AJR Am J Roentgenol. 2002;179:1545–50.
21. Lu JG, Lv B, Chen XB, Tang X, Jiang SL, Dai RP. What is the best contrast injection protocol for 64-row multi-detector cardiac computed tomography? Eur J Radiol. 2010;75:159–65.
22. Kerl JM, Ravenel JG, Nguyen SA, et al. Right heart: split-bolus injection of diluted contrast medium for visualization at coronary CT angiography. Radiology. 2008;247(2):356–64.
23. Budoff MJ, Shinbane JS, Child J, et al. Multiphase contrast medium injection for optimization of computed tomographic coronary angiography. Acad Radiol. 2006;13:159–65.
24. Sheiman RG, Raptopoulos V, Caruso P, Vrachliotis T, Pearlman J. Comparison of tailored and empiric scan delays for CT angiography of the abdomen. AJR Am J Roentgenol. 1996;167(3):725–9.
25. Cademartiri F, Nieman K, van der Lugt A, et al. Intravenous contrast material administration at 16-detector row helical CT coronary angiography: test bolus versus bolus-tracking technique. Radiology. 2004;233:817–23.
26. Mehnert F, Pereira PL, Trübenbach J, Kopp AF, Claussen CD. Automatic bolus tracking in monophasic spiral CT of the liver: liver-to-lesion conspicuity. Eur Radiol. 2001;11(4):580–4.
27. Tatsugami F, Awai K, Takada H, et al. Reduction of interpatient variability of arterial enhancement using a new bolus tracking system in 320-detector computed tomographic coronary angiography. J Comput Assist Tomogr. 2013;37:79–83.
28. Oda S, Utsunomiya D, Yuki H, et al. Low contrast and radiation dose coronary CT angiography using a 320-row system and a refined contrast injection and timing method. J Cardiovasc Comput Tomogr. 2015;9:19–27.
29. Hell MM, Bittner D, Schuhbaeck A, et al. Prospectively ECG-triggered high-pitch coronary angiography with third-generation dual-source CT at 70 kVp tube voltage: feasibility, image quality, radiation dose, and effect of iterative reconstruction. J Cardiovasc Comput Tomogr. 2014;8:418–25.
30. Scholtz JE, Wichmann JL, Hüsers K, et al. Third-generation dual-source CT of the neck using automated tube voltage adaptation in combination with advanced modeled iterative reconstruction: evaluation of image quality and radiation dose. Eur Radiol. 2016;26:2623–31.
31. Oda S, Utsunomiya D, Funama Y, et al. A hybrid iterative reconstruction algorithm that improves the image quality of low-tube-voltage coronary CT angiography. AJR Am J Roentgenol. 2012;198:1126–31.
32. Iyama Y, Nakaura T, Yokoyama K, Kidoh M, Yamashita Y. Cardiac helical CT involving a low-radiation-dose protocol with a 100-kVp setting: usefulness of hybrid iterative reconstruction and display preset optimization. Roever. L, ed. Medicine. 2016;95(46):e5459.
33. Wu Q, Wang Y, Kai H, et al. Application of 80-kVp tube voltage, low-concentration contrast agent and iterative reconstruction in coronary CT angiography: evaluation of image quality and radiation dose. Int J Clin Pract. 2016;70(Suppl 9B):B50–5.
34. Sinitsyn VE, Komarova MA, Mershina EA. Comparison of low- and high-concentration (270 and 320 mg I/ml) iso-osmolar iodinated contrast media in coronary CT angiography: a randomized prospective single-center blinded study. Vestn Rentgenol Radiol. 2014:5–12.
35. Yin WH, Lu B, Gao JB, et al. Effect of reduced x-ray tube voltage, low iodine concentration contrast medium, and sinogram-affirmed iterative reconstruction on image quality and radiation dose at coronary CT angiography: results of the prospective multicenter REALISE trial. J Cardiovasc Comput Tomogr. 2015;9:215–24.
36. Lacomis JM, Wigginton W, Fuhrman C, et al. Multi-detector row CT of the left atrium and pulmonary veins before radio-frequency catheter ablation for atrial fibrillation 1. Radiographics. 2003;23:S35–48.
37. Rajiah P, Saboo SS, Abbara S. Role of CT in congenital heart disease. Curr Treat Options Cardiovasc Med. 2017;19:6.
38. Orwat S, Diller GP, Baumgartner H. Imaging of congenital heart disease in adults: choice of modalities. Eur Heart J Cardiovasc Imaging. 2013;15(1):6–17.
39. Ntsinjana HN, Hughes ML, Taylor AM. The role of cardiovascular magnetic resonance in pediatric congenital heart disease. J Cardiovasc Magn Reson. 2011;13:51.
40. Dillman JR, Hernandez RJ. Role of CT in the evaluation of congenital cardiovascular disease in children. AJR Am J Roentgenol. 2009;192:1219–31.
41. Ghoshhajra BB, Sidhu MS, El-Sherief A, et al. Adult congenital heart disease imaging with second-generation dual-source computed tomography:

initial experiences and findings. Congenit Heart Dis. 2012;7:516–25.
42. Han BK, Rigsby CK, Hlavacek A, et al. Computed tomography imaging in patients with congenital heart disease part I: rationale and utility. An Expert Consensus Document of the Society of Cardiovascular Computed Tomography (SCCT): endorsed by the Society of Pediatric Radiology (SPR) and the North American Society of Cardiac Imaging (NASCI). J Cardiovasc Comput Tomogr. 2015;9:475–92.
43. Han BK, Rigsby CK, Leipsic J, et al. Computed tomography imaging in patients with congenital heart disease, part 2: technical recommendations. An Expert Consensus Document of the Society of Cardiovascular Computed Tomography (SCCT): endorsed by the Society of Pediatric Radiology (SPR) and the North American Society of Cardiac Imaging (NASCI). J Cardiovasc Comput Tomogr. 2015;9(6):493–513.
44. Durmus T, Rogalla P, Lembcke A, et al. Low-dose triple-rule-out using 320-row-detector volume MDCT–less contrast medium and lower radiation exposure. Eur Radiol. 2011;21:1416–23.
45. Azzalini L, Abbara S, Ghoshhajra BB. Ultra-low contrast computed tomographic angiography (CTA) with 20-mL total dose for transcatheter aortic valve implantation (TAVI) planning. J Comput Assist Tomogr. 2014;38:105–9.
46. Bittner DO, Arnold M, Klinghammer L, et al. Contrast volume reduction using third generation dual source computed tomography for the evaluation of patients prior to transcatheter aortic valve implantation. Eur Radiol. 2016;26:4497–504.
47. Moriarty JM, Finn JP, Fonseca CG. Contrast agents used in cardiovascular magnetic resonance imaging: current issues and future directions. Am J Cardiovasc Drugs. 2010;10(4):227–37.
48. Nacif MS, Arai AE, Lima JAC, Bluemke D. Gadolinium-enhanced cardiovascular magnetic resonance: administered dose in relationship to United States Food and Drug Administration (FDA) guidelines. J Cardiovasc Magn Reson. 2012;14:18.
49. Kramer CM, Barkhausen J, Flamm SD, Kim RJ, Nagel E. Standardized cardiovascular magnetic resonance (CMR) protocols 2013 update. J Cardiovasc Magn Reson. 2013;15:91.
50. Wolff SD, Schwitter J, Coulden R, et al. Myocardial first-pass perfusion magnetic resonance imaging: a multicenter dose-ranging study. Circulation. 2004;110:732–7.
51. Giang TH, Nanz D, Coulden R, et al. Detection of coronary artery disease by magnetic resonance myocardial perfusion imaging with various contrast medium doses: first European multi-centre experience. Eur Heart J. 2004;25:1657–65.
52. Paiman EHM, Lamb HJ. When should we use contrast material in cardiac MRI? J Magn Reson Imaging. 2017;46(6):1551–72.
53. Kim RJ, Chen E-L, Lima JAC, Judd RM. Myocardial Gd-DTPA kinetics determine MRI contrast enhancement and reflect the extent and severity of myocardial injury after acute reperfused infarction. Circulation. 1996;94:3318–26.
54. Doltra A, Amundsen BH, Gebker R, Fleck E, Kelle S. Emerging concepts for myocardial late gadolinium enhancement MRI. Curr Cardiol Rev. 2013;9(3):185–90.
55. Oshinski JN, Yang Z, Jones JR, et al. Imaging time after Gd-DTPA injection is critical in using delayed enhancement to determine infarct size accurately with magnetic resonance imaging. Circulation. 2001;104(23):2838–42.
56. Pereira RS, Prato FS, Wisenberg G, et al. The use of Gd-DTPA as a marker of myocardial viability in reperfused acute myocardial infarction. Int J Cardiovasc Imaging. 2001;17(5):395–404.
57. Varga-Szemes A, van der Geest RJ, Spottiswoode BS, et al. Myocardial late gadolinium enhancement: accuracy of T1 mapping–based synthetic inversion-recovery imaging. Radiology. 2016;278:374–82.
58. Hamirani YS, Kramer CM. Cardiac MRI assessment of myocardial perfusion. Futur Cardiol. 2014;10(3):349–58.
59. Gould KL, Lipscomb K. Effects of coronary stenoses on coronary flow reserve and resistance. Am J Cardiol. 1974;34:48–55.
60. Rieber J. Cardiac magnetic resonance perfusion imaging for the functional assessment of coronary artery disease: a comparison with coronary angiography and fractional flow reserve. Eur Heart J. 2005;27:1465–71.
61. Edelman RR. Contrast-enhanced MR imaging of the heart: overview of the literature. Radiology. 2004;232(3):653–68.
62. Treibel TA, Fontana M, Maestrini V, et al. Automatic measurement of the myocardial interstitium. JACC Cardiovasc Imaging. 2016;9:54–63.
63. White SK, Sado DM, Fontana M, Banypersad SM, Maestrini V, Flett AS, Piechnik SK, Robson MD, Hausenloy DJ, Sheikh AM, Hawkins PN, Moon JC. T1 mapping for myocardial extracellular volume measurement by CMR. JACC Cardiovasc Imaging. 2013;6:955–62.
64. Miller CA, Naish J, Bishop P, Coutts G, Clark D, Zhao S, Ray SG, Yonan N, Williams SG, Flett AS, Moon JC, Greiser A, Parker GJ, Schmitt M. Comprehensive validation of cardiovascular magnetic resonance techniques for the assessment of myocardial extracellular volume. Circ Cardiovasc Imaging. 2013;6:373–83.
65. Moon JC, Messroghli DR, Kellman P, et al. Myocardial T1 mapping and extracellular volume quantification: a Society for Cardiovascular Magnetic Resonance (SCMR) and CMR Working Group of the European Society of Cardiology consensus statement. J Cardiovasc Magn Reson. 2013;15(1):92. https://doi.org/10.1186/1532-429X-15-92.
66. Wagner M, Rosler R, Lembcke A, et al. Whole-heart coronary magnetic resonance angiography at 1.5 Tesla: does a blood-pool contrast agent improve diagnostic accuracy? Invest Radiol. 2011;46:152–9.
67. Kerwin WS, O'Brien KD, Ferguson MS, Polissar N, Hatsukami TS, Yuan C. Inflammation in carotid

atherosclerotic plaque: a dynamic contrast-enhanced MR imaging study. Radiology. 2006;241:459–68.
68. Kim RJ, Albert TSE, Wible JH, et al. Performance of delayed enhancement magnetic resonance imaging with gadoversetamide contrast for the detection and assessment of myocardial infarction: an international, multicenter, double-blinded, randomized trial. Circulation. 2008;117:629–37.
69. Wagner A, Mahrholdt H, Holly TA, et al. Contrast-enhanced MRI and routine single photon emission computed tomography (SPECT) perfusion imaging for detection of subendocardial myocardial infarcts: an imaging study. Lancet. 2003;361:374–9.
70. Ibrahim T, Bulow HP, Hackl T, et al. Diagnostic value of contrast enhanced magnetic resonance imaging and single-photon emission computed tomography for detection of myocardial necrosis early after acute myocardial infarction. J Am Coll Cardiol. 2007;49:208–16.
71. Ugander M, Oki AJ, Hsu L-Y, et al. Extracellular volume imaging by magnetic resonance imaging provides insights into overt and subclinical myocardial pathology. Eur Heart J. 2012;33:1268–78.
72. ACCF/ACR/AHA/NASCI/SCMR 2010 expert consensus document on cardiovascular magnetic resonance: a report of the American College of Cardiology Foundation Task Force on Expert Consensus Documents. J Am Coll Cardiol. 2010;55(23):2614–62.
73. Coelho-Filho OR, Rickers C, Kwong RY, et al. MR myocardial perfusion imaging. Radiology. 2013;266:701–15.
74. Ingkanisorn WP, Kwong RY, Bohme NS, et al. Prognosis of negative adenosine stress magnetic resonance in patients presenting to an emergency department with chest pain. J Am Coll Cardiol. 2006;47(7):1427–32.
75. Kwong RY, Schussheim AE, Rekhraj S, et al. Detecting acute coronary syndrome in the emergency department with cardiac magnetic resonance imaging. Circulation. 2003;107(4):531–7.
76. Steel K, Broderick R, Gandla V, et al. Complementary prognostic values of stress myocardial perfusion and late gadolinium enhancement imaging by cardiac magnetic resonance in patients with known or suspected coronary artery disease. Circulation. 2009;120(14):1390–400.
77. Schulz-Menger J, Abdel-Aty H, Busjahn A, et al. Left ventricular outflow tract planimetry by cardiovascular magnetic resonance differentiates obstructive from non-obstructive hypertrophic cardiomyopathy. J Cardiovasc Magn Reson. 2006;8:741–6.
78. Moon JC, McKenna WJ, McCrohon JA, et al. Toward clinical risk assessment in hypertrophic cardiomyopathy with gadolinium cardiovascular magnetic resonance. J Am Coll Cardiol. 2003;41:1561–7.
79. Matsunaka T, Hamada M, Matsumoto Y, et al. First-pass myocardial perfusion defect and delayed contrast enhancement in hypertrophic cardiomyopathy assessed with MRI. Magn Reson Med Sci. 2003;2:61–9.
80. Tandri H, Castillo E, Ferrari VA, et al. Magnetic resonance imaging of arrhythmogenic right ventricular dysplasia: sensitivity, specificity, and observer variability of fat detection versus functional analysis of the right ventricle. J Am Coll Cardiol. 2006;48:2277–84.
81. Sen-Chowdhry S, Prasad SK, Syrris P, et al. Cardiovascular magnetic resonance in arrhythmogenic right ventricular cardiomyopathy revisited: comparison with task force criteria and genotype. J Am Coll Cardiol. 2006;48:2132–40.
82. Nazarian S, Bluemke DA, Lardo AC, et al. Magnetic resonance assessment of the substrate for inducible ventricular tachycardia in nonischemic cardiomyopathy. Circulation. 2005;112:2821–5.
83. Assomull RG, Prasad SK, Lyne J, et al. Cardiovascular magnetic resonance, fibrosis, and prognosis in dilated cardiomyopathy. J Am Coll Cardiol. 2006;48:1977–85.
84. Schulz-Menger J, Wassmuth R, Abdel-Aty H, et al. Patterns of myocardial inflammation and scarring in sarcoidosis as assessed by cardiovascular magnetic resonance. Heart. 2006;92:399–400.
85. O'Donnell DH, Abbara S, Chaithiraphan V, et al. Cardiac tumors: optimal cardiac MR sequences and spectrum of imaging appearances. Am J Roentgenol. 2009;193:377–87.
86. Simonetti OP, Kim RJ, Fieno DS, et al. An improved MR imaging technique for the visualization of myocardial infarction. Radiology. 2001;218:215–23.
87. Buckley O, Madan R, Kwong R, et al. Cardiac masses, part 1: imaging strategies and technical considerations. Am J Roentgenol. 2011;197:W837–41.
88. Pazos-Lopez P, Pozo E, Siqueira ME, Garcia-Lunar I, Cham M, Jacobi A, Macaluso F, Fuster V, Narula J, Sanz J. Value of CMR for the differential diagnosis of cardiac masses. JACC Cardiovasc Imaging. 2014;7:896–905.

Contrast Agents in Vascular Interventional Radiology

24

F. Gonca Eldem and Bora Peynircioğlu

24.1 Introduction

Contrast agents are divided into two as positive contrast agents and negative contrast agents in general. Positive contrast agents attenuate X-rays more than the soft tissues. Negative contrast agents attenuate X-rays less than the soft tissues [1]. In interventional radiology positive contrast agents that can be used are iodinated contrast agents and gadolinium-based contrast agents while the only negative contrast agent that can be used through an intravascular route is carbon dioxide (CO_2).

24.2 Iodine-Based Contrast Agents

The numerous types of iodine contrast media (ICM) can be grouped physicochemically according to their: [1] osmolality into high osmolar CM (HOCM), low osmolar (LOCM), or iso-osmolar (IOCM); [2] ionicity (to ionic or nonionic CM); and [3] the number of benzene rings (either monomeric or dimeric CM). They share a common tri-iodinated benzene ring either as a monomer or dimer. HOCM have an osmolality of 2000 mOsm/kg, LOCM have an osmolality range of 600–800 mOsm/kg, and IOCM have an osmolality of 290 mOsm/kg which is isotonic to plasma. Development of ionic contrast agents in the 1920s and 1930s were with HOCM agents which allowed radiologists visualize vessels and organs. These first initiated HOCM have been replaced by lower osmolality contrast agents because of their toxicities and adverse reactions.

The role of contrast agents in interventional radiology carry some nuances than diagnostic imaging and every interventional radiologist should consider these small differences. First of all, the route of administration is more likely to be arterial except from the procedures involving veins. Secondly, patient population that has been administered ICM with DSA should be considered different in their clinical status. Therefore, when using ICM in vascular procedures quality of the images, nephrotoxicity, and other adverse effects may be different.

Previously many studies showed that intra-arterial use of ICM has a higher risk for developing contrast nephropathy than intravenous routes. However, in the last two decades the literature has been dominated by reports from cardiac angiography especially on the topic of contrast nephropathy. Instead, coronary angiography is different than other angiographic procedures and of course from intravenous route of administration. One should keep in mind that coronary angiography is an injection of ICM from a suprarenal position with the use of a catheter that may

F. G. Eldem (✉) · B. Peynircioğlu
Department of Radiology, Hacettepe University
Faculty of Medicine, Ankara, Turkey

S. M. Erturk et al. (eds.), *Medical Imaging Contrast Agents: A Clinical Manual*,
https://doi.org/10.1007/978-3-030-79256-5_24

dislodge an atherosclerotic plaque and the ICM dose delivered to kidney are more abrupt and concentrated [2–4]. Because of the possibility of various points of administration through an intra-arterial route, in the latest update of European Society of Urogenital Radiology (ESUR) guidelines the term intra-arterial administration has been broadened. The change is made based on the dilution factor of the ICM regarding points of administration. The terms intra-arterial ICM administration with first pass renal exposure and intra-arterial ICM administration with second pass renal exposure are now in use. Injections from catheters into the right heart, pulmonary arteries, carotid, subclavian, brachial, coronary, mesenteric arteries as well as into the infrarenal abdominal aorta, iliac, femoral, and crural arteries are now under the definition of intra-arterial ICM administration with second pass renal exposure as they undergo dilution by circulation. On the other hand, the term intra-arterial ICM administration with first pass renal exposure indicates that ICM reaches the renal arteries during its first pass in a relatively undiluted form depending on the distance of the site of injection from the renal arteries. This consists of injections into the left heart, thoracic and suprarenal abdominal aorta, and selectively into the renal arteries [5].

The choice of contrast agent in interventional radiology depends on their general and local tolerance, iodine content, injectability and image quality, and effects on renal function.

24.2.1 Contrast Enhancement in DSA Images

The contrast enhancement of the vessels in interventional procedures depend on the X-ray absorption by iodine content in the contrast media. A direct proportional relationship between iodine content and vascular enhancement has been established in previous CT studies [6, 7]. However, the effect of osmolality has also been pointed out that the contrast enhancement effect is lowered by intravascular dilution suggesting that agents with an osmolality higher than blood (290 mOsm/kg H_2O) will undergo dilution more than the iso-osmolar agents. Pannu et al. reported no statistical difference in mean aortic attenuations between IOCM iodixanol (320 mgI/mL) and LOCM iohexol (350 mgI/mL) although iodixanol has a lower iodine concentration and concluded that there is less dilution with IOCM [8]. However, another study has proven otherwise comparing iodixanol (320 mgI/mL) with iopamidol (370 mgI/mL). This study was a MDCT study and showed statistically significant greater vascular contrast with iopamidol-370 by measuring CNR values of the coronary arteries [6].

In clinical practice, many interventional radiologists use LOCM with 300 mg iodine per mL. It is believed that lowering the concentration may disrupt image quality, especially in peripheral angiography examinations. However, a clinical randomized non-inferiority trial done with 300, 240, and 140 mgI/mL content of iohexol among patients undergoing DSA for peripheral arterial disease showed results of non-inferiority in diagnosing and treating arterial stenosis and occlusions. Although the CNR values were higher for the control group of iohexol 300 as expected, the trial showed similar confidence scores in between groups. The image quality for femoropopliteal and crural angiographies were generally diagnostic however the negative side of using lowered iodine concentration caused using larger volumes of contrast [9].

On the other hand, a recent study done with DSA phantoms suggested that the molecular structure of the nonionic contrast media is another factor effecting the contrast enhancement. Iopamidol, iomeprol, iopromide, ioversol, iohexol, and iodixanol were evaluated in this study. The authors derived a formula for predicting the pixel value ratio of two different contrast media and called it "contrast enhancement ratio" (CER). This formula was based on weight factor and the results showed that iodixanol, iopamidol, and iomeprol have the same ability of contrast enhancement and iohexol showed the lowest ability [10].

All of these studies show that iodine content, plasma dilution, leak to the interstitium, and flow rates of contrast media are all responsible for contrast visualization in images. However, we should also keep in mind image quality is not only determined by the contrast agents and patient-related factors (weight, etc.) and technical factors (resolution of the DSA equipment, mAs and kVp values, etc.) are also responsible.

24.2.2 Adverse Effects of Contrast Agents Regarding Their Properties

24.2.2.1 Patient Discomfort Associated with Intra-arterial Injections

The intensity and severity of adverse events have been dramatically reduced with the shift from HOCM to LOCM. However, different than intravenous administration sensation of pain and discomfort and warmth are still seen in interventional procedures. These symptoms are caused by damage in the endothelium in combination with secondary local vasodilatation of the arteries and capillaries [11]. Other than these damage to erythrocytes, disturbed blood-brain barrier and depressed cardiac contractility are other osmolality-related adverse effects. General tolerance depends on osmolality and chemotoxicity. Additional to osmolality, local tolerance also depends on the site of injection, flow rate, volume and patient's age, and underlying disease and psychology. Pain worsens with the increasing intravascular concentration. Patients undergoing visceral angiography report less pain than patients undergoing extremity angiography procedures where injections are done into arteries supplying skeletal muscles [12]. Suprarenal aortic injections are slightly better tolerated than infrarenal aortic injections. Aorto-bifemoral angiography produces less discomfort than selective femoral angiography. Elimination of discomfort and pain is important as the advent use of DSA imaging. DSA is more susceptible to movement artifacts. High-quality visualization of below the knee vessels or arteries of the hand and digits require more volume of contrast or selective injections which both enhance the sensation of discomfort [13].

Earlier results were in favor of LOCM when compared to HOCM. Early studies done comparing LOCM within themselves showed a lower degree of pain and heat after iopromide when compared to iohexol [11]. In controversy, other larger populated studies have reported no statistically significant difference in between [14].

In the English literature, there are many trials comparing IOCM to LOCM. In general population, the incidence of pain and discomfort is seen in 20% of intra-arterial procedures [15–17]. A meta-analysis by McCullough reviewed 22 randomized control trials (RCT) to compare the discomfort rates associated with IOCM to those reported with various LOCM. Overall discomfort (regardless of severity) was significantly different between patients receiving IOCM and various LOCMs. IOCM was favored over all LOCMs combined for incidence of pain, regardless of severity. A greater reduction in the magnitude of pain was observed with IOCM, particularly with selective limb and carotid/intracerebral procedures. Similarly, the analysis of warmth sensation, regardless of severity, favored IOCM over LOCMs. LOCM included in the analyses were iohexol, ioxaglate, iopamidol, and iomeprol and the IOCM included in the analyses was iodixanol [18]. Another study done by Palena et al. prospectively compared IOCM iodixanol to LOCM ioversol in a diabetic patient population who underwent treatment for critical limb ischemia. This study also confirmed results in favor of IOCM [19]. Reduction in pain and discomfort is an important goal for the tolerability of procedures and also for image quality. The uncomfortable feelings will cause body motion which will jeopardize diagnostic accuracy and effect clinical decision-making and also prolong the procedure resulting in repeat examinations. This will expose patients to additional injections and higher doses of radiation [18].

Iodixanol is more viscose than other agents. When the viscosity of the CM increases it requires more pressure to maintain adequate flow rates during angiography [20]. Another issue is injectability; it is harder to inject with high viscosity agents when microcatheters are used. A study from the cardiology literature compared the effects of viscosity during balloon angioplasty with IOCM and LOCM. Balloon inflation times were found to be higher in coronary balloon catheters with IOCM (iodixanol) compared to LOCM (ioxaglate) [21]. This study is also valuable for vascular interventions as reducing inflation times will reduce limb discomfort seen in peripheral angioplasty. A new IOCM iosimenol is a dimeric, nonionic agent with lower molecular weight and viscosity than iodixanol at equal concentration. The early results showed an efficacy similar to that of iodixanol but with the advantage of having a higher iodine concentration and lower viscosity. However, further larger trials are needed [22].

24.2.2.2 Post-contrast Acute Kidney Injury in Vascular Interventional Radiology

The term contrast-induced nephropathy (CIN) is now replaced with the term post-contrast acute kidney injury (PC-AKI) by the suggestions of ACR Committee on Drugs and Contrast Media [4]. PC-AKI is a general term used to describe a sudden deterioration in renal function that occurs within 48 h following intravascular administration of ICM. PC-AKI is a correlative diagnosis and it can occur regardless of whether the contrast medium was the cause. The committee suggested the use of the term CIN in patients where only a causal relation between the administrated CM and deterioration of the renal function can be clearly shown. CIN is defined as a causative diagnosis and considered as a subgroup of PC-AKI. They suggested that the studies so far likely include the combination of both and do not permit separation of CIN from PC-AKI. This should be kept in my mind while reading further with this chapter. The studies in the literature with intra-arterial use of CM will further be discussed under the term PC-AKI as no study has been done with a suitable control group to separate these two terms.

In the latest update of ESUR guidelines, the committee suggested that the studies directly comparing intravenous to intra-arterial route and found no difference [2, 23–25] had selection bias and the new definitions of first pass and second pass renal exposure were not separated.

The incidence of PC-AKI following intra-arterial administration with first pass renal exposure is frequently reported higher than intravenous route. However, as mentioned before the literature is dominated by coronary interventions and in these studies the patients have many procedural variables (hypotension, etc.), co-morbidities, and catheter manipulations which can also be a cause of AKI therefore making the results confounding [3, 26, 27]. Nonetheless, AKI in general is a significant problem in this kind of critically ill patients. A meta-analyses done by Ghumman et al. showed that the incidence of AKI after peripheral angiography performed with carbon dioxide as a contrast agent remained high at 6.2% supporting the idea of other factors existing and causing renal impairment other than ICM [28].

The latest update brought new changes in the guidelines of ESUR. Intra-arterial administration of CM with a second pass is now considered as having no higher risk than intravenous CM administration. These include procedures of infrarenal abdominal aorta, iliac, femoral, crural arteries and subclavian, brachial, carotid, and selective mesenteric artery injections. Because of the difficulties in separating the effects of the procedure from CM, the committee decided to choose a higher cut-off eGFR level for patients undergoing interventional procedures with first pass renal exposure. They also decided to include coronary interventions in this category Taking preventive measurements are now recommended for patients with an eGFR value <45 mL/min/1.73 m^2 who will undergo a first pass renal exposure intervention. For patients undergoing intra-arterial administration with a second pass or intravenous administration the cut-off eGFR value was decided as 30 mL/min/1.73 m^2 and preventive measurements are suggested for the patients having lower eGFR values [5].

The results of the studies comparing PC-AKI incidence between LOCM to IOCM are controversial. One of the first trials the NEPHRIC trial randomized patients with diabetes and chronic kidney disease comparing LOCM and IOCM. The result was in favor of IOCM, they found the incidence of PK-AKI with iodixanol lower in this high-risk population [29]. After this many RCTs were done in high-risk populations and meta-analyses of these trials were published showing that the incidence of PC-AKI was similar between IOCM and LOCM [30–32]. The most recent meta-analyses including patients with renal insufficiency undergoing coroner angiography with or without PTA again confirmed the same results. However, in this latest analysis which was done in between iodixanol and iopromid a significant reduced risk for cardiovascular events were found in favor of iodixanol [32]. In the latest update, it is still accepted as there is no significant difference between IOCM and LOCM in PC-AKI risk and the guideline recalls the avoidance of HOCM and repeated CM injections in a short period of time (48–72 h). More recent studies published after the guideline still show no significant difference between IOCM and LOCM [33, 34].

Another important subject to consider is the volume of CM. Cigarroa et al. suggested the following formula of (5× body weight in kg) divided by serum creatinine (mg/dL) to calculate the maximum volume of contrast agent to be used. However, this was developed at the time when HOCM were in use and does not apply to date situations [35, 36]. To date ratios of CM dose to eGFR or CM volume to eGFR are used. When using intra-arterial administration CM dose (in grams Iodine) to absolute eGFR (in mL/min/1.73 m^2) should be below 1.1 or CM volume (in mL) to eGFR (in mL/min/1.73 m^2) should be below 3 [37–40].

There are only a few trials describing long-term effects of ICM with viscosity and osmolality. A recent study investigated the long-term effect of contrast volume with an incidence of 1 year major adverse cardiac and cerebrovascular events (MACCE) and all cause bleeding events. They divided the contrast volume amount into quartiles of <100 mL, 101–140 mL, 141–200 mL, and >200 mL. MACCE incidences were found 7.1%, 7.8%, 9.3%, and 11.7%, respectively with statistical significance [41].

24.3 CO_2 as a Contrast Agent

24.3.1 History

Room air was the first negative contrast that was used as an imaging agent in 1914 with an attempt to visualize the abdominal viscera with radiographs. After that visualization of retroperitoneal structures was done with room air, oxygen, and CO_2. Intravenous usage of CO_2 was first done in the 1950s for the evaluation of pericardial effusion [42]. Later in 1969 Hipona reported the use of CO_2 for the evaluation of inferior vena cava [43]. Hawkins a well-known pioneer of CO_2 angiography discovered the intra-arterial use of CO_2 by accident. In 1971 during a routine celiac axis injection, 70 cc of room air was inadvertently injected into a patient instead of iodinated contrast. Hawkins visualized the celiac axis and its branches as a negative image on cut film. Luckily no ill side effects were observed and he coupled this experience with his previous knowledge of CO_2 as an intravenous agent and pioneered it as a potential negative contrast agent for intra-arterial system. After studies with animals, he successfully applied the principles on humans however the imaging quality was scent because of technical limitations of angiography of that time. Later in the 1980s after introduction of digital subtraction angiography, safer and more reliable delivery systems, CO_2 evolved into a safe and valid vascular imaging agent [44]. Carbon dioxide was initially used only in patients with renal failure and contrast allergy. Today with the advent of imaging technologies and the many unique properties of CO_2 provides its use in multiple occasions alone or in combination with iodinated contrast agents.

24.3.2 Physical and Chemical Properties of CO_2

Understanding the basic principles and properties of CO_2 is essential for a safe use. CO_2 is a colorless, odorless, compressible nontoxic gas with high solubility and low viscosity properties. It is the only negative contrast agent that has proven to be safe and reliable in patients with renal insufficiency and iodinated contrast agent allergy. CO_2 is also an endogenous byproduct of the body. After injection, it rapidly dissolves in the blood and is transported to the lungs predominantly as bicarbonate ion which is reversed back into CO_2 and then exhaled. As it is also endogenously produced it has no hepatotoxicity, nephrotoxicity, or allergy which has been confirmed by multiple animal and human studies [45, 46]. Some of its unique physical properties contribute to the utility of its use as a contrast agent and in some occasions CO_2 has advantages over ICM.

24.3.2.1 High Solubility

Carbon dioxide is highly soluble in blood causing rapid intravascular clearance. It is more soluble than oxygen by 20–30 times. When administered intravenously it dissolves within 30–60 s. It is less occlusive than other gases.

24.3.2.2 Fluid Displacement

Iodinated contrast agents mix with blood when administered whereas CO_2 displaces blood instead of mixing with it. This miscibility feature of CO_2 provides better visualization of large caliper vessels as it does not suffer from dilution effects seen in ICM.

24.3.2.3 Low Viscosity

Viscosity of CO_2 is 1/400 than ICM. This provides high diffusibility among structures. It can be administered through small size catheters. CO_2 also passes through the space in between catheters and guidewires which facilitates interventional procedures by eliminating the need for guidewire catheter exchanges [47]. For diagnostic imaging 15–30 mL of CO_2 can be easily administered through 3F catheters, 20–25G needles, end hole catheters, in between catheter and guidewires, from side ports of vascular sheaths (Fig. 24.1).

24.3.2.4 Buoyancy

The density of CO_2 is lower than blood therefore when submerged into a fluid the gas bubble rises upward by the exerted force of the stronger fluid. This property is called as buoyancy meaning floating on blood [48]. CO_2 prefers the nondependent (anterior) portion of the vessel. Studies showed that the buoyancy of a CO_2 bubble has a parabolic flow profile along the nondependent portion of the vessel with incomplete fluid displacement along the dependent portion regardless of the vessel size [49]. This key feature affects image quality in angiography. In vessels originating from anterior portions of the aorta such as celiac artery, mesenteric arteries, and buoyancy is an advantage (Fig. 24.2); however, in vessels originating posteriorly this feature causes disadvantage in posterior vessels like left renal artery, internal iliac arteries making them difficult to visualize. Patient repositioning, tilting/rotation of the table, or selective injections can be done to overcome this disadvantage. Low viscosity and buoyancy of CO_2 enable excellent visualization of central veins and vena cava even with peripheral injections. In lower limb angiography buoyancy is used to improve the visualizations of below the knee vessels by tilting the table in Trendelenburg or elevating the limb by 15–20° to enhance infrageniculate vessel filling (Fig. 24.3).

24.3.2.5 Reflux

The gaseous nature of CO_2 causes bubbles to be formed at the catheter's tip and they move upwards. A central reflux forms (Fig. 24.4) from the point of administration [50]. This permits visualization of ostial pathologies without the need of catheter withdrawal and offers an advantage in visceral artery stenting procedures.

24.3.2.6 Compressibility

As all gases CO_2 is also compressible. During injection via a catheter pressure builds up and when exiting the tip of the catheter this will cause an expansion of the gas known as explosive delivery. This will cause discomfort to the patient and poor image quality and also carries a risk of vascular injury due to the local pressure rise in the elastic vascular chamber [50]. To decrease this explosion rate, catheters should be cleared from liquid or blood with a test injection of 3–5 mL of CO_2 [51].

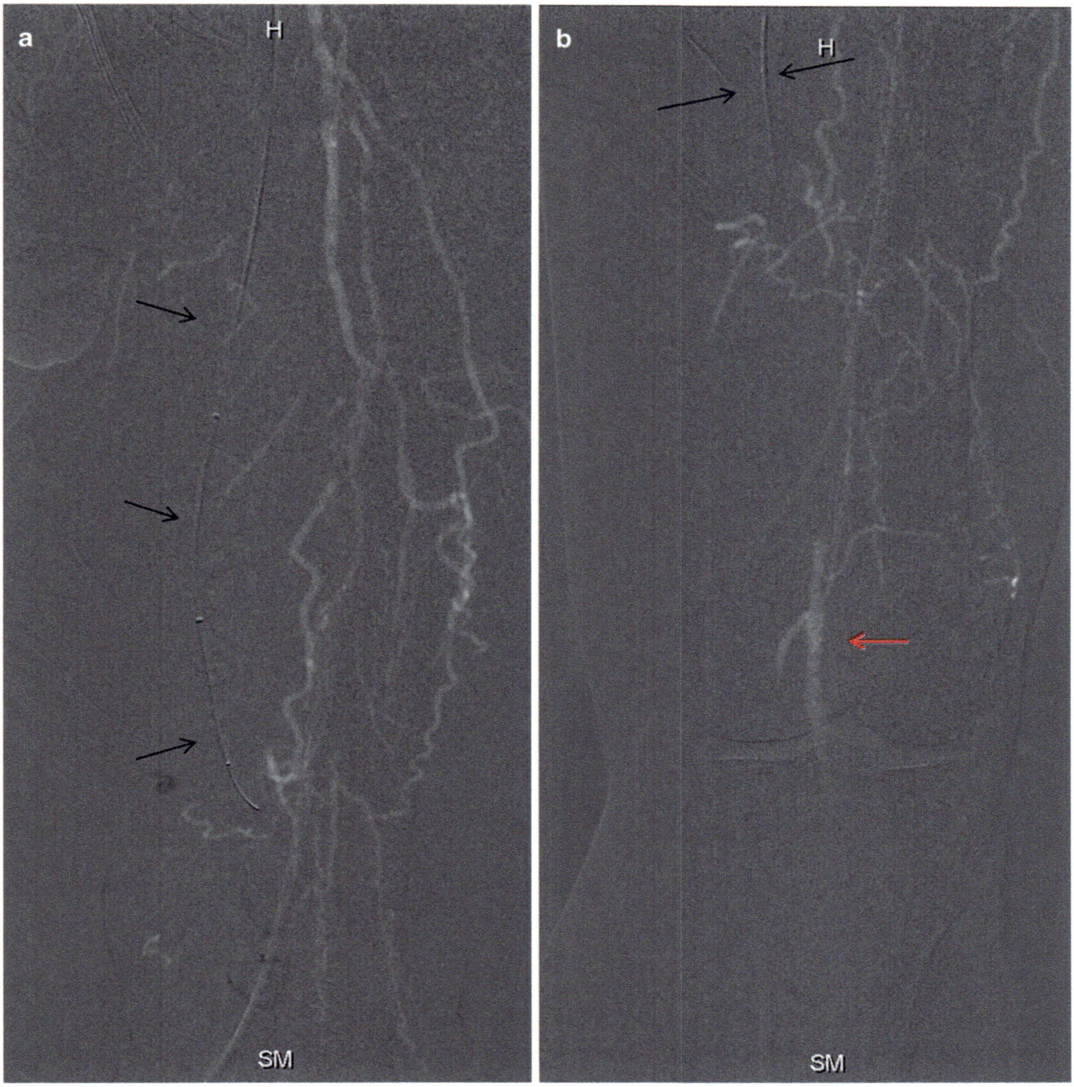

Fig. 24.1 A femoropopliteal angiography image with CO_2. The injection is done from the side port of the vascular sheath without exchanging the crossing-over catheter (black arrows in **a** and **b**). Red arrow in (**b**), points out the recanalization point of the popliteal artery

24.4 Delivery Systems

Different kinds of methods have been published for the delivery of CO_2 [52–54]. As a source of CO_2, medical/research grade high purified sources should be used. From this source, there should be a mechanism to deliver. Many commercial canisters contain three million of pressurized gas. First attempts were to apply CO_2 with a syringe directly from the source into the delivery catheter. This approach causes compressed pressurized volumes within the syringe resulting in explosive delivery therefore is not used.

The handheld syringe method has been used for decades and it is safe if properly used. One-way or three-way stopcock and a 30–60 mL luer-lock type syringe is required. Filling and injection are done manually. The blood is first washed out

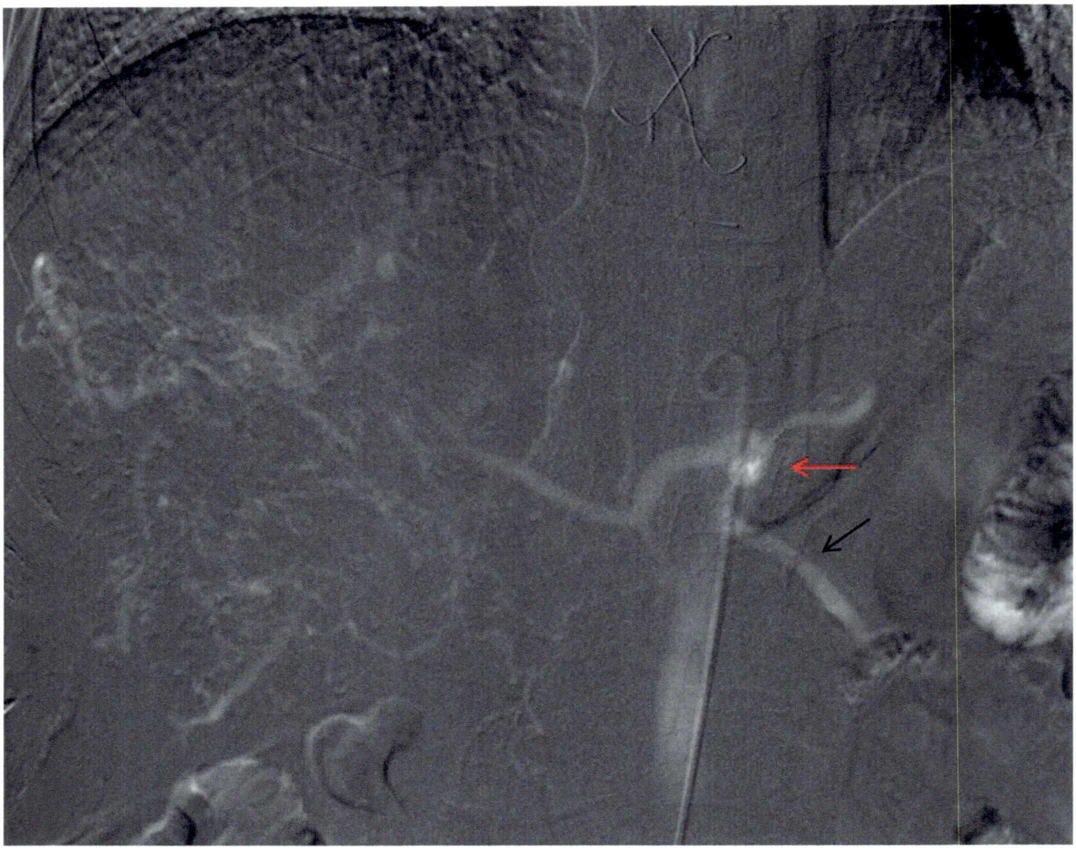

Fig. 24.2 Abdominal aortography with CO_2. Anterior positioned arteries celiac artery (red arrow) and superior mesenteric artery (black arrow) are easily visualized because of the buoyancy effect of CO_2

with 5 mL of CO_2. As it is controlled manually, it has the advantage of optimal timing, injection control, and ability to stop injection immediately. Low cost is also another advantage. However, air contamination is a potential risk and radiation exposure is higher [55].

The plastic bag systems were the method of choice by experts for many years [52]. Filters were used to remove particulates or bacterial contaminations from the cylinder, regulator, and connecting tubes. Commercially there were kits containing the tubes, stopcocks, and bags. However, they are now discontinued because of an unfortunate complication of inadvertent filing of the bag with O_2 instead of CO_2 [56].

A portable medical CO_2 delivery system the CO_2 Mmander is a FDA-approved system consisting of a small 10,000 cc canister of CO_2. It is used in conjunction with the AngiAssist delivery apparatus which consists of a K valve, one-way safety valves, preattached 60 mL reservoir syringe, and a 30 mL syringe. The system does not require complex assembly and therefore is user-friendly. It allows nonexplosive gas delivery [57].

Early in the 1990s, automated injectors were designed to offer more control over injection rates as they did in ICM. However, the first generations were bulky, cumbersome to use, and expensive and were not successful to replace the much cheaper and easy-to-use bag method. Recently new generation computerized automated injectors are designed. They offer several advantages as precise control of injection timing, pressure,

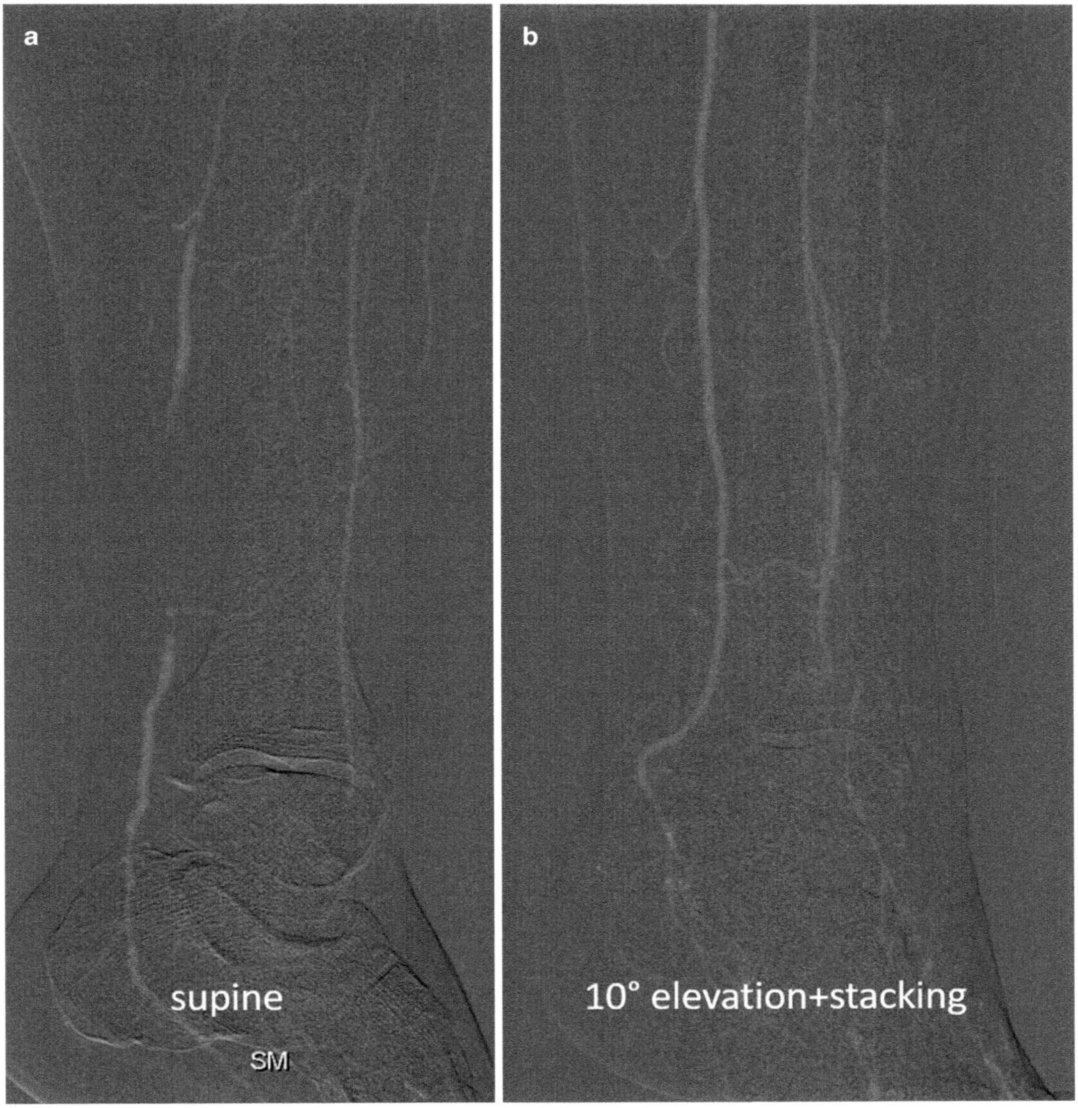

Fig. 24.3 Angiography of the crural arteries. Incomplete filling of posterior tibial artery (**a**) has improved after elevation of the limb (**b**) and a better image quality is achieved with stacking software

and volume. They significantly reduce the radiation exposure of the operator. The newest device the Angiodroid Injector (Angiodroid SRL, Italy) computes the amount of gas to be injected into the vessel and accordingly automatically purges air out, verifies CO_2 purity, and determines the delivered CO_2 volume and pressure [48]. Early results with this system are encouraging in efficacy and safety [58–60].

24.5 Injection of CO_2: Tips and Tricks

So far there are no standardized methods for dosing, injection rates or which catheter to choose, adjunct techniques, and safeguards, although some general principles for particular applications exist. CO_2 can be delivered through any lumen as told before but end hole catheters are

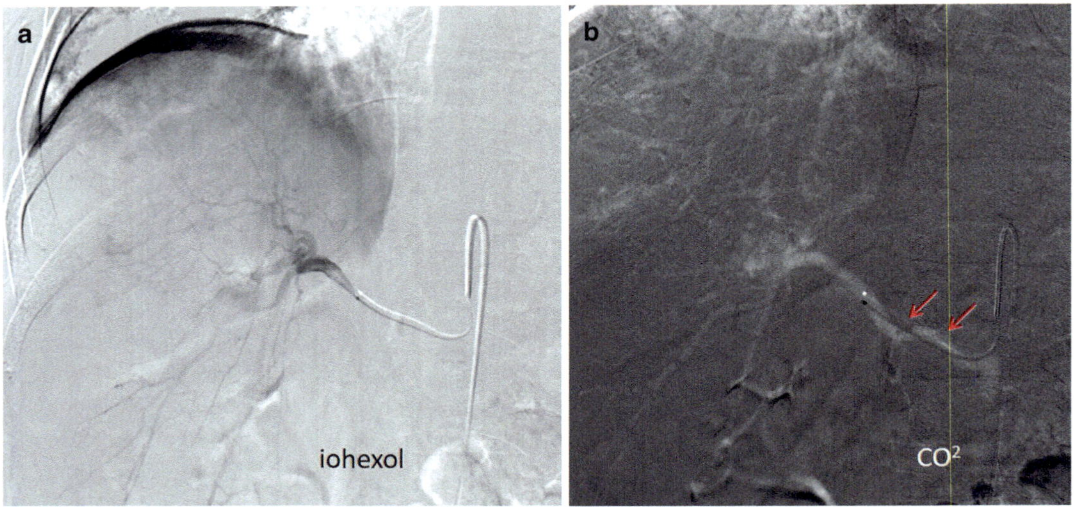

Fig. 24.4 Hepatic artery angiography during a TACE procedure. Injection with ICM (**a**) and CO_2 (**b**) with a 2.4 F microcatheter. The central reflux is visualized (red arrows in **b**) from the point of administration. Also, note that some visceral collaterals are seen with CO_2 (**b**) but not with ICM

sufficient. The operator should consider the volume of blood to be displaced and the vessel's origin of takeoff to be imaged. The injection rate should slightly exceed the rate of the blood flow in the vessel being studied [48]. With the automated injectors, this rate can usually be defined as [systolic pressure of the patient +30]. Too slow injections will not be enough to completely fill the vessel. Too rapid injections on the other hand will reflux. Reflux feature can be handy in undulating arteries, proximal vessels, or in the arteries in dependent areas. For example, an injection from the common femoral artery will reflux into the iliac arteries and distal aorta. An injection of CO_2 from the renal artery will result in filling of the renal orifice. Amounts of CO_2 for the aorta are 15–30 mL/s for 1.5 s. Amounts for mesenteric, renal, iliac, and femoral arteries are 10–20 mL/s. Regardless of the volume injected, CO_2 is delivered within 2 s. In small vessels such as tibial arteries, CO_2 is injected over 2–3 s [51] (Table 24.1).

Table 24.1 Adjustable parameters for a better image quality when CO_2 is used as a contrast agent

Tips and tricks for CO_2 Imaging	
Positioning	Elevation of region of interest 10–30° Use sedation to decrease motion Glucagon to decrease bowel gas Nitroglycerin for peripheral arteries
Imaging parameters	High-resolution DSA 5–7 frame/rates 60 ms pulse width
Injection	End hole catheter Selective injection Wait in between injections 30–60 s
Volume	Aorta 20–50 mL Visceral arteries 5–20 mL Peripheral lower extremity arteries 5–20 mL Inferior vena cava 20–50 mL Central veins 5–20 mL Portal vein 10–20 mL
Post imaging	Pixel shift Mask shift Stacking software

24.6 Advantages and Indications

All of the previously described features of CO_2 offer some advantages during vascular procedures. First of all, the main benefit is the lack of renal toxicity and allergic responses. All patients with renal insufficiency or under higher risk of developing CIN should be considered for CO_2 imaging.

All arterial structures below the diaphragm and all venous structures can be evaluated with

CO_2. It can be used instead of ICM or in conjunction with ICM. Low viscosity and buoyancy and the ability to image with reflux are the advantages that can be used in visceral artery stenting. By selective catheterization, the orifices of the vessels can be delineated and stented with lesser catheter exchanges. Advantage of its lack of nephrotoxicity is unquestionable especially in patients with renal vascular disease who have already compromised renal function [61].

The efficacy in iliofemoral imaging with CO_2 has been well documented with the highest diagnostic value being above the knee arterial segments [62]. However, due to its low viscosity CO_2 is superior to ICM in identifying collaterals which is very important in occlusive diseases (Fig. 24.1). Antegrade, retrograde, and even contralateral (cross-midline) collaterals are easily identified with CO_2 allowing the operator to assess the physiology of the disease, reconstituted segments distal to the occlusion, and better demonstration of revascularization options [51, 58]. Although infrapopliteal arteries are more challenging for CO_2 imaging, we believe that new computerized automated injectors will have better results.

Detection of bleeding is another area that CO_2 is advantageous over ICM. Because of its viscosity gas travels easier from small points of bleeding sources and when existing through a bleeding point it expands and a cloud-like image is formed and is easier to identify [63].

Another mostly used area of CO_2 is TIPSS procedure. The localization of the portal vein which is the most cumbersome step can be done from the hepatic veins with catheter wedged CO_2 injections [64]. The low viscosity and high diffusibility of CO_2 make it very easy to pass through the sinusoids into the portal system and will stay in the portal vein as a target (Fig. 24.5). Hawkins later modified the technique and used the TIPS needle for CO_2 injection within the hepatic parenchyma [44]. This modification prevents the rarely seen complication of capsular rupture.

24.7 Disadvantages and Contraindications

The fluid displacement and non-mixing feature of CO_2 causes fragmentation of bubbles in high turbulence flow areas like bifurcations. This causes a specific type of artifact called pseudo stenosis which is only seen in CO_2 imaging. This appearance resembles cobblestones and should be confirmed with additional views or by using diluted ICM (Fig. 24.6).

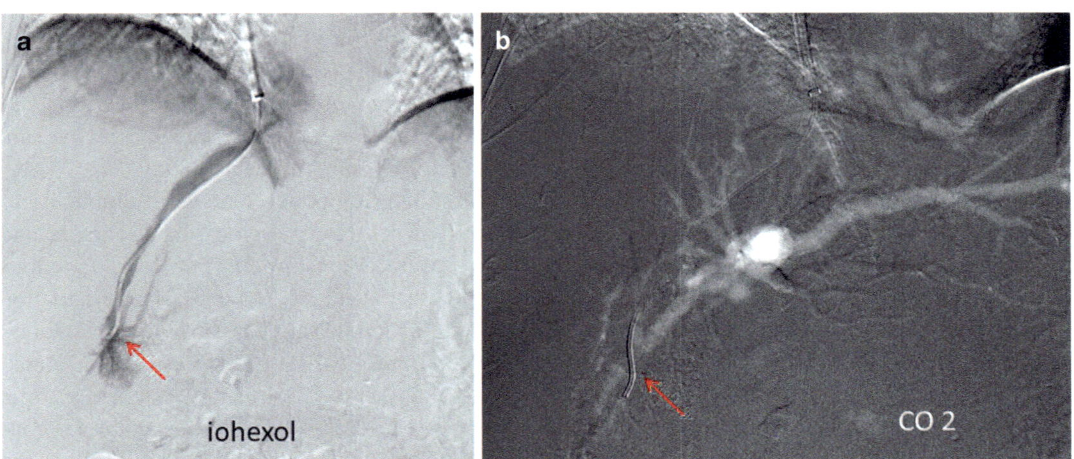

Fig. 24.5 Wedge hepatic venography during TIPS procedure. ICM allows visualization of only a limited segment of the portal vein (**a**) whereas with CO_2 injections from the same point (red arrow in **a** and **b**) the whole portal system can be visualized (**b**)

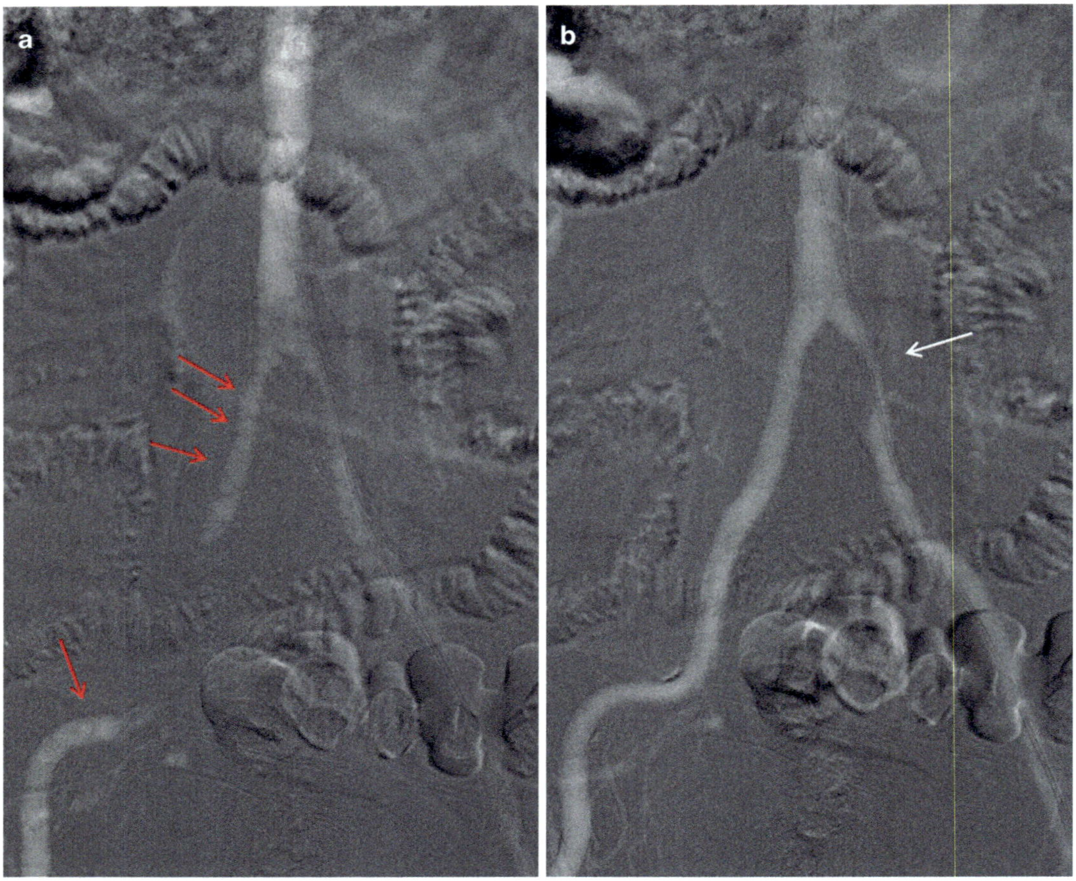

Fig. 24.6 Pelvic angiography with CO_2. After bifurcation, a cobblestone appearance (red arrows in **a**) is seen in the right iliac artery as pseudo stenosis. Reconstructed image with stacking software (**b**) shows that the right iliac artery has no stenosis and the real diseased segment is the left iliac artery (white arrow in **b**)

Imaging with CO_2 requires specific imaging parameters and software programs and also specific delivery systems to prevent air contamination and gas compression. As it is a negative contrast agent, subtracted imaging is required and high-resolution digital subtraction angiography (DSA) equipment is essential. To enhance contrast visualization high mA and low kV are needed which increase the radiation exposure. The gas bubbles of CO_2 need some time to cluster and displace the whole blood and to track this aggregation higher frame rates are used which also is another reason for higher radiation exposure. As DSA is required the images are very susceptible to motion artifacts (Fig. 24.7), bowel gas, and peristalsis causing degraded images with CO_2. Therefore, post-processing software such as masking, pixel shifting, and stacking software are required for optimum image quality (Fig. 24.8).

Although CO_2 bubbles are very soluble, it has been shown to cause myocardial ischemia and has a severe effect on left ventricular functions in animal studies [65]. In the cerebral circulation multiple injections of CO_2 cause break down on the blood-brain barrier therefore it is considered as neurotoxic [66–68]. Imaging of thoracic aorta, coronary arteries, and cerebral circulation is contraindicated with CO_2. Injections into the aorta with a prone positioned patient is also contraindicated because of the risk for spinal ischemia. In

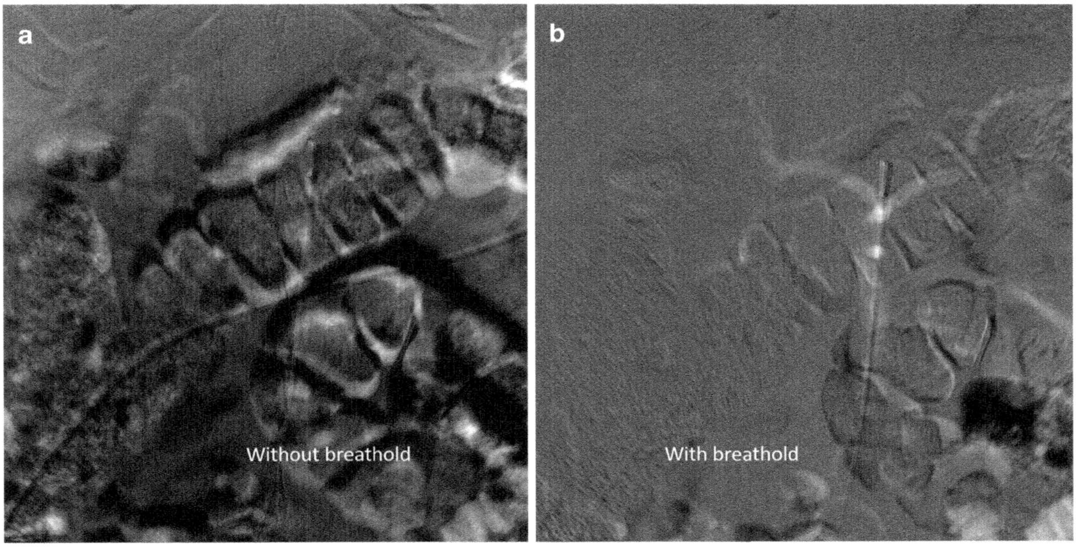

Fig. 24.7 Abdominal aortography with CO_2. Motion artifacts caused by breathing disrupt the image quality (**a**). Repeated injection with breath hold command (**b**) avoids motion artifacts caused by respiration

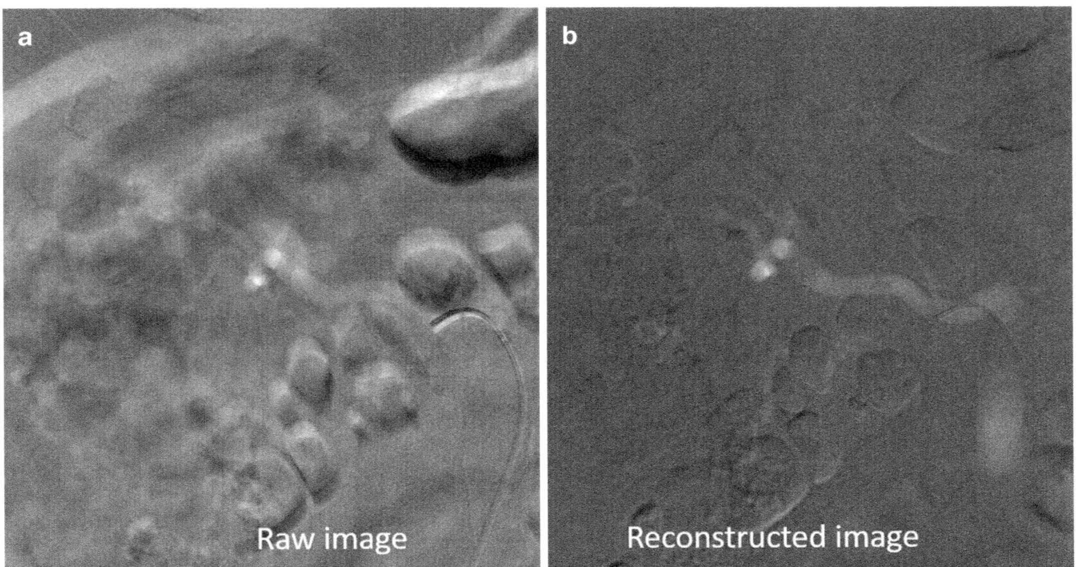

Fig. 24.8 Selective renal angiography with CO_2. The initial image obtained with CO_2 (**a**) has a low diagnostic quality because of a mismatch with the timing of the mask. It is not possible to evaluate the orifice of the renal artery. Reconstructed images with a replaced mask and pixel shift and stacking (**b**) show a significant improvement in image quality

patients who will undergo CO_2 imaging should not receive nitrous oxide anesthesia as it may cause volume expansion in the CO_2 bubble. In patients with pulmonary hypertension or severe chronic obstructive lung disease the duration in between the injections should be kept longer.

References

1. Aspelin P, Bellin MF, Jakobsen J, Webb JAW. Classification and terminology. In: Thomsen HS, Webb JAW, editors. Contrast media. Medical radiology (diagnostic imaging). Berlin, Heidelberg: Springer; 2009.
2. Karlsberg RP, Dohad SY, Sheng R, Iodixanol Peripheral Computed Tomographic Angiography Study Investigator Panel. Contrast medium-induced acute kidney injury: comparison of intravenous and intraarterial administration of iodinated contrast medium. J Vasc Interv Radiol. 2011;22(8):1159–65.
3. Nyman U, Almen T, Jacobsson B, Aspelin P. Are intravenous injections of contrast media really less nephrotoxic than intra-arterial injections? Eur Radiol. 2012;22(6):1366–71.
4. ACR Committee on Drugs and Contrast Media. ACR manual on contrast media, v10.3. American College of Radiology; 2018. https://www.acr.org/-/media/ACR/Files/Clinical-Resources/Contrast_Media.pdf. Accessed May 2019.
5. van der Molen AJ, Reimer P, Dekkers IA, Bongartz G, Bellin MF, Bertolotto M, et al. Post-contrast acute kidney injury—part 1: definition, clinical features, incidence, role of contrast medium and risk factors: recommendations for updated ESUR Contrast Medium Safety Committee guidelines. Eur Radiol. 2018;28(7):2845–55.
6. Christensen JD, Meyer LT, Hurwitz LM, Boll DT. Effects of iopamidol-370 versus iodixanol-320 on coronary contrast, branch depiction, and heart rate variability in dual-source coronary MDCT angiography. AJR Am J Roentgenol. 2011;197(3):W445–51.
7. Silvennoinen HM, Hamberg LM, Valanne L, Hunter GJ. Increasing contrast agent concentration improves enhancement in first-pass CT perfusion. AJNR Am J Neuroradiol. 2007;28(7):1299–303.
8. Pannu HK, Thompson RE, Phelps J, Magee CA, Fishman EK. Optimal contrast agents for vascular imaging on computed tomography: iodixanol versus iohexol. Acad Radiol. 2005;12(5):576–84.
9. Jens S, Schreuder SM, De Boo DW, van Dijk LC, van Overhagen H, Bipat S, et al. Lowering iodinated contrast concentration in infrainguinal endovascular interventions: a three-armed randomized controlled non-inferiority trial. Eur Radiol. 2016;26(8):2446–54.
10. Imai K, Ikeda M, Satoh Y, Fujii K, Kawaura C, Nishimoto T, et al. Contrast enhancement efficacy of iodinated contrast media: effect of molecular structure on contrast enhancement. Eur J Radiol Open. 2018;5:183–8.
11. Steiner RM, Grainger RG, Memon N, Weiss D, Kanofsky PB, Menduke H. The effect of contrast media of low osmolality on the peripheral arterial blood flow in the dog. Clin Radiol. 1980;31(6):621–7.
12. Gmeinwieser JK, Wenzel-Hora BI. Peripheral and penile angiography with iotrolan 280 versus non-ionic monomers: results of the European clinical phase II and III trials. Eur Radiol. 1995;5(2):S30–8.
13. Darcy MD. Lower-extremity arteriography: current approach and techniques. Radiology. 1991;178(3):615–21.
14. Ohlsén H, Albrechtsson U, Billström Å, Calissendorff B, Gustavsson S, Jensen R, Johnsson K, Nyberg P, Strindberg L. Comparison of iopromide versus iohexol in aortobifemoral arteriography: a Swedish multi-center study of 446 patients. Acta Radiol. 1991;32(2):130–3.
15. Justesen P, Downes M, Grynne BH, Lang H, Rasch W, Seim E. Injection-associated pain in femoral arteriography: a European multicenter study comparing safety, tolerability, and efficacy of iodixanol and iopromide. Cardiovasc Intervent Radiol. 1997;20(4):251–6.
16. Poirier VC, Monsein LH, Newberry PD, Kreps BJ. Double-blind, randomized comparison of iodixanol 320 and iohexol 300 for cerebral angiography. Invest Radiol. 1994;29(Suppl 2):S43–4.
17. Singh K, Sundgren R, Bolstad B, Björk L, Lie M. Iodixanol in abdominal digital subtraction angiography. Acta Radiol. 1993;34(3):242–5.
18. McCullough PA, Capasso P. Patient discomfort associated with the use of intra-arterial iodinated contrast media: a meta-analysis of comparative randomized controlled trials. BMC Med Imaging. 2011;11:12.
19. Palena LM, Sacco ZD, Brigato C, Sultato E, Barra D, Candeo A, et al. Discomfort assessment in peripheral angiography: randomized clinical trial of Iodixanol 270 versus Ioversol 320 in diabetics with critical limb ischemia. Catheter Cardiovasc Interv. 2014;84(6):1019–25.
20. Brunette J, Mongrain R, Rodes-Cabau J, Larose E, Leask R, Bertrand OF. Comparative rheology of low- and iso-osmolarity contrast agents at different temperatures. Catheter Cardiovasc Interv. 2008;71(1):78–83.
21. Mogabgab O, Patel VG, Michael TT, Kotsia A, Christopoulos G, Banerjee S, et al. Impact of contrast agent viscosity on coronary balloon deflation times: bench testing results. J Interv Cardiol. 2014;27(2):177–81.
22. Meurer K, Laniado M, Hosten N, Kelsch B, Hogstrom B. Intra-arterial and intravenous applications of Iosimenol 340 injection, a new non-ionic, dimeric, iso-osmolar radiographic contrast medium: phase 2 experience. Acta Radiol. 2015;56(6):702–8.
23. Kooiman J, Le Haen PA, Gezgin G, de Vries JP, Boersma D, Brulez HF, et al. Contrast-induced acute kidney injury and clinical outcomes after intra-arterial and intravenous contrast administration: risk comparison adjusted for patient characteristics by design. Am Heart J. 2013;165(5):793–99, 799.e1.
24. McDonald JS, Leake CB, McDonald RJ, Gulati R, Katzberg RW, Williamson EE, et al. Acute kidney injury after intravenous versus intra-arterial contrast material administration in a paired cohort. Invest Radiol. 2016;51(12):804–9.
25. Tong GE, Kumar S, Chong KC, Shah N, Wong MJ, Zimmet JM, et al. Risk of contrast-induced nephropa-

thy for patients receiving intravenous vs. intra-arterial iodixanol administration. Abdom Radiol (NY). 2016;41(1):91–9.
26. Stratta P, Izzo C, Canavese C, Quaglia M. Letter to the editor re: are intravenous injections of contrast media really less nephrotoxic than intra-arterial injections? Eur Radiol. 2013;23(5):1260–3.
27. Nyman U, Almen T, Jacobsson B, Aspelin P. Reply to letter to the editor re: are intravenous injections of contrast media really less nephrotoxic than intra-arterial injections? Eur Radiol. 2013;23(5):1264–5.
28. Ghumman SS, Weinerman J, Khan A, Cheema MS, Garcia M, Levin D, et al. Contrast induced-acute kidney injury following peripheral angiography with carbon dioxide versus iodinated contrast media: a meta-analysis and systematic review of current literature. Catheter Cardiovasc Interv. 2017;90(3):437–48.
29. Aspelin P, Aubry P, Fransson SG, Strasser R, Willenbrock R, Berg KJ. Nephrotoxic effects in high-risk patients undergoing angiography. N Engl J Med. 2003;348(6):491–9.
30. McCullough PA, Brown JR. Effects of intra-arterial and intravenous iso-osmolar contrast medium (iodixanol) on the risk of contrast-induced acute kidney injury: a meta-analysis. Cardiorenal Med. 2011;1(4):220–34.
31. Solomon R. Contrast media: are there differences in nephrotoxicity among contrast media? Biomed Res Int. 2014;2014:934947.
32. Zhang J, Jiang Y, Rui Q, Chen M, Zhang N, Yang H, et al. Iodixanol versus iopromide in patients with renal insufficiency undergoing coronary angiography with or without PCI. Medicine (Baltimore). 2018;97(18):e0617.
33. Azzalini L, Vilca LM, Lombardo F, Poletti E, Laricchia A, Beneduce A, et al. Incidence of contrast-induced acute kidney injury in a large cohort of all-comers undergoing percutaneous coronary intervention: comparison of five contrast media. Int J Cardiol. 2018;273:69–73.
34. Han XF, Zhang XX, Liu KM, Tan H, Zhang Q. Contrast-induced nephropathy in patients with diabetes mellitus between iso- and low-osmolar contrast media: a meta-analysis of full-text prospective, randomized controlled trials. PLoS One. 2018;13(3):e0194330.
35. Cigarroa RG, Lange RA, Williams RH, Hillis LD. Dosing of contrast material to prevent contrast nephropathy in patients with renal disease. Am J Med. 1989;86(6 Pt 1):649–52.
36. Solomon R, Briguori C, Bettmann M. Selection of contrast media. Kidney Int Suppl. 2006;100:S39–45.
37. Gurm HS, Dixon SR, Smith DE, Share D, Lalonde T, Greenbaum A, et al. Renal function-based contrast dosing to define safe limits of radiographic contrast media in patients undergoing percutaneous coronary interventions. J Am Coll Cardiol. 2011;58(9):907–14.
38. Nyman U, Bjork J, Aspelin P, Marenzi G. Contrast medium dose-to-GFR ratio: a measure of systemic exposure to predict contrast-induced nephropathy after percutaneous coronary intervention. Acta Radiol. 2008;49(6):658–67.
39. Nyman U. Contrast dose, estimated GFR, and techniques to reduce contrast dose in PCI—time to consider some basic principles! J Invasive Cardiol. 2016;28(10):E126–E7.
40. Kooiman J, Seth M, Share D, Dixon S, Gurm HS. The association between contrast dose and renal complications post PCI across the continuum of procedural estimated risk. PLoS One. 2014;9(3):e90233.
41. Feng YQ, He XY, Song FE, Chen JY. Association between contrast media volume and 1-year clinical outcomes in patients undergoing coronary angiography. Chin Med J (Engl). 2018;131(20):2424–32.
42. Scatliff JH, Kummer AJ, Janzen AH. The diagnosis of pericardial effusion with intracardiac carbon dioxide. Radiology. 1959;73:871–83.
43. Hipona FA, Ferris EJ, Pick R. Capnocavography: a new technic for examination of the inferior vena cava. Radiology. 1969;92(3):606–9.
44. Hawkins IF. Carbon dioxide digital subtraction arteriography. AJR Am J Roentgenol. 1982;139(1):19–24.
45. Hawkins IF, Caridi JG. Carbon dioxide (CO2) digital subtraction angiography: 26-year experience at the University of Florida. Eur Radiol. 1998;8(3):391–402.
46. Back MR, Caridi JG, Hawkins IF Jr, Seeger JM. Angiography with carbon dioxide (CO2). Surg Clin North Am. 1998;78(4):575–91.
47. Caridi JG, Hawkins IF Jr, Cho K, Sohn SY, Langham MR Jr, Weichmann BN, et al. CO2 splenoportography: preliminary results. AJR Am J Roentgenol. 2003;180(5):1375–8.
48. Sharafuddin MJ, Marjan AE. Current status of carbon dioxide angiography. J Vasc Surg. 2017;66(2):618–37.
49. Song K, Cho D, Shinn K, Charlton E, Cho K. Gas dynamics in CO2 angiography: in vitro evaluation in a circulatory system model. Invest Radiol. 1999;34(2):151–5.
50. Corazza I, Rossi PL, Feliciani G, Pisani L, Zannoli S, Zannoli R. Mechanical aspects of CO(2) angiography. Phys Med. 2013;29(1):33–8.
51. Cho KJ. Carbon dioxide angiography: scientific principles and practice. Vasc Specialist Int. 2015;31(3):67–80.
52. Hawkins IF Jr, Caridi JG, Kerns SR. Plastic bag delivery system for hand injection of carbon dioxide. AJR Am J Roentgenol. 1995;165(6):1487–9.
53. Cronin P, Patel JV, Kessel DO, Robertson I, McPherson SJ. Carbon dioxide angiography: a simple and safe system of delivery. Clin Radiol. 2005;60(1):123–5.
54. de Almeida Mendes C, Wolosker N, Krutman M. A simple homemade carbon dioxide delivery system for endovascular procedures in the iliofemoral arteries. Circ J. 2013;77(3):831.
55. Cho DR, Cho KJ, Hawkins IF Jr. Potential air contamination during CO2 angiography using a hand-held syringe: theoretical considerations and gas chromatography. Cardiovasc Intervent Radiol. 2006;29(4):637–41.

56. Cho KJ, Hawkins IF Jr. Discontinuation of the plastic bag delivery system for carbon dioxide angiography will increase radiocontrast nephropathy and life-threatening complications. AJR Am J Roentgenol. 2011;197(5):W940–1.
57. Caridi JG. Vascular imaging with carbon dioxide: confidence in a safe, efficacious, user-friendly system. Semin Intervent Radiol. 2015;32(4):339–42.
58. Micari A, Sbarzaglia P, Meeks MDME, Liso A, Riina M, Lunetto ML, et al. New imaging modalities in peripheral interventions. Eur Heart J Suppl. 2015;17(Suppl A):A18–22.
59. Scalise F, Novelli E, Auguadro C, Casali V, Manfredi M, Zannoli R. Automated carbon dioxide digital angiography for lower-limb arterial disease evaluation: safety assessment and comparison with standard iodinated contrast media angiography. J Invasive Cardiol. 2015;27(1):20–6.
60. Palena LM, Diaz-Sandoval LJ, Candeo A, Brigato C, Sultato E, Manzi M. Automated carbon dioxide angiography for the evaluation and endovascular treatment of diabetic patients with critical limb ischemia. J Endovasc Ther. 2016;23(1):40–8.
61. Caridi JG, Stavropoulos SW, Hawkins IF Jr. Carbon dioxide digital subtraction angiography for renal artery stent placement. J Vasc Interv Radiol. 1999;10(5):635–40.
62. Mendes CA, Martins AA, Teivelis MP, Kuzniec S, Varella AY, Fioranelli A, et al. Carbon dioxide contrast medium for endovascular treatment of ilio-femoral occlusive disease. Clinics. 2015;70(10):675–9.
63. Caridi JG, Cho KJ, Fauria C, Eghbalieh N. Carbon dioxide digital subtraction angiography (CO2 DSA): a comprehensive user guide for all operators. Vasc Dis Manag. 2014;11(10):E221–56.
64. Rees CR, Niblett RL, Lee SP, Diamond NG, Crippin JS. Use of carbon dioxide as a contrast medium for transjugular intrahepatic portosystemic shunt procedures. J Vasc Interv Radiol. 1994;5(2):383–6.
65. Lambert CR, de Marchena EJ, Bikkina M, Arcement BK. Effects of intracoronary carbon dioxide on left ventricular function in swine. Clin Cardiol. 1996;19(6):461–5.
66. Coffey R, Quisling RG, Mickle JP, Hawkins IF Jr, Ballinger WB. The cerebrovascular effects of intraarterial CO2 in quantities required for diagnostic imaging. Radiology. 1984;151(2):405–10.
67. Dimakakos PB, Stefanopoulos T, Doufas AG, Papasava M, Gouliamos A, Mourikis D, et al. The cerebral effects of carbon dioxide during digital subtraction angiography in the aortic arch and its branches in rabbits. AJNR Am J Neuroradiol. 1998;19(2):261–6.
68. Kozlov DB, Lang EV, Barnhart W, Gossler A, De Girolami U. Adverse cerebrovascular effects of intra-arterial CO2 injections: development of an in vitro/in vivo model for assessment of gas-based toxicity. J Vasc Interv Radiol. 2005;16(5):713–26.

Quo Vadis: An Epilog

25

Pablo R. Ros, Ibrahim Inan,
and Sukru Mehmet Erturk

Since the invention of x-rays, the use of contrast materials in radiological imaging continued to develop and evolve parallel to the technological advances in radiological devices. Technical developments in radiology have led to the creation of novel applications in imaging techniques and a decrease in using contrast agents. Considering that radiology is an area in which novel medical technology is most used, it is not surprising that it plays a lead role in medicine.

There have been recent developments in the use of contrast agents in radiological imaging. For instance, they are being utilized in perfusion MRI or CT for the diagnosis of acute stroke, and demonstration of salvageable tissue called penumbra in the brain parenchyma. The evaluation of contrast agent uptake kinetics by perfusion imaging enables quantitative evaluation of cerebral blood flow per unit time, cerebral blood volume, peak enhancement time, and mean blood transfer time, and allows the evaluation of ischemia or tumor vascularity in cerebral parenchyma. Perfusion imaging provides essential information in the analysis of ischemic stroke and the evaluation of recurrence after radiotherapy and characterization of brain tumors. Besides, simultaneous CT or MR angiography reveals pathological findings in intracranial arterial structures to explain stroke etiology. Recent advances in prostate imaging have enabled the imaging of clinically significant prostate cancer foci using multi-parametric MR imaging. Perfusion imaging plays an important role in multi-parametric prostate MR imaging. We can now evaluate not only the presence and pattern but also dynamic characteristics of contrast enhancement can in solid lesions and especially in breast and kidney masses [1].

Another current issue on the agenda is the use of iodinated contrast agents in mammography, which reduces the need for breast MRI. Contrast-enhanced mammography is used at a few centers worldwide; however, it is expected to become widespread due to the short imaging time and lower costs when compared to MRI [2].

New technological developments aim to reduce the need for and the dosage of contrast agents. Contrast enhancement can be evaluated using a lower amount of contrast material on dual-energy CT, and iodine maps obtained are employed for the demonstration of contrast material distribution [3]. In MR imaging devices, shorter T1 relaxation times allow adequate imaging at lower doses of contrast agents. MR angiography examinations without administration of contrast agents are routinely employed for the visualization of arteries and veins. Dual-head

P. R. Ros
Case Western Reserve University, Cleveland, OH, USA

I. Inan
Centermed Imaging Center, Istanbul, Turkey

S. M. Erturk (✉)
Department of Radiology, Istanbul University School of Medicine, Istanbul, Turkey

S. M. Erturk et al. (eds.), *Medical Imaging Contrast Agents: A Clinical Manual*,
https://doi.org/10.1007/978-3-030-79256-5_25

contrast agent injection systems, which allow the saline and contrast agent injection at the desired rate and dose, are also beneficial in reducing the dose of the drug. Perfusion maps of the cerebral parenchyma can be obtained without contrast agents using the arterial spin labeling technique.

The new drafting techniques aim to reduce not only the contrast agent but also the radiation dose in CT imaging. For example, with split bolus techniques, the contrast agents are administered stepwise. Thus, different tissues and organs can be visualized at a single imaging session by using less ionizing radiation and without increasing the total contrast agent dose [4].

By changing the molecular structure of contrast agents, not only the side effect profile but also the distribution of the agent in the body can be altered. This approach paved the way for the emergence of contrast agents specific to different tissues. Contrast agents specific to the hepatobiliary system produce specific contrast enhancement of the liver parenchyma on MR imaging and pass through the biliary tract to visualize the biliary system. Iron-containing hematopoietic system-specific contrast agents are also available, and atherosclerotic plaque-specific contrast agents are being investigated [1]. Contrast materials containing synthetic compounds of HDL and LDL imitations, and hydrophobic nanoparticles containing gadolinium forming micelles are developed to show atherosclerotic plaques [5]. With tissue-specific contrast agents using iodine-containing nanoparticles, metastatic tissues, pathological lymph nodes, specific inflammation, and infections can be visualized [6]. We are about the enter a new era of "smart molecules" that are used as contrast agents.

Chemical particles formed by elements other than iodine are also investigated as contrast agents. Gold is one of the leading elements. Gold-containing nanoparticles have low viscosity and osmolality and can provide higher x-ray absorption compared to iodized contrast media, and these nanoparticles provide advantages in imaging by remaining longer in blood compared to iodinated contrast media. It is argued that these nanoparticles have fewer side effects than conventional contrast agents. This is especially important in obese patients that need higher amounts of contrast media and for procedures such as angiography [6].

Conjugation of iron oxide-containing nanoparticles with various antibodies and molecules made the specific enhancement of colorectal cancers and glial tumors possible [7]. Bismuth, tantalum, tungsten, ytterbium, and gadolinium are elements that can be utilized as contrast-enhancing nanoparticles [8]. Increasing and diversifying tissue- and organ-related contrast can offer diagnostic convenience and have the potential to produce clinically important results in identifying and staging of lesions.

Micro-air bubbles containing a phospholipidic shell can be used as contrast media safely in ultrasonography. In fact, ultrasound contrast agents can be used for therapeutic purposes, as well [9]. For instance, tissue ablation and sonothrombolysis can be achieved by generating thermal energy from micro-air bubbles using low acoustic energy. Drug particles can be placed into these micro-air bubbles for targeted therapy. This method can be used for gene delivery in systemic gene therapies [10].

Another current issue in terms of contrast agents is the use of carbon dioxide as an alternative to iodinated contrast agents in digital subtraction angiography. The risk of renal impairment because of the use of high volumes of iodinated contrast media may cause a broader use of carbon dioxide [11]. Xenon is another gaseous contrast agent that can be used to demonstrate ventilation [6].

Thanks to the developments in information technology, nowadays, massive amounts of data are quickly recorded and complex analyses can easily be performed using approaches such as deep learning. Deep learning proves itself in analyzing radiological images. Using deep learning, radiologists will be able to reduce the contrast agent dose [12–15]. The artificial intelligence technology and the opportunities provided by it will most probably have unpredictable results. Through the automation of the radiological imaging process, it is envisaged that steps including the acquisition and analysis of images will improve by using artificial intelligence. Artificial intelligence will definitely affect the way we utilize contrast media. In conclusion, although recent developments in imaging technology appear to decrease the need of contrast media, "smarter" agents are expected to emerge in a near future. We believe that our fellow radiologists will adapt themselves quickly to new developments.

References

1. Lohrke J, Frenzel T, Endrikat J, et al. 25 years of contrast-enhanced MRI: developments, current challenges and future perspectives. Adv Ther. 2016;33(1):1–28.
2. Covington MF, Pizzitola VJ, Lorans R, et al. The future of contrast-enhanced mammography. Am J Roentgenol. 2018;210(2):292–300.
3. Faggioni L, Gabelloni M. Iodine concentration and optimization in computed tomography angiography: current issues. Invest Radiol. 2016;51(12):816–22.
4. Kekelidze M, Dwarkasing RS, Dijkshoorn ML, et al. Kidney and urinary tract imaging: triple-bolus multidetector CT urography as a one-stop shop—protocol design, opacification, and image quality analysis. Radiology. 2010;255(2):508–16.
5. Young VE, Degnan AJ, Gillard JH. Advances in contrast media for vascular imaging of atherosclerosis. Imaging Med. 2011;3(3):353.
6. Ahn S, Jung SY, Lee SJ. Gold nanoparticle contrast agents in advanced X-ray imaging technologies. Molecules. 2013;18(5):5858–90.
7. Khairnar S, More N, Mounika C, Kapusetti G. Advances in contrast agents for contrast-enhanced magnetic resonance imaging. J Med Imaging Radiat Sci. 2019;50(4):575–89.
8. Koç MM, Aslan N, Kao AP, Barber AH. Evaluation of X-ray tomography contrast agents: a review of production, protocols, and biological applications. Microsc Res Tech. 2019;82(6):812–48.
9. Stride E, Segers T, Lajoinie G, et al. Microbubble agents: new directions. Ultrasound Med Biol. 2020;46(6):1326–43.
10. Caschera L, Lazzara A, Piergallini L, et al. Contrast agents in diagnostic imaging: present and future. Pharmacol Res. 2016;110:65–75.
11. Pedersoli F, Bruners P, Kuhl C, Schmitz-Rode T. Current CO2 angiography. Radiologe. 2019;59(6):533–40.
12. Gong E, Pauly JM, Wintermark M, Zaharchuk G. Deep learning enables reduced gadolinium dose for contrast-enhanced brain MRI. J Magn Reson Imaging. 2018;48(2):330–40.
13. Liu F, Jang H, Kijowski R, Bradshaw T, McMillan AB. Deep learning MR imaging–based attenuation correction for PET/MR imaging. Radiology. 2017;286(2):676–84.
14. Nakao T, Hanaoka S, Nomura Y, et al. Deep neural network-based computer-assisted detection of cerebral aneurysms in MR angiography. J Magn Reson Imaging. 2018;47(4):948–53.
15. Zaharchuk G, Gong E, Wintermark M, Rubin D, Langlotz C. Deep learning in neuroradiology. Am J Neuroradiol. 2018;39(10):1776–84.

GPSR Compliance

The European Union's (EU) General Product Safety Regulation (GPSR) is a set of rules that requires consumer products to be safe and our obligations to ensure this.

If you have any concerns about our products, you can contact us on ProductSafety@springernature.com

In case Publisher is established outside the EU, the EU authorized representative is:

Springer Nature Customer Service Center GmbH
Europaplatz 3
69115 Heidelberg, Germany

Batch number: 10732801

Printed by Printforce, the Netherlands